W9-CEP-980

DO YOU REALLY *KNOW* WHAT YOU'RE EATING? LET CORINNE T. NETZER ENLIGHTEN YOU!

Now more than ever before, Americans are becoming aware of their diets, paying attention to their hearts and arteries as well as to their waistlines. A good diet can promote good health and well-being—and there's no better guide to eating right than *The Complete Book of Food Counts.* Everything you need to know is here: calorie, carbohydrate, cholesterol, sodium, protein, fat, and fiber values for thousands of foods, alphabetized for quick and easy reference.

So take control! You can do it with the help of this revised and updated edition of Corinne T. Netzer's portable classic:

THE COMPLETE BOOK OF FOOD COUNTS

YOUR GUIDE TO OPTIMUM HEALTH

Also by Corinne T. Netzer

THE BRAND-NAME CALORIE COUNTER
THE BRAND-NAME CARBOHYDRATE GRAM COUNTER
THE CHOLESTEROL CONTENT OF FOOD
THE CORINNE T. NETZER DIETER'S DIARY
THE CORINNE T. NETZER ENCYCLOPEDIA OF FOOD VALUES
THE CORINNE T. NETZER 1994 CALORIE COUNTER
THE DIETER'S CALORIE COUNTER
THE CORINNE T. NETZER FAT GRAM COUNTER
THE CORINNE T. NETZER FIBER COUNTER

THE CORINNE T. NETZER GOOD EATING SERIES:
101 HIGH FIBER RECIPES
101 LOW CALORIE RECIPES
101 LOW CHOLESTEROL RECIPES
101 LOW FAT RECIPES
101 LOW SODIUM RECIPES
101 VEGETARIAN RECIPES

Third Edition

THE
COMPLETE
BOOK
OF
FOOD COUNTS

Corinne T. Netzer

A DELL BOOK

Published by
Dell Publishing
a division of
Bantam Doubleday Dell Publishing Group, Inc.
1540 Broadway
New York, New York 10036

ISBN: 0-440-21271-5

Printed in the United States of America
Published simultaneously in Canada

March 1994

10 9 8 7 6 5

OPM

Introduction

The third edition of *The Complete Book of Food Counts* is the largest compilation of essential food data in this format. It contains data (calories, protein, carbohydrates, fat, cholesterol, sodium, and fiber) for basic generic foods, brand-name foods, and restaurant chains. Whether you are interested in dieting or nutrition—or both—you will find this book unique and invaluable as a reference. Should you need even more data, you may wish to consult *Corinne T. Netzer's Encyclopedia of Food Values.*

Since this book is alphabetized, you should have no difficulty finding whatever you wish to look up. There are, however, times when you may have to look in more than one place. If you are searching for a particular food and cannot find it immediately, look for it under a category, such as cakes, puddings, cookies, soups. Wherever sensible I have cross-referenced listings, but the pressure of space has made it impossible to do that for every item.

Compare only foods listed in similar measures. This rule particularly applies to the confusion between measures by capacity and measures by weight. Eight ounces is not necessarily equivalent to eight fluid ounces or one cup. Eight ounces is a measure of how much something weighs; one cup is a measure of how much space it occupies. For instance, a cup of lightweight food, such as puffed rice or popcorn, weighs about one ounce, and eight ounces of the same product would fill many cups. Naturally, you can convert a similar unit of measure into a smaller or larger amount. The following table may be useful in making such conversions.

Equivalents by Capacity
(all measures level)

1 quart	=	4 cups
1 cup	=	8 fluid ounces
	=	1/2 pint
	=	16 tablespoons
2 tablespoons	=	1 fluid ounce
1 tablespoon	=	3 teaspoons

Equivalents by Weight

1 pound	=	16 ounces
3.57 ounces	=	100 grams
1 ounce	=	28.35 grams

All the material contained in *The Complete Book of Food Counts* is based on information from the United States government, from producers and processors of brand-name foods, and from food chains. The data contained herein is the most complete and accurate information available as this book goes to press. Please bear in mind that seasonal and regional differences can affect the nutritional value of foods. Also, the food industry often changes recipes and sizes and may discontinue products or add new ones. In the future I will revise and update this book to keep you completely informed.

Good luck and good dieting.

CORINNE T. NETZER

Abbreviations and Symbols

c . . . . crude fiber*
cal. . . . . calories
carbo. . . . . carbohydrates
chol. . . . . cholesterol
cont. container
d . . . . dietary fiber
diam. diameter
fl. . . . . fluid
gms . . . . grams
″ . . . . inch
< . . . . less than
(0) . . . . may contain trace amounts
m.q. . . . . measurable quantity**
mgs . . . . milligrams
lb. . . . . pound
n.a. . . . . not available
oz. . . . . ounces
pkg. . . . . package
pkt. . . . . packet
prot. . . . . protein
sod. . . . . sodium
sq. . . . . square
tbsp. . . . . tablespoon
tsp. teaspoon
tr. . . . . trace
w/ . . . . with
* . . . . prepared according to basic
        package directions, except as noted

*Obtained through crude method of analysis; actual content may be higher.
**Believed to contain measurable quantities, but data is unavailable at this time.
(A "measurable quantity" may range from a trace to significant amounts.)

Note: Brand-name foods and restaurants listed in italics denote registered trademarks.

A

Food and Measure	cal.	prot. (gms)	carbo. (gms)	fat (gms)	chol. (mgs)	sod. (mgs)	fiber (gms)
Abalone, meat only, raw, 4 oz.	119	19.4	6.8	.9	96	341	0
Acerola, fresh:							
trimmed, 1/2 cup . . .	16	.2	3.8	.1	0	4	.2 c
juice, 6 fl. oz.	36	.7	8.7	.5	0	6	.5 c
Acorn squash:							
baked, cubed, 1/2 cup	57	1.1	14.9	.1	0	4	2.9 d
boiled, mashed, 1/2 cup	41	.8	10.7	.1	0	3	3.4 d
Adzuki beans:							
dry *(Arrowhead Mills),* 2 oz.	190	13.0	35.0	1.0	0	3	14.3 d
boiled, 1/2 cup	147	8.7	28.5	.1	0	9	2.3 c
canned, 1/2 cup:							
(Eden)	100	6.0	17.0	<1.0	0	20	4.3 d
sweetened	351	5.6	81.4	<.1	0	323	2.3 c
Agar, see "Seaweed"							
Agnoletti, cheese and basil, refrigerated *(Contadina),* 3 oz.	270	13.0	38.0	7.0	40	220	m.q.
Alfalfa seeds:							
(Arrowhead Mills), 1 cup	40	5.0	4.0	1.0	0	m.q.	m.q.
Alfalfa seeds, sprouted, raw:							
1/2 cup	5	.7	.6	.1	0	1	.4 d
1 tbsp.	1	.1	.1	<.1	0	tr.	.1 d
(Shaw's), 2 oz.	16	2.0	2.0	<1.0	0	3	<1.0 d

Food and Measure	cal.	prot. (gms)	carbo. (gms)	fat (gms)	chol. (mgs)	sod. (mgs)	fiber (gms)
Alfalfa and dill seeds, sprouted, raw *(Shaw's)*, 2 oz. . . .	8	2.0	<1.0	<1.0	0	55	3.0 d
Alfalfa and radish seeds, sprouted, raw *(Shaw's)*, 2 oz.	25	2.0	2.0	1.0	0	3	<1.0 d
Alfredo sauce:							
mix *(Lawry's)*, 1 pkg.	226	8.0	19.2	10.3	1	3222	.6 d
refrigerated *(Contadina Light)*, 3.3 oz. . . .	150	7.0	7.0	10.0	40	460	n.a.
Algae, see "Seaweed"							
Allspice *(Spice Islands)*, 1 tsp. . . .	5	.1	1.4	.2	0	1	.4 d
Almond, shelled, 1 oz., except as noted:							
(Beer Nuts)	170	6.0	6.0	14.0	0	65	3.0 d
(Dole) . :	170	6.0	5.0	14.0	0	4	m.q.
(Fisher)	170	6.0	6.0	15.0	0	0	m.q.
dried:							
1 oz.	167	5.7	5.8	14.8	0	3	3.1 d
slivered, 1 cup . . .	795	26.9	27.5	70.5	0	15	14.7 d
blanched	166	5.8	5.3	14.9	0	3	1.9 d
dry-roasted	167	4.6	6.9	14.7	0	3	3.9 d
dry-roasted, salted	167	4.6	6.9	14.7	0	221	3.9 d
honey-roasted	168	5.2	7.9	14.2	0	37	m.q.
oil-roasted:							
1 oz.	176	5.8	4.5	16.4	0	3	3.2 d
salted	176	5.8	4.5	16.4	0	221	3.2 d
salted *(Master Choice)*	180	6.0	5.0	16.0	0	200	m.q.
blanched	174	5.4	5.1	16.1	0	3	3.2 d
toasted	167	5.8	6.5	14.4	0	3	3.2 d
Almond butter:							
1 tbsp.	101	2.4	3.4	9.5	0	2	.5 d
(Erewhon), 1 tbsp. . .	90	3.0	2.0	8.0	0	18	m.q.
(Roaster Fresh), 1 oz.	184	5.0	6.0	16.0	0	4	m.q.

Food and Measure	cal.	prot. (gms)	carbo. (gms)	fat (gms)	chol. (mgs)	sod. (mgs)	fiber (gms)
raw *(Hain* Natural), 2 tbsp.	190	8.0	3.0	18.0	0	5	m.q.
blanched, toasted *(Hain)*, 2 tbsp.	210	8.0	3.0	19.0	0	5	m.q.
salted, 1 tbsp.	101	2.4	3.4	9.5	0	72	.5 d
honey cinnamon, 1 tbsp.	96	2.5	4.3	8.4	0	2	.5 d
Almond meal, partially defatted, 1 oz.	116	11.2	8.2	5.2	0	2	.7 c
Almond paste, 1 oz.	127	3.4	12.4	7.2	0	3	4.2 d
Amaranth, 1/2 cup:							
raw, trimmed	4	.3	.6	<.1	0	3	.1 c
boiled, drained	14	1.4	2.7	.1	0	14	.9 c
Amaranth, whole-grain, 1 oz.	106	4.1	18.8	1.8	0	6	4.3 d
Amaranth flakes *(Arrowhead Mills)*, 1 oz.	110	4.0	21.0	2.0	0	0	3.0 d
Amaranth flour or seeds *(Arrowhead Mills)*, 2 oz.	200	8.0	35.0	3.0	0	1	3.9 d
Anasazi beans, dry *(Arrowhead Mills)*, 2 oz.	200	13.0	35.0	1.0	0	3	12.1 d
Anchovy, meat only:							
fresh, European, raw 1 oz.	37	5.8	0	1.4	m.q.	29	0
canned, in olive oil:							
drained, 1 oz. . . .	60	8.2	0	2.8	m.q.	1040	0
5 medium, .7 oz.	42	5.8	0	1.9	m.q.	734	0
Angel hair pasta entree, frozen:							
(Lean Cuisine), 10 oz.	240	10.0	38.0	5.0	10	410	m.q.
(Weight Watchers Smart Ones), 8.55 oz.	120	8.0	18.0	<1.0	0	290	m.q.
Anise seed, 1 tsp.	7	.4	1.1	.3	0	tr.	.3 d

Food and Measure	cal.	prot. (gms)	carbo. (gms)	fat (gms)	chol. (mgs)	sod. (mgs)	fiber (gms)
Apple:							
raw, w/peel:							
2 3/4"-diam. apple	81	.3	21.1	.5	0	1	3.7 d
sliced, 1/2 cup . . .	32	.1	8.4	.2	0	tr.	3.0 d
raw, peeled:							
2 3/4"-diam. apple	72	.2	19.0	.4	0	tr.	2.4 d
sliced, 1/2 cup . . .	31	.1	8.2	.2	0	tr.	2.1 d
cooked, sliced, peeled:							
boiled, 1/2 cup . . .	46	.2	11.7	.3	0	1	2.1 d
microwaved, 1/2 cup	48	.2	12.3	.4	0	1	2.4 d
canned, sweetened, sliced, drained, 1/2 cup	68	.2	17.0	.5	0	3	1.7 d
dried, 2 oz.:							
sulfured, uncooked	138	.5	37.4	.2	0	49	4.9 d
chunks *(Sun-Maid/ Sunsweet)*	150	1.0	42.0	0	0	<40	m.q.
Apple, escalloped, frozen *(Stouffer's),* 6 oz.	200	<1.0	41.0	4.0	n.a.	15	m.q.
Apple butter, all varieties *(Smucker's),* 1 tsp.	12	0	3.0	0	0	0	m.q.
Apple cider, 6 fl. oz., except as noted:							
canned or frozen* *(Tree Top)*	90	0	22.0	0	0	10	n.a.
sparkling *(Welch's)* . .	100	0	24.0	0	0	5	n.a.
and spice *(R.W. Knudsen),* 8 fl. oz. . . .	110	<1.0	28.0	<1.0	0	(0)	n.a.
Apple crisp, frozen:							
(Pepperidge Farm Classic), 4 oz. . . .	240	2.0	41.0	8.0	38	125	1.0 d
(Weight Watchers Sweet Celebrations), 3.5 oz.	190	1.0	40.0	5.0	0	190	m.q.

Food and Measure	cal.	prot. (gms)	carbo. (gms)	fat (gms)	chol. (mgs)	sod. (mgs)	fiber (gms)
Apple drink, canned (Hi-C Jammin' Apple), 6 fl. oz.	90	0	23.0	0	0	20	(0)
Apple dumpling, frozen (Pepperidge Farm), 3 oz.	260	2.0	33.0	13.0	n.a.	230	n.a.
Apple fritter, frozen (Mrs. Paul's), 4 oz.	240	4.0	35.0	9.0	5	500	m.q.
Apple fruit roll, see "Fruit snack"							
Apple fruit square, frozen (Pepperidge Farm), 2.5 oz. . . .	220	2.0	27.0	12.0	m.q.	170	m.q.
Apple juice, 6 fl. oz., except as noted:							
unsweetened	87	.1	21.7	.2	0	6	.2 d
(Minute Maid)	80	0	21.0	0	0	30	m.q.
(Mott's/Mott's Natural)	80	<1.0	20.0	<1.0	0	10	m.q.
(Ocean Spray 100%)	90	0	23.0	0	0	15	m.q.
(R.W. Knudsen Clear), 8 fl. oz.	90	<1.0	22.0	<1.0	0	(0)	m.q.
(R.W. Knudsen Natural), 8 fl. oz.	85	<1.0	21.0	<1.0	0	(0)	m.q.
(Red Cheek/Red Cheek Natural) . .	80	<1.0	20.0	<1.0	0	10	m.q.
(Tropicana)	80	<1.0	20.0	<1.0	0	15	m.q.
(Welch's)	90	0	22.0	0	0	20	m.q.
blend (Juicy Juice) . .	90	0	21.0	0	0	5	m.q.
Gravenstein (R.W. Knudsen), 8 fl. oz.	110	<1.0	28.0	<1.0	0	(0)	m.q.
sparkling (Welch's) . .	100	0	24.0	0	0	5	0
canned or frozen* (Tree Top)	90	0	22.0	0	0	10	m.q.
chilled or frozen* (Sunkist), 8 fl. oz.	79	.2	19.4	.2	0	12	m.q.
frozen*	84	.3	20.7	.2	0	13	.2 d
Apple pie spice (Tone's), 1 tsp. . .	9	.2	2.4	.2	0	1	.7 d

Food and Measure	cal.	prot. (gms)	carbo. (gms)	fat (gms)	chol. (mgs)	sod. (mgs)	fiber (gms)
Apple punch:							
(Red Cheek), 10 fl. oz.	184	<1.0	47.0	<1.0	0	11	(0)
chilled *(Minute Maid)*,							
6 fl. oz.	90	0	23.0	0	0	20	(0)
Apple sticks, frozen							
(Farm Rich), 4 oz.	260	2.0	44.0	8.0	0	565	m.q.
Apple-apricot juice							
(R.W. Knudsen),							
8 fl. oz.	120	<1.0	29.0	<1.0	0	(0)	m.q.
Apple-banana juice							
(R.W. Knudsen),							
8 fl. oz.	85	<1.0	21.0	<1.0	0	(0)	m.q.
Apple-blackberry							
juice, 8 fl. oz.:							
(R.W. Knudsen) . . .	100	<1.0	24.0	<1.0	0	(0)	m.q.
(Santa Cruz Natural)	120	<1.0	29.0	1.0	0	(0)	m.q.
Apple-blueberry juice							
drink *(Boku)*, 6 fl.							
oz.	90	0	22.0	0	0	0	0
Apple-boysenberry							
juice, 8 fl. oz.:							
(R.W. Knudsen) . . .	110	<1.0	28.0	<1.0	0	(0)	m.q.
(Santa Cruz Natural)	120	<1.0	29.0	1.0	0	(0)	m.q.
Apple-cherry juice							
(Red Cheek), 10 fl.							
oz.	184	<1.0	47.0	<1.0	0	18	m.q.
Apple-citrus juice,							
canned or frozen*							
(Tree Top), 6 fl. oz.	90	1.0	22.0	0	0	10	m.q.
Apple-cranberry							
drink *(Mott's)*,							
11.5 fl. oz.	188	<1.0	47.0	<1.0	0	4	(0)
Apple-cranberry							
juice, 6 fl. oz., ex-							
cept as noted:							
(R.W. Knudsen),							
8 fl. oz.	110	<1.0	28.0	<1.0	0	(0)	m.q.
(Master Choice) . . .	80	0	19.0	0	0	<20	m.q.

Food and Measure	cal.	prot. (gms)	carbo. (gms)	fat (gms)	chol. (mgs)	sod. (mgs)	fiber (gms)
(Mott's)	83	<1.0	24.0	<1.0	0	17	m.q.
(Santa Cruz Natural),							
8 fl. oz.	115	<1.0	28.0	<1.0	0	(0)	m.q.
(Smucker's Naturally							
100%), 8 fl. oz. . .	120	0	32.0	0	0	10	m.q.
canned or frozen*							
(Tree Top)	100	0	25.0	0	0	10	m.q.
cocktail *(Welch's)* . .	110	0	27.0	0	0	20	m.q.
Apple-cranberry juice							
drink *(Tropicana)*,						·	
6 fl. oz.	110	<1.0	27.0	<1.0	0	15	(0)
Apple-grape juice:							
(Juicy Juice),							
8.45 fl. oz.	120	1.0	29.0	0	0	10	m.q.
(Mott's), 6 fl. oz. . . .	86	<1.0	23.0	<1.0	0	17	m.q.
(Red Cheek), 10 fl. oz.	180	<1.0	45.0	<1.0	0	15	m.q.
canned or frozen*							
(Tree Top), 6 fl. oz.	100	0	25.0	0	0	10	m.q.
cocktail *(Welch's*							
Orchard), 6 fl. oz.	110	0	27.0	0	0	20	(0)
cocktail, frozen*							
(Welch's Orchard),							
6 fl. oz.	110	0	27.0	0	0	0	(0)
Apple-grape-cherry							
juice cocktail:							
(Welch's), 6 fl. oz. . .	120	0	30.0	0	0	20	0
frozen* *(Welch's*							
Orchard), 6 fl. oz.	110	0	27.0	0	0	0	0
Apple-grape-rasp-							
berry juice cock-							
tail, 6 fl. oz.:							
(Welch's)	120	0	30.0	0	0	20	0
frozen* *(Welch's*							
Orchard)	110	0	27.0	0	0	0	0
Apple-orange-pine-							
apple juice cock-							
tail, 6 fl. oz.:							
(Welch's)	110	0	27.0	0	0	15	(0)

Food and Measure	cal.	prot. (gms)	carbo. (gms)	fat (gms)	chol. (mgs)	sod. (mgs)	fiber (gms)
Apple-orange-pineapple juice cocktail *(cont.)*							
frozen* *(Welch's/Welch's Orchard)*	110	0	27.0	0	0	0	(0)
Apple-peach juice *(R. W. Knudsen)*, 8 fl. oz.	140	<1.0	34.0	<1.0	0	(0)	m.q.
Apple-peach juice drink *(Boku)*, 6 fl. oz.	90	0	22.0	0	0	0	0
Apple-pear juice, canned or frozen* *(Tree Top)*, 6 fl. oz.	90	0	22.0	0	0	10	m.q.
Apple-raspberry drink *(Mott's)*, 11.5 fl. oz.	172	<1.0	43.0	<1.0	0	19	(0)
Apple-raspberry juice:							
(R.W. Knudsen), 8 fl. oz.	110	<1.0	28.0	<1.0	0	(0)	m.q.
(Mott's), 6 fl. oz. . . .	83	<1.0	22.0	<1.0	0	48	m.q.
(Santa Cruz Natural), 8 fl. oz.	120	<1.0	29.0	1.0	0	(0)	m.q.
canned or frozen* *(Tree Top)*, 6 fl. oz.	80	0	21.0	0	0	10	m.q.
Apple-raspberry juice drink *(Boku)*, 6 fl. oz.	90	0	22.0	0	0	0	0
Apple-strawberry juice, 8 fl. oz.:							
(R.W. Knudsen) . . .	110	<1.0	28.0	<1.0	0	(0)	m.q.
(Santa Cruz Natural)	120	<1.0	29.0	<1.0	0	(0)	m.q.
Apple-strawberry nectar *(Kern's)*, 6 fl. oz.	110	0	26.0	0	0	0	m.q.
Applesauce, 4 oz., except as noted:							
unsweetened, 1/2 cup	53	.2	13.8	.1	0	2	1.5 d
sweetened, 1/2 cup	97	.2	25.5	.2	0	32	1.5 d

8

Food and Measure	cal.	prot. (gms)	carbo. (gms)	fat (gms)	chol. (mgs)	sod. (mgs)	fiber (gms)
(Mott's/Mott's Chunky)	88	<1.0	22.0	<1.0	0	<1	m.q.
(Mott's Natural) . . .	48	<1.0	12.0	<1.0	0	<1	m.q.
(Stokely), 1/2 cup . . .	90	0	23.0	0	0	30	m.q.
(Tree Top Natural)							
1/2 cup	60	0	15.0	0	0	0	m.q.
regular or Gravenstein							
(Santa Cruz Natural)	60	<1.0	14.0	<1.0	0	(0)	m.q.
original or cinnamon							
(Tree Top), 1/2 cup	80	0	21.0	0	0	0	m.q.
cinnamon *(Mott's)* . .	90	<1.0	23.0	<1.0	0	25	m.q.
Dutch, spice *(Mott's)*	84	<1.0	21.0	<1.0	0	<1	m.q.
Applesauce blend:							
all blends *(Santa Cruz*							
Natural), 4 oz.	60	<1.0	14.0	<1.0	0	(0)	m.q.
w/mixed fruit *(Mott's*							
Fruit Pak), 3.9 oz.	75	<1.0	18.0	<1.0	0	0	m.q.
w/peach *(Mott's* Fruit							
Pak), 3.9 oz.	72	<1.0	18.0	<1.0	0	7	m.q.
w/pineapple *(Mott's*							
Fruit Pak)*, 3.9 oz.	84	<1.0	21.0	<1.0	0	2	m.q.
w/strawberry *(Mott's*							
Fruit Pak)*, 3.9 oz.	72	<1.0	18.0	<1.0	0	10	m.q.
Apricot:							
fresh:							
3 medium, 12 per							
lb.	51	1.5	11.8	.4	0	1	2.5 d
pitted, halves,							
1/2 cup	37	1.1	8.6	.3	0	1	1.9 d
canned, 1/2 cup:							
in water *(Libby's)*	35	0	9.0	0	0	5	m.q.
in juice	60	.8	15.3	<.1	0	5	1.6 d
in heavy syrup,							
w/skin	107	.7	27.7	.1	0	5	1.7 d
in heavy syrup							
(Libby's)	110	0	28.0	0	0	15	m.q.
dried, 2 oz.:							
sulfured	135	2.1	35.0	.3	0	6	5.1 d
(Del Monte)	140	2.0	35.0	0	0	<10	m.q.

Food and Measure	cal.	prot. (gms)	carbo. (gms)	fat (gms)	chol. (mgs)	sod. (mgs)	fiber (gms)
Apricot *(cont.)*							
frozen, sweetened,							
1/2 cup	119	.9	30.4	.1	0	5	2.1 d
Apricot fruit snack,							
see "Fruit snack"							
Apricot nectar:							
6 fl. oz.	106	.7	27.1	.2	0	6	1.1 d
(Kern's), 6 fl. oz. . . .	110	1.0	27.0	0	0	0	m.q.
(R.W. Knudsen),							
8 fl. oz.	105	<1.0	24.0	<1.0	0	(0)	m.q.
(Libby's), 6 fl. oz. . .	110	0	26.0	0	0	0	m.q.
Apricot-pineapple							
nectar *(Kern's)*,							
6 fl. oz.	110	0	27.0	0	0	5	m.q.
Arby's, 1 serving:							
breakfast:							
biscuit:							
plain	280	6.0	34.0	14.9	0	730	m.q.
w/bacon	318	6.8	35.5	17.9	8	904	m.q.
w/ham	323	13.0	34.3	16.6	21	1169	m.q.
w/sausage . . .	460	12.0	35.0	31.9	60	1000	m.q.
croissant:							
plain	260	6.0	28.0	15.6	49	300	m.q.
bacon and egg	430	17.4	28.8	30.0	245	720	m.q.
ham and cheese	345	16.0	29.3	20.7	90	939	m.q.
mushroom and							
cheese	493	13.0	34.0	37.7	116	935	m.q.
sausage and egg	519	17.5	29.3	39.2	271	632	m.q.
danish, cinnamon							
nut	360	6.0	60.0	11.0	0	105	m.q.
muffin, blueberry	240	4.0	40.0	7.0	22	200	m.q.
platters:							
scrambled egg	460	15.0	44.9	24.0	346	591	m.q.
w/bacon	593	21.8	51.0	33.0	458	880	m.q.
w/ham	518	24.4	45.3	26.2	374	1177	m.q.
w/sausage . . .	640	21.0	45.9	41.0	406	861	m.q.
Toastix	420	8.0	43.0	25.0	20	440	m.q.

Food and Measure	cal.	prot. (gms)	carbo. (gms)	fat (gms)	chol. (mgs)	sod. (mgs)	fiber (gms)
sandwiches:							
ArbyQ	389	17.6	48.2	15.2	29	1268	m.q.
Bac'N Cheddar							
Deluxe	512	21.2	38.9	31.5	38	1094	m.q.
Beef'N Cheddar . .	508	24.6	43.2	26.5	52	1166	m.q.
chicken barbeque,							
grilled	386	23.4	46.7	13.1	43	1002	m.q.
chicken breast fillet	445	22.2	52.1	22.5	45	958	m.q.
chicken Cordon							
Bleu	518	30.0	52.1	27.1	92	1463	m.q.
chicken deluxe,							
grilled	430	23.6	41.8	19.9	44	901	m.q.
fish fillet	526	23.0	50.0	27.0	44	872	m.q.
French dip	368	22.0	35.0	15.4	43	1018	m.q.
French Dip'N Swiss	429	28.7	35.5	19.0	67	1438	m.q.
Ham'N Cheese . .	355	24.6	34.5	14.2	55	1400	m.q.
Italian sub	671	34.1	47.4	38.8	69	2062	m.q.
Philly Beef'N Swiss	467	24.1	38.2	25.3	53	1144	m.q.
roast beef, giant . .	544	33.2	45.6	26.3	72	1433	m.q.
roast beef, junior	233	11.5	22.8	10.8	22	519	m.q.
roast beef, regular	383	22.0	35.4	18.2	43	936	m.q.
roast beef, super	552	23.7	54.1	28.3	43	1174	m.q.
roast beef sub . . .	623	37.7	46.8	32.0	73	1847	m.q.
roast chicken club	503	30.5	36.6	27.0	46	1143	m.q.
tuna sub	663	74.0	50.2	37.0	43	1342	m.q.
turkey sub	486	32.8	46.5	19.0	51	2033	m.q.
light sandwiches:							
roast beef deluxe	294	18.0	33.0	10.0	42	826	m.q.
roast chicken deluxe	276	24.0	33.0	7.0	33	777	m.q.
roast turkey deluxe	260	20.0	33.0	6.0	33	1262	m.q.
side dishes:							
cheddar fries . . .	399	6.2	46.2	21.9	9	443	m.q.
curly fries	337	4.2	43.2	17.7	0	167	m.q.
french fries	246	2.1	29.8	13.2	0	114	m.q.
potato, baked:							
plain	240	5.8	50.2	1.9	0	58	m.q.
w/butter and sour							
cream	463	7.7	52.7	25.2	40	203	m.q.

Food and Measure	cal.	prot. (gms)	carbo. (gms)	fat (gms)	chol. (mgs)	sod. (mgs)	fiber (gms)
Arby's, potato baked (cont.)							
Broccoli'N Ched-							
dar	417	10.5	55.0	17.9	22	361	m.q.
deluxe	621	17.2	58.9	36.4	58	605	m.q.
Mushroom'N							
Cheese	515	15.0	57.5	26.7	47	923	m.q.
potato cakes . . .	204	1.8	19.8	12.0	0	397	m.q.
soups, 8 oz.:							
Boston clam chow-							
der	193	8.3	17.5	10.0	26	1032	n.a.
cream of broccoli	166	7.7	18.0	7.2	24	1050	m.q.
lumberjack mixed							
vegetable	89	2.3	12.6	3.6	4	1075	m.q.
old fashioned							
chicken noodle	99	6.0	14.8	1.8	25	929	n.a.
potato w/bacon . .	184	6.5	20.0	8.8	20	1068	m.q.
Wisconsin cheese	281	9.0	19.7	18.0	32	1084	m.q.
salads:							
chef	205	18.5	13.0	9.5	126	796	m.q.
garden	117	7.0	11.4	5.2	12	134	m.q.
roast chicken . . .	204	24.0	12.2	7.2	43	508	m.q.
side	25	2.0	4.0	.3	0	30	m.q.
salad dressing, 2 oz.:							
blue cheese	295	2.3	2.5	31.2	50	489	n.a.
buttermilk ranch . .	349	.3	1.9	38.5	6	471	n.a.
honey French . . .	322	.2	21.8	26.9	0	486	n.a.
light Italian	23	0	3.5	1.1	0	1110	n.a.
Thousand Island . .	298	.5	9.8	29.2	24	493	n.a.
sauces:							
au jus, 4 oz.	7	1.0	1.0	0	0	750	n.a.
Arby's Sauce, .5 oz.	15	.1	3.3	.2	0	113	n.a.
Horsey Sauce, .5 oz.	55	.1	2.6	5.0	<1	105	n.a.
desserts:							
apple turnover . . .	303	4.4	27.5	18.3	0	178	m.q.
blueberry turnover	320	3.0	32.0	19.0	0	240	m.q.
cheesecake	306	5.2	21.3	22.8	94	220	n.a.
cherry turnover . .	280	4.6	25.4	17.8	0	200	m.q.

Food and Measure	cal.	prot. (gms)	carbo. (gms)	fat (gms)	chol. (mgs)	sod. (mgs)	fiber (gms)
chocolate chip cookie	130	2.0	17.0	4.0	0	95	m.q.
Polar Swirl:							
Butterfinger . . .	457	12.1	61.6	18.1	28	318	n.a.
Heath	543	10.6	76.3	21.8	39	346	n.a.
Oreo	482	10.5	65.8	19.7	35	521	n.a.
peanut butter cup	517	14.0	61.4	24.0	34	385	n.a.
Snickers	511	12.2	73.3	18.8	33	351	n.a.
shake, chocolate	451	10.2	76.5	11.6	36	341	(0)
shake, jamocha . .	368	9.3	59.1	10.5	35	262	(0)
shake, vanilla . . .	330	10.5	46.2	11.5	32	281	0
Arrowhead:							
raw, 25/8"-diam. corm	12	.6	2.4	<.1	0	3	.1 c
boiled, 1"-diam. corm	9	.5	1.9	<.1	0	2	.2 c
Arrowroot flour,							
1 cup	457	.4	112.8	.1	0	2	4.4 d
Artichoke, globe:							
fresh, boiled:							
1 medium, 10.6 oz.	60	4.2	13.4	.2	0	114	6.5 d
hearts, 1/2 cup . . .	42	2.9	9.4	.1	0	80	4.5 d
canned, hearts, 1/2 cup:							
w/liquid *(Progresso)*	20	1.0	5.0	0	0	490	2.0 d
drained *(Progresso)*	16	2.0	4.0	<1.0	0	300	3.0 d
marinated, w/liquid *(Progresso)* . . .	190	1.0	16.0	15.0	0	460	2.0 d
frozen, hearts, 3 oz.:							
(Birds Eye Deluxe)	30	2.0	7.0	0	0	40	m.q.
(Seabrook)	25	3.0	4.0	0	0	6	1.0 c
Artichoke, Jerusalem, see "Jerusalem artichoke"							
Arugula:							
trimmed, 1 oz.	7	.7	1.0	.2	0	8	m.q.
trimmed, 1/2 cup . . .	2	.3	.4	.1	0	3	m.q.

Food and Measure	cal.	prot. (gms)	carbo. (gms)	fat (gms)	chol. (mgs)	sod. (mgs)	fiber (gms)
Asparagus:							
fresh:							
raw, 4 spears,							
3.8 oz.	14	1.3	2.6	.1	0	1	1.2 d
boiled, 4 spears,							
1/2″-diam. base	14	1.6	2.5	.2	0	7	1.3 d
boiled, drained,							
cuts, 1/2 cup . .	22	2.3	3.8	.3	0	10	1.9 d
canned, 1/2 cup:							
(Stokely)	20	2.0	3.0	0	0	380	m.q.
spears, white (Green							
Giant)	16	2.0	3.0	0	0	410	1.0 d
spears or cut (Green							
Giant)	18	2.0	3.0	0	0	420	1.0 d
cut (Green Giant							
50% Less Salt)	18	2.0	3.0	0	0	210	1.0 d
frozen, 3.3 oz., except							
as noted:							
boiled, 4 spears, ap-							
prox. 2.1 oz. . .	17	1.8	2.9	.3	0	2	1.2 d
spears (Frosty							
Acres)	25	3.0	4.0	0	0	4	1.0 c
cuts and spears							
(Frosty Acres) . .	25	3.0	4.0	0	0	6	m.q.
cuts (Green Giant							
Harvest Fresh),							
1/2 cup	25	3.0	4.0	0	0	95	2.0 d
Asparagus bean, see							
"Winged bean"							
Asparagus pilaf, fro-							
zen:							
(Green Giant Garden							
Gourmet Right for							
Lunch), 9.5 oz. . .	190	5.0	37.0	4.0	10	610	3.0 d
Au jus gravy:							
canned (Franco-Ameri-							
can), 2 oz.	10	0	2.0	0	n.a.	330	n.a.

14

Food and Measure	cal.	prot. (gms)	carbo. (gms)	fat (gms)	chol. (mgs)	sod. (mgs)	fiber (gms)
canned *(Heinz HomeStyle)*, 2 oz. or ¼ cup	18	0	2.0	1.0	0	350	n.a.
mix:							
(French's), ⅛ pkt.	8	0	1.0	0	0	200	n.a.
(Lawry's), 1 pkt. . .	89	4.8	11.7	2.5	2	2790	.1 c
(McCormick/Schilling), ¼ cup* . .	20	1.0	3.5	.3	n.a.	262	n.a.
Au jus sauce mix *(Knorr)*, 1 serving	15	.3	2.6	.1	n.a.	m.q.	n.a.
Au jus seasoning mix *(French's* Roasting Bag)*, ⅛ pkg. . . .	10	0	2.0	0	0	270	n.a.
Avocado, California:							
1 medium, 8 oz. . . .	306	3.6	12.0	30.0	0	21	4.7 d
trimmed, 1 oz.	50	.6	2.0	4.9	0	3	.8 d
cocktail *(Frieda's)*, 1 oz.	47	.8	1.8	4.6	0	1	m.q.
Avocado dip *(Kraft)*, 2 tbsp.	50	1.0	3.0	4.0	0	210	n.a.

B

Food and Measure	cal.	prot. (gms)	carbo. (gms)	fat (gms)	chol. (mgs)	sod. (mgs)	fiber (gms)
Bacon, cooked:							
4.5 oz. (1 lb. raw) . .	732	38.7	.8	62.5	107	2026	0
(Black Label), 1 oz.	142	3.0	<2.0	14.0	18	192	0
(Black Label Low Salt),							
1.8 oz.	250	5.0	<2.0	25.0	32	260	0
(Hormel Microwave),							
1 oz.	142	3.0	<2.0	14.0	18	192	0
(Jones Dairy Farm),							
1 slice	130	2.0	tr.	13.0	18	230	0
(Oscar Mayer), 2 slices	60	4.0	0	5.0	10	290	0
(Oscar Mayer Center							
Cut), 3 slices . . .	70	5.0	<1.0	5.0	15	320	0
(Oscar Mayer Lower							
Salt), 2 slices . . .	80	5.0	0	7.0	15	220	0
(Range Brand Thick							
Slice), 1 oz.	152	2.0	<1.0	16.0	17	199	0
turkey, see "Turkey							
bacon"							
Bacon, Canadian:							
unheated, 1 oz. . . .	45	5.9	.5	2.0	14	399	0
(Jones Dairy Farm)							
.5-oz. slice	30	3.0	tr.	1.0	7	140	0
(Oscar Mayer), 2 slices	50	9.0	0	2.0	25	600	0
"Bacon," vegetarian:							
.2-oz. strip	25	.9	.5	2.4	0	117	.2 d
frozen *(Morningstar*							
Farms Breakfast							
Strips), 3 strips . .	80	3.0	4.0	6.0	0	350	m.q.
frozen *(Worthington*							
Stripples), 4 strips	120	4.0	6.0	9.0	0	460	m.q.

Food and Measure	cal.	prot. (gms)	carbo. (gms)	fat (gms)	chol. (mgs)	sod. (mgs)	fiber (gms)
Bacon bits, real or imitation:							
(Bac*Os), 2 tsp. . . .	25	2.0	2.0	1.0	0	90	n.a.
(Hormel), 1 oz.	117	12.0	1.0	7.0	16	1008	0
(McCormick/Schilling Bac'N Pieces), 1 tbsp.	26	2.0	2.0	.5	n.a.	205	n.a.
(Oscar Mayer), 1 tbsp.	20	3.0	0	1.0	5	190	0
pieces (Hormel), 1 oz.	94	12.0	<2.0	5.0	26	654	0
Bacon breakfast bis-cuit, frozen (Swan-son), 3.2 oz.	340	10.0	22.0	23.0	m.q.	990	m.q.
Bacon horseradish dip, 2 tbsp.:							
(Breakstone's/Sealtest)	70	1.0	2.0	6.0	15	270	n.a.
(Kraft)	60	1.0	3.0	5.0	0	200	n.a.
(Kraft Premium) . . .	50	1.0	2.0	5.0	15	270	n.a.
Bacon and onion dip, 2 tbsp.:							
(Breakstone's Gour-met)	70	1.0	2.0	6.0	15	210	n.a.
(Kraft Premium) . . .	60	1.0	2.0	5.0	15	170	n.a.
Bagel, 1 piece:							
plain (Thomas') . . .	170	9.0	34.0	<1.0	0	200	1.0 d
cinnamon raisin (Thomas')	160	8.0	36.0	<1.0	0	180	1.0 d
egg (Thomas')	180	9.0	33.0	<1.0	35	200	1.0 d
onion (Thomas') . . .	180	9.0	35.0	<1.0	0	200	1.0 d
Bagel, frozen, 1 piece:							
plain:							
(Lender's)	150	6.0	30.0	1.0	0	320	2.0 d
(Lender's Bagelet-tes)	70	3.0	14.0	<1.0	0	130	1.0 d
(Lender's Big'N Crusty)	210	8.0	43.0	2.0	0	430	3.0 d

Food and Measure	cal.	prot. (gms)	carbo. (gms)	fat (gms)	chol. (mgs)	sod. (mgs)	fiber (gms)
Bagel, frozen (cont.)							
blueberry (Lender's)	190	7.0	38.0	2.0	0	320	2.0 d
cinnamon raisin:							
(Lender's)	190	6.0	39.0	2.0	0	310	2.0 d
(Lender's Big'N							
Crusty)	230	8.0	47.0	2.0	0	330	2.0 d
egg:							
(Lender's)	150	6.0	30.0	1.0	0	310	1.0 d
(Lender's Big'N							
Crusty)	210	8.0	44.0	1.0	0	400	2.0 d
oat (Lender's)	170	7.0	36.0	2.0	0	300	4.0 d
onion:							
(Lender's)	150	6.0	30.0	1.0	0	300	2.0 d
(Lender's Big'N							
Crusty)	210	8.0	43.0	1.0	0	410	m.q.
poppy (Lender's) . . .	140	6.0	30.0	1.0	0	290	2.0 d
pumpernickel							
(Lender's)	140	5.0	31.0	1.0	0	330	2.0 d
rye (Lender's)	140	5.0	30.0	1.0	0	320	2.0 d
sesame (Lender's) . .	150	6.0	29.0	1.0	0	280	2.0 d
soft (Lender's Original)	200	7.0	38.0	3.0	10	340	2.0 d
Bagel chips (Pepper-							
idge Farm):							
cheese, 1/2 oz.	70	2.0	10.0	3.0	0	100	m.q.
onion, toasted, and							
garlic, 1/2 oz. . . .	60	2.0	10.0	2.0	0	105	m.q.
Bagel sandwich, see							
specific listings							
Baked beans,							
canned:							
(Allens), 1/2 cup . . .	170	6.0	21.0	1.0	n.a.	330	5.0 d
(Campbell's Home							
Style), 4 oz.	130	6.0	24.0	2.0	n.a.	430	13.0 d
(Grandma Brown's),							
1/2 cup	150	7.3	27.0	1.5	<1	328	7.8 d
(Grandma Brown's							
Saucepan), 1/2 cup	154	6.8	26.2	2.4	<1	296	7.4 d

Food and Measure	cal.	prot. (gms)	carbo. (gms)	fat (gms)	chol. (mgs)	sod. (mgs)	fiber (gms)
(Green Giant/Joan of Arc), 1/2 cup	130	6.0	30.0	1.0	2	570	6.0 d
barbecue, 4 oz.:							
(Campbell's)	130	5.0	22.0	2.0	n.a.	430	6.0 d
(Campbell's Old Fashioned) . . .	150	6.0	26.0	2.0	n.a.	400	m.q.
brown sugar and bacon:							
(Campbell's), 4 oz.	150	5.0	25.0	3.0	m.q.	430	m.q.
(Hanover), 1/2 cup	140	6.0	27.0	1.0	m.q.	530	6.0 d
brown sugar and molasses *(Campbell's* Old Fashioned), 4 oz.	150	5.0	27.0	3.0	n.a.	340	6.0 d
w/franks, in sauce *(Libby's Diner)*, 7.75 oz.	330	15.0	38.0	15.0	55	930	m.q.
w/honey *(B&M Brick Oven)*, 8 oz.	240	14.0	50.0	3.0	0	890	11.0 d
w/honey, Boston *(Health Valley Fat Free)*, 7.5 oz. . . .	190	8.0	41.0	<1.0	0	290	5.0 d
maple *(B&M Brick Oven/Friends)*, 8 oz.	240	14.0	52.0	2.0	<5	890	11.0 d
New England style *(Campbell's)*, 4 oz.	150	5.0	m.q.	3.0	n.a.	340	m.q.
w/onions *(Bush's Best)*, 4 oz.	126	6.0	27.0	1.0	n.a.	554	7.0 d
pea *(B&M Brick Oven)*, 8 oz.	270	14.0	50.0	6.0	5	750	11.0 d
w/pork:							
(Crest Top), 1/2 cup	110	6.0	18.0	1.0	m.q.	430	5.0 d
(Heinz), 8 oz. . . .	250	12.0	44.0	5.0	m.q.	740	m.q.
(Hunt's), 4 oz. . . .	135	6.0	26.0	1.0	1	430	8.0 d
(Wagon Master), 1/2 cup	130	5.0	24.0	1.0	m.q.	540	5.0 d
pea, small *(Friends)*, 8 oz.	260	14.0	53.0	5.0	<5	890	11.0 d

Food and Measure	cal.	prot. (gms)	carbo. (gms)	fat (gms)	chol. (mgs)	sod. (mgs)	fiber (gms)
Baked beans, w/pork *(cont.)*							
red kidney *(Friends),* 8 oz.	270	14.0	55.0	4.0	4	990	11.0 d
tomato *(B&M* Brick Oven), 8 oz. . . .	230	12.0	48.0	3.0	n.a.	1010	10.0 d
in tomato sauce *(Campbell's),* 4 oz.	120	5.0	21.0	2.0	n.a.	370	5.0 d
in tomato sauce *(Green Giant/Joan of Arc),* 1/2 cup	90	5.0	21.0	1.0	0	420	5.0 d
red kidney *(B&M* Brick Oven), 8 oz.	240	12.0	48.0	4.0	5	680	11.0 d
vegetarian:							
4 oz.	105	5.4	23.3	.5	0	450	8.7 d
(B&M 50% Less Sodium), 8 oz. . . .	230	14.0	50.0	3.0	0	370	11.0 d
(Bush's Deluxe), 4 oz.	110	5.0	25.0	<1.0	0	350	6.0 d
(Heinz), 8 oz. . . .	250	9.0	50.0	2.0	0	890	m.q.
honey baked, w/miso *(Health Valley),* 7.5 oz.	180	8.0	38.0	<1.0	0	60	5.4 d
in tomato sauce *(Campbell's),* 4 oz.	110	6.0	20.0	1.0	0	400	5.0 d
yellow eye *(B&M* Brick Oven), 8 oz.	250	14.0	50.0	5.0	5	810	11.0 d
Baking mix:							
(Bisquick), 1/2 cup . .	240	4.0	37.0	8.0	0	700	m.q.
(Bisquick Reduced Fat), 1/2 cup	210	5.0	39.0	4.0	0	660	m.q.
whole wheat *(Hain),* 1/3 cup	150	6.0	30.0	1.0	n.a.	680	5.0 d
Baking powder *(Davis),* 1 tsp.	8	0	2.0	0	0	330	0
Baking soda *(Tone's),* 1 tsp.	0	0	0	0	0	821	0

Food and Measure	cal.	prot. (gms)	carbo. (gms)	fat (gms)	chol. (mgs)	sod. (mgs)	fiber (gms)
Balsam pear, fresh:							
leafy-tips, 1/2 cup:							
raw	7	1.3	.8	.2	0	3	.6 c
boiled, drained . .	10	1.0	2.0	.1	0	4	.6 d
pods, 1/2 cup:							
raw, 1/2″ pieces . .	8	.5	1.7	.1	0	3	1.3 d
boiled, drained,							
1/2″ pieces . . .	12	.5	2.7	.1	0	4	1.2 d
Bamboo shoots:							
fresh, 1/2 cup:							
raw, slices	21	2.0	4.0	.2	0	3	1.7 d
boiled, drained,							
1/2″ slices	8	.9	1.2	.1	0	3	1.0 c
canned:							
drained, 1/2 cup . .	13	1.1	2.1	.3	0	5	2.0 d
(La Choy), 1/4 cup	6	<1.0	1.0	<1.0	0	2	<1.0 d
Banana:							
fresh:							
whole, 1 lb.	271	3.1	69.1	1.4	0	3	7.1 d
1 medium,							
8 3/4″ long	105	1.2	26.7	.6	0	1	2.7 d
mashed, 1/2 cup . .	104	1.2	26.4	.5	0	1	2.7 d
dehydrated, 1/4 cup	87	1.0	22.1	.5	0	1	1.9 d
Banana, baking, see							
"Plantain"							
Banana, manzano							
(Frieda's), 1 oz. . .	24	.3	6.3	.1	0	<1	m.q.
Banana, red, 1 me-							
dium, 7 1/4″ long . .	118	1.6	30.7	.3	0	1	m.q.
Banana berry drink							
(Hi-C Stompin' Ba-							
nana Berry), 6 fl. oz.	90	0	22.0	0	0	25	(0)
Banana flavor drink							
mix *(Nestlé Quik),*							
2 1/2 heaping tsp.	90	0	21.0	0	0	0	n.a.
Banana nectar							
(Libby's), 6 fl. oz.	110	0	26.0	0	0	15	m.q.

Food and Measure	cal.	prot. (gms)	carbo. (gms)	fat (gms)	chol. (mgs)	sod. (mgs)	fiber (gms)
Banana squash,							
baked *(Frieda's)*,							
1 oz.	18	.5	4.4	.1	0	3	m.q.
Banana-pineapple							
nectar *(Kern's)*,							
6 fl. oz.	110	1.0	27.0	0	0	0	m.q.
Barbecue sauce,							
2 tbsp., except as							
noted:							
(Enrico's Original) . .	36	2.0	6.0	2.0	0	8	n.a.
(Heinz Select), 1 oz.	40	0	9.0	0	0	275	n.a.
(Heinz Thick & Rich							
Chunky), 1 oz. . . .	30	1.0	6.0	0	0	380	n.a.
(Heinz Thick & Rich							
Old Fashioned),							
1 oz.	35	0	8.0	0	0	350	n.a.
(Heinz Thick & Rich							
Original), 1 oz. . . .	35	0	8.0	0	0	390	n.a.
(Hunt's Homestyle),							
1 tbsp.	20	<1.0	6.0	<1.0	0	170	<1.0 d
(Hunt's Original),							
1 tbsp.	20	<1.0	5.0	<1.0	0	160	<1.0 d
(Kraft)	45	0	10.0	1.0	0	460	n.a.
(Kraft Thick 'N Spicy							
Original)	50	0	12.0	1.0	0	430	n.a.
(Luzianne)	110	0	19.0	4.0	0	350	<1.0 d
(Maull's)	40	0	10.0	0	0	320	(0)
(Maull's Lite)	25	0	6.0	0	n.a.	170	(0)
(Ott's Original)	29	0	7.0	0	0	380	0
beer flavor *(Maull's)*	45	0	9.0	0	0	310	(0)
Cajun style *(Heinz*							
Thick & Rich), 1 oz.	35	0	8.0	0	0	360	n.a.
chunky *(Kraft Thick 'N*							
Spicy)	60	0	13.0	1.0	0	420	n.a.
country style *(Hunt's)*,							
1 tbsp.	20	<1.0	5.0	<1.0	0	140	<1.0 d
Dijon and honey							
(Lawry's), 1/4 cup	203	4.7	27.0	1.2	0	1768	.4 c

Food and Measure	cal.	prot. (gms)	carbo. (gms)	fat (gms)	chol. (mgs)	sod. (mgs)	fiber (gms)
fajita (Lawry's), 1 oz.	38	2.2	5.1	1.0	<1	534	n.a.
garlic (Kraft)	40	0	9.0	0	0	420	n.a.
Hawaiian style (Heinz Thick & Rich), 1 oz.	40	0	10.0	0	0	210	n.a.
hickory smoke:							
(Heinz Select), 1 oz.	35	0	8.0	0	0	260	n.a.
(Heinz Thick & Rich), 1 oz.	35	0	8.0	0	0	380	n.a.
(Hunt's), 1 tbsp. . . .	20	<1.0	5.0	<1.0	0	160	<1.0 d
(Kraft)	45	0	10.0	1.0	0	440	n.a.
(Kraft Thick 'N Spicy)	50	0	12.0	1.0	0	430	n.a.
or original (Lea & Perrins), 1 tbsp.	30	0	7.0	0	0	150	0
w/honey:							
(Hain), 1 tbsp. . . .	14	0	1.0	1.0	0	120	n.a.
(Kraft Thick 'N Spicy)	60	0	13.0	1.0	0	340	n.a.
hot:							
(Kraft)	45	0	9.0	1.0	0	520	n.a.
hickory smoke (Kraft)	45	0	9.0	1.0	0	360	n.a.
Texas (Heinz Thick & Rich), 1 oz. . . .	30	0	7.0	0	0	390	n.a.
hot and spicy (Master Choice), 1 tbsp.	30	0	7.0	0	0	140	n.a.
Italian seasonings (Kraft)	50	0	10.0	1.0	0	280	n.a.
Kansas City style:							
(Hunt's), 1 tbsp. . . .	20	<1.0	5.0	<1.0	0	85	<1.0 d
(Kraft)	50	0	11.0	1.0	0	270	n.a.
(Kraft Thick 'N Spicy)	60	0	13.0	1.0	0	270	n.a.
(Maull's)	60	0	15.0	0	0	320	(0)
mesquite:							
(Enrico's), 1 tbsp.	18	1.0	3.0	1.0	0	4	n.a.

Food and Measure	cal.	prot. (gms)	carbo. (gms)	fat (gms)	chol. (mgs)	sod. (mgs)	fiber (gms)
Barbecue sauce, mesquite *(cont.)*							
smoke *(Heinz* Thick & Rich), 1 oz. . . .	30	0	7.0	0	0	380	n.a.
smoke *(Kraft)* . . .	45	0	10.0	1.0	0	410	n.a.
smoke *(Kraft Thick 'N Spicy)*	50	0	12.0	1.0	0	430	n.a.
mushroom *(Heinz* Thick & Rich), 1 oz.	30	1.0	6.0	0	0	460	n.a.
New Orleans style *(Hunt's)*, 1 tbsp. . . .	20	<1.0	5.0	<1.0	0	150	<1.0 d
onion:							
(Heinz Thick & Rich), 1 oz.	30	0	7.0	0	0	420	n.a.
(Maull's)	45	0	9.0	0	0	310	(0)
bits, plain or hickory smoke *(Kraft)* . .	50	0	11.0	1.0	0	340	n.a.
Oriental:							
(La Choy), 1 tbsp.	16	.7	3.8	<.1	0	304	<.1 d
stir-fry *(Lawry's)*, 1/4 cup	120	1.9	19.6	3.8	0	1128	.2 c
Ozark recipe *(Ott's)*	53	0	14.0	0	0	319	0
Silver Dollar City *(Ott's)*	38	0	10.0	0	0	364	0
sloppy Joe, w/beef *(Libby's)*, 1/3 cup	110	5.0	7.0	7.0	m.q.	190	n.a.
smoky *(Maull's)* . . .	40	0	10.0	0	0	310	(0)
smoky *(Ott's)*	28	0	7.0	0	0	382	0
Southern or Western *(Hunt's)*, 1 tbsp. . . .	20	<1.0	5.0	<1.0	0	170	<1.0 d
sweet:							
(Maull's Sweet-N-Mild)	60	0	12.0	0	0	280	(0)
(Maull's Sweet-N-Smokey)	60	0	13.0	0	0	300	(0)
(Ott's Sweet-n-Mild)	39	0	10.0	0	0	379	0
sweet and sour *(Lawry's)*, 1/4 cup	549	3.4	11.7	7.5	0	4056	.4 c
teriyaki *(Lawry's)*, 1 oz.	63	.7	14.1	.4	<1	568	n.a.

Food and Measure	cal.	prot. (gms)	carbo. (gms)	fat (gms)	chol. (mgs)	sod. (mgs)	fiber (gms)
Texas style *(Hunt's)*,							
1 tbsp.	25	<1.0	6.0	<1.0	0	150	<1.0 d
Barley:							
dry, 1 cup	651	23.0	135.2	4.2	0	22	31.8 d
dry *(Arrowhead Mills)*,							
2 oz.	200	5.0	45.0	1.0	0	<1	7.2 d
hull-less *(Arrowhead*							
Mills), 2 oz.	180	6.0	43.0	1.0	0	0	8.0 d
pearled:							
dry, 1 cup	704	19.8	155.5	2.3	0	18	31.2 d
cooked, 1 cup . . .	193	3.6	44.3	.7	0	5	6.0 d
Barley flakes *(Arrow-*							
head Mills), 2 oz.	200	5.0	45.0	1.0	0	1	7.4 d
Barley flour *(Arrow-*							
head Mills), 2 oz.	200	7.0	35.0	1.0	0	1	7.2 d
Barley malt *(Eden)*,							
1/2 tsp.	10	0	2.0	0	0	1	n.a.
Basella, see "Vine-spinach"							
Basil:							
fresh:							
1 oz.	8	.7	1.2	.2	0	0	m.q.
5 medium leaves	1	.1	.1	<.1	0	0	m.q.
chopped, 2 tbsp.	1	.1	.2	<.1	0	0	m.q.
dried, ground, 1 tsp.	4	.2	.9	.1	0	tr.	.2 d
Baskin-Robbins:							
ice cream, 1 regular scoop:							
chocolate, world							
class	280	5.0	35.0	14.0	36	145	n.a.
chocolate raspberry							
truffle *International*							
Creams	310	4.0	35.0	17.0	45	115	n.a.
strawberry, very							
berry	220	3.0	30.0	10.0	30	95	n.a.
vanilla	240	4.0	24.0	14.0	52	115	0

Food and Measure	cal.	prot. (gms)	carbo. (gms)	fat (gms)	chol. (mgs)	sod. (mgs)	fiber (gms)
Baskin-Robbins *(cont.)*							
Chilly Burger, vanilla,							
1 piece	240	4.0	32.0	11.0	29	130	n.a.
Tiny Toon Adventures,							
1 piece:							
mint chocolate chip	230	3.0	19.0	15.0	17	35	n.a.
vanilla	210	3.0	18.0	14.0	18	35	n.a.
Toonwiches:							
chocolate	330	4.0	46.0	14.0	33	105	n.a.
vanilla	340	5.0	45.0	16.0	34	65	n.a.
cones, unfilled:							
sugar, 1 piece . . .	60	1.0	11.0	1.0	0	45	m.q.
waffle, 1 piece . . .	140	3.0	28.0	2.0	0	5	m.q.
Bass, meat only:							
freshwater:							
raw, 4 oz.	129	21.4	0	4.2	77	79	0
baked, broiled, or							
microwaved, 4 oz.	166	27.4	0	5.4	99	102	0
sea, see "Sea bass"							
striped:							
raw, 4 oz.	110	20.1	0	2.7	91	78	0
baked, broiled, or							
microwaved, 4 oz.	141	25.8	0	3.4	117	100	0
Batter mix (see also							
specific listings):							
(Golden Dipt), 1 oz.	100	3.0	21.0	0	0	740	m.q.
(Golden Dipt Corny							
Dog), 1 oz.	100	3.0	22.0	0	0	490	m.q.
Bay leaf, dried, crum-							
bled *(Spice Islands),*							
1 tsp.	5	.1	.3	.1	0	<1	.3 c
Bean dip:							
(Chi-Chi's Fiesta),							
1 oz.	30	1.0	4.0	1.0	3	126	m.q.
hot *(Hain),* 2 tbsp. . .	40	2.0	5.0	1.0	0	120	m.q.
jalapeño:							
(Frito-Lay's), 1 oz.	30	1.0	4.0	1.0	0	115	m.q.

Food and Measure	cal.	prot. (gms)	carbo. (gms)	fat (gms)	chol. (mgs)	sod. (mgs)	fiber (gms)
(Old El Paso), 1 tbsp.	14	1.0	2.0	0	0	53	1.0 d
Mexican (Hain), 2 tbsp.	35	2.0	5.0	1.0	0	120	m.q.
onion (Hain), 2 tbsp.	35	2.0	5.0	1.0	0	115	m.q.
Bean dishes, canned, see specific bean listings							
Bean dishes, mix* (see also specific listings):							
(Hunt's Big John's Beans'n Fixin's), 4 oz.	170	5.0	26.0	6.0	6	490	6.0 d
Cajun, and sauce (Lipton), 1/2 cup	150	5.0	28.0	3.0	n.a.	440	m.q.
Bean salad, three bean, canned (Green Giant), 1/2 cup	70	2.0	18.0	<1.0	0	470	3.0 d
Bean sprouts, see "Sprouts" and specific listings							
Beans, see specific listings							
Beans, snap, see "Green bean"							
Beans and frankfurters, frozen (Morton), 8.5 oz.	300	9.0	39.0	11.0	25	1270	m.q.
Bearnaise sauce mix:							
dry, .9-oz. pkt.	90	3.5	14.8	2.2	tr.	841	.1 c
(McCormick/Schilling McCormick Collection), 1/4 cup* . . .	129	3.0	6.0	11.0	n.a.	450	n.a.
Beechnuts, dried, shelled, 1 oz. . . .	164	1.8	9.5	14.2	0	m.q.	1.1 c

Food and Measure	cal.	prot. (gms)	carbo. (gms)	fat (gms)	chol. (mgs)	sod. (mgs)	fiber (gms)
Beef, choice, meat only[1], 4 oz.:							
brisket, whole:							
braised, lean w/fat	437	26.6	0	35.8	107	69	0
braised, lean only	274	33.7	0	14.5	105	79	0
chuck, arm pot roast:							
braised, lean w/fat	395	30.6	0	29.2	112	67	0
braised, lean only	255	37.4	0	10.5	115	75	0
chuck, blade roast:							
braised, lean w/fat	412	29.7	0	31.5	117	73	0
braised, lean only	298	35.2	0	16.3	120	81	0
flank steak[2]:							
braised, lean only	269	31.8	0	14.7	81	82	0
broiled, lean only	256	30.0	0	14.2	77	92	0
ground, raw:							
extra lean	265	21.1	0	19.3	78	75	0
lean	298	20.0	0	23.4	85	78	0
regular	351	18.8	0	30.0	96	77	0
ground, broiled, medium:							
extra lean	290	28.8	0	18.5	95	79	0
lean	308	28.0	0	20.9	99	87	0
regular	328	27.3	0	23.5	102	94	0
porterhouse steak:							
broiled, lean w/fat	346	28.2	0	25.1	94	69	0
broiled, lean only	247	31.9	0	12.2	91	75	0
rib, whole:							
roasted, lean w/fat	426	25.1	0	35.4	96	71	0
roasted, lean only	276	30.9	0	15.9	91	82	0
rib, large end (ribs 6–9):							
roasted, lean w/fat	434	25.3	0	36.2	96	71	0
roasted, lean only	284	31.2	0	16.7	92	83	0

[1] *Trimmed to 1/4″ fat, except as noted.*

[2] *Trimmed to 0″ fat.*

Food and Measure	cal.	prot. (gms)	carbo. (gms)	fat (gms)	chol. (mgs)	sod. (mgs)	fiber (gms)
rib, small end (ribs 10–12):							
broiled, lean w/fat	376	26.7	0	31.3	95	70	0
broiled, lean only	264	31.8	0	14.3	91	78	0
round, bottom:							
braised, lean w/fat	322	32.5	0	20.3	109	57	0
braised, lean only	249	35.8	0	10.7	109	58	0
round, eye of:							
roasted, lean w/fat	273	30.2	0	16.0	82	67	0
roasted, lean only	198	32.9	0	6.5	78	70	0
round, full cut:							
broiled, lean w/fat	272	31.0	0	15.4	91	69	0
broiled, lean only	217	33.1	0	8.3	88	73	0
round, tip:							
roasted, lean w/fat	280	30.1	0	16.9	94	70	0
roasted, lean only	213	32.6	0	8.3	92	74	0
round, top:							
broiled, lean w/fat	254	34.2	0	12.0	96	68	0
broiled, lean only	214	35.9	0	6.7	95	69	0
fried, lean w/fat . .	314	36.7	0	17.4	110	77	0
fried, lean only . .	257	39.8	0	9.7	110	81	0
shank, crosscuts:							
braised, lean w/fat	298	34.8	0	16.6	91	69	0
braised, lean only	228	38.2	0	7.2	88	73	0
shortribs:							
braised, lean w/fat	534	24.5	0	47.6	107	57	0
braised, lean only	335	34.9	0	20.6	105	66	0
sirloin, top:							
broiled, lean w/fat	305	31.3	0	19.0	102	70	0
broiled, lean only	229	34.4	0	9.1	101	75	0
fried, lean w/fat . .	370	31.9	0	25.9	111	79	0
fried, lean only . .	270	36.8	0	12.4	112	87	0
T-bone steak:							
broiled, lean w/fat	338	28.3	0	24.0	94	69	0
broiled, lean only	243	31.9	0	11.8	91	75	0
tenderloin:							
broiled, lean w/fat	345	28.4	0	24.8	98	67	0
broiled, lean only	252	32.0	0	12.7	95	71	0

Food and Measure	cal.	prot. (gms)	carbo. (gms)	fat (gms)	chol. (mgs)	sod. (mgs)	fiber (gms)
Beef *(cont.)*							
top loin:							
broiled, lean w/fat	338	28.8	0	23.8	90	71	0
broiled, lean only	243	32.5	0	11.5	86	77	0
Beef, corned (see also "Beef luncheon meat") brisket, cooked, 4 oz. . . .	285	20.6	.5	21.5	111	1286	0
Beef, corned, hash, canned:							
(Dinty Moore Cup), 7.5 oz.	350	19.0	22.0	9.0	65	850	m.q.
(Libby's), 7.5 oz. . . .	400	18.0	20.0	27.0	m.q.	1260	m.q.
(Mary Kitchen), 1 oz.	47	3.0	2.0	3.0	9	111	m.q.
Beef, dried:							
cured, 1 oz.	47	8.3	.4	1.1	m.q.	984	0
sliced *(Hormel),* 1 oz.	45	8.0	1.0	1.0	20	1137	0
Beef, roast, hash, canned *(Mary Kitchen),* 1 oz. . . .	46	3.0	3.0	3.0	8	97	m.q.
"Beef," vegetarian (see also " 'Hamburger,' vegetarian"):							
canned:							
(Worthington Savory Slices), 2 slices	100	8.0	4.0	6.0	0	340	m.q.
steak *(Worthington Prime Steaks),* 3.25-oz. piece . .	160	10.0	7.0	10.0	0	410	m.q.
steak *(Worthington Vegetable Steaks),* 2 1/2 pieces . . .	110	17.0	5.0	2.0	0	400	m.q.
stew *(Worthington Country Stew),* 9.5 oz.	220	10.0	23.0	10.0	0	760	m.q.
Swiss steak *(LaLoma),* 1 piece	170	14.0	7.0	10.0	0	360	m.q.

Food and Measure	cal.	prot. (gms)	carbo. (gms)	fat (gms)	chol. (mgs)	sod. (mgs)	fiber (gms)
frozen:							
(Worthington Beef Style Meatless), 4 slices	130	12.0	7.0	6.0	0	750	m.q.
(Worthington Stakelets), 1 piece	150	13.0	7.0	8.0	0	460	m.q.
corned *(Worthington),* 4 slices . .	120	9.0	8.0	6.0	0	740	m.q.
pie *(Worthington),* 1 pie	360	9.0	44.0	16.0	0	1940	m.q.
smoked *(Worthington),* 3 slices . .	120	10.0	7.0	6.0	0	790	m.q.
steak *(LaLoma Griddle Steaks),* 1 piece	140	14.0	4.0	7.0	0	390	m.q.
Beef dinner, frozen:							
(Banquet Extra Helping), 15.5 oz. . . .	430	36.0	42.0	13.0	100	1220	m.q.
in barbecue sauce *(Swanson),* 11 oz.	460	30.0	51.0	15.0	m.q.	850	m.q.
champignon *(Tyson Premium),* 10.5 oz.	370	27.0	31.0	15.0	51	830	m.q.
chopped *(Banquet Meals),* 9.5 oz.	270	9.0	24.0	15.0	35	1060	m.q.
chopped steak *(Swanson Hungry Man),* 16.75 oz.	640	35.0	41.0	37.0	m.q.	1600	m.q.
enchilada, see "Enchilada dinner"							
marinated, slow-cooked *(Le Menu New American Cuisine),* 10.25 oz. . .	310	19.0	28.0	14.0	m.q.	710	m.q.
meat loaf, see "Meat loaf dinner"							
patty, charbroiled *(Freezer Queen),* 9.5 oz.	266	13.0	20.0	14.0	24	800	m.q.

Food and Measure	cal.	prot. (gms)	carbo. (gms)	fat (gms)	chol. (mgs)	sod. (mgs)	fiber (gms)
Beef dinner, frozen *(cont.)*							
pepper steak:							
(Armour Classics Lite), 11.25 oz.	220	17.0	29.0	4.0	35	970	m.q.
(Healthy Choice), 11 oz.	260	20.0	40.0	5.0	40	500	m.q.
pot roast:							
(The Budget Gourmet Light and Healthy), 10 oz.	230	25.0	19.0	7.0	60	510	m.q.
old fashioned *(Le Menu New American Cuisine)*, 10 oz.	250	24.0	22.0	7.0	m.q.	600	m.q.
Yankee *(Freezer Queen)*, 9.25 oz.	240	15.0	35.0	4.0	20	680	m.q.
Yankee *(Healthy Choice)*, 11 oz.	260	19.0	36.0	4.0	55	400	m.q.
Yankee *(Swanson)*, 11.5 oz.	270	18.0	35.0	7.0	m.q.	670	m.q.
Yankee *(Swanson Hungry Man)*, 16 oz.	420	30.0	49.0	11.0	m.q.	920	m.q.
roast, sandwich *(Swanson)*, 10.25 oz.	340	13.0	50.0	10.0	25	690	m.q.
Salisbury steak:							
(Armour Classics), 11.25 oz.	350	22.0	26.0	17.0	55	1430	m.q.
(Armour Classics Lite), 11.5 oz. . . .	300	21.0	29.0	11.0	40	980	m.q.
(Banquet Extra Helping), 16.25 oz.	590	33.0	57.0	28.0	85	2760	m.q.
(Freezer Queen), 9.5 oz.	260	14.0	19.0	14.0	20	980	m.q.
(Healthy Choice), 11.5 oz.	280	19.0	45.0	7.0	50	550	m.q.
(Swanson), 10.5 oz.	390	18.0	42.0	17.0	m.q.	890	m.q.

Food and Measure	cal.	prot. (gms)	carbo. (gms)	fat (gms)	chol. (mgs)	sod. (mgs)	fiber (gms)
(Swanson Hungry Man), 16.25 oz.	630	35.0	50.0	32.0	m.q.	1620	m.q.
char-grilled (Le Menu New American Cuisine), 10.5 oz.	360	21.0	30.0	17.0	m.q.	680	m.q.
old fashioned (Le Menu New American Cuisine Healthy), 10.25 oz.	270	19.0	37.0	5.0	25	480	m.q.
parmigiana (Armour Classics), 11.5 oz.	410	22.0	32.0	21.0	60	1120	m.q.
sirloin (The Budget Gourmet Light and Healthy), 11 oz.	280	21.0	30.0	9.0	40	530	m.q.
short ribs (Tyson Premium), 11 oz. . . .	470	25.0	38.0	24.0	70	950	m.q.
sirloin:							
w/barbecue sauce (Healthy Choice), 11 oz.	280	17.0	44.0	4.0	25	240	m.q.
chopped (Swanson), 10.5 oz.	340	20.0	29.0	17.0	m.q.	750	m.q.
smothered (Le Menu New American Cuisine), 10 oz.	430	16.0	60.0	14.0	m.q.	780	m.q.
special recipe (The Budget Gourmet Light and Healthy), 11 oz.	250	18.0	29.0	9.0	60	560	m.q.
tips (Healthy Choice), 11.25 oz.	270	22.0	29.0	7.0	65	360	m.q.
tips (Le Menu New American Cuisine), 7.7 oz.	290	23.0	25.0	11.0	m.q.	750	m.q.

Food and Measure	cal.	prot. (gms)	carbo. (gms)	fat (gms)	chol. (mgs)	sod. (mgs)	fiber (gms)
Beef dinner, frozen, sirloin *(cont.)*							
tips *(Swanson)*,							
7 oz.	190	14.0	18.0	7.0	m.q.	430	m.q.
tips *(Swanson Hungry Man)*,							
15.75 oz.	450	30.0	50.0	14.0	m.q.	1260	m.q.
wine sauce *(The Budget Gourmet Light and Healthy)*, 11 oz.	280	21.0	36.0	8.0	25	560	m.q.
sliced:							
(Banquet Meals),							
9 oz.	230	26.0	19.0	7.0	70	660	m.q.
(Swanson), 11.25 oz.	330	27.0	37.0	8.0	m.q.	690	m.q.
gravy and *(Freezer Queen)*, 9 oz. . .	140	12.0	18.0	3.0	20	770	m.q.
Stroganoff *(Armour Classics Lite)*,							
11.25 oz.	250	18.0	33.0	6.0	55	510	m.q.
Swiss steak *(Swanson)*, 10 oz.	350	27.0	36.0	11.0	m.q.	690	m.q.
teriyaki *(The Budget Gourmet Light and Healthy)*, 10.75 oz.	260	19.0	37.0	7.0	30	530	m.q.
Beef entree, canned or packaged:							
chow mein, 3/4 cup:							
(La Choy)	40	5.0	5.0	2.0	16	960	2.0 d
(La Choy Bi-Pack)	70	7.0	8.0	1.0	20	840	1.0 d
pepper, 3/4 cup:							
(La Choy Bi-Pack)	80	7.0	10.0	2.0	17	950	2.0 d
Oriental *(La Choy)*	100	7.0	12.0	4.0	9	1340	2.0 d
roast, 10 oz.:							
and gravy, w/potatoes *(Dinty Moore American Classics)*	260	26.0	26.0	6.0	45	910	m.q.

Food and Measure	cal.	prot. (gms)	carbo. (gms)	fat (gms)	chol. (mgs)	sod. (mgs)	fiber (gms)
tender *(Hormel Top Shelf)*	240	28.0	19.0	6.0	60	880	m.q.
Salisbury steak *(Hormel Top Shelf)*, 10 oz.	320	25.0	22.0	15.0	70	910	m.q.
stew, 7.5 oz., except as noted:							
(Dinty Moore Cup)	180	11.0	15.0	9.0	30	830	m.q.
(Healthy Choice) . .	140	15.0	16.0	2.0	35	540	m.q.
(Hormel Micro Cup)	230	13.0	11.0	15.0	45	1140	m.q.
(Libby's)	200	11.0	17.0	9.0	m.q.	1020	m.q.
(Libby's Diner), 7.75 oz.	240	12.0	22.0	12.0	40	790	m.q.
Beef entree, freeze-dried *(Mountain House)*, 1 cup*:							
Bourguignon	280	20.0	20.0	13.0	m.q.	880	n.a.
and rice, w/onions . .	330	11.0	42.0	12.0	m.q.	1300	m.q.
and rice, pepper and onion sauce	230	10.0	32.0	7.0	m.q.	1200	m.q.
stew	260	16.0	26.0	9.0	m.q.	820	m.q.
Stroganoff	250	9.0	27.0	12.0	m.q.	750	n.a.
Beef entree, frozen:							
Cantonese:							
(The Budget Gourmet), 9.1 oz. . .	270	15.0	31.0	9.0	40	880	m.q.
w/rice *(Weight Watchers Stir-Fry)*, 9 oz.	200	14.0	27.0	4.0	15	530	m.q.
champignon *(Tyson Gourmet Selection)*, 10.5 oz.	370	27.0	31.0	15.0	m.q.	830	m.q.
cheeseburger:							
(Hormel Quick Meal), 4.8 oz. . .	400	21.0	35.0	20.0	75	600	m.q.
(MicroMagic), 4.75 oz.	450	17:0	29.0	25.0	80	790	m.q.

Food and Measure	cal.	prot. (gms)	carbo. (gms)	fat (gms)	chol. (mgs)	sod. (mgs)	fiber (gms)
Beef entree, frozen, cheeseburger *(cont.)*							
bacon *(Hormel Quick Meal)*, 5 oz.	440	24.0	32.0	24.0	80	800	m.q.
bacon *(MicroMagic)*, 4 oz.	396	17.0	31.0	20.0	36	711	m.q.
chili *(Hormel Quick Meal)*, 6 oz. . . .	450	23.0	39.0	22.0	90	700	m.q.
double *(Hormel Quick Meal)*, 7.5 oz.	590	35.0	47.0	29.0	120	780	m.q.
mini *(Jimmy Dean)*, 1 burger	120	6.0	11.0	5.0	m.q.	310	m.q.
creamed, chipped:							
(Banquet Cookin' Bag), 4 oz. . . .	100	7.0	9.0	4.0	m.q.	m.q.	n.a.
(Freezer Queen Cook-in-Pouch), 4 oz.	80	5.0	9.0	3.0	10	460	n.a.
(Stouffer's), 5.5 oz.	230	9.0	9.0	17.0	m.q.	850	n.a.
(Swanson), 9 oz. . . .	290	19.0	17.0	16.0	m.q.	1140	n.a.
enchilada, see "Enchilada entree"							
hamburger:							
(Hormel Quick Meal), 4.3 oz. . . .	350	18.0	34.0	16.0	60	360	m.q.
(MicroMagic), 4 oz.	350	13.0	26.0	18.0	55	500	m.q.
jade garden *(Weight Watchers Stir-Fry)*, 9 oz.	150	13.0	17.0	3.0	20	490	m.q.
London broil *(Weight Watchers Ultimate 200)*, 7.5 oz.	110	17.0	4.0	3.0	25	320	n.a.
meat loaf, see "Meat loaf entree"							
and noodles, w/gravy, vegetables *(Stouffer's Home-style)*, 8 3/8 oz. . . .	230	16.0	26.0	7.0	m.q.	720	m.q.

Food and Measure	cal.	prot. (gms)	carbo. (gms)	fat (gms)	chol. (mgs)	sod. (mgs)	fiber (gms)
Oriental:							
(The Budget Gourmet Light and Healthy), 10 oz.	290	18.0	36.0	8.0	30	840	m.q.
w/vegetables and rice *(Lean Cuisine)*, 8⅝ oz. . .	290	20.0	31.0	9.0	40	590	m.q.
patty:							
charbroiled *(Freezer Queen* Family), 7 oz..	180	12.0	9.0	11.0	m.q.	1050	n.a.
charbroiled *(On-Cor)*, 8 oz..	277	18.0	12.0	18.0	m.q.	1180	n.a.
charbroiled, mushroom gravy and *(Banquet* Family), 7 oz..	260	11.0	12.0	18.0	m.q.	m.q.	m.q.
Italian, tomato sauce and *(On-Cor)*, 8 oz..	316	21.0	17.0	18.0	m.q.	1410	m.q.
and mushroom gravy *(Banquet Entree Express)*, 7 oz..	350	17.0	12.0	26.0	m.q.	1190	m.q.
onion gravy and *(Banquet* Family), 7 oz..	260	11.0	13.0	19.0	m.q.	m.q.	n.a.
onion gravy and *(Freezer Queen* Family), 7 oz. . .	200	13.0	10.0	12.0	m.q.	960	n.a.
pepper Oriental *(Chun King)*, 13 oz.	310	17.0	53.0	3.0	40	1300	m.q.
pepper steak:							
(Healthy Choice), 9.5 oz..	250	18.0	36.0	4.0	40	560	m.q.
green, w/rice *(Stouffer's)*, 10.5 oz.	310	20.0	35.0	10.0	m.q.	700	m.q.

Food and Measure	cal.	prot. (gms)	carbo. (gms)	fat (gms)	chol. (mgs)	sod. (mgs)	fiber (gms)
Beef entree, frozen, pepper steak *(cont.)*							
w/rice *(The Budget Gourmet)*, 10 oz.	300	18.0	40.0	8.0	35	720	m.q.
and peppers *(Freezer Queen)*, 9 oz. . . .	210	17.0	30.0	2.0	20	880	m.q.
pie:							
(Stouffer's), 10 oz.	460	18.0	37.0	27.0	m.q.	1130	m.q.
(Swanson), 7 oz. . .	370	12.0	38.0	19.0	m.q.	730	m.q.
(Swanson Hungry Man), 14 oz. . . .	600	34.0	51.0	29.0	m.q.	1310	m.q.
pot roast:							
w/browned potatoes *(Stouffer's Home-style)*, 8⅞ oz. . .	280	20.0	24.0	11.0	m.q.	690	m.q.
Yankee *(Freezer Queen)*, 9 oz. . .	170	17.0	20.0	3.0	30	320	m.q.
ribs, barbecue *(Healthy Choice Homestyle Classics)*, 11 oz.	330	28.0	40.0	6.0	70	530	m.q.
Salisbury steak:							
(Banquet Healthy Balance), 10.5 oz.	260	17.0	31.0	8.0	35	790	m.q.
(Banquet Meals), 9.5 oz.	290	14.0	28.0	16.0	35	910	m.q.
(Dining Lite), 9 oz.	200	18.0	14.0	8.0	55	1000	m.q.
(Freezer Queen), 9 oz.	300	17.0	21.0	16.0	25	890	n.a.
(On-Cor), 8 oz. . .	281	18.0	10.0	19.0	m.q.	1339	n.a.
and gravy *(Banquet Entree Express)*, 7 oz.	300	16.0	13.0	21.0	m.q.	1310	n.a.
gravy and *(Banquet Cookin' Bag)*, 5 oz.	190	9.0	8.0	14.0	m.q.	m.q.	n.a.
gravy and *(Banquet Family)*, 7 oz. . .	260	11.0	11.0	19.0	m.q.	m.q.	n.a.

Food and Measure	cal.	prot. (gms)	carbo. (gms)	fat (gms)	chol. (mgs)	sod. (mgs)	fiber (gms)
gravy and (Freezer Queen Family), 7 oz.	200	13.0	9.0	13.0	m.q.	1110	n.a.
gravy and (Freezer Queen Cook-in-Pouch), 5 oz. . .	160	10.0	4.0	12.0	15	760	n.a.
w/macaroni and cheese (Lean Cuisine), 9.5 oz. . .	270	27.0	22.0	8.0	50	500	m.q.
w/macaroni and cheese (Stouffer's Homestyle), 9 5/8 oz.	350	25.0	23.0	17.0	m.q.	1130	m.q.
w/mushroom gravy (Healthy Choice Homestyle Classics), 11 oz.	280	21.0	35.0	6.0	55	500	m.q.
w/mashed potatoes (Swanson), 9 oz.	340	20.0	23.0	19.0	m.q.	970	m.q.
sirloin (The Budget Gourmet Light and Healthy), 9 oz.	220	16.0	24.0	8.0	25	730	m.q.
sandwich, see "Beef sandwich"							
sirloin:							
cheddar melt (The Budget Gourmet), 9.4 oz.	380	18.0	29.0	21.0	85	950	m.q.
in herb sauce (The Budget Gourmet Light and Healthy), 9.5 oz.	250	20.0	21.0	9.0	30	860	m.q.
roast, supreme (The Budget Gourmet), 9 oz.	320	19.0	28.0	15.0	85	630	m.q.

Food and Measure	cal.	prot. (gms)	carbo. (gms)	fat (gms)	chol. (mgs)	sod. (mgs)	fiber (gms)
Beef entree, frozen, sirloin *(cont.)*							
tips *(Weight Watchers Ultimate 200)*, 7.5 oz.	200	20.0	20.0	6.0	30	560	m.q.
tips w/mushroom gravy *(Healthy Choice)*, 9.5 oz.	260	20.0	34.0	6.0	35	580	m.q.
tips and noodles, w/gravy *(Swanson)*, 7 oz.	190	14.0	18.0	7.0	m.q.	430	m.q.
tips and country vegetables *(The Budget Gourmet)*, 10 oz.	290	17.0	19.0	17.0	40	810	m.q.
sliced:							
(On-Cor), 8 oz. . .	90	12.0	7.0	2.0	m.q.	1453	n.a.
gravy and *(Banquet Cookin' Bag)*, 4 oz.	100	8.0	5.0	5.0	m.q.	m.q.	n.a.
gravy and *(Banquet Family)*, 7 oz. . . .	140	17.0	8.0	5.0	m.q.	m.q.	n.a.
gravy and *(Freezer Queen Cook-in-Pouch)*, 4 oz. . .	70	8.0	6.0	2.0	15	470	n.a.
gravy and *(Freezer Queen Family)*, 7 oz.	130	15.0	10.0	3.0	m.q.	870	n.a.
stew:							
(Banquet Family), 7 oz.	140	6.0	18.0	5.0	m.q.	m.q.	m.q.
(Freezer Queen), 7 oz.	150	9.0	15.0	6.0	m.q.	820	m.q.
(On-Cor), 8 oz. . .	134	13.0	15.0	2.0	m.q.	1080	m.q.
Stroganoff:							
(The Budget Gourmet Light and Healthy), 8.75 oz.	260	19.0	27.0	10.0	50	480	m.q.

Food and Measure	cal.	prot. (gms)	carbo. (gms)	fat (gms)	chol. (mgs)	sod. (mgs)	fiber (gms)
w/parsley noodles *(Stouffer's)*, 9.75 oz.	390	23.0	30.0	20.0	m.q.	1140	m.q.
Beef entree mix:							
pepper steak *(La Choy Dinner Classics)*, 3/4 cup*	180	17.0	9.0	9.0	60	760	1.0 d
stew, hearty *(Stew Starter)*, 1/8 mix . .	90	2.0	20.0	<1.0	0	740	m.q.
Beef entree sauce, see "Entree sauce"							
Beef gravy, canned:							
1/4 cup	31	2.2	2.8	1.4	2	326	0
(Franco-American), 2 oz.	35	1.0	4.0	2.0	m.q.	300	n.a.
(Pepperidge Farm Hearty), 2 oz. . . .	25	2.0	3.0	1.0	m.q.	350	n.a.
Beef jerky (see also "Sausage stick"), 1 piece, except as noted:							
(Frito-Lay's), .21 oz.	25	3.0	1.0	1.0	10	200	0
(Frito-Lay's Tender), .7 oz.	120	5.0	2.0	10.0	25	370	0
(Pemmican Arrowhead)	70	8.0	2.0	3.0	m.q.	580	0
(Pemmican Steakers)	40	5.0	2.0	1.0	m.q.	160	0
(Pemmican Tender Brave/Chief/Trail/ Tribe Packs), 1 oz.	90	13.0	2.0	3.0	m.q.	920	0
(Slim Jim)	20	2.0	1.0	1.0	<5	130	0
(Slim Jim Big Jerk) . .	20	3.0	1.0	1.0	5	170	0
(Slim Jim Giant Jerk)	50	7.0	2.0	2.0	15	420	0
plain, peppered, jalapeño or *Tabasco (Pemmican Natural)*, 1 oz.	80	14.0	2.0	2.0	m.q.	660	0

Food and Measure	cal.	prot. (gms)	carbo. (gms)	fat (gms)	chol. (mgs)	sod. (mgs)	fiber (gms)
Beef jerky (cont.)							
plain or Tabasco (Slim Jim Super Jerk) . .	30	4.0	1.0	1.0	10	250	0
teriyaki (Pemmican Natural), 1 oz.	80	14.0	2.0	2.0	m.q.	550	0
Beef luncheon meat, 1 oz., except as noted:							
corned:							
(Healthy Deli St. Paddy's)	25	3.9	1.1	.5	9	290	0
(Hillshire Farm Deli Select)	31	6.0	<1.0	.4	m.q.	230	0
(Hormel)	62	8.0	<2.0	3.0	21	248	0
cooked (Healthy Deli)	35	5.7	.7	1.0	14	230	0
canned (Libby's), 2.4 oz.	160	17.0	2.0	9.0	m.q.	750	0
roast:							
(Healthy Deli) . . .	30	5.9	.4	.4	13	170	0
(Hormel Bread Ready)	31	5.0	1.0	1.0	13	434	0
(Oscar Mayer Deli-Thin), 5 slices . .	70	12.0	<1.0	2.0	30	600	0
Black Forest (Healthy Deli) . .	35	6.0	.7	.8	12	170	0
Italian (Healthy Deli)	33	5.6	.3	.8	16	160	0
oven-roasted (Weight Watchers)	35	5.0	<1.0	1.0	15	220	0
oven-roasted, cured (Hillshire Farm Deli Select) . . .	31	6.0	<1.0	.5	m.q.	270	0
smoked:							
(Healthy Deli) . . .	37	6.1	.7	1.0	12	240	0
(Hillshire Farm Deli Select)	31	6.0	<1.0	.5	m.q.	270	0

Food and Measure	cal.	prot. (gms)	carbo. (gms)	fat (gms)	chol. (mgs)	sod. (mgs)	fiber (gms)
Beef marinade seasoning mix *(Lawry's Seasoning Blends)*, 1 pkg.	49	1.2	10.7	.2	<1	7284	<.1 c
Beef pie, see "Beef entree, frozen"							
Beef roll or stick, see "Beef jerky" and "Sausage stick"							
Beef sandwich, frozen:							
barbecue *(Hormel Quick Meal)*, 4.3 oz.	370	15.0	40.0	17.0	55	590	m.q.
barbecue *(Tyson Microwave)*, 1 piece	200	15.0	29.0	2.7	30	600	m.q.
pocket *(Hot Pockets)*, 4.5 oz.:							
in BBQ sauce . . .	330	11.0	47.0	11.0	30	890	m.q.
and broccoli	260	9.0	31.0	10.0	25	950	m.q.
and cheddar	350	14.0	36.0	16.0	45	750	m.q.
Beef sandwich mix *(Swift Premium Quick Fixin's)*, 3.5 oz.:							
and gravy	100	12.0	7.0	3.0	30	590	n.a.
Italian sauce and . .	80	10.0	4.0	3.0	25	850	n.a.
Beef stew, see "Beef entree"							
Beef seasoning mix:							
stew:							
(French's), 1/7 pkg.	16	1.0	3.0	0	0	480	n.a.
(Lawry's Seasoning Blends), 1 pkg.	131	5.4	25.7	.7	0	3181	1.2 c
(McCormick/Schilling), 1/4 pkg. . .	33	1.3	6.0	.3	n.a.	806	n.a.
(McCormick/Schilling Bag'n Season), 1 pkg. . . .	87	7.5	11.0	1.0	n.a.	4320	n.a.

Food and Measure	cal.	prot. (gms)	carbo. (gms)	fat (gms)	chol. (mgs)	sod. (mgs)	fiber (gms)
Beef seasoning mix (cont.)							
Stroganoff (McCormick/Schilling),							
1/4 pkg.	32	1.0	6.0	.3	n.a.	1078	n.a.
Beefalo, meat only,							
roasted, 4 oz. . . .	213	34.8	0	7.2	66	93	0
Beer, 12 fl. oz.:							
regular	146	.9	13.2	0	0	19	.7 d
light	100	.7	4.8	0	0	10	0
Beer batter mix							
(Golden Dipt), 1 oz.	100	2.0	22.0	0	0	650	n.a.
Beerwurst, see "Salami, beer"							
Beet:							
fresh, raw:							
trimmed, sliced,							
1/2 cup	29	1.1	6.5	.1	0	53	1.9 d
2 medium, 2" diam.,							
approx. 8.6 oz.	70	2.6	15.6	.3	0	126	4.6 d
fresh, boiled, drained:							
sliced, 1/2 cup . . .	38	1.4	8.5	.2	0	65	1.4 d
2 medium, 2" diam.,							
approx. 3.5 oz.	44	1.7	10.0	.2	0	77	1.7 d
canned, 1/2 cup:							
w/liquid	36	1.0	8.3	.1	0	324	1.4 d
drained, sliced . . .	27	.8	6.1	.1	0	m.q.	1.5 d
cut and sliced							
(Stokely)	40	1.0	8.0	0	0	300	m.q.
Harvard, w/liquid	89	1.0	22.4	.1	0	199	m.q.
pickled, w/liquid . .	74	.9	18.5	.1	0	299	.7 c
Beet greens, 1/2 cup:							
raw, 1" pieces	4	.4	.8	<.1	0	38	.7 d
boiled, drained,							
1" pieces	20	1.9	3.9	.1	0	173	2.1 d
Berliner, pork and							
beef, 1 oz.	65	4.3	.7	4.9	13	368	0

Food and Measure	cal.	prot. (gms)	carbo. (gms)	fat (gms)	chol. (mgs)	sod. (mgs)	fiber (gms)
Berry drink:							
canned, 6 fl. oz.:							
(Hawaiian Punch Very Berry) . . .	90	0	22.0	0	0	30	(0)
(Hi-C Boppin' Berry)	90	0	23.0	0	0	25	(0)
wild *(Hi-C)*	90	0	22.0	0	0	20	(0)
mix*, 8 fl. oz.:							
(Wyler's Bunch 'O Berries)	80	(0)	20.0	(0)	0	15	(0)
mountain berry punch *(Kool-Aid)*	100	0	25.0	0	0	15	0
mountain berry punch *(Kool-Aid Presweetened)*	70	0	18.0	0	0	0	0
Berry juice:							
(Juicy Juice), 6 fl. oz.	90	1.0	22.0	0	0	10	m.q.
(R.W. Knudsen Razzleberry), 8 fl. oz.	90	<1.0	21.0	<1.0	0	(0)	m.q.
Berry juice drink:							
(Tropicana Berries & Berries), 6 fl. oz. . .	90	<1.0	23.0	<1.0	0	20	(0)
blend *(Tang Fruit Box)*, 8.45 fl. oz.	140	0	36.0	0	0	10	(0)
Berry nectar *(Santa Cruz Natural)*, 8 fl. oz.	90	<1.0	22.0	<1.0	0	(0)	m.q.
Berry punch *(Minute Maid)*, 6 fl. oz. . . .	90	0	23.0	0	0	20	(0)
Berry-grape juice drink, mixed berry *(Boku)*, 8 fl. oz. . .	120	0	29.0	0	0	65	0
Biscuit, 1 piece, except as noted:							
(Arnold Old Fashioned)	60	1.0	8.0	3.0	m.q.	100	m.q.
(Wonder)	80	2.0	14.0	1.0	n.a.	140	.6 d
breakfast, whole wheat *(LaLoma Ruskets)*, 2 pieces . . .	110	4.0	22.0	0	0	95	m.q.

Food and Measure	cal.	prot. (gms)	carbo. (gms)	fat (gms)	chol. (mgs)	sod. (mgs)	fiber (gms)
Biscuit *(cont.)*							
country *(Awrey's 3")*, 2 oz.	160	4.0	23.0	5.0	0	530	1.0 d
round or square *(Awrey's 2")*, 1 oz. . . .	80	2.0	12.0	3.0	0	260	0
sliced or unsliced *(Awrey's)*, 2 oz.	160	4.0	23.0	5.0	0	520	1.0 d
square *(Awrey's 3")*, 2 oz.	160	4.0	23.0	5.0	0	520	1.0 d
frozen *(Bridgford)*, 2 oz.	180	4.0	28.0	6.0	1	632	m.q.
mix* (see also "Baking Mix") *(Robin Hood/ Gold Medal)*	90	2.0	14.0	3.0	0	270	m.q.
refrigerated:							
(Big Country Butter Tastin')	100	2.0	13.0	4.0	0	320	m.q.
(1869 Brand Butter Tastin')	100	2.0	12.0	5.0	0	300	m.q.
(Grands! Butter Tastin')	190	4.0	22.0	9.0	0	560	m.q.
(Pillsbury Big Premium Heat 'N Eat), 2 pieces . .	280	5.0	32.0	15.0	0	610	m.q.
(Pillsbury Country)	50	1.0	10.0	1.0	0	180	m.q.
plain or buttermilk *(Ballard Extra Lights Ovenready)*	50	1.0	10.0	<1.0	0	180	m.q.
baking powder *(1869 Brand)* . .	100	2.0	12.0	5.0	0	310	m.q.
butter *(Pillsbury)* . .	50	1.0	10.0	<1.0	0	180	m.q.
buttermilk:							
(Big Country) . .	100	2.0	14.0	4.0	0	320	m.q.
(1869 Brand) . .	100	2.0	12.0	5.0	0	310	m.q.
(Hungry Jack Extra Rich)	50	1.0	9.0	1.0	0	180	m.q.
(Hungry Jack Flaky)	90	2.0	12.0	4.0	0	300	m.q.

Food and Measure	cal.	prot. (gms)	carbo. (gms)	fat (gms)	chol. (mgs)	sod. (mgs)	fiber (gms)
(Hungry Jack Fluffy)	90	2.0	12.0	4.0	0	280	m.q.
(Pillsbury)	50	1.0	10.0	1.0	0	180	m.q.
(Pillsbury Heat 'N Eat), 2 pieces . .	170	4.0	27.0	5.0	0	530	m.q.
(Pillsbury Tender Layer)	50	1.0	9.0	1.0	0	170	m.q.
cinnamon raisin *(Grands!)*	190	3.0	27.0	7.0	0	540	m.q.
flaky:							
(Grands!)	190	4.0	23.0	8.0	0	530	m.q.
(Hungry Jack) . .	80	2.0	12.0	4.0	0	300	m.q.
(Hungry Jack Butter Tastin')	100	2.0	11.0	4.0	0	280	m.q.
(Hungry Jack Honey Tastin') . .	90	2.0	13.0	4.0	0	290	m.q.
fluffy *(Pillsbury Good 'N Buttery)* . . .	90	1.0	11.0	5.0	0	270	m.q.
grain, mixed *(Roman Meal)*, 2 pieces	180	4.2	33.6	3.8	0	456	1.4 d
honey nut oat bran *(Roman Meal)* . .	131	2.4	20.6	4.7	0	278	.9 d
Southern style:							
(Big Country) . .	100	2.0	14.0	4.0	0	320	m.q.
(Hungry Jack Flaky)	80	2.0	12.0	4.0	0	300	m.q.
white *(Roman Meal)*	127	2.4	18.8	4.7	0	308	0
Bitter melon, see "Balsam pear"							
Black bean dishes:							
canned, 5 oz.:							
w/tofu wieners *(Health Valley Tofu Fast Menu)* . . .	160	16.0	14.0	3.0	0	250	13.6 d
Western, w/vegetables *(Health Valley Fast Menu Fat Free)*	70	9.0	9.0	<1.0	0	115	9.6 d

Food and Measure	cal.	prot. (gms)	carbo. (gms)	fat (gms)	chol. (mgs)	sod. (mgs)	fiber (gms)
Black bean dishes *(cont.)*							
mix*:							
w/butter *(Fantastic Instant)*, 1/2 cup	176	8.0	23.0	6.0	m.q.	373	12.0 d
and rice *(Fantastic Caribbean)*, 10 oz.	190	9.0	41.0	2.0	0	490	8.0 d
Black beans:							
dry:							
(Frieda's), 1 oz. . .	40	2.7	6.8	.2	0	79	3.7 d
boiled, 1/2 cup . . .	113	7.6	20.4	.5	0	1	7.5 d
canned:							
(Eden No Salt Added), 1/2 cup	70	7.0	17.0	<1.0	0	15	6.0 d
(Green Giant/Joan of Arc), 1/2 cup	90	7.0	21.0	0	0	580	6.0 d
(Progresso), 4 oz.	90	9.0	19.0	1.0	0	350	6.5 d
turtle soup:							
dry, 1/2 cup	312	19.6	58.2	.8	0	8	22.9 d
dry *(Arrowhead Mills)*, 2 oz. . . .	190	13.0	35.0	1.0	0	9	11.3 d
boiled, 1/2 cup . . .	120	7.5	22.4	.3	0	3	4.9 d
canned *(Hain)*, 4 oz.	70	6.0	15.0	1.0	0	310	6.0 d
Blackberry, 1/2 cup:							
fresh, trimmed	37	.5	9.2	.3	0	tr.	3.6 d
canned:							
in water *(Allens)* . .	25	1.0	4.0	<1.0	0	15	m.q.
in heavy syrup . . .	118	1.7	29.6	.2	0	3	4.4 d
frozen, unsweetened	49	.9	11.8	.3	0	1	3.8 d
Black-eyed peas, see "Cowpeas"							
Blintz, frozen, 2 pieces, except as noted:							
apple-raisin *(Golden)*	160	5.0	32.0	3.0	20	290	m.q.
blueberry *(Golden)* . .	180	4.0	37.0	2.0	20	300	m.q.
cheese:							
(Golden)	160	12.0	25.0	2.0	25	270	m.q.
(King Kold), 1 piece	113	6.0	18.9	1.6	m.q.	272	m.q.

Food and Measure	cal.	prot. (gms)	carbo. (gms)	fat (gms)	chol. (mgs)	sod. (mgs)	fiber (gms)
(King Kold No Salt)							
1 piece	96	6.4	18.6	.5	m.q.	78	m.q.
cherry *(Golden)* . . .	190	5.0	37.0	3.0	10	290	m.q.
potato *(Golden)* . . .	210	6.0	29.0	9.0	10	340	m.q.
Blood sausage, 1 oz.	107	4.1	.4	9.8	34	m.q.	0
Bloody Mary mixer, 6 fl. oz.:							
(Libby's)	40	2.0	8.0	0	0	1120	n.a.
(Tabasco)	56	2.4	11.0	.3	0	1548	1.0 d
extra spicy *(Tabasco)*	56	2.7	11.1	.4	0	1645	1.6 d
Blueberry, 1/2 cup:							
fresh	41	.5	10.2	.3	0	5	2.0 d
canned in heavy syrup	112	.8	28.2	.4	0	4	1.9 d
frozen, unsweetened	39	.3	9.4	.5	0	1	2.1 d
frozen, sweetened . .	94	.5	25.2	.2	0	2	2.4 d
Blueberry nectar *(R.W. Knudsen),* 8 fl. oz.	135	<1.0	34.0	<1.0	0	(0)	m.q.
Blueberry-cranberry drink *(Ocean Spray Cran•Blueberry),* 6 fl. oz.	120	0	31.0	0	0	10	(0)
Bluefish, meat only:							
raw, 4 oz.	141	22.7	0	4.8	67	68	0
baked, broiled, or microwaved, 4 oz. . .	180	29.1	0	6.2	86	87	0
Boar, wild, meat only, roasted, 4 oz. . . .	181	32.1	0	5.0	m.q.	m.q.	0
Bockwurst, raw, 1 oz.	87	3.8	.1	7.8	m.q.	m.q.	0
Bok-choy, see "Cabbage, Chinese"							
Bologna (see also "Chicken bologna," etc.), 1 slice, except as noted:							
(Healthy Deli), 1 oz.	40	3.8	1.6	2.0	11	200	0
(Hillshire Farm Large), 1 oz.	90	3.0	<1.0	8.0	m.q.	m.q.	0

Food and Measure	cal.	prot. (gms)	carbo. (gms)	fat (gms)	chol. (mgs)	sod. (mgs)	fiber (gms)
Bologna (cont.)							
(Hillshire Farm Ring), 1 oz.	89	3.0	<1.0	8.0	m.q.	m.q.	0
(Kahn's Deluxe Club/ Giant Deluxe) . . .	90	3.0	1.0	8.0	m.q.	290	0
(Kahn's Deluxe Club Family Pack)	70	2.0	1.0	6.0	m.q.	220	0
(Kahn's Giant Thick Deluxe)	110	4.0	1.0	10.0	m.q.	330	0
(Kahn's Thick Deluxe)	140	5.0	1.0	13.0	m.q.	450	0
(Kahn's Thin Sliced Deluxe)	60	2.0	1.0	5.0	m.q.	190	0
(Oscar Mayer)	90	3.0	<1.0	8.0	15	310	0
(Oscar Mayer Healthy Favorites), 3 slices	60	8.0	4.0	1.0	15	720	0
(Oscar Mayer Light)	60	3.0	2.0	4.0	15	310	0
(Oscar Mayer Wisconsin Ring), 2 oz. . .	180	7.0	1.0	16.0	35	470	0
beef:							
(Kahn's/Kahn's Giant)	90	3.0	1.0	8.0	m.q.	300	0
(Kahn's Family Pack)	70	2.0	1.0	6.0	m.q.	230	0
(Oscar Mayer) . . .	90	3.0	<1.0	8.0	15	300	0
(Oscar Mayer Light)	50	3.0	2.0	4.0	10	310	0
beef and cheddar (Kahn's)	90	4.0	1.0	8.0	m.q.	320	0
garlic (Kahn's)	90	3.0	1.0	8.0	m.q.	290	0
garlic (Oscar Mayer)	130	5.0	1.0	12.0	25	470	0
"Bologna," vegetarian, frozen (Worthington Bolono), 2 slices	60	7.0	2.0	2.0	0	390	m.q.
Bonito, meat only, raw, 4 oz. . . . . . :	146	29.3	.5	2.3	m.q.	50	0
Borage:							
raw, 1" pieces, 1/2 cup	9	.8	1.4	.3	0	35	.4 c
boiled, drained, 4 oz.	28	2.4	4.0	.9	0	98	1.2 c
Bouillon (see also "Soup"):							

Food and Measure	cal.	prot. (gms)	carbo. (gms)	fat (gms)	chol. (mgs)	sod. (mgs)	fiber (gms)
dry, all varieties (Herb-Ox Very Low Sodium), 1 pkt.	12	<1.0	2.0	<1.0	m.q.	10	(0)
dry, beef:							
(Herb-Ox), 1 cube	10	<1.0	1.0	<1.0	m.q.	860	(0)
(Herb-Ox Instant), 1 tsp.	10	<1.0	1.0	<1.0	m.q.	900	(0)
(Knorr Granulated), 1 serving	10	.4	1.2	.4	2	1010	(0)
flavor (Knorr), 1 serving	14	.7	.3	1.1	<1	1250	(0)
dry, chicken:							
(Herb-Ox), 1 cube	10	<1.0	<1.0	<1.0	m.q.	890	(0)
(Herb-Ox Instant), 1 tsp.	12	<1.0	2.0	<1.0	n.a.	900	(0)
(Knorr Granulated) 1 serving	10	.4	1.4	.3	0	1070	(0)
flavor (Knorr), 1 serving	16	.7	.6	1.2	<1	1210	(0)
dry, fish flavor (Knorr), 1 serving	10	1.0	.4	.4	n.a.	1130	(0)
dry, vegetable, vegetarian (Knorr), 1 serving	16	.3	.9	1.2	0	990	(0)
liquid, 2 tsp.:							
beef (Knorr)	16	<1.0	3.0	.0	0	900	(0)
chicken (Knorr) . .	16	<1.0	3.0	.0	0	800	(0)
Boysenberry, 1/2 cup:							
fresh, see "Blackberry"							
canned in heavy syrup	113	1.3	28.6	.2	0	4	3.3 d
frozen, unsweetened	33	.7	8.1	.1	0	1	2.6 d
Boysenberry juice (Smucker's Naturally 100%), 8 fl. oz. . .	120	0	30.0	0	0	10	m.q.
Boysenberry nectar (R.W. Knudsen), 8 fl. oz.	110	<1.0	33.0	<1.0	0	(0)	m.q.

Food and Measure	cal.	prot. (gms)	carbo. (gms)	fat (gms)	chol. (mgs)	sod. (mgs)	fiber (gms)
Brains, 4 oz.:							
beef, fried	222	14.3	0	18.0	2262	179	0
lamb, fried	310	19.2	0	25.2	2840	178	0
pork, braised	156	13.8	0	10.8	2894	103	0
veal, fried	242	16.4	0	19.0	2404	200	0
Bran, see "Cereal" and specific listings							
Bratwurst:							
(Hillshire Farm Fully Cooked), 2 oz. . . .	170	7.0	1.0	16.0	m.q.	380	0
(Kahn's), 1 link	190	7.0	2.0	17.0	m.q.	490	0
fresh *(Hillshire Farm),* 2 oz.	190	7.0	1.0	17.0	m.q.	410	0
pork, cooked, 1 oz.	85	4.0	.6	7.3	17	158	0
smoked *(Hillshire Farm),* 2 oz.	190	8.0	1.0	17.0	m.q.	540	0
spicy *(Hillshire Farm),* 2 oz.	180	8.0	1.0	17.0	m.q.	m.q.	0
Braunschweiger:							
(Oscar Mayer German Brand), 2 oz. . . .	200	8.0	<1.0	18.0	90	650	0
(Oscar Mayer Sliced), 1 slice	100	4.0	<1.0	9.0	50	320	0
(Oscar Mayer Tube), 2 oz.	190	8.0	2.0	17.0	100	610	0
Brazil nuts, shelled, 1 oz., 6 large or 8 medium kernels	186	4.1	3.6	18.8	0	tr.	1.6 d
Bread, 1 slice, except as noted:							
apple walnut swirl *(Pepperidge Farm)*	80	3.0	14.0	1.0	0	130	2.0 d
(Arnold/Brownberry Bran'nola)	90	3.0	16.0	2.0	0	150	3.0 d
bran:							
(Arnold Bakery Light Country)	40	2.0	7.0	<1.0	0	80	3.0 d

Food and Measure	cal.	prot. (gms)	carbo. (gms)	fat (gms)	chol. (mgs)	sod. (mgs)	fiber (gms)
(Brownberry Light Country)	40	2.0	10.0	<1.0	0	80	3.0 d
honey *(Pepperidge Farm)*	90	3.0	18.0	1.0	0	160	1.0 d
whole *(Brownberry Natural)*	60	2.0	10.0	1.0	0	170	2.0 d
brown, see "Bread, brown"							
brown and serve:							
Austrian wheat *(Bread du Jour),* 1 oz.	70	3.0	12.0	1.0	0	140	1.2 d
French *(Bread du Jour),* 1 oz. . . .	70	3.0	13.0	1.0	0	150	.7 d
French *(DiCarlo Parisian),* 1 oz.	70	2.0	12.0	1.0	0	170	.8 d
French, petite *(Bread du Jour),* 1 loaf	230	10.0	44.0	2.0	0	540	2.4 d
grain, mixed:							
stick, soft *(Roman Meal),* 2.7 oz. . . .	184	7.1	31.8	2.9	0	375	3.2 d
mini *(Roman Meal),* 1/2 loaf . .	138	5.3	23.8	2.2	0	281	2.4 d
cinnamon:							
chip *(Arnold)*	80	2.0	13.0	2.0	0	90	<1.0 d
raisin *(Wonder)* . .	60	3.0	12.0	1.0	0	95	.9 d
swirl *(Pepperidge Farm)*	90	2.0	15.0	3.0	0	110	2.0 d
corn or date nut, see "Bread, sweet"							
French:							
(Pepperidge Farm Fully Baked), 1 oz.	80	3.0	15.0	1.0	0	140	0
(Wonder)	70	3.0	13.0	1.0	0	150	.7 d
sliced or twin *(Pepperidge Farm),* 1 oz.	80	3.0	15.0	1.0	0	160	0

Food and Measure	cal.	prot. (gms)	carbo. (gms)	fat (gms)	chol. (mgs)	sod. (mgs)	fiber (gms)
Bread, French *(cont.)*							
stick *(Francisco)* . .	70	3.0	12.0	1.0	0	110	m.q.
stick *(Savoni)*, 1 oz.	80	3.0	15.0	<1.0	0	m.q.	1.0 d
twin *(Francisco)*, 2 oz.	150	5.0	27.0	2.0	0	280	m.q.
grain, mixed:							
(Roman Meal Round Top)	68	2.8	11.9	.9	0	141	1.2 d
(Roman Meal Sandwich)	55	2.3	9.6	.7	0	114	1.0 d
w/oat bran *(Roman Meal)*	69	2.8	11.9	1.0	0	140	1.1 d
nutty *(Arnold/ Brownberry Bran'nola)*	90	3.0	14.0	2.0	0	120	3.0 d
7 *(Home Pride* Butter-Top)	70	3.0	12.0	1.0	<5	135	1.2 d
7 *(Pepperidge Farm* Hearty)	90	2.5	18.0	1.0	0	170	1.0 d
7 *(Pepperidge Farm* Light Style) . . .	40	2.0	10.0	0	0	135	2.0 d
7 *(Roman Meal)* . .	68	2.9	11.9	.9	0	142	1.2 d
7 *(Roman Meal* Light)	42	2.2	7.1	.5	0	103	2.6 d
w/sunflower seeds *(Roman Meal* Sun Grain)	70	3.1	10.8	1.5	0	140	1.4 d
12 *(Arnold* Natural)	60	2.0	10.0	1.0	0	100	1.0 d
12 *(Brownberry* Natural)	60	2.0	11.0	1.0	0	110	1.0 d
12 *(Roman Meal)*	73	2.7	11.6	1.7	0	143	1.0 d
12 *(Roman Meal* Light)	42	2.2	6.9	.6	0	106	2.7 d
whole *(Roman Meal* 100%)*	93	4.3	16.1	1.3	0	198	2.2 d
health nut *(Brownberry* Natural)	70	2.0	11.0	2.0	0	170	2.0 d

Food and Measure	cal.	prot. (gms)	carbo. (gms)	fat (gms)	chol. (mgs)	sod. (mgs)	fiber (gms)
(Hollywood Special Formula):							
dark	40	2.0	9.0	<1.0	0	90	.4 d
Fitness Blend . . .	50	4.0	8.0	<.5	0	90	1.0 d
light	40	2.0	9.0	<1.0	0	125	.3 d
Italian:							
(Arnold Bakery Light)	40	2.0	7.0	<1.0	0	90	2.0 d
(Brownberry Bakery Light)	40	2.0	9.0	<1.0	0	90	2.0 d
(Francisco Sliced)	70	3.0	12.0	1.0	0	110	m.q.
(Pepperidge Farm Sliced)	70	2.0	12.0	1.0	0	125	m.q.
(Wonder Family) . .	70	3.0	13.0	1.0	0	170	.7 d
(Wonder Light) . . .	40	2.0	6.0	0	0	115	3.0 d
sliced stick or loaf *(Francisco)* . . .	70	3.0	12.0	1.0	0	110	m.q.
stick *(Francisco),* 1 oz.	90	3.0	17.0	1.0	0	110	m.q.
oat:							
(Arnold/Brownberry Bran'nola Country)	90	3.0	16.0	3.0	0	130	3.0 d
(Roman Meal) . . .	71	2.6	12.5	1.0	0	145	.8 d
crunchy *(Pepperidge Farm* Hearty) . .	95	4.0	17.0	2.0	0	145	1.5 d
oat bran:							
(Roman Meal Light)	42	2.3	7.2	.4	0	103	2.4 d
honey *(Roman Meal)*	72	3.0	11.8	1.2	0	137	1.0 d
honey nut *(Roman Meal)*	74	3.1	11.2	1.7	0	129	1.0 d
oatmeal:							
(Arnold)	60	2.0	12.0	1.0	0	95	2.0 d
(Arnold Bakery Light)	40	2.0	8.0	<1.0	0	100	2.0 d
(Brownberry Bakery Light)	40	2.0	10.0	<1.0	0	100	2.0 d
(Brownberry Natural)	60	2.0	11.0	1.0	0	140	1.0 d
(Pepperidge Farm)	90	3.0	17.0	1.0	0	200	1.0 d

Food and Measure	cal.	prot. (gms)	carbo. (gms)	fat (gms)	chol. (mgs)	sod. (mgs)	fiber (gms)
Bread, oatmeal *(cont.)*							
(Pepperidge Farm Light Style) . . .	45	2.0	9.0	0	0	95	1.0 d
(Pepperidge Farm Thin)	35	1.0	6.0	.5	0	80	.5 d
w/bran *(Oatmeal Goodness* Light)	40	2.0	6.0	<1.0	0	95	2.8 d
w/bran, sunflower or wheat *(Oatmeal Goodness)* . . .	80	4.0	14.0	1.0	0	150	1.3 d
raisin *(Arnold)* . . .	60	2.0	12.0	<1.0	0	90	2.0 d
raisin *(Brownberry)*	60	2.0	12.0	1.0	0	90	2.0 d
sandwich *(Brownberry* Natural)	70	2.0	11.0	2.0	0	120	2.0 d
soft *(Brownberry)*	60	2.0	12.0	1.0	0	95	2.0 d
soft *(Pepperidge Farm)*	60	2.0	11.0	0	0	95	m.q.
w/wheat *(Oatmeal Goodness* Light)	40	2.0	6.0	<1.0	0	90	2.8 d
orange raisin *(Brownberry)*	70	2.0	13.0	1.0	0	90	1.0 d
pan de aqua *(Arnold Augusto)*, 1 oz. . .	80	3.0	14.0	1.0	0	150	1.0 d
pita or pocket:							
oat bran *(Sahara)*, 1/2 piece	80	2.0	15.0	<1.0	0	160	2.0 d
wheat or white *(Arnold)*, 1/2 piece	71	3.0	16.0	0	0	m.q.	m.q.
wheat, whole *(Sahara)*, 1 piece . .	130	7.0	23.0	1.0	0	310	5.0 d
wheat, whole, mini *(Sahara)*, 1 piece	70	3.0	12.0	<1.0	0	150	2.0 d
white *(Pepperidge Farm* Wholesome Choice), 1 piece	140	5.0	30.0	1.0	0	410	2.0 d

Food and Measure	cal.	prot. (gms)	carbo. (gms)	fat (gms)	chol. (mgs)	sod. (mgs)	fiber (gms)
white, mini (Pepper-idge Farm Whole-some Choice), 1 piece	70	3.0	15.0	0	0	200	1.0 d
white (Sahara), 1 mini or 1/2 regu-lar	80	3.0	16.0	1.0	0	150	1.0 d
white (Sahara), 1/2 large	120	4.0	23.0	1.0	0	220	2.0 d
white (Toufayan Pitettes), 1 piece	70	3.0	16.0	0	0	190	1.0 d
pumpernickel:							
(Arnold)	70	3.0	15.0	1.0	0	200	1.0 d
(August Bros. 1 lb.)	80	3.0	14.0	1.0	0	210	1.0 d
(August Bros. 24 oz.)	90	3.0	18.0	1.0	0	220	1.0 d
(Pepperidge Farm Family)	80	3.0	15.0	1.0	0	230	2.0 d
(Pepperidge Farm Party), 4 slices	60	2.0	12.0	1.0	0	160	1.0 d
raisin (Arnold Sun-Maid)	70	2.0	13.0	1.0	0	85	1.0 d
raisin cinnamon:							
(Arnold)	70	2.0	13.0	1.0	0	85	1.0 d
(Brownberry)	70	2.0	12.0	1.0	0	85	1.0 d
(Monk's), 1 oz. . . .	70	3.0	10.0	2.0	0	85	m.q.
swirl (Pepperidge Farm)	90	2.0	16.0	2.0	0	100	1.0 d
raisin walnut (Brownberry)	70	2.0	10.0	3.0	0	100	2.0 d
rye:							
(Arnold Real Jewish Melba Thin) . . .	40	2.0	9.0	<1.0	0	95	1.0 d
(Beefsteak Hearty/ Soft)	60	2.0	11.0	1.0	0	170	.8 d
(Beefsteak Mild) . .	70	3.0	12.0	1.0	0	180	.9 d
(Pepperidge Farm Party), 4 slices	60	2.0	12.0	1.0	0	250	1.0 d

Food and Measure	cal.	prot. (gms)	carbo. (gms)	fat (gms)	chol. (mgs)	sod. (mgs)	fiber (gms)
Bread, rye *(cont.)*							
caraway *(Arnold Real Jewish)* . .	70	3.0	13.0	<1.0	0	150	1.0 d
caraway *(Brownberry Natural)*	70	3.0	15.0	1.0	0	180	1.0 d
Dijon *(Arnold Real Jewish)*	70	3.0	15.0	<1.0	0	210	1.0 d
Dijon *(Pepperidge Farm)*	50	2.0	9.0	1.0	0	180	1.0 d
dill *(Arnold)*	60	2.0	10.0	1.0	0	140	1.0 d
dill *(Brownberry Natural)*, 2 slices . .	150	5.0	28.0	2.0	0	170	1.0 d
onion *(August Bros.)*	80	3.0	14.0	1.0	0	210	1.0 d
onion *(Beefsteak)*	60	2.0	11.0	1.0	0	170	.8 d
pumpernickel *(Brownberry Natural)*	70	3.0	13.0	1.0	0	150	1.0 d
seeded *(Pepperidge Farm Family)* . .	80	3.0	16.0	1.0	0	220	2.0 d
seeded or seedless *(August Bros. 1 lb.)*	80	3.0	14.0	1.0	0	210	1.0 d
seeded or seedless *(August Bros. 24 oz.)*	90	3.0	18.0	1.0	0	220	1.0 d
seeded or seedless *(Levy's Real Jewish)*	80	3.0	16.0	<1.0	0	180	1.0 d
seedless *(Arnold Real Jewish)* . .	70	3.0	15.0	<1.0	0	150	1.0 d
seedless *(August Bros. Thin)* . . .	40	2.0	8.0	<2.0	0	110	1.0 d
seedless *(Brownberry Natural)*, 2 slices . . .	150	5.0	28.0	2.0	0	180	1.0 d

Food and Measure	cal.	prot. (gms)	carbo. (gms)	fat (gms)	chol. (mgs)	sod. (mgs)	fiber (gms)
seedless (*Brownberry* Natural Thin)	50	3.0	9.0	1.0	0	180	1.0 d
seedless (*Pepperidge Farm* Family)	80	3.0	16.0	1.0	0	210	2.0 d
soft (*Arnold Bakery* Light)	40	2.0	7.0	<1.0	0	90	2.0 d
soft (*Brownberry Bakery* Light) . .	40	2.0	10.0	<1.0	0	100	2.0 d
soft, seeded or unseeded (*Arnold Bakery*)	70	2.0	14.0	1.0	0	170	1.0 d
rye and pumpernickel (*August Bros.*) . . .	90	3.0	18.0	1.0	0	220	1.0 d
sandwich, dark (*Brownberry* Natural)	60	2.0	12.0	1.0	0	170	2.0 d
sourdough:							
(*Francisco*)	90	3.0	19.0	1.0	0	250	1.0 d
(*Roman Meal Light*)	41	2.3	7.0	.4	0	143	2.6 d
(*Wonder Light*) . . .	40	2.0	6.0	0	0	115	3.0 d
whole grain (*Roman Meal*)	67	2.9	11.5	.9	0	219	1.3 d
whole grain (*Roman Meal Light*) . . .	41	2.3	6.9	.4	0	138	2.7 d
sunflower and bran (*Monk's*), 1 oz. . . .	70	3.0	12.0	1.0	0	80	2.0 d
Vienna (*Pepperidge Farm Light Style*)	45	2.0	10.0	0	0	100	1.0 d
wheat:							
(*Arnold Brick Oven* 1 lb.)	60	2.0	9.0	2.0	0	105	2.0 d
(*Arnold Brick Oven* 2 lb.)	90	3.0	14.0	2.0	0	130	2.0 d
(*Arnold* Natural) . .	80	3.0	15.0	1.0	0	180	2.0 d
(*Beefsteak* Hearty)	70	3.0	12.0	1.0	0	160	1.4 d
(*Brownberry* Hearth)	70	3.0	12.0	1.0	0	150	2.0 d
(*Brownberry* Natural)	80	3.0	14.0	1.0	0	190	2.0 d
(*Fresh & Natural*)	70	4.0	11.0	1.0	0	130	1.6 d

Food and Measure	cal.	prot. (gms)	carbo. (gms)	fat (gms)	chol. (mgs)	sod. (mgs)	fiber (gms)
Bread, wheat *(cont.)*							
(Home Pride Butter Top)	70	3.0	12.0	1.0	<5	170	1.4 d
(Home Pride Honey ButterTop)	100	3.0	17.0	2.0	<5	210	1.8 d
(Home Pride Light)	40	2.0	7.0	<1.0	<5	115	2.4 d
(Pepperidge Farm 1½ lb.)	90	3.0	18.0	2.0	0	190	2.0 d
(Pepperidge Farm Light Style) . . .	45	2.0	9.0	0	0	90	1.0 d
(Pepperidge Farm Family 2 lb.) . . .	70	2.0	13.0	1.0	0	130	2.0 d
(Pepperidge Farm Very Thin), 2 slices	35	2.0	7.0	0	0	75	0
(Roman Meal Light)	42	2.2	7.2	.4	0	104	2.6 d
(Thomas' Light) . .	40	2.0	6.0	1.0	0	75	2.0 d
(Wonder Country Style/Golden) . .	70	3.0	12.0	1.0	0	160	1.0 d
(Wonder Family) . .	70	2.0	13.0	1.0	0	150	.9 d
(Wonder Light) . . .	40	2.0	7.0	0	0	115	2.0 d
apple honey *(Brownberry)* . .	60	2.0	11.0	1.0	0	130	2.0 d
cracked *(Pepperidge Farm* Thin), 2 slices	70	2.0	13.0	1.0	0	140	1.0 d
cracked *(Roman Meal)*	93	4.3	15.3	1.5	0	196	2.2 d
cracked *(Wonder)*	70	3.0	13.0	1.0	0	180	.8 d
dark *(Arnold/ Brownberry Bran'nola)*	90	4.0	15.0	3.0	0	150	3.0 d
golden *(Arnold Bakery* Light) . .	40	2.0	7.0	<1.0	0	90	2.0 d
golden *(Brownberry* Light)	40	2.0	8.0	<1.0	0	80	2.0 d

Food and Measure	cal.	prot. (gms)	carbo. (gms)	fat (gms)	chol. (mgs)	sod. (mgs)	fiber (gms)
hearty (Arnold/ Brownberry Bran'nola)	100	3.0	15.0	3.0	0	160	3.0 d
hearty (Roman Meal Light)	42	2.2	7.3	.4	0	104	2.5 d
honey wheatberry (Arnold)	80	3.0	13.0	2.0	0	140	2.0 d
honey wheatberry (Roman Meal) . .	69	2.8	12.3	.9	0	141	1.0 d
sesame (Pepperidge Farm Hearty) . .	95	3.5	18.0	1.5	0	170	1.5 d
soft (Brownberry)	70	3.0	14.0	1.0	0	115	1.0 d
sprouted (Pepperidge Farm), 2 slices	70	3.0	11.0	2.0	0	100	2.0 d
wheatberry (Roman Meal Light) . . .	42	2.2	7.3	.4	0	105	2.5 d
wheat, whole:							
(Arnold Brick Oven Light 100%) . . .	40	2.0	6.0	<1.0	0	85	3.0 d
(Arnold Stone Ground 100%)	50	2.0	8.0	1.0	<5	100	2.0 d
(Monk's 100% Stone Ground), 1 oz.	70	3.0	13.0	1.0	0	110	m.q.
(Pepperidge Farm Thin), 2 slices . .	60	2.0	12.0	1.0	0	110	2.0 d
(Roman Meal light 100%)	42	2.7	6.8	.4	0	104	2.4 d
(Roman Meal 100%)	64	3.0	10.8	.9	0	140	2.1 d
(Wonder Stone- ground 100%) . .	80	4.0	13.0	1.0	0	160	2.2 d
regular or soft (Won- der 100%)	60	4.0	10.0	1.0	0	130	1.7 d
white:							
(Arnold Bakery Light Premium)	40	2.0	7.0	<1.0	0	90	2.0 d

Food and Measure	cal.	prot. (gms)	carbo. (gms)	fat (gms)	chol. (mgs)	sod. (mgs)	fiber (gms)
Bread, white *(cont.)*							
(Arnold Brick Oven							
1 lb.)	60	2.0	11.0	1.0	0	135	1.0 d
(Arnold Brick Oven							
2 lb.)	90	3.0	14.0	2.0	0	160	1.0 d
(Arnold Brick Oven							
Light)	40	2.0	10.0	<1.0	0	95	2.0 d
(Arnold Brick Oven							
Thin)	40	1.0	7.0	<1.0	0	75	<1.0 d
(Arnold Country) . .	100	3.0	18.0	2.0	0	200	1.0 d
(Beefsteak Robust)	70	3.0	12.0	1.0	0	140	.7 d
(Brownberry Coun-							
try)	100	3.0	19.0	2.0	0	200	1.0 d
(Brownberry Natural)	60	2.0	11.0	1.0	0	135	<1.0 d
(Home Pride Butter-							
Top)	70	3.0	12.0	1.0	<5	170	1.4 d
(Home Pride Light)	40	2.0	7.0	<1.0	<5	115	2.4 d
(Monk's)	60	3.0	10.0	1.0	0	95	m.q.
(Pepperidge Farm							
Country), 2 slices	190	7.0	38.0	2.0	0	340	2.0 d
(Pepperidge Farm							
Large Family)* . .	70	2.0	13.0	1.0	0	150	0
(Pepperidge Farm							
Thin)	80	2.0	14.0	2.0	0	130	0
(Pepperidge Farm							
Thin 8 oz.)	70	2.0	13.0	1.0	0	120	0
(Pepperidge Farm							
Very Thin)	20	.5	4.0	0	0	40	0
(Roman Meal Light)	42	2.1	7.4	.4	0	106	2.6 d
(Wonder)	70	2.0	13.0	1.0	0	150	.7 d
(Wonder Light) . . .	40	2.0	7.0	0	0	115	2.0 d
w/buttermilk *(Won-*							
der)*	70	2.0	13.0	1.0	0	150	.7 d
extra fiber *(Arnold*							
Brick Oven)* . . .	50	2.0	10.0	<1.0	0	90	2.0 d
sandwich							
(Brownberry) . .	60	2.0	12.0	1.0	0	120	<1.0 d

Food and Measure	cal.	prot. (gms)	carbo. (gms)	fat (gms)	chol. (mgs)	sod. (mgs)	fiber (gms)
sandwich (Pepperidge Farm),							
2 slices	130	4.0	24.0	2.0	0	260	0
soft (Brownberry)	80	2.0	13.0	2.0	0	130	1.0 d
toasting (Pepperidge Farm)	90	3.0	17.0	1.0	0	200	1.0 d
Bread, brown, canned, 1/2″ slice:							
(B&M/Friends)	92	2.0	21.0	0	0	345	2.0 d
raisin (B&M/Friends)	94	2.0	22.0	0	0	320	2.0 d
Bread, frozen, garlic (Pepperidge Farm),							
1 oz.	100	2.0	11.0	6.0	15	140	m.q.
Bread, sweet, date nut:							
(Dromedary), 1/2″ slice	80	1.0	13.0	2.0	0	160	m.q.
(Thomas'), 1-oz. slice	90	1.0	18.0	2.0	<5	170	1.0 d
Bread, sweet, mix*, 1/12 loaf, except as noted:							
apple cinnamon (Pillsbury)	180	2.0	31.0	6.0	20	170	m.q.
banana (Pillsbury) . .	170	3.0	27.0	5.0	35	200	m.q.
blueberry (Pillsbury)	180	2.0	30.0	6.0	20	160	m.q.
cornbread:							
(Ballard)	150	4.0	25.0	3.0	30	580	m.q.
(Dromedary), 2″ sq.	130	3.0	20.0	3.0	n.a.	480	m.q.
white (Robin Hood/ Gold Medal							
Pouch), 1/6 recipe	140	4.0	22.0	4.0	m.q.	490	m.q.
yellow (Robin Hood/ Gold Medal							
Pouch), 1/6 recipe	150	4.0	23.0	5.0	m.q.	500	m.q.
cranberry (Pillsbury)	160	2.0	30.0	4.0	20	150	m.q.
date (Pillsbury)	160	2.0	31.0	3.0	20	150	m.q.
date nut (Dromedary)	183	2.0	26.0	8.0	n.a.	248	m.q.
gingerbread, see "Cake mix"							

Food and Measure	cal.	prot. (gms)	carbo. (gms)	fat (gms)	chol. (mgs)	sod. (mgs)	fiber (gms)
Bread, sweet, mix *(cont.)*							
nut *(Pillsbury)*	170	3.0	27.0	6.0	20	190	m.q.
oatmeal raisin *(Pillsbury)*	190	3.0	30.0	7.0	20	180	m.q.
Bread crumbs,							
1/2 oz., except as noted:							
plain *(Arnold)*	50	2.0	8.0	<1.0	0	80	<1.0 d
plain *(Progresso)* . . .	60	2.0	11.0	<1.0	0	110	m.q.
Italian *(Arnold)*	50	2.0	8.0	<1.0	0	200	<1.0 d
Italian *(Progresso)* . .	60	2.0	11.0	<1.0	0	240	m.q.
seasoned *(Contadina)*, 1 rounded tbsp. . . .	35	1.0	7.0	<1.0	n.a.	250	.1 d
Bread dough:							
frozen, honey wheat *(Bridgford)*, 1 oz.	80	3.0	14.0	1.0	0	150	m.q.
frozen, white:							
(Bridgford), 1 oz.	80	3.0	14.0	1.0	0	160	m.q.
(Rich's), 2 slices . .	120	5.0	24.0	1.0	0	210	.8 d
refrigerated, 1″ slice, except as noted:							
(Roman Meal), 1 oz.	85	2.3	13.2	2.8	0	199	.6 d
French, crusty *(Pillsbury)*	60	2.0	11.0	<1.0	0	120	m.q.
twists, 1 piece:							
cornbread *(Pillsbury)*	70	1.0	8.0	3.0	0	150	m.q.
oatmeal, country *(Hearty Grains)*	80	2.0	15.0	1.0	0	120	1.0 d
wheat, cracked, and honey *(Hearty Grains)*	80	2.0	14.0	1.0	0	120	1.0 d
wheat *(Pipin' Hot)* . .	70	2.0	12.0	2.0	0	170	m.q.
white *(Pipin' Hot)* . .	70	3.0	12.0	2.0	0	170	m.q.
Bread shell, Italian:							
(Boboli 6″), 1 piece	300	13.0	49.0	7.0	5	620	2.0 d
(Boboli 12″), 1 piece	1200	52.0	196.0	28.0	20	2480	8.0 d

Food and Measure	cal.	prot. (gms)	carbo. (gms)	fat (gms)	chol. (mgs)	sod. (mgs)	fiber (gms)
Bread snacks, 1/2 oz.:							
cinnamon raisin swirl *(Pepperidge Farm* Bread Crisps) . . .	70	2.0	9.0	2.0	0	90	m.q.
nacho cheese and corn *(Pepperidge Farm* Bread Bites)	70	2.0	9.0	2.0	10	160	m.q.
Breadfruit:							
1/2 cup	114	1.2	29.8	.3	0	2	5.4 d
1/4 small, 3.4 oz. . . .	99	1.0	26.0	.2	0	2	4.7 d
Breadfruit seeds, 1 oz.:							
raw[1], shelled	54	2.1	8.3	1.6	0	n.a.	.5 c
boiled[2], shelled . . .	48	1.5	9.1	.7	0	n.a.	.5 c
roasted[1], shelled . . .	59	1.8	11.4	.8	0	n.a.	.6 c
Breading mix, frying *(Golden Dipt),* 1 oz.	90	3.0	20.0	0	0	630	m.q.
Breadsticks, 1 piece, except as noted:							
plain *(Stella D'Oro)* . .	40	1.0	7.0	1.0	0	55	m.q.
plain *(Stella D'Oro* Dietetic)	45	1.0	7.0	1.0	0	<10	m.q.
cheddar *(Pepperidge Farm* Thin), 1/2 oz.	60	2.0	9.0	2.0	5	115	1.0 d
garlic and herb *(Master Choice)*	14	<1.0	2.0	<1.0	0	30	m.q.
onion *(Stella D'Oro)*	40	1.0	6.0	1.0	0	m.q.	m.q.
onion *(Pepperidge Farm* Thin), 1/2 oz.	60	2.0	10.0	1.0	0	75	1.0 d
pizza *(Stella D'Oro)*	45	1.0	7.0	1.0	0	m.q.	m.q.
sesame:							
(Pepperidge Farm Thin), 1/2 oz. . . .	60	2.0	10.0	2.0	0	90	m.q.
(Stella D'Oro) . . .	50	1.0	6.0	2.0	0	45	m.q.

[1] *South American cultivar.*
[2] *Pacific area cultivar.*

Food and Measure	cal.	prot. (gms)	carbo. (gms)	fat (gms)	chol. (mgs)	sod. (mgs)	fiber (gms)
Breadsticks, sesame *(cont.)*							
(Stella D'Oro Dietetic)	50	1.0	6.0	2.0	0	<10	m.q.
wheat *(Stella D'Oro)*	40	1.0	6.0	1.0	0	m.q.	m.q.
refrigerated, soft:							
(Pillsbury)	100	3.0	17.0	2.0	0	230	m.q.
(Roman Meal) . . .	117	3.1	18.2	3.9	0	274	.8 d
Breakfast, see specific listings							
Broad beans:							
raw, 1/2 cup	40	3.1	6.4	.4	0	28	2.3 d
boiled, drained, 4 oz.	64	5.4	11.5	.6	0	47	2.2 c
Broad beans, mature, dry *(Frieda's* Fava Beans), 1 oz. . . .	15	1.6	1.9	.2	0	14	m.q.
dry, boiled, 1/2 cup	93	6.5	16.7	.3	0	4	4.6 d
canned, 1/2 cup:							
w/liquid	91	7.0	15.9	.3	0	580	.5 c
(Progresso Fava Beans)	90	7.0	15.0	<1.0	0	420	12.0 d
Broccoli:							
fresh:							
raw, chopped, 1/2 cup	12	1.3	2.3	.2	0	12	1.3 d
raw, 1 spear, 8.7 oz.	42	4.5	7.9	.5	0	40	4.5 d
boiled, drained:							
chopped, 1/2 cup	22	2.3	3.9	.2	0	20	2.3 d
1 spear, 6.3 oz.	51	5.4	9.1	.6	0	46	5.2 d
frozen, 3.3 oz., except as noted:							
spears, 10-oz. pkg.	84	8.7	15.2	1.0	0	49	8.5 d
spears *(Green Giant Harvest Fresh),* 1/2 cup	20	2.0	4.0	0	0	115	2.0 d
spears *(Green Giant Select),* 1/2 cup	18	2.0	5.0	0	0	25	3.0 d
spears *(Seabrook)*	25	3.0	5.0	0	0	20	1.0 c

Food and Measure	cal.	prot. (gms)	carbo. (gms)	fat (gms)	chol. (mgs)	sod. (mgs)	fiber (gms)
spears, baby *(Seabrook)*	30	3.0	5.0	0	0	14	1.0 c
spears, cuts or chopped *(Stilwell)*, 1/2 cup	25	2.0	4.0	0	0	20	2.0 d
florets *(Frosty Acres)*	30	3.0	5.0	0	0	14	1.0 c
cuts *(Green Giant Polybag)*, 1/2 cup	18	2.0	5.0	0	0	25	4.0 d
cuts *(Green Giant Harvest Fresh)*, 1/2 cup	16	2.0	3.0	0	0	95	2.0 d
cuts *(Seabrook)* . .	25	3.0	5.0	0	0	50	1.0 c
chopped, 10-oz. pkg. . . .	75	8.0	13.6	.8	0	68	8.5 d
chopped *(Seabrook)*	25	3.0	5.0	0	0	18	1.0 c
frozen, in butter sauce:							
cut *(Green Giant One Serving)*, 4.5 oz.	45	3.0	7.0	2.0	5	420	3.0 d
spears *(Green Giant)*, 1/2 cup . . .	40	2.0	6.0	2.0	5	350	2.0 d
frozen, in cheese sauce:							
(Bird's Eye), 1/2 cup	70	4.0	7.0	3.0	10	410	2.0 d
(Freezer Queen Family), 4.5 oz.	50	3.0	8.0	1.0	m.q.	900	m.q.
(Green Giant), 1/2 cup	60	3.0	9.0	2.0	2	530	2.0 d
cut *(Green Giant One Serving)*, 5 oz.	80	4.0	13.0	2.0	5	700	2.0 d
Broccoli combinations, frozen:							
carrots and rotini, in cheese sauce *(Green Giant One Serving)*, 5.5 oz. . . .	100	5.0	17.0	2.0	5	440	3.0 d

Food and Measure	cal.	prot. (gms)	carbo. (gms)	fat (gms)	chol. (mgs)	sod. (mgs)	fiber (gms)
Broccoli combinations, frozen *(cont.)*							
and cauliflower:							
(*Frosty Acres* Swiss Mix), 3 oz.	25	2.0	5.0	0	0	36	1.0 c
medley (*Green Giant Valley Combinations*), 1/2 cup . .	60	2.0	9.0	2.0	0	340	3.0 d
cauliflower and carrots:							
(*Green Giant* One Serving), 4 oz. . .	30	3.0	7.0	0	0	40	3.0 d
in butter sauce (*Green Giant*), 1/2 cup	30	2.0	4.0	1.0	5	240	3.0 d
in cheese sauce (*Bird's Eye*), 1/2 cup	60	4.0	8.0	2.0	5	300	2.0 d
in cheese sauce (*Green Giant* One Serving), 5 oz. . .	80	3.0	13.0	2.0	5	650	2.0 d
in cheese sauce (*Green Giant*), 1/2 cup	60	3.0	9.0	2.0	2	490	2.0 d
fanfare (*Green Giant Valley Combinations*), 1/2 cup . . .	80	3.0	14.0	2.0	0	340	3.0 d
pasta, cauliflower, carrots, cheese sauce (*Freezer Queen Family*), 4.5 oz. . .	80	3.0	13.0	1.0	m.q.	930	m.q.
and red peppers (*Green Giant Select*), 1/2 cup	25	2.0	4.0	0	0	15	2.0 d
Broccoli and cheese pastry, frozen *(Pepperidge Farm*), 1 piece	230	5.0	18.0	16.0	m.q.	380	m.q.
Broth, see "Soup"							

Food and Measure	cal.	prot. (gms)	carbo. (gms)	fat (gms)	chol. (mgs)	sod. (mgs)	fiber (gms)
Brown gravy:							
canned or in jars:							
(Heinz HomeStyle), 2 oz. or 1/4 cup	25	1.0	3.0	1.0	1	320	.3 d
(La Choy), 1/2 tsp.	15	<1.0	4.0	<1.0	0	15	<1.0 d
w/onions *(Heinz* HomeStyle), 2 oz. or 1/4 cup	25	1.0	3.0	1.0	<1	330	n.a.
mix:							
(French's), 1/4 pkg.	18	0	3.0	0	0	220	n.a.
(Hain), 1/4 pkg. . . .	16	<1.0	3.0	0	0	600	n.a.
(Lawry's), 1 pkg. . . .	96	2.8	13.2	3.6	3	1710	.2 c
(McCormick/Schilling), 1/4 cup* . .	23	.5	3.5	.8	n.a.	313	n.a.
(McCormick/Schilling Lite), 1/4 cup*	10	<1.0	2.0	1.0	n.a.	450	n.a.
(Pillsbury), 1/4 cup*	16	0	3.0	0	0	180	0
(Spatini), 1 cup* . .	93	3.7	16.4	1.3	3	1494	.1 c
vegetarian *(LaLoma Gravy Quik)*, 2 tbsp.*	45	<1.0	2.0	4.0	0	150	n.a.
Brownie, 1 piece, except as noted:							
(Drake's Old Fashion)	160	2.0	20.0	3.0	10	100	m.q.
(Tastykake)	340	4.0	53.0	14.0	20	220	5.0 d
all varieties *(Hostess Brownie Bites)*, 5 pieces	260	4.0	31.0	15.0	50	140	1.8 d
butterscotch *(Rachel's)*, 2.1 oz. . . .	270	3.0	36.0	13.0	40	170	m.q.
chocolate, double *(Rachel's)*, 2.1 oz. . . .	290	3.0	29.0	17.0	30	135	m.q.
chocolate, double, w/nuts *(Rachel's)*, 2.1 oz.	290	4.0	30.0	17.0	30	150	m.q.
fudge:							
(Drake's)	380	4.0	60.0	15.0	10	102	m.q.
(Little Debbie) . . .	270	3.0	38.0	13.0	11	95	m.q.

Food and Measure	cal.	prot. (gms)	carbo. (gms)	fat (gms)	chol. (mgs)	sod. (mgs)	fiber (gms)
Brownie (cont.)							
fudge nut:							
(Awrey's Sheet Cake), 1.2 oz. . . .	150	2.0	16.0	9.0	25	115	1.0 d
(Frito-Lay's), 3 oz.	360	3.0	56.0	14.0	8	225	m.q.
iced (Awrey's Sheet Cake), 2.5 oz. . . .	300	3.0	36.0	17.0	40	210	1.0 d
Brownie, frozen, 1 piece:							
à la mode (Weight Watchers Sweet Celebrations) . . .	180	5.0	35.0	4.0	5	150	m.q.
chocolate (Weight Watchers Sweet Celebrations) . . .	100	3.0	16.0	3.0	5	150	m.q.
hot fudge (Pepperidge Farm Classic) . . .	370	4.0	46.0	18.0	75	150	m.q.
mint frosted (Weight Watchers Sweet Celebrations) . . .	100	2.0	18.0	2.0	5	130	m.q.
peanut butter fudge (Weight Watchers Sweet Celebrations)	100	2.0	18.0	3.0	5	140	m.q.
Swiss mocha fudge (Weight Watchers Sweet Celebrations)	90	2.0	18.0	2.0	5	140	m.q.
Brownie mix*, 1 piece:							
(Betty Crocker Supreme Original) . .	140	1.0	22.0	5.0	20	95	m.q.
(Betty Crocker Supreme Party)	160	1.0	26.0	6.0	10	105	m.q.
caramel (Betty Crocker Supreme)	120	1.0	21.0	4.0	10	115	m.q.
chocolate:							
double (Pillsbury Great Additions)	140	1.0	19.0	6.0	10	75	m.q.

Food and Measure	cal.	prot. (gms)	carbo. (gms)	fat (gms)	chol. (mgs)	sod. (mgs)	fiber (gms)
German (Betty Crocker Supreme)	160	1.0	24.0	7.0	10	120	m.q.
milk (Duncan Hines Brownies Plus)	160	1.0	20.0	8.0	n.a.	95	m.q.
chocolate chip (Betty Crocker Supreme)	130	1.0	20.0	5.0	10	90	m.q.
frosted:							
(Betty Crocker Supreme)	160	1.0	26.0	6.0	10	105	m.q.
(Betty Crocker MicroRave) . . .	180	2.0	27.0	7.0	0	130	m.q.
fudge:							
(Betty Crocker Family Size)	140	1.0	22.0	5.0	10	100	m.q.
(Betty Crocker Light)	100	1.0	21.0	1.0	0	90	m.q.
(Duncan Hines) . .	130	1.0	18.0	5.0	n.a.	90	m.q.
(Pillsbury, 15 oz.)	140	2.0	21.0	6.0	15	95	m.q.
(Pillsbury, 21.5 oz.)	150	1.0	20.0	7.0	10	90	m.q.
(Pillsbury Lovin' Lites)	100	1.0	19.0	2.0	0	85	m.q.
(Pillsbury Microwave)	190	2.0	25.0	9.0	0	110	m.q.
(Robin Hood/Gold Medal Pouch) . .	100	1.0	15.0	4.0	m.q.	70	m.q.
w/chocolate fudge frosting (Pillsbury Microwave) . . .	240	2.0	32.0	11.0	0	140	m.q.
double (Duncan Hines Brownies Plus)	150	2.0	22.0	6.0	n.a.	105	m.q.
Funfetti, frosted (Pillsbury Great Additions)	160	1.0	23.0	7.0	10	100	m.q.
w/hot fudge topping (Betty Crocker Micro-Rave Singles)	340	5.0	54.0	12.0	0	270	m.q.

Food and Measure	cal.	prot. (gms)	carbo. (gms)	fat (gms)	chol. (mgs)	sod. (mgs)	fiber (gms)
Brownie mix *(cont.)*							
peanut butter *(Duncan Hines Brownies Plus)*	150	3.0	16.0	8.0	n.a.	105	m.q.
turtle *(Duncan Hines Gourmet)*	200	2.0	27.0	9.0	n.a.	125	m.q.
walnut:							
(Betty Crocker Supreme)	130	1.0	18.0	6.0	10	85	m.q.
(Duncan Hines Brownies Plus)	150	1.0	19.0	7.0	n.a.	90	m.q.
(Pillsbury Great Additions)	140	2.0	16.0	8.0	10	70	m.q.
Browning sauce							
(Gravymaster), 1 tsp.	12	.5	2.4	tr.	0	<1	tr.c
Brussels sprouts:							
fresh:							
raw, 1/2 cup	19	1.5	3.9	.1	0	11	1.8 d
boiled, drained, 1 sprout, .7 oz.	8	.5	1.8	.1	0	4	.9 d
boiled, drained, 1/2 cup	30	2.0	6.8	.4	0	17	3.4 d
frozen, 1/2 cup, except as noted:							
boiled, drained . .	33	2.8	6.5	.3	0	18	1.4 d
(Bird's Eye), 3.3 oz.	35	3.0	7.0	0	0	15	3.0 d
(Seabrook), 3.3 oz.	35	3.0	7.0	0	0	12	1.0 c
baby *(Seabrook)*, 3.3 oz.	40	4.0	7.0	0	0	5	1.0 c
in butter sauce *(Green Giant)* . .	40	3.0	8.0	1.0	5	280	4.0 d
Buckwheat:							
whole-grain, 1 oz. . . .	97	3.8	20.3	1.0	0	<1	2.8 d
whole-grain, 1 cup . .	584	22.5	121.6	5.8	0	1	17.0 d
Buckwheat flour:							
1 oz.	95	3.6	20.0	.9	0	n.a.	11.4 d
1 cup	402	15.1	84.7	3.7	0	n.a.	12.0 d

Food and Measure	cal.	prot. (gms)	carbo. (gms)	fat (gms)	chol. (mgs)	sod. (mgs)	fiber (gms)
(Arrowhead Mills), 2 oz.	190	7.0	41.0	1.0	0	0	7.1 d
Buckwheat groats:							
brown or white *(Arrowhead Mills),* 2 oz.	190	7.0	41.0	1.0	0	<1	7.1 d
roasted:							
dry, 1 oz.	98	3.3	21.2	.8	0	3	.5 c
cooked, 1 cup . . .	182	6.7	39.5	1.2	0	8	1.0 c
Bulgur (see also "Tabbouleh mix"):							
dry, 1 oz.	97	3.5	21.5	.4	0	5	5.2 d
dry, 1 cup	479	17.2	106.2	1.9	0	23	25.6 d
cooked, 1 cup	152	5.6	33.8	.4	0	9	8.2 d
Bun, see "Rolls"							
Bun, sweet (see also "Roll, sweet"), 1 piece:							
honey:							
(Aunt Fanny's) . . .	360	4.0	42.0	20.0	10	150	m.q.
apple bear *(Aunt Fanny's)*	460	6.0	50.0	26.0	5	220	m.q.
creme-filled *(Aunt Fanny's Bogie)*	460	6.0	49.0	27.0	10	200	m.q.
glazed *(Tastykake)*	360	6.0	42.0	20.0	0	220	4.0 d
iced *(Tastykake)* . .	350	5.0	50.0	15.0	0	250	1.0 d
jelly-filled *(Aunt Fanny's Birdie)*	450	6.0	53.0	24.0	5	210	m.q.
lemon bear *(Aunt Fanny's)*	440	5.0	52.0	23.0	5	200	m.q.
snow bear *(Aunt Fanny's)*	480	6.0	60.0	24.0	5	220	m.q.
frozen, cinnamon *(Rich's Ever Fresh)*	310	3.0	34.0	19.0	10	90	1.9 d
frozen, honey *(Rich's Ever Fresh)*	270	3.0	29.0	16.0	5	600	1.0 d
Burbot, meat only:							
raw, 4 oz.	102	21.9	0	.9	68	110	0

Food and Measure	cal.	prot. (gms)	carbo. (gms)	fat (gms)	chol. (mgs)	sod. (mgs)	fiber (gms)
Burbot *(cont.)*							
baked, broiled, or microwaved, 4 oz. . . .	130	28.1	0	1.2	87	141	0
Burdock root:							
raw, pieces, 1/2 cup	43	.9	10.3	.1	0	3	1.9 d
raw, 1 medium, 7.3 oz.	112	1.3	13.6	.1	0	4	5.1 d
boiled, drained, 1" pieces, 1/2 cup . .	55	1.3	13.2	.1	0	3	1.1 d
"Burger," vegetarian, see " 'Hamburger,' vegetarian"							
Burger King, 1 serving:							
breakfast:							
blueberry mini muffins	292	4.0	37.0	14.0	72	244	m.q.
Breakfast Buddy w/sausage and cheese	255	11.0	15.0	16.0	127	492	m.q.
Croissan'wich:							
w/bacon	353	16.0	19.0	23.0	230	780	m.q.
w/ham	351	19.0	20.0	22.0	236	1373	m.q.
w/sausage . . .	534	21.0	22.0	40.0	258	985	m.q.
French toast sticks	440	4.0	60.0	27.0	0	490	m.q.
hash browns	213	2.0	25.0	12.0	0	318	m.q.
burgers, chicken, and sandwiches:							
bacon double cheeseburger . .	470	30.0	26.0	28.0	100	800	m.q.
bacon double cheeseburger deluxe	570	32.0	26.0	38.0	110	990	m.q.
BK Broiler chicken	280	20.0	29.0	10.0	50	770	m.q.
cheeseburger . . .	300	16.0	28.0	14.0	45	660	m.q.
chicken sandwich	700	27.0	54.0	42.0	60	1440	m.q.
Chicken Specialty:							
American	682	31.0	57.0	37.0	75	1659	m.q.

Food and Measure	cal.	prot. (gms)	carbo. (gms)	fat (gms)	chol. (mgs)	sod. (mgs)	fiber (gms)
French	686	35.0	55.0	36.0	78	2080	m.q.
Italian	570	30.0	61.0	23.0	49	1551	m.q.
Chicken Tenders,							
6 pieces	236	16.0	14.0	13.0	38	541	m.q.
double cheese-							
burger	450	27.0	29.0	25.0	90	840	m.q.
Double Whopper	860	46.0	44.0	55.0	170	950	m.q.
Double Whopper, w/							
cheese	950	51.0	46.0	63.0	195	1260	m.q.
hamburger	260	14.0	28.0	10.0	30	500	m.q.
BK Big Fish	710	24.0	58.0	43.0	60	1110	m.q.
Whopper	630	27.0	44.0	38.0	90	880	m.q.
Whopper, w/cheese	720	32.0	46.0	46.0	115	1190	m.q.
Whopper Jr.	330	14.0	28.0	19.0	40	500	m.q.
Whopper Jr.,							
w/cheese	380	16.0	29.0	22.0	50	660	m.q.
side dishes:							
french fries, medium	372	5.0	43.0	20.0	0	238	m.q.
onion rings	339	5.0	38.0	19.0	0	628	m.q.
salad, w/out dressing:							
chef salad	178	17.0	7.0	9.0	103	568	m.q.
chunky chicken							
salad	142	20.0	8.0	4.0	49	443	m.q.
garden salad . . .	95	6.0	8.0	5.0	15	125	m.q.
dinner/side salad	20	1.0	4.0	0	0	10	m.q.
salad dressings,							
1.2 oz.:							
bleu cheese	150	1.0	1.0	16.0	29	256	n.a.
French	145	0	12.0	11.0	0	200	n.a.
light Italian	15	0	3.0	1.0	0	355	n.a.
ranch	175	1.0	2.0	18.0	10	158	n.a.
Thousand Island . .	145	1.0	8.0	13.0	18	202	n.a.
sauces, 1 oz., except							
as noted:							
A.M. Express dip	84	0	21.0	0	0	18	n.a.
barbecue dipping	36	0	9.0	0	0	397	n.a.
BK Broiler, .4 oz.	37	0	1.0	4.0	5	74	n.a.
Bulls Eye, .5 oz. . . .	22	0	5.0	0	0	47	n.a.

Food and Measure	cal.	prot. (gms)	carbo. (gms)	fat (gms)	chol. (mgs)	sod. (mgs)	fiber (gms)
Burger King, sauces (cont.)							
honey dipping . . .	91	0	23.0	0	0	12	n.a.
ranch dipping . . .	171	0	2.0	18.0	0	208	n.a.
sweet & sour dip-							
ping	45	0	11.0	0	0	52	n.a.
desserts:							
apple pie	320	3.0	45.0	14.0	0	420	m.q.
Snickers ice cream	220	5.0	20.0	14.0	15	65	n.a.
shakes, medium:							
chocolate	320	9.0	54.0	7.0	20	230	(0)
chocolate (w/syrup)	400	10.0	68.0	9.0	20	350	(0)
strawberry (w/syrup)	370	10.0	67.0	6.0	20	240	(0)
vanilla	310	9.0	53.0	6.0	20	230	(0)
Burrito, frozen (see							
also "Burrito en-							
tree"):							
beef (*Hormel*), 4 oz.	300	9.0	37.0	13.0	35	620	m.q.
beef, nacho (*Patio*							
Britos), 3 oz.	220	7.0	25.0	11.0	25	350	m.q.
beef and bean:							
(*Patio Britos*), 3 oz.	210	4.0	28.0	9.0	15	290	m.q.
hot, red chili (*Patio*),							
5 oz.	340	11.0	44.0	13.0	20	810	m.q.
medium (*Patio*),							
5 oz.	370	11.0	43.0	16.0	25	830	m.q.
mild, green chili (*Pa-*							
tio), 5 oz.	330	12.0	43.0	12.0	30	770	m.q.
red hot, red chili							
(*Patio*), 5 oz. . .	360	12.0	43.0	15.0	25	800	m.q.
cheese:							
(*Hormel*), 4 oz.	250	9.0	43.0	5.0	30	670	m.q.
nacho (*Patio Britos*),							
3.63 oz.	250	7.0	32.0	10.0	20	330	m.q.
chicken and cheese,							
spicy (*Patio Britos*),							
3 oz.	210	4.0	28.0	9.0	25	280	m.q.
chili, red (*Hormel*),							
4 oz.	280	9.0	40.0	10.0	35	620	m.q.

Food and Measure	cal.	prot. (gms)	carbo. (gms)	fat (gms)	chol. (mgs)	sod. (mgs)	fiber (gms)
Burrito, breakfast,							
frozen:							
(Swanson Original),							
3.5 oz.	200	8.0	25.0	7.0	m.q.	510	m.q.
bacon *(Swanson)*,							
3.5 oz.	250	10.0	27.0	11.0	m.q.	540	m.q.
w/home fries *(Swanson Fiesta)*, 5.75 oz.	330	10.0	31.0	18.0	m.q.	610	m.q.
sausage *(Swanson)*,							
3.15 oz.	250	9.0	24.0	13.0	m.q.	500	m.q.
Burrito dinner mix							
(Tio Sancho Dinner Kit):							
seasoning, 3.25 oz.	265	12.3	49.3	2.1	n.a.	5031	5.5 c
1 tortilla	125	3.3	24.0	1.9	n.a.	569	.1 c
Burrito entree, frozen:							
bean and cheese *(Old El Paso)*, 1 piece	330	14.0	44.0	11.0	m.q.	680	m.q.
beef and bean:							
hot *(Old El Paso)*, 1 piece	310	12.0	41.0	11.0	m.q.	710	m.q.
medium *(Old El Paso)*, 1 piece . .	330	13.0	41.0	13.0	29	630	m.q.
medium or mild *(Healthy Choice Quick Meal)*, 5.4 oz.	270	12.0	42.0	7.0	15	520	m.q.
mild *(Old El Paso)*, 1 piece	320	13.0	42.0	11.0	m.q.	500	m.q.
chicken *con queso*, mild *(Healthy Choice Quick Meal)*, 5.4 oz.	280	15.0	40.0	8.0	20	500	m.q.
Burrito seasoning mix:							
(Lawry's Seasoning Blends), 1 pkg. . .	132	6.0	23.3	1.7	3	2516	.9 c
(Old El Paso), 1/8 pkg.	17	1.0	3.0	0	0	275	1.0 d

Food and Measure	cal.	prot. (gms)	carbo. (gms)	fat (gms)	chol. (mgs)	sod. (mgs)	fiber (gms)
Butter:							
regular, unsalted:							
1 stick or 4 oz. . . .	813	1.0	0	92.0	248	12	0
1 tbsp.	100	.1	0	11.4	31	1	0
1 tsp.	34	<.1	0	3.8	10	<1	0
regular, salted:							
1 stick or 4 oz. . . .	813	1.0	0	92.0	248	937	0
1 tbsp.	100	.1	0	11.4	31	115	0
1 tsp.	34	<.1	0	3.8	10	39	0
1 pat, 90 per lb. . . .	36	<.1	0	4.1	11	41	0
whipped, unsalted:							
1/2 cup or 1 stick	542	.6	<.1	61.3	165	8	0
1 tbsp.	67	.1	tr.	7.6	20	1	0
1 tsp.	23	tr.	tr.	2.6	7	<1	0
whipped, salted:							
1/2 cup or 1 stick	542	.6	<.1	61.3	165	625	0
1 tbsp.	67	.1	tr.	7.6	20	78	0
1 tsp.	23	tr.	tr.	2.6	7	26	0
Butter beans, see "Lima beans"							
Butter flavor seasoning *(McCormick/ Schilling Best O' Butter),* 1/2 tsp.:							
cheddar flavor	6	<1.0	<1.0	<1.0	n.a.	75	0
garlic flavor	4	<1.0	<1.0	<1.0	n.a.	67	0
original or sour cream flavor	4	<1.0	<1.0	<1.0	n.a.	65	0
Butterbur:							
fresh:							
raw, 1/2 cup	7	.2	1.7	<.1	0	4	.6 c
raw, 1 stalk, .2 oz.	1	<.1	.2	tr.	0	tr.	.1 c
boiled, drained, 4 oz.	9	.3	2.4	<.1	0	5	.9 c
canned:							
chopped, 1/2 cup	2	.1	.2	.1	0	3	.6 c
3 stalks, 1.6 oz. . . .	1	<.1	.2	<.1	0	2	.4 c

Food and Measure	cal.	prot. (gms)	carbo. (gms)	fat (gms)	chol. (mgs)	sod. (mgs)	fiber (gms)
Butterfish, meat only:							
raw, 4 oz.	166	19.6	0	9.1	74	100	0
baked, broiled, or microwaved, 4 oz. . . .	212	25.1	0	11.7	94	129	0
Buttermilk, see "Milk" and "Milk, dry"							
Butternut squash:							
fresh, 1/2 cup:							
raw, cubed	32	.7	8.1	.1	0	3	1.1 d
baked, cubed . . .	41	.9	10.7	.1	0	4	2.9 d
frozen:							
12-oz. pkg.	192	6.0	49.0	.3	0	8	4.4 d
boiled, drained:							
4 oz.	44	1.4	11.4	.1	0	2	1.0 c
mashed, 1/2 cup . .	47	1.5	12.1	.1	0	2	1.0 c
Butternuts, dried:							
in shell, 1 lb.	750	30.5	14.8	69.8	0	1	5.8 d
shelled, 1 oz.	174	7.1	3.4	16.2	0	tr.	1.3 d
Butterscotch chips, baking (Nestlé Toll House Morsels), 1 oz.	150	1.0	19.0	8.0	n.a.	25	(0)
Butterscotch topping:							
(Kraft), 1 tbsp.	60	0	13.0	1.0	0	70	(0)
(Smucker's), 2 tbsp.	140	0	33.0	1.0	0	75	(0)
(Smucker's Special Recipe), 2 tbsp. . .	160	1.0	33.0	3.0	n.a.	40	(0)

C

Food and Measure	cal.	prot. (gms)	carbo. (gms)	fat (gms)	chol. (mgs)	sod. (mgs)	fiber (gms)
Cabbage:							
raw:							
5¾"-diam. head,							
2.5 lb.	228	13.1	49.3	2.4	0	164	20.9 d
shredded, ½ cup	9	.5	1.9	.1	0	6	.8 d
boiled, drained, shred-							
ded, ½ cup	17	.8	3.4	.3	0	6	2.1 d
Cabbage, Chinese:							
bok-choy:							
raw, whole, 1 lb.	52	6.0	8.7	.8	0	257	4.0 d
raw, shredded,							
½ cup	5	.5	.8	.1	0	23	.4 d
boiled, drained,							
shredded, ½ cup	10	1.3	1.5	.1	0	29	1.4 d
napa, raw *(Frieda's)*,							
1 oz.	4	.3	.9	<.1	0	7	m.q.
pe-tsai:							
raw, whole, 1 lb.	68	5.1	13.6	.8	0	38	4.2 d
raw, shredded,							
½ cup	6	.5	1.2	.1	0	3	.4 d
boiled, drained,							
shredded, ½ cup	8	.9	1.4	.1	0	6	1.0 d
Cabbage, red:							
raw, whole, 1 lb. . . .	100	5.0	22.2	.9	0	38	7.3 d
raw, shredded, ½ cup	10	.5	2.1	.1	0	4	.7 d
boiled, drained, shred-							
ded, ½ cup	16	.8	3.5	.2	0	6	1.5 d
Cabbage, savoy:							
raw, whole, 1 lb. . . .	100	7.3	22.1	.4	0	102	11.2 d
raw, shredded, ½ cup	10	.7	2.1	<.1	0	10	1.1 d

Food and Measure	cal.	prot. (gms)	carbo. (gms)	fat (gms)	chol. (mgs)	sod. (mgs)	fiber (gms)
boiled, drained, shredded, 1/2 cup	18	1.3	4.0	.1	0	17	.5 c
Cabbage, stuffed, frozen:							
(On-Cor), 8 oz.	170	10.0	15.0	8.0	n.a.	1010	m.q.
w/meat, in tomato sauce *(Lean Cuisine),* 9.5 oz.	210	13.0	26.0	6.0	30	560	m.q.
Cactus pear, see "Prickly pear"							
Cajun sauce, see "Creole sauce"							
Cajun seasoning *(Tone's),* 1 tsp. . .	9	.4	2.1	.2	0	215	.5 d
Cake (see also "Cake, snack" and "Cake, mix"), 1/12 cake, except as noted:							
apple streusel *(Awrey's),* 2″ sq.	160	2.0	18.0	9.0	15	120	0
banana, iced *(Awrey's),* 2″ sq.	140	1.0	17.0	8.0	20	120	0
Black Forest torte *(Awrey's),* 1/14 cake	350	3.0	38.0	21.0	50	330	1.0 d
carrot, iced:							
supreme *(Awrey's),* 2″ sq.	210	3.0	23.0	12.0	25	170	0
3-layer *(Awrey's)* . .	390	5.0	44.0	23.0	45	310	1.0 d
chocolate:							
double, iced *(Awrey's),* 2″ sq. . .	130	2.0	21.0	6.0	15	150	1.0 d
double, 2-layer *(Awrey's)*	250	3.0	38.0	11.0	35	260	1.0 d
double, 3-layer *(Awrey's)*	310	3.0	48.0	14.0	35	290	2.0 d
double torte *(Awrey's),* 1/14 cake	340	3.0	51.0	15.0	35	300	2.0 d

Food and Measure	cal.	prot. (gms)	carbo. (gms)	fat (gms)	chol. (mgs)	sod. (mgs)	fiber (gms)
Cake, chocolate (cont.)							
German, iced (Awrey's), 2″ sq. . .	160	2.0	19.0	9.0	20	150	0
German, 3-layer (Awrey's)	350	3.0	46.0	18.0	40	300	1.0 d
milk, yellow, 2-layer (Awrey's)	290	3.0	33.0	17.0	50	320	0
white iced, 2-layer (Awrey's)	270	3.0	34.0	15.0	40	290	1.0 d
coconut:							
butter cream (Awrey's), 2″ sq. . .	160	1.0	19.0	9.0	25	180	0
yellow, 3-layer (Awrey's)	350	3.0	40.0	21.0	50	340	0
coffee:							
caramel nut (Awrey's)	140	2.0	15.0	8.0	5	150	0
long John (Awrey's)	160	2.0	19.0	8.0	10	130	0
devil's food, iced (Awrey's), 2″ sq.	150	1.0	17.0	8.0	25	160	1.0 d
lemon:							
3-layer (Awrey's) . .	320	2.0	38.0	19.0	45	310	0
yellow, 2-layer (Awrey's)	290	2.0	33.0	17.0	45	310	0
Neapolitan torte (Awrey's), 1/14 cake . .	380	3.0	43.0	22.0	55	370	0
orange, iced:							
frosty (Awrey's), 2″ sq.	150	1.0	19.0	8.0	20	170	0
three-layer (Awrey's)	320	2.0	40.0	17.0	35	320	0
peanut butter torte (Awrey's), 1/14 cake	380	7.0	44.0	22.0	40	340	1.0 d
pistachio torte (Awrey's), 1/14 cake . .	370	3.0	41.0	22.0	35	370	1.0 d
pound, golden (Awrey's)	130	2.0	19.0	5.0	20	150	0
raisin spice, iced (Awrey's), 2″ sq.	160	1.0	21.0	8.0	20	120	0

Food and Measure	cal.	prot. (gms)	carbo. (gms)	fat (gms)	chol. (mgs)	sod. (mgs)	fiber (gms)
raspberry nut (Awrey's), 1/16 cake . .	310	3.0	39.0	16.0	30	220	0
sponge (Awrey's), 2″ sq.	80	1.0	11.0	3.0	15	125	0
strawberry supreme, torte (Awrey's), 1/14 cake	270	3.0	38.0	12.0	45	310	1.0 d
walnut torte (Awrey's), 1/14 cake	320	2.0	38.0	19.0	30	290	0
yellow, iced (Awrey's), 2″ sq.	150	1.0	18.0	9.0	25	180	0
Cake, frozen (see also "Cake, snack, frozen"), 1.7 oz., except as noted:							
Boston cream:							
(Mrs. Smith's 8″), 1/8 cake	170	2.0	29.0	5.0	25	140	0
(Pepperidge Farm Special recipe), 2 oz.	190	2.0	28.0	8.0	30	80	m.q.
cheesecake:							
French (Sara Lee), 1/8 cake	250	4.0	23.0	16.0	20	120	n.a.
New York (Master Choice), 1/6 cake	280	6.0	19.0	20.0	83	225	.n.a.
chocolate:							
double, layer (Sara Lee), 1/8 cake . .	270	3.0	33.0	14.0	30	140	m.q.
fudge layer (Pepperidge Farm) . . .	180	1.0	23.0	10.0	20	140	m.q.
fudge stripe (Pepperidge Farm) . .	170	2.0	20.0	9.0	20	140	m.q.
German, layer (Pepperidge Farm) . .	180	1.0	22.0	10.0	20	170	m.q.
chocolate mousse:							
(Pepperidge Farm Special Recipe), 2 oz.	190	2.0	25.0	9.0	20	90	m.q.

Food and Measure	cal.	prot. (gms)	carbo. (gms)	fat (gms)	chol. (mgs)	sod. (mgs)	fiber (gms)
Cake, frozen, chocolate mousse (cont.)							
(Sara Lee), 1/8 cake	260	3.0	23.0	17.0	20	100	m.q.
coconut layer:							
(Pepperidge Farm)	180	1.0	24.0	8.0	20	120	m.q.
(Sara Lee Flaky),							
1/8 cake	270	2.0	33.0	14.0	20	110	m.q.
devil's food layer							
(Pepperidge Farm)	180	1.0	24.0	9.0	20	135	m.q.
golden layer (Pep-							
peridge Farm) . .	180	1.0	24.0	9.0	20	110	m.q.
lemon mousse (Pep-							
peridge Farm							
Special Recipe),							
1.6 oz.	170	2.0	21.0	9.0	20	120	m.q.
pineapple cream							
(Pepperidge Farm							
Special Recipe),							
2 oz.	190	2.0	28.0	7.0	20	130	m.q.
pound:							
all butter (Sara Lee),							
1/15 cake	130	2.0	14.0	7.0	m.q.	85	m.q.
chocolate (Pepper-							
idge Farm Fat							
Free), 1 oz. . . .	70	2.0	15.0	1.0	0	85	m.q.
golden (Pepperidge							
Farm Fat Free),							
1 oz.	70	1.0	15.0	0	0	80	m.q.
strawberry:							
cream (Pepperidge							
Farm Special							
Recipe), 2 oz. . .	190	1.0	30.0	7.0	20	120	m.q.
stripe layer (Pepper-							
idge Farm),							
1.5 oz.	160	1.0	21.0	8.0	20	120	m.q.
vanilla layer (Pep-							
peridge Farm) . .	190	1.0	25.0	8.0	20	120	m.q.

Food and Measure	cal.	prot. (gms)	carbo. (gms)	fat (gms)	chol. (mgs)	sod. (mgs)	fiber (gms)
Cake, mix*, 1/12 cake or pkg., except as noted:							
angel food:							
(Betty Crocker Traditional)	130	3.0	30.0	0	0	170	m.q.
(Duncan Hines) . .	140	3.0	30.0	0	0	130	m.q.
(Pillsbury Lovin' Loaf), 1/8 cake . .	90	2.0	20.0	0	0	210	m.q.
confetti, lemon custard, or white *(Betty Crocker)*	150	3.0	34.0	0	0	300	m.q.
banana:							
(Duncan Hines) . .	260	3.0	36.0	11.0	65	295	m.q.
(Pillsbury Plus) . . .	250	3.0	35.0	11.0	55	280	m.q.
Black Forest cherry *(Pillsbury Bundt),* 1/16 cake	270	3.0	41.0	12.0	40	320	m.q.
blueberry *(Streusel Swirl),* 1/16 cake . .	260	3.0	39.0	11.0	40	200	m.q.
Boston cream:							
(Betty Crocker Classics), 1/8 cake . .	270	4.0	50.0	6.0	30	390	m.q.
(Pillsbury Bundt), 1/16 cake	260	3.0	42.0	10.0	40	290	m.q.
butter pecan *(Betty Crocker SuperMoist)*	250	3.0	35.0	11.0	55	320	m.q.
butter recipe:							
(Pillsbury Plus) . . .	260	3.0	35.0	12.0	75	370	m.q.
chocolate *(Betty Crocker SuperMoist)* . . .	280	4.0	35.0	14.0	75	400	m.q.
chocolate *(Pillsbury Plus)*	250	4.0	32.0	13.0	75	420	m.q.
fudge[1] *(Duncan Hines)*	270	3.0	34.0	13.0	65	350	m.q.

[1] Prepared with margarine.

Food and Measure	cal.	prot. (gms)	carbo. (gms)	fat (gms)	chol. (mgs)	sod. (mgs)	fiber (gms)
Cake, mix, butter recipe *(cont.)*							
golden[1] *(Duncan Hines)*	270	3.0	36.0	13.0	65	270	m.q.
yellow *(Betty Crocker SuperMoist)* . . .	260	3.0	37.0	11.0	75	340	m.q.
carrot:							
(Betty Crocker SuperMoist) . . .	250	3.0	36.0	10.0	55	300	m.q.
(Dromedary)	232	3.0	23.0	15.0	m.q.	292	m.q.
(Pillsbury Plus) . . .	260	3.0	34.0	12.0	55	300	m.q.
cherry chip *(Betty Crocker SuperMoist)*	190	3.0	37.0	3.0	0	270	m.q.
chocolate:							
(Simply Splendid), 3 oz.	268	3.0	43.0	10.0	0	275	1.0 d
dark *(Pillsbury Plus)*	250	3.0	32.0	12.0	55	340	m.q.
fudge *(Betty Crocker SuperMoist)* . . .	260	3.0	35.0	12.0	55	450	m.q.
fudge *(Pillsbury Bundt Tunnel of Fudge)*, 1/16 cake	310	3.0	42.0	16.0	40	340	m.q.
fudge, dark Dutch *(Duncan Hines)*	280	4.0	33.0	15.0	65	470	m.q.
German *(Betty Crocker Super-Moist)*	260	3.0	35.0	12.0	55	420	m.q.
German *(Pillsbury Plus)*	250	3.0	34.0	11.0	55	280	m.q.
German, w/frosting *(Betty Crocker MicroRave)*, 1/6 cake	320	3.0	37.0	18.0	35	250	m.q.
milk *(Betty Crocker SuperMoist)* . . .	260	4.0	34.0	12.0	55	340	m.q.

[1] *Prepared with margarine.*

Food and Measure	cal.	prot. (gms)	carbo. (gms)	fat (gms)	chol. (mgs)	sod. (mgs)	fiber (gms)
mousse *(Pillsbury Bundt)*, 1/16 cake	260	3.0	37.0	12.0	40	310	m.q.
pudding *(Betty Crocker* Classic), 1/6 cake	230	3.0	44.0	5.0	35	250	m.q.
Swiss *(Duncan Hines)*	280	4.0	33.0	15.0	65	375	m.q.
chocolate caramel *(Pillsbury Bundt)*, 1/16 cake	290	3.0	43.0	13.0	45	370	m.q.
chocolate chip:							
(Betty Crocker SuperMoist) . . .	290	3.0	35.0	15.0	55	300	m.q.
(Pillsbury Plus) . . .	240	3.0	34.0	10.0	35	280	m.q.
chocolate *(Betty Crocker SuperMoist)* . . .	260	3.0	34.0	12.0	55	400	m.q.
chocolate eclair *(Pillsbury Bundt)*, 1/16 cake	260	3.0	42.0	10.0	40	290	m.q.
chocolate macaroon *(Pillsbury Bundt)*, 1/16 cake	280	3.0	37.0	14.0	40	340	m.q.
cinnamon *(Streusel Swirl)*, 1/16 cake	260	3.0	38.0	11.0	40	200	m.q.
devil's food:							
(Betty Crocker SuperMoist) . . .	260	4.0	35.0	12.0	55	430	m.q.
(Betty Crocker SuperMoist Light)	200	4.0	36.0	4.0	55	340	m.q.
(Duncan Hines) . .	280	4.0	33.0	15.0	65	375	m.q.
(Pillsbury Lovin' Lites)	160	4.0	32.0	2.0	0	380	m.q.
(Pillsbury Plus) . . .	270	4.0	32.0	14.0	55	350	m.q.
chocolate frosted *(Betty Crocker MicroRave)*, 1/6 cake	310	3.0	36.0	17.0	35	250	m.q.

Food and Measure	cal.	prot. (gms)	carbo. (gms)	fat (gms)	chol. (mgs)	sod. (mgs)	fiber (gms)
Cake, mix *(cont.)*							
fudge marble:							
(Betty Crocker							
SuperMoist) . . .	260	3.0	36.0	11.0	55	290	m.q.
(Duncan Hines) . .	260	3.0	36.0	11.0	65	295	m.q.
fudge swirl *(Pillsbury*							
Plus)	270	3.0	36.0	12.0	55	300	m.q.
Funfetti (Pillsbury Plus)	230	3.0	35.0	9.0	0	290	m.q.
funnel cake *(Golden*							
Dipt), 1/8 mix . . .	100	2.0	20.0	1.0	0	170	m.q.
gingerbread:							
(Betty Crocker Clas-							
sic), 1/9 cake . .	220	3.0	35.0	7.0	30	330	m.q.
(Dromedary), 2″ sq.	100	1.0	19.0	2.0	n.a.	190	m.q.
(Pillsbury), 1/9 cake	180	2.0	32.0	5.0	0	300	m.q.
lemon:							
(Betty Crocker							
SuperMoist) . . .	260	3.0	37.0	11.0	55	280	m.q.
(Pillsbury Bundt Tun-							
nel of Lemon),							
1/16 cake	270	2.0	44.0	9.0	40	280	m.q.
(Pillsbury Plus) . . .	240	3.0	34.0	10.0	55	280	m.q.
chiffon *(Betty*							
Crocker Classic)	200	4.0	36.0	5.0	35	200	m.q.
pudding *(Betty*							
Crocker Classic),							
1/6 cake	230	2.0	45.0	5.0	35	270	m.q.
supreme *(Streusel*							
Swirl), 1/16 cake	260	3.0	37.0	11.0	40	300	m.q.
lemon, orange, or							
pineapple supreme							
(Duncan Hines) . .	260	3.0	36.0	11.0	65	295	m.q.
lemon-poppyseed							
(Simply Splendid),							
3 oz.	268	3.0	37.0	12.0	0	277	1.0 d
orange-walnut *(Simply*							
Splendid), 3 oz. . . .	276	3.0	37.0	13.0	0	276	1.0 d

Food and Measure	cal.	prot. (gms)	carbo. (gms)	fat (gms)	chol. (mgs)	sod. (mgs)	fiber (gms)
pineapple:							
creme *(Pillsbury Bundt)*, 1/16 cake	280	2.0	42.0	11.0	40	280	m.q.
upside-down *(Betty Crocker Classic)*, 1/9 cake	270	2.0	43.0	10.0	25	240	m.q.
pound:							
(Dromedary), 1/2" slice	150	2.0	21.0	6.0	n.a.	160	m.q.
golden *(Betty Crocker Classic)*	200	2.0	28.0	9.0	35	170	m.q.
rainbow chip *(Betty Crocker Super-Moist)*	250	3.0	35.0	11.0	55	320	m.q.
sour cream:							
chocolate *(Betty Crocker Super-Moist)*	260	3.0	35.0	12.0	55	430	m.q.
white *(Betty Crocker SuperMoist)* . . .	180	3.0	36.0	3.0	0	290	m.q.
spice *(Betty Crocker SuperMoist)*	260	3.0	36.0	11.0	55	320	m.q.
spice or strawberry supreme *(Duncan Hines)*	260	3.0	36.0	11.0	65	295	m.q.
strawberry *(Pillsbury Plus)*	250	3.0	35.0	11.0	55	310	m.q.
swirl *(Betty Crocker SuperMoist)*	260	3.0	36.0	11.0	55	280	m.q.
vanilla:							
French *(Duncan Hines)*	260	3.0	36.0	11.0	65	295	m.q.
golden *(Betty Crocker Super-Moist)*	280	3.0	36.0	14.0	55	270	m.q.
sunshine *(Pillsbury Plus)*	260	3.0	34.0	12.0	55	300	m.q.

Food and Measure	cal.	prot. (gms)	carbo. (gms)	fat (gms)	chol. (mgs)	sod. (mgs)	fiber (gms)
Cake, mix *(cont.)*							
white:							
(Betty Crocker							
SuperMoist) . . .	230	2.0	34.0	10.0	0	320	m.q.
(Betty Crocker							
SuperMoist Light)	180	2.0	37.0	3.0	0	330	m.q.
(Duncan Hines) . .	250	3.0	36.0	10.0	65	260	m.q.
(Pillsbury Lovin'							
Lites)	170	3.0	35.0	2.0	0	310	m.q.
(Pillsbury Plus) . . .	220	3.0	34.0	9.0	0	290	m.q.
yellow:							
(Betty Crocker							
SuperMoist) . . .	260	3.0	36.0	11.0	55	300	m.q.
(Betty Crocker							
SuperMoist Light)	200	3.0	37.0	4.0	55	310	m.q.
(Duncan Hines) . .	260	3.0	36.0	11.0	65	295	m.q.
(Pillsbury Lovin'							
Lites)	170	3.0	35.0	2.0	0	310	m.q.
(Pillsbury Plus) . . .	260	3.0	34.0	12.0	55	300	m.q.
butter *(Betty*							
Crocker Super-							
Moist)	260	3.0	37.0	11.0	75	340	m.q.
w/frosting *(Betty*							
Crocker Micro-							
wave), 1/6 cake	300	2.0	36.0	17.0	35	220	m.q.
Cake, snack (see also							
specific listings),							
1 piece:							
apple:							
pastry pocket *(Tas-*							
tykake)	320	4.0	38.0	18.0	10	220	1.0 d
spice *(Hostess Light)*	130	2.0	29.0	1.0	0	150	.5 d
strudel *(Aunt*							
Fanny's), 3 oz.	330	4.0	38.0	18.0	n.a.	210	m.q.
banana:							
(Hostess Suzy Q's)	240	2.0	38.0	9.0	20	200	m.q.
(Hostess Twinkies)	150	2.0	26.0	5.0	20	200	.5 d
(Tastykake Creamie)	170	2.0	25.0	7.0	10	90	1.0 d

Food and Measure	cal.	prot. (gms)	carbo. (gms)	fat (gms)	chol. (mgs)	sod. (mgs)	fiber (gms)
twins (Little Debbie)	130	1.0	18.0	6.0	5	70	m.q.
butterscotch (Tastykake Krimpets)	100	1.0	19.0	3.0	20	85	0
cheese pastry pocket (Tastykake)	330	4.0	38.0	19.0	10	230	1.0 d
cherry:							
cordial (Little Debbie)	170	1.0	23.0	9.0	0	100	m.q.
pastry (Tastykake)	330	4.0	41.0	17.0	10	230	1.0 d
strudel (Aunt Fanny's), 3 oz.	320	4.0	39.0	16.0	5	190	m.q.
chocolate:							
(Hostess Choco Bliss)	200	2.0	29.0	9.0	5	210	1.2 d
(Hostess Choco-Diles)	240	2.0	32.0	11.0	20	180	1.5 d
(Hostess Ding Dongs)	170	2.0	21.0	9.0	5	115	1.0 d
(Hostess Grizzly Chomps)	110	2.0	23.0	1.0	0	140	.8 d
(Hostess Ho Hos)	120	1.0	16.0	6.0	10	70	.6 d
(Hostess Suzy Q's)	250	2.0	37.0	10.0	15	300	2.0 d
(Little Debbie) . . .	150	1.0	22.0	7.0	0	100	m.q.
(Little Debbie Choco-Cake) . .	250	2.0	35.0	12.0	0	190	m.q.
(Little Debbie Choc-o-Jels)	140	1.0	20.0	7.0	0	85	m.q.
(Tastykake Creamie)	170	2.0	24.0	8.0	10	125	1.0 d
(Tastykake Junior)	340	4.0	57.0	12.0	60	220	4.0 d
(Tastykake Kandy Kakes)	80	1.0	13.0	3.0	0	35	1.0 d
cream filled (Drake's Devil Dog)	180	2.0	25.0	8.0	0	120	m.q.
cream filled (Drake's Ring Ding)	180	2.0	23.0	10.0	0	65	m.q.
roll, cream filled (Drake's Yodel)	150	2.0	16.0	9.0	5	65	m.q.
twins (Little Debbie)	120	1.0	16.0	6.0	5	85	m.q.

Food and Measure	cal.	prot. (gms)	carbo. (gms)	fat (gms)	chol. (mgs)	sod. (mgs)	fiber (gms)
Cake, snack *(cont.)*							
chocolate chip *(Little Debbie)*	150	0	21.0	7.0	0	95	m.q.
coconut:							
(Little Debbie) . . .	270	2.0	38.0	13.0	5	180	m.q.
(Tastykake Junior)	300	4.0	60.0	6.0	50	300	3.0 d
(Tastykake Kandy Kake)	80	1.0	11.0	4.0	0	40	1.0 d
covered *(Hostess Sno Balls)*	150	1.0	26.0	4.0	2	160	1.0 d
rounds *(Little Debbie)*	140	1.0	21.0	7.0	0	80	m.q.
coffee:							
(Drake's Small) . .	250	3.0	37.0	9.0	15	180	m.q.
(Tastykake Koffee Kake Junior) . . .	260	3.0	44.0	8.0	40	210	1.0 d
apple streusel *(Little Debbie)*	100	1.0	16.0	4.0	5	90	m.q.
blueberry *(Little Debbie)*	130	1.0	23.0	3.0	5	95	m.q.
cherry *(Little Debbie)*	110	1.0	18.0	3.0	5	55	m.q.
cinnamon crumb *(Hostess* 97% Fat Free)	80	1.0	19.0	1.0	0	95	.4 d
cream filled *(Tastykake* Koffee Kake)	110	1.0	18.0	4.0	15	80	0
crumb *(Hostess)* . .	120	1.0	19.0	5.0	10	80	.7 d
crisp, Dutch *(Little Debbie)*	100	0	13.0	6.0	0	45	m.q.
cupcake:							
butter cream, cream filled *(Tastykake)*	120	1.0	20.0	4.0	5	120	1.0 d
chocolate *(Hostess)*	180	2.0	30.0	6.0	5	290	.9 d
chocolate *(Tastykake)*	100	2.0	19.0	3.0	5	120	1.0 d
chocolate *(Tastykake Royale)*	170	2.0	28.0	7.0	5	130	2.0 d

Food and Measure	cal.	prot. (gms)	carbo. (gms)	fat (gms)	chol. (mgs)	sod. (mgs)	fiber (gms)
chocolate, cream filled (Drake's Yankee Doodle) . . .	100	1.0	16.0	4.0	0	110	m.q.
chocolate, cream filled (Tastykake)	130	2.0	21.0	5.0	5	130	1.0 d
chocolate, cream filled (Tastykake Tasty Too)	100	1.0	21.0	1.0	0	115	1.0 d
chocolate, creme filled (Hostess Lights)	130	2.0	26.0	2.0	0	190	.9 d
creme (Tastykake Kreme Kup) . . .	90	1.0	15.0	3.0	5	115	1.0 d
golden, cream filled (Drake's Sunny Doodle)	100	1.0	16.0	3.0	10	100	m.q.
orange (Aunt Fanny's)	334	3.0	54.0	12.0	n.a.	363	m.q.
orange (Hostess)	160	1.0	27.0	5.0	10	150	.5 d
vanilla, cream filled (Tastykake Tasty Too)	100	1.0	21.0	1.0	0	120	1.0 d
date nut pastry (Awrey's), 1.6 oz. . . .	230	2.0	35.0	10.0	15	150	1.0 d
devil's food:							
creme filled (Little Debbie)	150	1.0	23.0	7.0	5	130	m.q.
finger (Aunt Fanny's)	288	4.0	49.0	9.0	n.a.	438	m.q.
squares (Little Debbie)	130	1.0	19.0	6.0	0	85	m.q.
(Drake's Funny Bone)	150	3.0	18.0	8.0	0	110	m.q.
fudge:							
crispy bar (Little Debbie)	170	1.0	20.0	10.0	5	55	m.q.
macaroon (Little Debbie)	140	1.0	18.0	8.0	0	60	m.q.
rounds (Little Debbie)	140	1.0	23.0	5.0	0	80	m.q.

Food and Measure	cal.	prot. (gms)	carbo. (gms)	fat (gms)	chol. (mgs)	sod. (mgs)	fiber (gms)
Cake, snack *(cont.)*							
golden, cream filled:							
(Hostess Twinkies)	150	2.0	27.0	5.0	20	200	.5 d
(Hostess Twinkies							
Lights)	110	2.0	21.0	2.0	0	160	.4 d
(Little Debbie) . . .	150	2.0	24.0	6.0	5	140	m.q.
(Hostess Dessert							
Cup)	90	2.0	18.0	2.0	15	170	.4 d
(Hostess Lil Angels)	90	1.0	14.0	2.0	2	95	m.q.
(Hostess Tiger Tails)	240	4.0	38.0	8.0	25	290	1.3 d
jelly:							
(Tastykake Krimpets)	90	1.0	19.0	1.0	20	80	1.0 d
roll *(Little Debbie)*	230	1.0	41.0	7.0	15	160	m.q.
lemon *(Tastykake Ju-*							
nior)	310	3.0	64.0	7.0	75	330	1.0 d
lemon stix *(Little Deb-*							
bie)	100	1.0	15.0	5.0	5	25	m.q.
marshmallow supreme							
(Little Debbie) . . .	130	1.0	22.0	5.0	0	75	m.q.
mint *(Little Debbie*							
Sprints)	120	1.0	13.0	7.0	5	45	m.q.
oatmeal *(Little Debbie*							
Oatmeal II)	140	2.0	27.0	4.0	0	190	m.q.
orange *(Tastykake Ju-*							
nior)	340	3.0	61.0	9.0	50	240	1.0 d
peanut butter:							
(Tastykake Kandy							
Kakes)	90	2.0	11.0	4.0	5	40	1.0 d
bar *(Little Debbie)*	130	2.0	16.0	7.0	5	100	m.q.
and jelly sandwich							
(Little Debbie) . .	130	2.0	21.0	5.0	0	100	m.q.
wafer *(Little Debbie*							
Nutty Bar)	140	2.0	17.0	8.0	0	60	m.q.
peanut cluster *(Little*							
Debbie)	190	3.0	22.0	11.0	0	125	m.q.
pound, all butter							
(Drake's)	270	4.0	37.0	12.0	15	220	m.q.

Food and Measure	cal.	prot. (gms)	carbo. (gms)	fat (gms)	chol. (mgs)	sod. (mgs)	fiber (gms)
pumpkin (Little Debbie Delights)	130	1.0	21.0	5.0	5	115	m.q.
raspberry finger (Aunt Fanny's)	303	3.0	53.0	9.0	0	337	m.q.
spice:							
(Little Debbie) . . .	150	1.0	21.0	7.0	5	115	m.q.
finger (Aunt Fanny's)	290	3.0	49.0	9.0	n.a.	433	m.q.
strawberry:							
(Tastykake Krimpet)	100	1.0	20.0	2.0	20	85	0
filled (Hostess Twinkies Fruit N Creme), 1.5 oz.	140	1.0	27.0	3.0	20	180	.5 d
Swiss roll (Little Debbie)	130	0	19.0	6.0	5	80	m.q.
vanilla:							
(Hostess Grizzly Chomps)	110	2.0	23.0	1.0	0	140	.8 d
(Little Debbie) . . .	160	1.0	22.0	8.0	0	90	m.q.
(Tastykake Creamie)	180	1.0	25.0	9.0	25	115	1.0 d
creme (Little Debbie)	160	1.0	23.0	7.0	5	90	m.q.
finger (Aunt Fanny's)	250	3.0	50.0	9.0	25	380	m.q.
zebra cake (Little Debbie)	160	1.0	22.0	8.0	0	90	m.q.
Cake, snack, frozen (see also specific listings), 1 piece:							
caramel fudge à la mode (Weight Watchers Sweet Celebrations) . . .	180	4.0	35.0	3.0	5	170	m.q.
cheesecake:							
brownie (Weight Watchers Sweet Celebrations) . .	200	9.0	34.0	5.0	10	260	m.q.
strawberry (Pepper- idge Farm) . . .	250	5.0	41.0	8.0	125	210	m.q.

Food and Measure	cal.	prot. (gms)	carbo. (gms)	fat (gms)	chol. (mgs)	sod. (mgs)	fiber (gms)
Cake, snack, frozen, cheesecake *(cont.)*							
strawberry *(Weight Watchers Sweet Celebrations)* . .	180	7.0	28.0	4.0	20	210	m.q.
chocolate, German *(Pepperidge Farm)*	250	2.0	29.0	13.0	45	230	m.q.
coffee, cinnamon streusel *(Weight Watchers)*	160	3.0	27.0	4.0	5	190	m.q.
fudge, double *(Weight Watchers Sweet Celebrations)* . . .	180	4.0	33.0	4.0	5	150	m.q.
strawberry shortcake à la mode *(Weight Watchers Sweet Celebrations)* . . .	170	3.0	33.0	2.0	5	150	m.q.
Cake, snack, mix* (see also "Dessert bar mix" and specific listings), 1 piece:							
applesauce raisin *(Robin Hood/Gold Medal Snackin Cake)*	140	1.0	28.0	3.0	0	160	m.q.
banana vanilla frosted *(Pillsbury Microwave)*	170	1.0	26.0	7.0	10	160	m.q.
banana walnut *(Robin Hood/Gold Medal Snackin Cake)* . . .	150	1.0	27.0	4.0	0	200	m.q.
carrot, cream cheese frosting *(Pillsbury Microwave)*	170	1.0	25.0	7.0	10	200	m.q.
chocolate, chocolate fudge frosted *(Pillsbury Microwave)* . .	160	2.0	24.0	7.0	10	210	m.q.

Food and Measure	cal.	prot. (gms)	carbo. (gms)	fat (gms)	chol. (mgs)	sod. (mgs)	fiber (gms)
chocolate chip, golden (Robin Hood/Gold Medal Snackin Cake)	140	1.0	26.0	4.0	0	190	m.q.
chocolate chip fudge (Robin Hood/Gold Medal Snackin Cake)	150	2.0	25.0	5.0	0	210	m.q.
cupcake, frosted: chocolate (Pillsbury Funfetti Microwave)	160	1.0	24.0	7.0	10	190	m.q.
yellow (Pillsbury Funfetti Microwave)	180	1.0	28.0	7.0	10	160	m.q.
devil's food, w/chocolate frosting (Betty Crocker MicroRave Singles), 1 cake . .	450	5.0	65.0	19.0	50	520	m.q.
yellow, w/chocolate frosting (Betty Crocker MicroRave Singles), 1 cake . .	460	4.0	65.0	20.0	50	510	m.q.
Calamansi punch (R.W. Knudsen Rain Forest), 8 fl. oz. . . .	115	<1.0	27.0	<1.0	0	(0)	m.q.
Calves liver, see "Liver, veal"							
Candy, 1 oz., except as noted:							
almond, candy coated (Brach's Jordan) . .	120	2.0	23.0	2.0	n.a.	0	m.q.
(Baby Ruth), 2.2 oz.	300	5.0	37.0	15.0	0	140	m.q.
(Boyer Smoothie), .5-oz. pkg.	75	2.5	12.5	7.5	n.a.	n.a.	n.a.
bridge mix (Brach's)	130	1.0	19.0	6.0	n.a.	40	m.q.
butter rum (Pearson Nips), 1 piece . . .	30	<1.0	6.0	<1.0	n.a.	20	0

Food and Measure	cal.	prot. (gms)	carbo. (gms)	fat (gms)	chol. (mgs)	sod. (mgs)	fiber (gms)
Candy *(cont.)*							
(Butterfinger), 2.1 oz.	280	4.0	41.0	11.0	0	110	m.q.
butterscotch *(Callard &*							
Bowser)	115	0	25.2	1.9	n.a.	n.a.	0
candy corn *(Heide/*							
Heide Indian) . . .	110	0	27.0	0	0	40	0
caramel:							
(Kraft), 1 piece . . .	30	0	6.0	1.0	0	25	n.a.
(Pearson Nips),							
1 piece	30	<1.0	6.0	<1.0	n.a.	20	n.a.
(Sugar Babies),							
15/8-oz. pkg. . .	180	1.0	40.0	2.0	n.a.	85	n.a.
(Sugar Daddy),							
13/8-oz. pop . . .	150	1.0	33.0	1.0	n.a.	85	n.a.
chocolate coated							
(Pom Poms) . . .	100	1.0	15.0	3.0	n.a.	70	(0)
chocolate coated,							
w/cookies *(Twix)*,							
1-oz. piece . . .	140	2.0	19.0	7.0	n.a.	60	m.q.
milk chocolate							
coated *(Rolo)*,							
1.93 oz.	270	3.0	37.0	12.0	15	110	(0)
w/peanut, chocolate							
coated *(Oh*							
Henry!), 2 oz. . .	250	7.0	34.0	10.0	m.q.	135	m.q.
carob, 4 sections:							
almond *(Caroby)* . .	150	4.0	12.0	10.0	0	50	m.q.
milk or mint							
(Caroby)	150	4.0	13.0	9.0	n.a.	55	n.a.
milk-free *(Caroby)*	160	4.0	11.0	11.0	0	25	n.a.
cherry:							
chocolate cream							
(Brach's)	110	1.0	21.0	2.0	n.a.	20	m.q.
dark/milk chocolate							
coated *(Brach's)*	110	1.0	22.0	2.0	n.a.	20	m.q.
chocolate:							
(Heide Chocolate							
Babies)	110	0	27.0	<1.0	n.a.	40	n.a.

Food and Measure	cal.	prot. (gms)	carbo. (gms)	fat (gms)	chol. (mgs)	sod. (mgs)	fiber (gms)
(Hershey's Special Dark), 1.45 oz.	230	2.0	24.0	14.0	n.a.	0	m.q.
w/almonds *(Golden Almond Solitaires)*, 1.4 oz. . .	230	5.0	18.0	15.0	5	25	m.q.
w/almonds, candy coated *(Holidays)*	150	3.0	17.0	8.0	n.a.	20	m.q.
candy coated *(M&M's)*, 1.69 oz.	240	3.0	33.0	10.0	n.a.	65	m.q.
candy coated *(Holidays)*	140	2.0	19.0	6.0	n.a.	35	m.q.
chips, see "Chocolate, baking"							
French vanilla, semi-sweet *(Guittard)*	135	1.0	17.0	9.0	0	0	<1.0 c
parfait *(Pearson Nips)*, 1 piece . .	30	<1.0	5.0	<1.0	n.a.	15	(0)
w/peanut butter, candy coated *(M&M's)*	140	3.0	18.0	7.0	n.a.	40	m.q.
w/peanuts, candy coated *(Holidays)*	140	3.0	17.0	7.0	n.a.	30	m.q.
w/peanuts, candy coated *(M&M's)*, 1.7 oz.	250	6.0	29.0	13.0	n.a.	55	m.q.
white, w/almonds *(Nestlé Alpine)*, 1.25 oz.	200	4.0	16.0	13.0	m.q.	25	m.q.
chocolate, milk:							
(Cadbury's Dairy Milk)	150	2.0	17.0	8.0	m.q.	45	m.q.
(Guittard Old Dutch)	150	2.0	17.0	9.0	<5	20	<1.0 c
(Hershey's), 1.55 oz.	240	4.0	25.0	14.0	10	40	m.q.
(Hershey's Kisses), 1 oz., 6 pieces	150	2.0	16.0	9.0	5	25	m.q.
(Nabisco Stars) . .	160	2.0	19.0	8.0	n.a.	35	m.q.
(Nestlé), 1.45 oz.	220	3.0	25.0	13.0	m.q.	25	m.q.
(Symphony), 1.4 oz.	220	3.0	22.0	13.0	10	35	m.q.

Food and Measure	cal.	prot. (gms)	carbo. (gms)	fat (gms)	chol. (mgs)	sod. (mgs)	fiber (gms)
Candy, chocolate, milk *(cont.)*							
w/almonds *(Cadbury's Roasted Almond)*	150	3.0	15.0	9.0	n.a.	40	m.q.
w/almonds *(Hershey's)*, 1.45 oz.	230	5.0	20.0	14.0	10	55	m.q.
w/almonds *(Hershey's Kisses)*, 1 oz., 6 pieces	160	3.0	14.0	10.0	n.a.	25	m.q.
w/almonds *(Nestlé)*, 1.45 oz.	220	4.0	19.0	14.0	m.q.	25	m.q.
w/almonds and toffee chips *(Symphony)*, 1.5 oz.	240	4.0	22.0	15.0	n.a.	40	m.q.
w/caramel *(Cadbury's Caramello)*	140	2.0	18.0	7.0	m.q.	55	m.q.
w/crisps *(Krackel)*, 1.45 oz.	220	3.0	25.0	12.0	10	75	m.q.
w/crisps *(Nestlé Crunch)*, 1.4 oz.	200	3.0	24.0	10.0	m.q.	45	m.q.
w/crisps and peanuts *(100 Grand)*, 1.5 oz.	200	2.0	31.0	8.0	m.q.	55	m.q.
w/fruit and nuts *(Chunky)*, 1.4 oz.	170	4.0	21.0	12.0	m.q.	20	m.q.
w/peanuts *(Mr. Goodbar)*, 1.75 oz.	260	5.0	23.0	17.0	n.a.	10	m.q.
w/pecan and caramel *(Demet's Turtles)*, 1 piece . .	90	1.0	10.0	5.0	m.q.	15	m.q.
w/raisins and almonds *(Cadbury's Fruit & Nut)* . . .	150	2.0	17.0	8.0	m.q.	40	m.q.
chocolate mint: *(Pearson Nips)*, 1 piece	30	<1.0	6.0	<1.0	n.a.	20	(0)

Food and Measure	cal.	prot. (gms)	carbo. (gms)	fat (gms)	chol. (mgs)	sod. (mgs)	fiber (gms)
candy coated (M&M's)	140	1.0	20.0	6.0	n.a.	35	m.q.
coconut, chocolate coated:							
(Mounds), 1.9 oz.	260	2.0	31.0	14.0	0	85	m.q.
dark chocolate (Bounty), 2.12 oz.	150	1.0	18.0	8.0	n.a.	50	m.q.
milk chocolate (Bounty), 2.12 oz.	150	1.0	18.0	8.0	n.a.	35	m.q.
w/almonds (Almond Joy), 1.76 oz. . .	250	3.0	28.0	14.0	0	70	m.q.
coconut, toasted (Andes Thins), 8 pieces	210	2.0	21.0	13.0	<5	35	0
coffee (Pearson Nips), 1 piece	30	<1.0	6.0	<1.0	n.a.	20	0
cough drops, 1 piece:							
(Beech-Nut)	10	0	3.0	0	0	0	0
(Halls Tablets) ...	15	tr.	3.7	tr.	0	tr.	0
cream (Heide Harvest Creams)	110	0	27.0	0	0	40	0
fruit flavored, all flavors:							
(Skittles), 2.3 oz. . . .	270	0	60.0	2.0	0	30	0
chews (Starburst), 2.07 oz.	240	0	48.0	5.0	0	30	0
fudge (Kraft Fudgies), 1 piece	35	0	6.0	1.0	0	25	(0)
grape (Heide Cool Grape)	110	0	28.0	0	0	0	0
gum, chewing, all flavors:							
(Beech-Nut)	10	0	2.0	0	0	0	0
(Big Red/Juicy Fruit)	10	tr.	2.3	tr.	0	0	0
(Care*Free)	8	0	2.0	0	0	0	0
(Doublemint/Wrigley's Spearmint)	10	tr.	2.3	tr.	0	0	0
(Extra Winter Fresh)	8	tr.	tr.	tr.	0	0	0
(Freedent)	10	0	2.3	0	0	0	0

Food and Measure	cal.	prot. (gms)	carbo. (gms)	fat (gms)	chol. (mgs)	sod. (mgs)	fiber (gms)
Candy, gum, chewing (cont.)							
(Freshen-Up) . . .	13	tr.	3.1	tr.	0	tr.	0
bubble (Bubble Yum)	25	0	7.0	0	0	0	0
bubble (Bubblicious)	25	tr.	6.2	tr.	0	tr.	0
bubble (Care*Free)	10	0	2.0	0	0	0	0
bubble (Hubba Bubba)	23	0	5.8	0	0	0	0
candy coated (Chiclets)	6	tr.	1.5	tr.	0	tr.	0
hard, all flavors (Jolly Rancher Kisses), 1 piece	23	0	5.7	0	0	<6	0
honey (Bit-O-Honey), 1.7 oz.	200	1.0	39.0	4.0	n.a.	125	n.a.
hot (Heide Hawaii) . .	110	0	28.0	0	0	0	0
hot (Heide Red Hot Dollars)	100	0	25.0	0	0	0	0
(Hot Tamales), 1 piece	9	<.1	2.1	tr.	0	1	0
jellied and gummed:							
(Chuckles)	100	0	25.0	0	0	10	0
(Heide Gummi Bears)	90	2.0	21.0	0	0	0	0
(Jujubes)	110	0	26.0	0	0	10	0
(Jujyfruits)	100	0	25.0	0	0	0	0
eggs (Heide)	110	0	28.0	0	0	0	0
spice (Heide Mexican Hats)	100	0	25.0	0	0	0	0
spearmint leaves (Brach's)	100	0	24.0	0	0	10	0
tropical (Amazin' Fruit Gummy Bears)	90	2.0	21.0	<1.0	0	20	0
licorice:							
(Diamond)	110	0	26.0	0	0	10	0
(Panda), 1.1 oz. bar	110	1.0	25.0	<1.0	0	100	0
(Pearson Nips), 1 piece	30	<1.0	6.0	<1.0	n.a.	20	0

Food and Measure	cal.	prot. (gms)	carbo. (gms)	fat (gms)	chol. (mgs)	sod. (mgs)	fiber (gms)
(Switzer)	94	1.4	22.0	.3	0	126	0
candy coated (Good & Fruity)	106	.6	26.0	(0)	0	8	0
candy coated (Good & Plenty)	106	1.1	26.0	(0)	0	52	0
cherry (Y&S Twizzlers Bites) . . .	100	1.0	23.0	<1.0	0	85	0
cherry (Y&S Cherry Nibs)	100	1.0	23.0	<1.0	0	80	0
raspberry (Panda), 1.1 oz. bar . . .	110	1.0	25.0	<1.0	0	90	0
soft (Heide)	100	0	25.0	0	0	0	0
strawberry (Y&S Twizzlers)	100	1.0	23.0	<1.0	0	95	0
lollipop:							
all flavors, except chocolate (Tootsie Pop)	111	.1	26.4	.6	tr.	1	(0)
chocolate (Tootsie Pop)	110	.1	26.2	.6	tr.	2	(0)
lozenge (Listerine), 1 piece	9	tr.	2.0	tr.	0	tr.	0
malted milk balls (Whoppers)	136	.9	20.0	5.6	n.a.	m.q.	n.a.
(Mars Bar), 1.76 oz.	240	4.0	30.0	11.0	n.a.	85	m.q.
marshmallow:							
(Funmallows), 1 piece	30	0	7.0	0	0	15	0
(Kraft Jet-Puffed), 1 piece	25	0	6.0	0	0	5	0
miniature (Kraft), 10 pieces	18	0	5.0	0	0	5	0
(Mike & Ikes), 1 piece	9	<.1	2.1	tr.	n.a.	1	0
(Milky Way), 2.15 oz.	280	3.0	42.0	11.0	n.a.	150	m.q.
(Milky Way Dark), 1.76 oz.	220	1.0	36.0	8.0	n.a.	115	m.q.
mint:							
(Mint Meltaway), .33-oz. piece . .	50	0	5.0	3.0	0	10	0

Food and Measure	cal.	prot. (gms)	carbo. (gms)	fat (gms)	chol. (mgs)	sod. (mgs)	fiber (gms)
Candy, mint *(cont.)*							
all flavors *(Breath Savers)*, 1 piece	8	0	2.0	0	0	0	0
butter or party *(Kraft)*, 1 piece	8	0	2.0	0	0	0	0
buttermint *(Andes Thins)*, 8 pieces	210	2.0	21.0	13.0	<5	25	0
w/chocolate *(Andes Creme de Menthe)*, 8 pieces	200	2.0	21.0	12.0	<5	25	0
chocolate coated *(After Eight)*, 1 piece	35	0	6.0	1.0	m.q.	0	m.q.
chocolate coated *(York Peppermint Pattie)*, 1.5 oz.	180	1.0	34.0	4.0	0	20	m.q.
crunch *(Andes Frost Mint)*, 8 pieces	200	2.0	22.0	12.0	<5	20	0
orange *(Andes Thins)*, 8 pieces	200	2.0	21.0	13.0	<5	25	0
parfait *(Andes Thins)*, 8 pieces	210	2.0	22.0	13.0	<5	25	0
(Munch), 1.42 oz. . .	220	6.0	19.0	14.0	n.a.	110	n.a.
nonpareils *(Nestlé Sno-Caps)*	140	1.0	21.0	5.0	m.q.	0	m.q.
nougat, chocolate coated, all flavors *(Charleston Chew!)*	120	1.0	22.0	3.0	n.a.	40	m.q.
(Pay Day), 1.85 oz. . .	250	9.0	28.0	12.0	n.a.	200	m.q.
peanut:							
(Tom's Peanut Plank), 1.7 oz. . .	250	8.0	28.0	12.0	0	30	m.q.
chocolate coated *(Goobers)*, 1³/₈ oz.	200	6.0	16.0	13.0	m.q.	15	3.0 d
French burnt *(Brach's)*	130	4.0	18.0	5.0	0	5	m.q.
roll *(Tom's)*, 1.75 oz.	240	6.0	29.0	11.0	n.a.	120	m.q.

Food and Measure	cal.	prot. (gms)	carbo. (gms)	fat (gms)	chol. (mgs)	sod. (mgs)	fiber (gms)
peanut brittle (Kraft)	130	3.0	20.0	5.0	0	135	m.q.
peanut butter:							
(Snickers), 1.76 oz.	280	6.0	23.0	18.0	n.a.	135	m.q.
(Tom's Peanut Butter Pals), 1.3 oz.	210	5.0	19.0	12.0	n.a.	120	m.q.
candy coated (Reese's Pieces), 1.63 oz.	230	7.0	28.0	10.0	0	80	m.q.
chocolate coated, w/cookie (Twix), .9-oz. piece . . .	130	3.0	13.0	7.0	n.a.	70	m.q.
cup, chocolate coated (Reese's), 1.6 oz.	250	6.0	23.0	15.0	5	160	m.q.
cup, chocolate coated, crunchy (Reese's), 1.8 oz.	280	7.0	24.0	18.0	5	130	m.q.
parfait (Pearson), 1 piece	30	<1.0	5.0	1.0	n.a.	20	m.q.
popcorn, caramel, see "Popcorn"							
raisins, chocolate coated:							
(Nabisco)	130	1.0	21.0	5.0	n.a.	15	m.q.
(Raisinets), 1 3/8 oz.	180	2.0	28.0	6.0	m.q.	10	m.q.
rock (Brach's Cut Rock)	110	0	27.0	0	0	10	0
(Snickers), 2.07 oz.	280	6.0	35.0	14.0	n.a.	160	m.q.
sesame, all varieties (Joyva), ...	178	3.0	25.0	9.0	0	60	m.q.
sour:							
(Heide Silly Sours)	110	0	28.0	0	0	0	0
balls (Brach's) . . .	110	0	27.0	0	0	15	0
taffy, all flavors (Brach's Salt Water)	100	0	24.0	1.0	0	30	0
(3 Musketeers), 2.13 oz.	260	2.0	44.0	9.0	n.a.	120	m.q.

Food and Measure	cal.	prot. (gms)	carbo. (gms)	fat (gms)	chol. (mgs)	sod. (mgs)	fiber (gms)
Candy *(cont.)*							
toffee:							
(Callard & Bowser)	135	.5	19.2	6.5	0	n.a.	0
crunch *(Andes Thins)*, 8 pieces	200	2.0	23.0	12.0	<5	50	0
English *(Heath)*, 1.4-oz. bar . . .	200	1.0	25.0	12.0	n.a.	180	m.q.
(Tootsie Roll)	112	.3	22.8	2.5	tr.	6	(0)
Cane syrup, 1 tbsp.	52	0	13.4	0	0	<1	0
Cannelloni, see "Kidney beans"							
Cannelloni entree, frozen:							
beef, w/tomato sauce *(Lean Cuisine)*, 9⅝ oz.	200	14.0	28.0	3.0	25	490	m.q.
cheese:							
(Dining Lite), 9 oz.	310	19.0	38.0	9.0	70	650	m.q.
w/tomato sauce *(Lean Cuisine)*, 9⅛ oz.	270	23.0	27.0	8.0	25	590	m.q.
Florentine *(Celentano)*, 12 oz.	350	21.0	48.0	8.0	n.a.	620	m.q.
Cantaloupe:							
pulp, cubed, ½ cup	29	.7	6.7	.2	0	7	.6 d
½ of 5″ melon	94	2.3	22.3	.7	0	23	2.1 d
Caper, 1 tbsp.:							
(Krinos)	0	0	0	0	0	170	0
(Progresso)	0	0	0	0	0	150	0
Capon, see "Chicken"							
Caponata, see "Eggplant appetizer"							
Capocollo *(Healthy Deli* Cappy*)*, 1 oz.	31	4.7	1.1	.9	12	270	0
Cappuccino, bottled:							
hot							
(Maxwell House), 6 fl. oz.:							
cinnamon	60	2.0	11.0	1.0	0	100	0

Food and Measure	cal.	prot. (gms)	carbo. (gms)	fat (gms)	chol. (mgs)	sod. (mgs)	fiber (gms)
coffee	60	1.0	12.0	1.0	0	110	0
mocha	70	2.0	12.0	2.0	0	80	0
iced, 8 fl. oz.:							
cinnamon (Chock o'ccino)	100	1.0	22.0	1.5	5	30	0
cinnamon (Maxwell House Cappio)	130	2.0	25.0	3.0	15	70	0
coffee (Chock o'ccino)	100	2.0	23.0	1.5	5	35	0
coffee (Maxwell House Cappio)	120	2.0	23.0	3.0	15	75	0
decaf (Chock o'ccino)	100	2.0	20.0	1.5	5	30	0
mocha (Chock o'ccino)	120	2.0	24.0	2.0	5	35	0
mocha (Maxwell House Cappio)	130	2.0	25.0	2.0	15	65	0
mocha (Nescafé Mocha Cooler)	150	7.0	23.0	4.0	17	210	0
vanilla nut (Chock o'ccino)	110	1.0	23.0	1.5	5	30	0
Captain D's, 1 serving:							
dinner[1], w/salad:							
chicken	414	30.0	54.8	7.6	71	2615	3.9 d
fish, baked	659	35.8	61.9	29.8	54	1767	4.4 d
orange roughy . . .	537	34.5	55.6	19.0	39	2156	3.9 d
dinner[1], shrimp, w/slaw	457	34.4	56.2	9.9	191	2194	3.9 d
side dishes:							
breadstick, 1 piece	91	3.0	17.0	1.2	0	210	m.q.
cole slaw, 4 oz. . .	158	2.6	11.8	11.8	16	246	1.9 d
crackers, 4 pieces	50	1.0	8.0	1.0	3	147	.2 d
cracklins, 1 oz. . .	218	1.3	15.7	16.8	0	741	0
dinner salad, no dressing	27	1.4	3.3	1.0	1	67	1.4 d

[1] Includes rice, green beans, and breadstick.

Food and Measure	cal.	prot. (gms)	carbo. (gms)	fat (gms)	chol. (mgs)	sod. (mgs)	fiber (gms)
Captain D's, side dishes (cont.)							
french fries, 3.5 oz.	302	3.4	49.6	9.9	0	152	m.q.
green beans, sea-soned, 4 oz. . . .	46	2.3	4.9	2.3	4	752	1.4 d
hushpuppy, 1 piece	126	2.1	19.9	4.1	0	465	.1 d
okra, fried, 4 oz. . .	300	6.8	34.1	15.6	0	445	m.q.
rice, 4 oz.	124	2.8	27.5	0	0	9	1.1 d
white beans, 4 oz.	126	8.1	22.2	.5	2	99	3.0 d
dressings, 1 pkt.:							
blue cheese	105	.2	.2	11.7	14	101	0
French	111	.2	4.0	10.7	7	187	0
Italian, low calorie	9	0	2.2	0	0	568	0
ranch	92	.4	.4	10.0	15	230	0
sauces, side portion:							
cocktail	34	.4	8.4	.1	0	252	0
sweet and sour . .	52	0	13.1	0	0	5	0
tartar.	75	.2	3.2	6.9	10	158	0
desserts, 1 slice:							
carrot cake	434	7.5	49.1	22.8	32	414	0
cheesecake	420	7.0	30.0	31.0	141	480	0
chocolate cake . .	303	3.8	48.9	10.2	20	259	0
lemon pie	351	7.0	59.0	10.0	45	135	0
pecan pie	458	5.0	64.2	19.8	4	373	4.4 d
Carambola:							
fresh:							
1 medium, 4.7 oz.	42	.7	9.9	.4	0	2	3.4 d
(Frieda's), 1 oz. . .	10	.2	2.3	.1	0	1	m.q.
dried (Frieda's), 1 oz.	22	.2	5.6	.1	0	1	m.q.
Caramel topping:							
(Kraft), 1 tbsp.	60	1.0	13.0	0	0	45	0
(Smucker's), 2 tbsp.	140	1.0	33.0	0	0	110	0
hot (Smucker's), 2 tbsp.	150	1.0	28.0	4.0	0	75	0
Caraway seed, 1 tsp.	7	.4	1.1	.3	0	tr.	.8 d
Cardamom, 1 tsp.:							
ground (Tone's) . . .	6	.2	1.3	.1	0	<1	.2 d
seed (Spice Islands)	6	.2	1.3	.1	0	tr.	.2 c

Food and Measure	cal.	prot. (gms)	carbo. (gms)	fat (gms)	chol. (mgs)	sod. (mgs)	fiber (gms)
Cardoon:							
raw, shredded, 1/2 cup	18	.6	4.4	.1	0	151	1.4 d
boiled, drained, 4 oz.	25	.9	6.0	.1	0	200	m.q.
Carissa:							
1 medium, .8 oz. . .	12	.1	2.7	.3	0	1	.2 c
sliced, 1/2 cup	46	.4	10.2	1.0	0	2	.7 c
Carl's Jr., 1 serving:							
breakfast:							
bacon, 2 strips . .	45	3.0	0	4.0	5	150	0
breakfast burrito . .	430	22.0	29.0	26.0	285	740	m.q.
English muffin							
w/margarine . . .	190	6.0	30.0	5.0	0	280	m.q.
French toast dips,							
w/out syrup . . .	450	10.0	59.0	20.0	4	570	m.q.
hash brown nuggets	270	3.0	27.0	17.0	5	410	m.q.
hot cakes w/marga-							
rine, no syrup . .	510	11.0	61.0	24.0	10	950	m.q.
sausage, 1 patty	190	8.0	0	18.0	30	520	0
scrambled eggs . .	120	9.0	2.0	9.0	245	105	0
Sunrise Sandwich	300	15.0	31.0	13.0	160	550	m.q.
chicken strips,							
6 pieces	260	19.0	11.0	19.0	25	600	n.a.
sandwiches:							
Carl's Catch Fish							
Sandwich	560	17.0	54.0	30.0	5	1220	m.q.
Carl's Original Ham-							
burger	460	25.0	46.0	20.0	50	810	m.q.
Charbroiled BBQ							
Chicken Sandwich	310	25.0	34.0	6.0	30	680	m.q.
Charbroiled Chicken							
Club Sandwich	570	35.0	42.0	29.0	60	1160	m.q.
Double Western Ba-							
con Cheeseburger	1030	56.0	58.0	63.0	145	1810	m.q.
Famous Star Ham-							
burger	610	26.0	42.0	38.0	50	890	m.q.
hamburger	320	17.0	33.0	14.0	35	590	m.q.
roast beef deluxe	540	28.0	46.0	26.0	40	1340	m.q.

Food and Measure	cal.	prot. (gms)	carbo. (gms)	fat (gms)	chol. (mgs)	sod. (mgs)	fiber (gms)
Carl's Jr., sandwiches *(cont.)*							
Santa Fe Chicken							
Sandwich	530	30.0	36.0	29.0	85	1230	m.q.
Super Star ham-							
burger	820	43.0	41.0	53.0	105	1210	m.q.
turkey club	530	30.0	50.0	23.0	60	2890	m.q.
Western Bacon							
Cheeseburger . .	730	34.0	59.0	39.0	90	1490	m.q.
"Great Stuff" pota-							
toes:							
bacon and cheese	730	26.0	60.0	43.0	45	1670	m.q.
broccoli and cheese	590	18.0	60.0	31.0	25	830	m.q.
cheese	690	23.0	70.0	36.0	40	1160	m.q.
chili	500	18.0	50.0	26.0	50	630	m.q.
lite	290	9.0	60.0	1.0	0	60	m.q.
sour cream and							
chive	470	11.0	64.0	19.0	20	180	m.q.
Entree Salads-To-Go:							
chicken	200	24.0	8.0	8.0	70	300	m.q.
garden	50	3.0	4.0	3.0	5	75	m.q.
salad dressing, 1 oz.:							
blue cheese	150	1.0	0	15.0	20	250	n.a.
French or Italian, re-							
duced calorie . .	40	0	5.0	2.0	0	290	n.a.
house	110	1.0	2.0	11.0	10	170	n.a.
Thousand Island . .	110	0	4.0	11.0	5	200	n.a.
side dishes:							
CrissCut Fries, regu-							
lar	330	4.0	27.0	22.0	tr.	890	m.q.
fries, regular	420	4.0	54.0	20.0	0	200	m.q.
onion rings	520	9.0	63.0	26.0	0	960	m.q.
salsa, 1 oz.	8	0	2.0	0	0	210	m.q.
zucchini	390	7.0	38.0	23.0	0	1040	m.q.
bakery products:							
blueberry muffin . .	340	5.0	61.0	9.0	45	300	m.q.
bran muffin	310	6.0	52.0	7.0	60	370	m.q.
cheese Danish . . .	520	7.0	75.0	16.0	0	230	m.q.
cheesecake	310	7.0	32.0	17.0	60	200	n.a.

Food and Measure	cal.	prot. (gms)	carbo. (gms)	fat (gms)	chol. (mgs)	sod. (mgs)	fiber (gms)
chocolate cake . .	300	3.0	49.0	11.0	25	262	m.q.
chocolate chip cookie	330	4.0	41.0	17.0	5	170	m.q.
cinnamon roll . . .	460	7.0	70.0	18.0	0	230	m.q.
fudge moussecake	400	5.0	42.0	23.0	110	85	n.a.
shake, regular	350	11.0	61.0	7.0	15	230	n.a.
Carob drink mix, powder, 3 tsp. . . .	45	.2	11.2	tr.	0	12	.2 c
Carob flour, 1 cup	395	4.8	91.6	.7	0	36	41.0 d
Carp, meat only: raw, 4 oz.	144	20.2	0	6.4	75	58	0
baked, broiled, or microwaved, 4 oz. . .	184	25.9	0	8.1	95	71	0
Carrot: fresh, raw: whole, 7¹/₂″ long, 2.8 oz.	31	.7	7.3	.1	0	25	2.2 d
shredded, ¹/₂ cup	24	.6	5.6	.1	0	19	1.7 d
baby, 1 medium, 2³/₄″ long	4	.1	.8	.1	0	3	m.q.
mini (Frieda's), 1 oz.	12	.3	2.7	.1	0	13	m.q.
fresh, boiled, drained, sliced, ¹/₂ cup . . .	35	.9	8.2	.1	0	52	2.6 d
canned, ¹/₂ cup: (Stokely)	35	1.0	7.0	0	0	300	m.q.
sliced, w/liquid . .	28	.8	6.2	.2	0	297	1.1 d
sliced, drained . . .	17	.5	4.0	.1	0	176	1.1 d
sliced (Allen)	30	1.0	7.0	<1.0	0	250	m.q.
frozen, ¹/₂ cup, except as noted: boiled, drained, sliced	26	.9	6.0	.1	0	43	2.6 d
(Seabrook), 3.3 oz.	40	1.0	9.0	0	0	44	1.0 c
whole, baby (Green Giant Harvest Fresh)	18	1.0	5.0	0	0	75	2.0 d
whole, baby (Green Giant Select) . .	20	1.0	7.0	0	0	35	2.0 d

Food and Measure	cal.	prot. (gms)	carbo. (gms)	fat (gms)	chol. (mgs)	sod. (mgs)	fiber (gms)
Carrot, frozen *(cont.)*							
sliced *(Frosty Acres)*,							
3.3 oz.	40	1.0	9.0	0	0	44	1.0 c
Carrot chips, 1 oz.:							
(Hain)	150	2.0	16.0	9.0	0	160	m.q.
(Hain No Salt)	150	2.0	16.0	7.0	0	30	m.q.
Carrot juice, canned:							
6 fl. oz.	73	1.7	17.1	.3	0	54	1.5 d
(Hollywood), 6 fl. oz.	60	1.0	13.0	0	0	135	m.q.
Casaba:							
1/10 of 73/4″ melon . .	43	1.5	10.2	.2	0	20	1.3 d
pulp, cubed, 1/2 cup	23	.8	5.3	.1	0	10	.7 d
Cashew, 1 oz., except							
as noted:							
(Beer Nuts)	170	5.0	8.0	13.0	0	80	1.0 d
(Frito-Lay's)	170	4.0	9.0	14.0	0	115	m.q.
(Tom's)	180	6.0	7.0	14.0	0	140	m.q.
dry-roasted:							
1 oz. or 18 medium	163	4.4	9.3	13.2	0	4	.9 d
whole or halves, 1 cup	787	21.0	44.8	63.5	0	21	4.1 d
(Flavor House)	160	6.0	9.0	12.0	0	200	2.0 d
whole *(Fisher)*	160	5.0	8.0	13.0	0	100	m.q.
honey-roasted, whole							
(Fisher)	150	4.0	7.0	13.0	0	90	m.q.
oil-roasted:							
1 oz. or 18 medium	163	4.6	8.1	13.7	0	5	1.1 d
whole or halves,							
1 cup	748	21.0	37.1	62.7	0	22	4.9 d
(Flavor House) . . .	160	6.0	8.0	12.0	0	125	1.0 d
(Master Choice) . .	170	5.0	8.0	14.0	0	150	m.q.
whole *(Fisher)* . . .	170	5.0	8.0	14.0	0	110	m.q.
halves *(Fisher)* . . .	170	5.0	8.0	14.0	0	155	m.q.
Cashew butter:							
1 oz.	167	5.0	7.8	14.0	0	4	.6 d
(Roaster Fresh), 1 oz.	165	4.0	9.0	14.0	0	4	m.q.
raw *(Hain)*, 2 tbsp. . . .	190	6.0	8.0	15.0	0	5	m.q.
toasted *(Hain)*, 2 tbsp.	190	6.0	8.0	16.0	0	5	m.q.

Food and Measure	cal.	prot. (gms)	carbo. (gms)	fat (gms)	chol. (mgs)	sod. (mgs)	fiber (gms)
Cassava (see also "Yuca"), trimmed, 1 oz.	34	.9	7.6	.1	0	2	<.1 d
Catfish, channel:							
farmed, meat only:							
raw, 4 oz.	153	17.7	0	8.6	15	60	0
baked, broiled, or							
microwaved, 4 oz.	172	21.2	0	9.1	73	91	0
wild, meat only:							
raw, 4 oz.	108	18.6	0	3.2	66	49	0
baked, broiled, or							
microwaved, 4 oz.	119	20.9	0	3.2	82	57	0
Catfish, frozen, (Delta Pride), 4 oz.	132	18.0	4.8	4.9	62	<1	0
Catfish entree, Cajùn, frozen (Gorton's), 1 piece	190	20.0	3.0	11.0	60	890	0
Catjang, boiled, 1/2 cup	100	7.0	17.5	.6	0	16	1.4 c
Catsup, 1 tbsp.:							
(Hain Natural)	16	0	4.0	0	0	155	m.q.
(Hain Natural No Salt)	16	0	4.0	0	0	5	m.q.
(Heinz)	16	0	4.0	0	0	200	m.q.
(Heinz Hot)	14	0	3.0	0	0	185	m.q.
(Heinz Lite)	8	0	2.0	0	0	115	m.q.
(Hunt's)	15	<1.0	4.0	<1.0	0	160	<1.0 d
(Hunt's No Salt Added)	20	<1.0	5.0	<1.0	0	0	<1.0 d
(Smucker's)	24	0	6.0	0	0	90	m.q.
(Stokely)	20	0	5.0	0	0	190	m.q.
Cauliflower:							
fresh:							
raw, 3 flowerets . .	14	1.1	2.9	.1	0	17	1.4 d
raw, 1" pieces, 1/2 cup	13	1.0	2.6	.1	0	15	1.3 d
boiled, drained, 1" pieces, 1/2 cup	14	1.1	2.6	.3	0	9	1.7 d

Food and Measure	cal.	prot. (gms)	carbo. (gms)	fat (gms)	chol. (mgs)	sod. (mgs)	fiber (gms)
Cauliflower *(cont.)*							
frozen:							
boiled, drained,							
1″ pieces, 1/2 cup	17	1.5	3.4	.2	0	16	2.0 d
(Frosty Acres),							
3.3 oz.	25	2.0	5.0	0	0	16	1.0 c
cuts *(Green Giant),*							
1/2 cup	12	1.0	3.0	0	0	25	2.0 d
frozen, breaded							
(Stilwell), 13 pieces	80	3.0	16.0	1.0	0	180	3.0 d
frozen, in cheese							
sauce:							
(Birds Eye), 5 oz.	90	5.0	8.0	5.0	n.a.	480	1.0 d
(Green Giant),							
1/2 cup	60	2.0	10.0	2.0	2	500	2.0 d
(Green Giant One							
Serving), 5.5 oz.	80	3.0	14.0	2.0	5	640	2.0 d
Cauliflower, pickled,							
sweet *(Vlasic),* 1 oz.	35	0	9.0	0	0	260	m.q.
Cavatelli, frozen							
(Celentano), 3.2 oz.	400	16.0	79.0	1.5	15	15	9.0 d
Caviar, granular (see							
also "Roe"):							
black or red, 1 oz. . .	71	6.9	1.1	5.0	165	420	0
black or red, 1 tbsp.	40	3.9	.6	2.9	94	240	0
Caviar spread, see							
"Taramosalata"							
Cayenne, see "Pep-							
per"							
Ceci, see "Chick-							
peas"							
Celeriac, fresh:							
raw, 1/2 cup	31	1.2	7.2	.2	0	78	1.4 d
boiled, drained, 4 oz.	28	1.1	6.7	.2	0	69	.9 c
Celery:							
raw:							
71/2″ stalk, 1.6 oz.	6	.3	1.5	.1	0	35	.7 d
diced, 1/2 cup . . .	10	.5	2.2	.1	0	52	1.0 d

Food and Measure	cal.	prot. (gms)	carbo. (gms)	fat (gms)	chol. (mgs)	sod. (mgs)	fiber (gms)
boiled, drained, diced, 1/2 cup . .	13	.6	3.0	.1	0	68	1.2 d
Celery, dried, 1 tsp.:							
flakes or seed *(Tone's)*	9	.4	.9	.5	0	4	.3 d
seed, 1 tsp.	8	.4	.8	.5	0	3	.2 d
Celery salt *(Tone's)*, 1 tsp.	6	.3	.6	.4	0	1584	.2 d
Cellophane noodles, see "Noodle, Chinese"							
Celtus, raw, trimmed, 1 oz.	6	.2	1.0	.1	0	3	.1 c
Cereal, ready-to-eat (see also specific grains), 1 oz., except as noted:							
bran (see also "oat bran," below):							
(All Bran)	70	4.0	21.0	1.0	0	260	9.0 d
(Arrowhead Mills Bran Flakes) . . .	100	4.0	20.0	1.0	0	1	4.1 d
(Bran Buds)	70	3.0	23.0	1.0	0	200	11.0 d
(Bran Chex)	90	2.0	24.0	0	0	200	4.0 d
(Kellogg's Bran Flakes)	90	3.0	22.0	0	0	220	5.0 d
(Kellogg's Fiberwise)	90	3.0	23.0	1.0	0	140	5.0 d
(Nabisco 100% Bran)	70	3.0	22.0	2.0	0	190	10.0 d
(Post Bran Flakes)	90	3.0	23.0	0	0	210	5.0 d
extra fiber *(Kellogg's All Bran)*	50	4.0	22.0	0	0	140	14.0 d
w/fruit *(Kellogg's Fruitful Bran)*, w/.4 oz. fruit . .	120	3.0	31.0	0	0	240	5.0 d
bran, w/raisins:							
(Erewhon Raisin Bran)	100	3.0	22.0	0	0	75	3.0 d

Food and Measure	cal.	prot. (gms)	carbo. (gms)	fat (gms)	chol. (mgs)	sod. (mgs)	fiber (gms)
Cereal, ready-to-eat, bran, w/raisins *(cont.)*							
(General Mills Raisin Nut Bran)	100	3.0	21.0	2.0	0	140	2.5 d
(Kellogg's Raisin Bran), w/.4 oz. raisins	120	3.0	31.0	1.0	0	210	5.0 d
(Malt-O-Meal Raisin Bran), 1.4 oz. . .	130	3.0	30.0	2.0	0	200	5.0 d
(Nutri-Grain), w/.4 oz. raisins	130	4.0	31.0	1.0	0	200	5.0 d
(Post Raisin Bran), 1.4 oz.	120	3.0	31.0	1.0	0	200	6.0 d
(Skinner's Raisin Bran)	110	3.0	19.0	2.0	0	45	4.0 d
(Total Raisin Bran), 1.5 oz.	140	3.0	33.0	1.0	0	190	4.0 d
corn:							
(Arrowhead Mills Flakes)	110	2.0	25.0	1.0	0	4	2.8 d
(Cocoa Puffs) . . .	110	1.0	25.0	1.0	0	180	m.q.
(Corn Pops)	110	1.0	26.0	0	0	90	1.0 d
(Country Corn Flakes)	110	2.0	25.0	<1.0	0	270	m.q.
(Honeycomb) . . .	110	1.0	25.0	0	0	180	tr.d
(Kellogg's Corn Flakes)	100	2.0	24.0	0	0	290	1.0 d
(Kellogg's Frosted Flakes)	110	1.0	26.0	0	0	200	1.0 d
(Malt-O-Meal) . . .	110	2.0	25.0	0	0	290	1.0 d
(Nut & Honey Crunch)	110	2.0	24.0	1.0	0	200	0
(Nutri-Grain)	100	2.0	24.0	1.0	0	170	3.0 d
(Post Toasties) . . .	110	2.0	25.0	0	0	280	tr.d
(Total Corn Flakes)	110	2.0	24.0	<1.0	0	200	m.q.
apple *(Arrowhead Mills Apple Corns)*	100	3.0	23.0	1.0	0	20	3.0 d

Food and Measure	cal.	prot. (gms)	carbo. (gms)	fat (gms)	chol. (mgs)	sod. (mgs)	fiber (gms)
golden (Health Valley Fruit Lites), .5 oz.	50	1.0	12.0	0	0	0	.8 d
maple (Arrowhead Mills Maple Corns)	100	3.0	23.0	1.0	0	21	3.0 d
puffed (Arrowhead Mills), .5 oz.	50	3.0	11.0	0	0	<1	.4 d
sugar frosted (Malt-O-Meal) . .	110	1.0	26.0	0	0	170	1.0 d
granola:							
(C.W. Post Hearty)	120	2.0	21.0	4.0	0	60	tr.d
all varieties (Health Valley Fat Free)	90	2.0	21.0	<1.0	0	20	2.5 d
apple, spiced (Erewhon)	130	3.0	17.0	6.0	0	55	m.q.
banana almond (Sunbelt)	130	3.0	20.0	4.0	0	25	m.q.
w/bran (Erewhon #9)	130	3.0	17.0	6.0	0	10	4.0 d
date nut (Erewhon)	130	3.0	17.0	6.0	0	45	m.q.
fruit and nut (Sunbelt)	120	3.0	19.0	5.0	0	20	m.q.
honey almond (Erewhon)	130	3.0	17.0	6.0	0	65	m.q.
maple (Erewhon)	130	3.0	17.0	5.0	0	55	m.q.
maple nut (Arrowhead Mills) . . .	250	8.0	36.0	9.0	0	4	11.9 d
sunflower crunch (Erewhon)	130	3.0	18.0	4.0	0	60	m.q.
kamut flakes (Erewhon)	90	4.0	18.0	0	0	60	4.0 d
kashi, puffed (Kashi), .75 oz.	70	3.0	16.0	<1.0	0	0	2.0 d
millet, puffed (Arrowhead Mills), .5 oz.	50	2.0	11.0	0	0	<1	.5 d
mixed grain and natural style:							
(Almond Delight) . .	110	2.0	23.0	2.0	0	200	1.0 d

Food and Measure	cal.	prot. (gms)	carbo. (gms)	fat (gms)	chol. (mgs)	sod. (mgs)	fiber (gms)
Cereal, ready-to-eat, mixed grain and natural style *(cont.)*							
(Apple Jacks) . . .	110	2.0	26.0	0	0	125	1.0 d
(Arrowhead Mills Arrowhead Crunch)	120	3.0	18.0	3.0	0	11	3.5 d
(Basic 4), 1.3 oz.	130	3.0	28.0	2.0	0	210	2.0 d
(Cinnamon Toast Crunch)	120	1.0	22.0	3.0	0	210	1.0 d
(Clusters)	110	3.0	22.0	2.0	0	140	2.0 d
(Crispix)	110	2.0	25.0	0	0	220	1.0 d
(Crunchy Nut Oh!s)	127	1.7	21.5	4.2	0	164	.9 d
(Double Dip Crunch)	120	2.0	23.0	2.0	0	160	0
(Erewhon Aztec) . .	100	2.0	24.0	0	0	65	1.0 d
(Erewhon Right Start)	90	3.0	24.0	0	0	80	5.0 d
(Erewhon Super-O's)	110	3.0	24.0	<1.0	0	5	4.0 d
(Fiber One)	60	2.0	23.0	1.0	0	140	13.0 d
(Froot Loops) . . .	110	2.0	25.0	1.0	0	125	1.0 d
(Fruit & Frosted O's)	110	2.0	25.0	1.0	0	120	1.0 d
(Grape Nuts)	110	3.0	23.0	0	0	170	3.0 d
(Grape Nuts Flakes)	100	3.0	23.0	1.0	0	130	3.0 d
(Honey Graham Chex)	110	1.0	25.0	1.0	0	180	m.q.
(Honey Graham Oh!s)	122	1.4	22.6	3.2	0	217	.7 d
(Just Right)	100	3.0	23.0	1.0	0	190	2.0 d
(Kix)	110	2.0	24.0	<1.0	0	260	m.q.
(Multi Grain Cheerios)	100	2.0	23.0	1.0	0	220	2.0 d
(Product 19)	100	3.0	24.0	0	0	320	1.0 d
(Quaker 100% Natural)	127	3.3	18.0	5.5	0	14	2.0 d
(Special K)	110	6.0	20.0	0	0	230	1.0 d
(Sunflakes MultiGrain)	100	2.0	24.0	1.0	0	240	3.0 d
(Total)	100	2.0	23.0	1.0	0	190	2.0 d
(Triples)	110	2.0	24.0	1.0	0	200	m.q.
(Uncle Sam)	110	4.0	20.0	1.0	0	65	7.0 d

Food and Measure	cal.	prot. (gms)	carbo. (gms)	fat (gms)	chol. (mgs)	sod. (mgs)	fiber (gms)
all varieties:							
(Health Valley Fiber Flakes) . . .	90	3.0	20.0	0	0	5	5.0 d
(Health Valley O's Fat Free)	90	3.0	19.0	<1.0	0	5	5.0 d
w/almonds *(Honey Bunches of Oats)*	120	2.0	22.0	3.0	0	160	1.0 d
almond raisin *(Nutri-Grain)*, w/.4 oz. nuts and fruit . .	140	3.0	31.0	2.0	0	220	3.0 d
w/apple *(Erewhon Apple Stroodles)*	90	3.0	23.0	0	0	15	3.0 d
apple and almond *(Kellogg's Mueslix Golden Crunch)*	120	3.0	25.0	2.0	0	170	3.0 d
apple raisin *(Apple Raisin Crisp)*, w/.3 oz. fruit . .	130	2.0	32.0	0	0	230	3.0 d
w/banana *(Erewhon Banana-O's)* . . .	110	2.0	24.0	0	0	15	2.0 d
w/bananas and Hawaiian fruit *(Sprouts 7)* . . .	90	3.0	16.0	<1.0	0	0	4.3 d
cinnamon *(Kellogg's Mini Buns)*	110	2.0	25.0	1.0	0	220	1.0 d
cinnamon and raisin *(Nature Valley)* . .	120	2.0	20.0	4.0	0	50	1.0 d
dates, raisins, walnuts *(Fruit & Fibre)*, 1.25 oz. . .	120	3.0	27.0	2.0	0	160	5.0 d
w/fiber nuggets *(Just Right)* . . .	100	2.0	24.0	1.0	0	200	2.0 d
w/fruit and nuts *(Kellogg's Mueslix Crispy Blend)*, 1.5 oz.	160	3.0	33.0	2.0	0	150	3.0 d
fruit and nut *(Nature Valley)*	130	2.0	19.0	5.0	0	45	1.0 d

Food and Measure	cal.	prot. (gms)	carbo. (gms)	fat (gms)	chol. (mgs)	sod. (mgs)	fiber (gms)
Cereal, ready-to-eat, mixed grain and natural style *(cont.)*							
honey roasted *(Honey Bunches of Oats)*	110	2.0	24.0	2.0	0	180	1.0 d
peaches, raisins, almonds *(Fruit & Fibre)*, 1.25 oz. . .	120	3.0	26.0	2.0	0	160	5.0 d
pecan, double *(Post Great Grains)*, 1.25 oz.	120	3.0	20.0	3.0	0	60	3.0 d
pineapple, banana, and coconut *(Fruit & Fibre)*, 1.25 oz.	120	3.0	27.0	3.0	0	170	5.0 d
plain or raisin *(Heartland)* . . .	130	3.0	18.0	4.0	0	80	2.0 d
w/raisins *(Erewhon Right Start)* . . .	90	3.0	22.0	0	0	80	5.0 d
raisin *(Grape Nuts)*	100	3.0	23.0	0	0	150	2.0 d
w/raisins *(Sprouts 7)*	90	4.0	16.0	<1.0	0	0	4.7 d
raisins, dates, nuts *(Just Right)*, w/.3 oz. fruit and nuts	140	3.0	30.0	1.0	0	190	2.0 d
raisin, date, pecan *(Post Great Grains)*, 1.25 oz.	140	3.0	27.0	3.0	0	70	3.0 d
trail mix *(Heartland)*	120	3.0	19.0	4.0	0	80	m.q.
muesli: *(Master Choice)*, 2 oz.	200	5.0	40.0	4.0	0	270	5.0 d
(Sunbelt)	100	3.0	22.0	1.0	0	70	m.q.
oat: *(Alpha-Bits)*	110	2.0	24.0	1.0	0	180	1.0 d
(Cheerios)	110	4.0	20.0	2.0	0	290	2.0 d
(Cinnamon Life) . .	101	5.0	18.9	1.7	0	182	2.5 d
(General Mills Oatmeal Crisp)	110	3.0	21.0	2.0	0	180	1.0 d

Food and Measure	cal.	prot. (gms)	carbo. (gms)	fat (gms)	chol. (mgs)	sod. (mgs)	fiber (gms)
(Honey Bunches of Oats)	110	2.0	23.0	2.0	0	160	2.0 d
(Honey Nut Cheerios)	110	3.0	23.0	1.0	0	250	1.5 d
(Life)	101	5.1	18.7	1.7	0	186	2.5 d
(Nut & Honey Crunch O's) . . .	110	2.0	22.0	2.0	0	190	1.0 d
(Toasty O's)	110	4.0	20.0	2.0	0	240	2.0 d
w/almonds *(Honey Bunches of Oats)*	110	2.0	23.0	2.0	0	150	2.0 d
apple cinnamon *(Cheerios)*	110	2.0	22.0	2.0	0	180	1.5 d
apple and cinnamon *(Toasty O's)* . . .	110	2.0	22.0	2.0	0	180	1.0 d
honey bran *(Kellogg's Oatbake)*	110	2.0	21.0	3.0	0	190	3.0 d
honey and nut *(Toasty O's)* . . .	110	3.0	23.0	1.0	0	180	2.0 d
marshmallow *(Alpha-Bits)*	110	2.0	25.0	1.0	0	150	1.0 d
w/raisins *(General Mills Oatmeal Raisin Crisp),* 1.2 oz.	130	3.0	25.0	2.0	0	170	1.5 d
raisin nut *(Kellogg's Oatbake)*	110	2.0	21.0	3.0	0	190	3.0 d
toasted *(Nature Valley)*	130	2.0	20.0	5.0	0	50	1.0 d
toasted, rings *(Skinner's)*	90	4.0	22.0	1.0	0	290	3.0 d
oat bran:							
(Arrowhead Mills Flakes)	110	4.0	20.0	2.0	0	9	3.4 d
(Common Sense)	100	4.0	22.0	1.0	0	250	3.0 d
(Cracklin' Oat Bran)	110	3.0	21.0	3.0	0	140	4.0 d
(Post Oat Flakes)	110	5.0	21.0	1.0	0	130	2.0 d
(Skinner's)	110	6.0	18.0	2.0	0	5	4.0 d

Food and Measure	cal.	prot. (gms)	carbo. (gms)	fat (gms)	chol. (mgs)	sod. (mgs)	fiber (gms)
Cereal, ready-to-eat, oat bran (cont.)							
w/raisins (Common Sense), w/.3 oz. raisins	130	4.0	29.0	1.0	0	250	3.0 d
w/toasted wheat germ (Erewhon)	115	5.0	18.0	2.0	0	15	m.q.
oatmeal, toasted:							
(Quaker)	100	3.0	22.0	1.0	0	160	2.0 d
honey nut (Quaker)	120	3.0	20.0	3.0	0	110	2.0 d
rice:							
(Erewhon Poppets)	110	2.0	24.0	1.0	0	10	1.0 d
(Frosted Krispies)	110	1.0	26.0	0	0	220	0
(Rice Krispies) . . .	110	2.0	25.0	0	0	290	0
chocolate (Cocoa Krispies)	110	1.0	25.0	0	0	190	0
rice, brown (Health Valley Fruit Lites), .5 oz.	50	<1.0	12.0	0	0	0	.5 d
rice, brown, crispy:							
(Erewhon)	110	2.0	24.0	<1.0	0	170	1.0 d
(Erewhon Low Sodium)	110	2.0	24.0	1.0	0	10	1.0 d
(Kellogg's Kenmei)	110	2.0	24.0	1.0	0	230	1.0 d
rice, puffed, .5 oz.:							
(Arrowhead Mills)	50	1.0	11.0	0	0	<1	.4 d
(Malt-O-Meal) . . .	50	1.0	12.0	0	0	0	0
(Quaker)	54	1.0	12.5	.1	0	1	.2 d
wheat:							
(Kellogg's Smacks)	110	2.0	25.0	1.0	0	70	1.0 d
(Malt-O-Meal Sugar Puffs)	110	2.0	25.0	0	0	25	1.0 d
(Nutri-Grain)	90	3.0	23.0	0	0	170	3.0 d
(Total)	100	3.0	22.0	1.0	0	140	3.0 d
(Wheat Chex) . . .	100	3.0	23.0	0	0	230	2.0 d
(Wheaties)	100	3.0	23.0	<1.0	0	200	3.0 d
(Wheaties Honey Gold)	100	2.0	25.0	<1.0	0	200	1.0 d

Food and Measure	cal.	prot. (gms)	carbo. (gms)	fat (gms)	chol. (mgs)	sod. (mgs)	fiber (gms)
apple cinnamon filled *(Kellogg's Apple Cinnamon Squares)*	90	2.0	23.0	0	0	5	2.0 d
blueberry filled *(Kellogg's Blueberry Squares)*	90	2.0	23.0	0	0	5	3.0 d
flakes *(Erewhon)* . .	110	3.0	22.0	0	0	75	3.0 d
w/fruit *(Erewhon Fruit'n Wheat)* . .	100	3.0	21.0	1.0	0	70	3.0 d
golden *(Health Valley Fruit Lites)*, .5 oz.	50	2.0	11.0	0	0	0	1.0 d
w/raisins:							
(Crispy Wheat 'N Raisins)	100	2.0	23.0	1.0	0	140	2.0 d
raisin filled *(Kellogg's Raisin Squares)*	90	2.0	23.0	0	0	0	2.0 d
strawberry filled *(Kellogg's Strawberry Squares)*	90	2.0	23.0	0	0	5	3.0 d
wheat, puffed, .5 oz.:							
(Arrowhead Mills)	50	2.0	11.0	0	0	<1	.9 d
(Malt-O-Meal) . . .	50	2.0	10.0	0	0	0	1.0 d
wheat, shredded:							
(Kellogg's Frosted Mini-Wheats) . .	100	3.0	24.0	0	0	0	3.0 d
(Nabisco), 1 piece	80	2.0	19.0	<1.0	0	0	3.0 d
(Nutri-Grain)	90	4.0	22.0	0	0	0	4.0 d
(S.W. Graham) . . .	100	3.0	23.0	0	0	190	3.0 d
(Sunshine), 1 piece	90	2.0	19.0	1.0	0	0	m.q.
bite size *(Sunshine)*, 2/3 cup	110	3.0	22.0	1.0	0	0	m.q.
bran *(Nabisco Shredded Wheat'n Bran)* . .	90	3.0	23.0	<1.0	0	0	4.0 d

Food and Measure	cal.	prot. (gms)	carbo. (gms)	fat (gms)	chol. (mgs)	sod. (mgs)	fiber (gms)
Cereal, ready-to-eat, wheat, shredded *(cont.)*							
cinnamon *(S. W. Graham)*	100	2.0	24.0	0	0	160	2.0 d
mini *(Nabisco Spoon Size)*	90	3.0	23.0	<1.0	0	0	3.0 d
whole grain *(Kellogg's)*	90	3.0	23.0	0	0	0	4.0 d
Cereal, cooking[1] (see also specific grains), 1 oz., except as noted:							
bran *(H-O Brand Super Bran)*, 1/3 cup	110	4.0	18.0	2.0	0	0	8.0 d
farina, see "wheat," below							
granola *(H-O Brand)*, 1/2 cup	200	6.0	43.0	3.0	0	45	5.0 d
mixed grain:							
(Arrowhead Mills Seven Grain) . . .	100	4.0	17.0	1.0	0	<1	4.0 d
(Erewhon Organic Barley Plus) . . .	110	3.0	22.0	1.0	0	0	1.0 d
(Roman Meal Original)	86	4.0	15.3	.7	0	<1	4.9 d
apple cinnamon *(Roman Meal)*, 1.2 oz.	112	3.5	18.2	2.0	0	6	6.4 d
w/oats *(Roman Meal Original)*, 1.2 oz.	114	5.1	18.7	1.4	0	1	4.8 d
oat bran:							
(Arrowhead Mills)	110	6.0	17.0	1.0	0	1	7.9 d
(Roman Meal) . . .	101	4.9	12.7	2.6	0	3	4.7 d
w/toasted wheat germ *(Erewhon Oat Bran)*	115	5.0	18.0	2.0	0	15	3.0 d

[1] *Uncooked, except as noted.*

Food and Measure	cal.	prot. (gms)	carbo. (gms)	fat (gms)	chol. (mgs)	sod. (mgs)	fiber (gms)
oatmeal and oats:							
(Arrowhead Mills Instant)	100	5.0	18.0	2.0	0	0	4.3 d
(H-O Brand Quick), 1/3 cup	100	5.0	18.0	2.0	0	0	3.0 d
(H-O Brand Instant), 1 pkt.	110	4.0	18.0	2.0	0	230	3.0 d
(H-O Brand Instant Box), 1/3 cup . .	100	5.0	18.0	2.0	0	0	3.0 d
(Instant Quaker), 1 pkt.	100	4.0	18.0	2.0	0	160	2.8 d
apple cinnamon *(Erewhon* Instant), 1.25 oz.	145	4.0	25.0	3.0	0	100	m.q.
apple cinnamon *(Instant Quaker),* 1 pkt.	120	4.0	26.0	2.0	0	100	3.0 d
apple cinnamon *(Quaker Oat Cups),* 5.5 oz. cont.	130	4.0	27.0	2.0	0	85	2.9 d
apple, date, and almond *(Arrowhead Mills* Instant) . .	130	5.0	23.0	3.0	0	3	3.7 d
apple raisin *(Erewhon* Instant), 1.3 oz.	150	4.0	27.0	3.0	0	100	m.q.
apple spice *(Arrowhead Mills* Instant)	130	5.0	23.0	2.0	0	1	3.4 d
bananas and cream *(Instant Quaker),* 1 pkt.	130	4.0	26.0	2.0	0	160	2.0 d
blueberries and cream *(Instant Quaker),* 1 pkt.	130	4.0	26.0	2.0	0	150	1.9 d
cinnamon raisin and almond *(Arrowhead Mills* Instant)	140	6.0	23.0	3.0	0	3	4.3 d

Food and Measure	cal.	prot. (gms)	carbo. (gms)	fat (gms)	chol. (mgs)	sod. (mgs)	fiber (gms)
Cereal, ready-to-eat, oatmeal and oats *(cont.)*							
w/fiber *(H-O Brand Instant),* 1 pkt.	110	5.0	18.0	2.0	0	140	3.0 d
w/fiber *(H-O Brand Instant Box),* 1/3 cup	100	5.0	15.0	2.0	0	5	3.0 d
w/fiber, apple and bran *(H-O Brand Instant),* 1 pkt.	130	3.0	26.0	2.0	0	140	3.0 d
w/fiber, raisin and bran *(H-O Brand Instant),* 1 pkt.	150	4.0	32.0	2.0	0	140	3.0 d
maple brown sugar *(H-O Brand In-stant),* 1 pkt. . .	160	4.0	32.0	2.0	0	285	3.0 d
maple brown sugar *(Instant Quaker),* 1 pkt.	140	4.0	31.0	2.0	0	240	2.9 d
maple spice *(Er-ewhon* Instant), 1.2 oz.	140	4.0	24.0	3.0	0	100	m.q.
w/oat bran *(Erewhon* Instant), 1.25 oz.	125	6.0	23.0	3.0	0	0	4.0 d
peaches and cream *(Instant Quaker),* 1 pkt.	130	3.0	26.0	2.0	0	150	2.3 d
raisin, date, and walnut *(Erewhon* Instant), 1.2 oz.	130	3.0	24.0	3.0	0	60	3.0 d
strawberries and cream *(Instant Quaker),* 1 pkt.	130	3.0	26.0	2.0	0	160	2.2 d
sweet'n mellow *(H-O Brand In-stant),* 1 pkt. . .	150	4.0	30.0	2.0	0	270	3.0 d
w/wheat, date, rai-sin, almond *(Ro-man Meal),* 1.3 oz.	134	4.5	23.9	1.7	0	3	3.0 d

Food and Measure	cal.	prot. (gms)	carbo. (gms)	fat (gms)	chol. (mgs)	sod. (mgs)	fiber (gms)
w/wheat, honey, coconut, almond (Roman Meal), 1.3 oz.	159	4.4	22.0	5.5	0	8	2.7 d
rice, brown (Arrowhead Mills Rice & Shine), 1/4 cup . . .	160	3.0	35.0	1.0	0	tr.	1.6 d
rice cream, brown (Erewhon Organic) . .	110	3.0	23.0	1.0	0	20	m.q.
rye, cream of (Roman Meal), 1.3 oz. . . .	112	5.4	20.3	.9	0	2	5.4 d
wheat:							
(Arrowhead Mills Bear Mush) . . .	100	3.0	21.0	0	0	1	1.3 d
(Malt-O-Meal) . . .	100	4.0	21.0	0	0	0	1.0 d
(Wheatena)	100	3.0	21.0	1.0	0	0	4.0 d
bulgur (Arrowhead Mills), 2 oz. . . .	200	6.0	43.0	1.0	0	0	5.4 d
chocolate (Malt-O-Meal)	100	3.0	22.0	0	0	0	1.0 d
cracked (Arrowhead Mills), 2 oz. . . .	180	7.0	40.0	1.0	0	1	2.3 d
farina (Pillsbury), 2/3 cup cooked	80	3.0	18.0	0	0	270	m.q.
farina, cream (H-O Brand), 3 tbsp.	120	3.0	26.0	0	0	0	3.0 d
maple and brown sugar (Malt-O-Meal)	100	3.0	22.0	0	0	0	1.0 d
w/oat bran (Malt-O-Meal Plus 40%), 1.3 oz.	130	6.0	25.0	2.0	0	0	3.0 d
Cereal, freeze-dried, granola, w/blueberries and milk (Mountain House), 1/2 cup	270	8.0	38.0	10.0	m.q.	60	m.q.
Cereal bar, see "Granola and cereal bar"							

Food and Measure	cal.	prot. (gms)	carbo. (gms)	fat (gms)	chol. (mgs)	sod. (mgs)	fiber (gms)
Cereal beverage, see "Coffee substitute"							
Cervelat, see "Thuringer cervelat"							
Chayote:							
raw:							
1 medium, 7.2 oz.	49	1.8	11.0	.6	0	8	6.1 d
1" pieces, 1/2 cup	16	.6	3.6	.2	0	3	2.0 d
(Frieda's), 1 oz. . . .	8	.2	2.0	<.1	0	1	m.q.
boiled, drained,							
1" pieces, 1/2 cup	19	.5	4.1	.4	0	1	.5 c
Cheddarwurst, 2 oz.:							
(Hillshire Farm Bun							
Size)	200	8.0	1.0	18.0	m.q.	480	0
links (Hillshire Farm)	190	8.0	1.0	17.0	m.q.	480	0
Cheese, 1 oz., except as noted:							
American, processed:							
(Alpine Lace) . . .	80	6.0	2.0	6.0	20	200	0
(Alpine Lace Free'N							
Lean)	40	8.0	1.0	0	5	290	0
(Heluva Good) . . .	110	6.0	1.0	9.0	m.q.	440	0
(Land O'Lakes) . .	110	6.0	1.0	9.0	30	450	0
plain or sharp (Borden Premium) . .	110	6.0	1.0	9.0	25	490	0
loaf (Kraft Deluxe)	110	6.0	1.0	9.0	25	430	0
hot pepper (Sargento)	110	6.0	<.5	9.0	27	410	(0)
sharp (Land O'Lakes)	100	6.0	1.0	9.0	30	360	0
sharp (Old English Loaf)	110	6.0	1.0	9.0	30	400	0
sharp (Old English Slices)	110	6.0	1.0	9.0	30	440	0
slices (Kraft Deluxe)	110	6.0	1.0	9.0	25	450	0
American and Swiss, processed (Land O'Lakes)	100	7.0	1.0	8.0	25	400	0

Food and Measure	cal.	prot. (gms)	carbo. (gms)	fat (gms)	chol. (mgs)	sod. (mgs)	fiber (gms)
asiago (Frigo)	110	7.0	1.0	9.0	m.q.	400	0
Babybel (Laughing Cow)	90	7.0	0	7.0	10	220	0
Babybel, mini (Laughing Cow), 3/4 oz. . .	70	5.0	0	6.0	15	170	0
(Bel Paese)	110	5.0	0	10.0	5	90	1.0 d
blue:							
(Frigo)	100	6.0	1.0	8.0	m.q.	400	0
(Kraft)	100	6.0	1.0	9.0	30	330	0
(Sargento)	100	6.0	1.0	8.0	21	400	0
Bonbel:							
(Laughing Cow) . .	100	6.0	0	8.0	25	230	0
mini (Laughing Cow), 3/4 oz. . .	70	5.0	0	6.0	15	170	0
mini (Laughing Cow Light), 3/4 oz. . .	45	6.0	0	3.0	10	160	0
brick:							
(Heluva Good) . . .	100	6.0	1.0	6.0	m.q.	160	0
(Kraft)	110	7.0	0	9.0	30	180	0
(Land O'Lakes) . .	110	7.0	1.0	8.0	25	160	0
Brie (Sargento)	100	6.0	<.5	8.0	28	180	0
burger (Sargento) . .	110	6.0	<.5	9.0	27	410	0
Cajun (Sargento) . . .	110	7.0	<.5	9.0	28	165	0
Camembert (Sargento)	90	6.0	<.5	7.0	20	240	0
cheddar:							
(Alpine Lace Ched-R-Lo) . . .	80	7.0	1.0	5.0	20	95	0
(Frigo)	110	7.0	1.0	9.0	30	200	0
(Frigo Lite)	80	8.0	1.0	5.0	17	190	0
(Heluva Good) . . .	100	7.0	1.0	9.0	m.q.	176	0
(Kraft)	110	7.0	1.0	9.0	30	180	0
(Land O'Lakes) . .	110	7.0	<1.0	9.0	30	180	0
(Land O'Lakes Chedarella) . . .	100	7.0	<1.0	8.0	25	180	0
(Sargento)	110	7.0	<.5	9.0	30	180	0
extra sharp, processed (Land O'Lakes)	100	6.0	1.0	9.0	30	370	0

Food and Measure	cal.	prot. (gms)	carbo. (gms)	fat (gms)	chol. (mgs)	sod. (mgs)	fiber (gms)
Cheese, cheddar (cont.)							
mild (Kraft Light Naturals)	80	9.0	0	5.0	20	220	0
processed (Alpine Lace Free'N Lean)	40	8.0	1.0	0	5	290	0
sharp, New York (Master Choice Special Reserve)	110	7.0	0	9.0	30	180	0
cheddar and bacon, processed (Land O'Lakes)	110	6.0	1.0	9.0	25	350	0
Cheshire	110	6.6	1.4	8.7	29	198	0
colby:							
(Alpine Lace Colbi-Lo)	80	7.0	1.0	5.0	20	85	0
(Heluva Good) . . .	110	7.0	1.0	9.0	m.q.	171	0
(Kraft)	110	7.0	1.0	9.0	30	180	0
(Kraft Light Naturals)	80	9.0	0	5.0	20	220	0
(Land O'Lakes) . .	110	7.0	1.0	9.0	25	170	0
(Sargento)	110	7.0	1.0	9.0	27	170	0
colby jack (Sargento)	110	7.0	<.5	9.0	27	160	0
colby and Monterey Jack, shredded (Kraft Light Naturals)	80	8.0	1.0	5.0	20	220	0
cottage cheese, 4% fat, creamed, 4 oz. or 1/2 cup:							
(Bison)	120	14.0	4.0	5.0	18	420	0
(Breakstone's) . . .	110	13.0	3.0	5.0	25	370	0
(Friendship California)	120	14.0	4.0	5.0	17	380	0
large curd (Knudsen)	120	14.0	4.0	5.0	20	340	0
small curd (Knudsen)	120	14.0	4.0	5.0	20	370	0
w/pineapple (Breakstone's)	140	10.0	14.0	5.0	25	260	m.q.
w/pineapple (Friendship)	140	11.0	15.0	4.0	17	300	m.q.

Food and Measure	cal.	prot. (gms)	carbo. (gms)	fat (gms)	chol. (mgs)	sod. (mgs)	fiber (gms)
cottage cheese, dry curd (Breakstone's), 4 oz.	90	16.0	6.0	0	10	65	0
cottage cheese, lowfat, 4 oz. or 1/2 cup, except as noted:							
2% (Breakstone's)	100	14.0	4.0	2.0	15	510	0
2% (Friendship Pot Style)	100	14.0	4.0	2.0	9	405	0
2% (Knudsen) . . .	100	14.0	4.0	2.0	15	370	0
2% (Sealtest) . . .	100	14.0	4.0	2.0	15	340	0
1% (Bison)	90	14.0	4.0	1.0	5	350	0
1% (Friendship No Salt)	90	14.0	4.0	1.0	5	31	0
1% (Friendship Lactose reduced/ Whipped)	90	14.0	4.0	1.0	5	350	0
1% (Light n' Lively)	80	14.0	4.0	2.0	10	370	0
apple, spiced, 2% (Knudsen), 6 oz.	180	16.0	20.0	2.0	15	280	m.q.
fruit cocktail, 2% (Knudsen)	130	11.0	16.0	2.0	10	330	m.q.
garden salad, 1% (Light n' Lively)	80	18.0	5.0	2.0	10	350	m.q.
mandarin orange, 2% (Knudsen) . .	110	11.0	11.0	2.0	10	320	m.q.
peach, 2% (Knudsen), 6 oz.	170	16.0	19.0	2.0	15	270	m.q.
peach and pineapple, 1% (Light n' Lively)	100	11.0	12.0	1.0	10	320	m.q.
pear, 2% (Knudsen)	110	11.0	12.0	2.0	10	320	m.q.
pineapple, 1% (Friendship) . . .	110	11.0	15.0	1.0	5	300	m.q.
pineapple, 2% (Knudsen), 6 oz.	170	16.0	18.0	2.0	15	300	m.q.

Food and Measure	cal.	prot. (gms)	carbo. (gms)	fat (gms)	chol. (mgs)	sod. (mgs)	fiber (gms)
Cheese, cottage, lowfat *(cont.)*							
strawberry, 2%							
(Knudsen), 6 oz.	170	16.0	19.0	2.0	15	320	m.q.
cottage cheese,							
nonfat:							
(Bison), 1/2 cup . .	80	13.0	4.0	<1.0	5	350	0
(Friendship), 1/2 cup	70	13.0	5.0	0	0	350	0
(Knudsen), 4 oz. . . .	70	15.0	3.0	0	5	420	0
cream cheese:							
(Heluva Good)	100	2.0	1.0	10.0	m.q.	84	0
(Philadelphia Brand)	100	2.0	1.0	10.0	30	90	0
w/chives *(Philadel-*							
phia Brand) . . .	90	2.0	1.0	9.0	30	125	(0)
w/pimiento *(Phila-*							
delphia Brand)	90	2.0	1.0	9.0	30	150	(0)
cream cheese, soft							
(Philadelphia Brand):							
plain	100	1.0	2.0	10.0	30	100	0
w/chives and onion	100	2.0	2.0	9.0	30	100	(0)
w/herb and garlic	100	1.0	2.0	9.0	25	160	(0)
w/olives and pi-							
miento	90	2.0	2.0	8.0	25	160	(0)
w/pineapple	90	1.0	4.0	8.0	25	90	(0)
w/smoked salmon	90	2.0	1.0	9.0	25	180	0
w/strawberries . . .	90	1.0	4.0	8.0	20	75	(0)
cream cheese,							
whipped							
(Philadelphia Brand):							
plain	100	2.0	1.0	10.0	30	85	0
w/chives	90	2.0	1.0	8.0	30	150	(0)
w/onions	90	2.0	2.0	8.0	25	170	(0)
w/smoked salmon	90	2.0	2.0	8.0	30	170	0
Edam:							
(Kraft)	90	8.0	0	7.0	20	310	0
(Land O'Lakes) . .	100	7.0	<1.0	8.0	25	270	0
(Laughing Cow) . .	100	6.0	0	8.0	25	230	0
(Sargento)	100	7.0	<.5	8.0	25	270	0

Food and Measure	cal.	prot. (gms)	carbo. (gms)	fat (gms)	chol. (mgs)	sod. (mgs)	fiber (gms)
farmer, 1/2 cup:							
(Friendship)	160	16.0	4.0	12.0	40	356	0
(Friendship No Salt)	160	16.0	4.0	12.0	40	8	0
feta:							
(Frigo)	100	6.0	1.0	8.0	m.q.	400	0
(Sargento)	80	4.0	1.0	6.0	25	320	0
imported (Krinos)	90	5.0	0	8.0	25	430	0
fontina (Sargento) . .	110	7.0	<.5	9.0	33	m.q.	0
gjetost (Sargento) . .	130	3.0	12.0	8.0	m.q.	170	0
goat:							
hard type	128	8.7	.6	10.1	30	98	0
semisoft type . . .	103	6.1	.7	8.5	22	146	0
soft type	76	5.3	.3	6.0	13	104	0
Gouda:							
(Kraft)	110	7.0	0	9.0	30	200	0
(Land O'Lakes) . .	100	7.0	1.0	8.0	30	230	0
(Laughing Cow) . .	110	7.0	0	9.0	30	230	0
(Sargento)	100	7.0	1.0	8.0	32	230	0
mini (Laughing Cow), 3/4 oz. . . .	80	5.0	0	6.0	20	170	0
Gruyère	117	8.5	.1	9.2	31	95	0
havarti (Casino) . . .	120	6.0	0	11.0	35	140	0
havarti (Sargento) . .	120	5.0	<.5	11.0	31	200	0
hoop (Friendship), 1/2 cup	84	18.0	2.0	1.0	8	10	0
Impastata (Frigo) . . .	60	4.0	1.0	5.0	15	50	0
Italian style, grated (Sargento)	110	8.0	1.0	8.0	26	105	0
jalapeño jack, processed (Land O'Lakes)	90	5.0	1.0	8.0	20	430	0
Jarlsberg:							
(Sargento)	100	7.0	1.0	7.0	16	130	0
smoked (Norseland)	97	7.0	1.0	7.0	18	135	0
limburger:							
(Mohawk Valley Little Gem)	90	6.0	0	8.0	25	250	0
(Sargento)	90	6.0	<.5	8.0	26	230	0

Food and Measure	cal.	prot. (gms)	carbo. (gms)	fat (gms)	chol. (mgs)	sod. (mgs)	fiber (gms)
Cheese *(cont.)*							
mascarpone *(Galbani Imported)*	128	1.5	1.2	13.1	39	17	0
Monterey Jack:							
(Alpine Lace Monti-Jack-Lo)	80	7.0	1.0	5.0	15	75	0
(Heluva Good) . . .	110	7.0	1.0	9.0	m.q.	152	0
(Kraft)	110	6.0	0	9.0	30	190	0
(Kraft Light Naturals)	80	9.0	0	5.0	20	220	0
(Sargento)	110	7.0	<.5	9.0	25	150	0
w/caraway *(Kraft)*	100	7.0	1.0	8.0	30	180	(0)
w/jalapeños *(Kraft)*	110	7.0	1.0	9.0	30	190	(0)
plain or hot pepper *(Land O'Lakes)*	110	7.0	<1.0	9.0	20	150	0
w/peppers *(Kraft* Light Naturals)	80	8.0	1.0	5.0	20	220	(0)
mozzarella:							
(Alpine Lace Free'N Lean)	40	9.0	0	0	5	185	0
(Heluva Good) . . .	90	6.0	1.0	7.0	m.q.	118	0
(Kraft)	90	6.0	1.0	7.0	20	190	0
(Kraft Light Naturals)	80	1.0	4.0	0	15	200	0
(Polly-O Free) . . .	40	8.0	1.0	0	5	240	0
(Polly-O Lite)	60	7.0	1.0	3.0	10	240	0
whole milk *(Polly-O)*	90	6.0	1.0	6.0	20	240	0
whole milk *(Sargento)*	90	6.0	1.0	7.0	25	120	0
whole milk *(Frigo)*	90	6.0	1.0	7.0	15	190	0
part skim *(Alpine Lace)*	70	7.0	1.0	5.0	15	75	0
part skim *(Frigo)* . .	80	7.0	1.0	5.0	10	190	0
part skim *(Frigo* Lite)	60	9.0	1.0	2.0	8	140	0
part skim *(Kraft)* . .	80	8.0	1.0	5.0	15	200	0
part skim *(Land O'Lakes)*	80	8.0	1.0	5.0	15	150	0
part skim *(Polly-O)*	80	6.0	1.0	5.0	15	240	0
part skim *(Sargento)*	80	8.0	1.0	5.0	15	150	0

Food and Measure	cal.	prot. (gms)	carbo. (gms)	fat (gms)	chol. (mgs)	sod. (mgs)	fiber (gms)
processed (Alpine Lace Free'N Lean)	40	9.0	0	0	5	290	0
Muenster:							
(Alpine Lace) . . .	100	7.0	1.0	9.0	25	85	0
(Heluva Good) . . .	100	7.0	1.0	8.0	m.q.	178	0
(Land O'Lakes) . .	100	7.0	<1.0	9.0	25	180	0
red rind (Sargento)	100	7.0	<.5	9.0	27	180	0
Neufchâtel (Philadelphia Brand Light)	80	3.0	1.0	7.0	25	115	0
Parmesan:							
(Kraft)	100	9.0	1.0	7.0	20	290	0
fresh (Sargento) . .	110	10.0	1.0	7.0	19	450	0
grated, 1 tbsp. . . .	23	2.1	.2	1.5	4	93	0
grated (Frigo) . . .	130	12.0	1.0	9.0	25	510	0
grated (Frigo Lite)	100	15.0	1.0	4.0	15	410	0
grated (Kraft) . . .	130	12.0	1.0	9.0	30	430	0
grated (Progresso), 1 tbsp.	23	2.0	<1.0	2.0	4	94	0
grated (Sargento)	130	12.0	2.0	9.0	22	530	0
Reggiano (Galbani Imported)	105	10.1	n.a.	7.1	21	188	0
wheel or fresh grated (Frigo) . .	110	10.0	1.0	7.0	m.q.	350	0
Parmesan and Romano:							
grated (Sargento)	110	10.0	1.0	7.0	24	400	0
grated, dry (Frigo)	130	12.0	1.0	9.0	m.q.	510	0
grated, fresh (Frigo)	110	10.0	1.0	7.0	m.q.	350	0
pimiento, processed (Kraft Deluxe) . . .	100	6.0	1.0	8.0	25	440	(0)
pizza, shredded (Frigo)	65	9.0	1.0	3.0	10	150	0
Port du Salut	100	6.7	.2	8.0	35	151	0
pot cheese (Sargento)	25	5.0	1.0	<.5	m.q.	1	0
provolone:							
(Alpine Lace Provo-Lo)	70	7.0	1.0	5.0	15	85	0
(Frigo)	100	7.0	1.0	7.0	20	230	0
(Frigo Lite)	70	8.0	1.0	4.0	10	205	0

Food and Measure	cal.	prot. (gms)	carbo. (gms)	fat (gms)	chol. (mgs)	sod. (mgs)	fiber (gms)
Cheese, provolone (cont.)							
(Heluva Good) . . .	100	7.0	1.0	8.0	m.q.	248	0
(Kraft)	100	7.0	1.0	7.0	25	260	0
(Land O'Lakes) . .	100	7.0	1.0	8.0	20	250	0
(Sargento)	100	7.0	1.0	8.0	20	250	0
queso blanco							
(Sargento)	100	7.0	.3	9.0	27	180	0
queso de papa							
(Sargento)	110	7.0	.4	9.0	30	180	0
ricotta:							
(Polly-O Free) . . .	25	4.0	1.0	0	<1	35	0
(Polly-O Lite)	35	4.0	1.0	2.0	5	35	0
(Sargento Lite) . . .	23	3.0	1.0	1.0	4	20	0
whole milk, 1/2 cup	216	14.0	3.8	16.1	63	104	0
whole milk (Frigo)	60	3.0	1.0	5.0	15	40	0
whole milk (Polly-O)	50	3.0	1.0	4.0	15	35	0
part skim (Frigo) . .	40	3.0	1.0	3.0	10	30	0
part skim (Polly-O)	45	4.0	1.0	3.0	10	35	0
low fat/salt (Frigo)	30	3.0	1.0	1.0	5	10	0
fat free (Frigo) . . .	20	4.0	2.0	0	3	15	0
Romano:							
(Kraft Natural) . . .	100	8.0	1.0	7.0	20	250	0
(Sargento)	110	9.0	1.0	8.0	29	340	0
grated (Kraft) . . .	130	11.0	1.0	9.0	30	350	0
grated (Polly-O) . .	130	11.0	1.0	10.0	30	530	0
grated (Progresso),							
1 tbsp.	23	2.0	<1.0	2.0	6	70	0
grated, dry (Frigo)	130	12.0	1.0	9.0	35	510	0
Pecorino, grated							
(Krinos), 1 tbsp.	25	1.0	0	2.0	5	135	0
wheel and fresh							
grated (Frigo) . .	110	9.0	1.0	8.0	30	350	0
Roquefort	105	6.1	.6	8.7	26	513	0
smoked (Sargento							
Smokestick)	100	7.0	1.0	7.0	24	390	0
string:							
(Frigo)	80	7.0	1.0	5.0	10	190	0
(Frigo Lite)	60	9.0	1.0	2.0	8	140	0

Food and Measure	cal.	prot. (gms)	carbo. (gms)	fat (gms)	chol. (mgs)	sod. (mgs)	fiber (gms)
(Polly-O Stick) . . .	90	7.0	2.0	6.0	15	200	0
part skim, w/jalape-							
ños (Kraft)	80	8.0	1.0	5.0	20	230	(0)
plain or smoked							
(Sargento)	80	8.0	1.0	5.0	15	150	0
Swiss:							
(Alpine Lace Swiss-							
Lo)	90	8.0	1.0	6.0	20	35	0
(Casino)	110	8.0	1.0	8.0	30	35	0
(Frigo)	110	8.0	1.0	8.0	m.q.	80	0
(Heluva Good) . . .	110	8.0	1.0	8.0	m.q.	74	0
(Kraft)	110	8.0	1.0	8.0	25	40	0
(Kraft Light Naturals)	90	10.0	1.0	5.0	20	70	0
(Kraft Very Low So-							
dium)	110	8.0	1.0	8.0	25	10	0
(Land O'Lakes) . .	110	8.0	1.0	8.0	25	75	0
(Sargento)	110	8.0	1.0	8.0	26	75	0
aged (Kraft)	110	8.0	1.0	8.0	25	45	0
baby (Cracker Barrel							
Natural)	110	7.0	0	9.0	25	65	0
Finland (Sargento)	110	8.0	<.5	8.0	26	75	0
processed (Borden							
Premium)	100	7.0	1.0	8.0	20	380	0
processed (Kraft							
Deluxe)	90	7.0	1.0	7.0	25	420	0
taco:							
(Sargento)	110	7.0	<.5	9.0	27	160	0
shredded (Frigo) . .	110	7.0	1.0	9.0	m.q.	200	0
shredded (Kraft) . .	110	7.0	1.0	9.0	30	190	0
taleggio (Tal-Fino							
Brand Imported) . .	89	5.4	.2	7.4	m.q.	176	0
Tilsit (Sargento) . . .	100	7.0	1.0	7.0	29	210	0
Tybo, red wax							
(Sargento)	100	7.0	<.5	7.0	23	200	0

Food and Measure	cal.	prot. (gms)	carbo. (gms)	fat (gms)	chol. (mgs)	sod. (mgs)	fiber (gms)
Cheese, imitation and substitute, 1 oz., except as noted:							
(Smartbeat Low Sodium), 1 slice . . .	35	4.0	2.0	2.0	0	90	0
American:							
(Heluva Good) . . .	80	6.0	1.0	6.0	2	310	0
(Smartbeat Fat Free), 1 slice . .	30	4.0	2.0	0	0	180	0
cheddar:							
imitation *(Frigo)* . .	90	5.0	1.0	7.0	n.a.	280	0
imitation *(Sargento)*	90	7.0	<.5	6.0	2	350	0
mellow *(Smartbeat),* 1 slice	30	4.0	2.0	0	0	180	0
cheese food							
(Cheeztwin)	90	5.0	3.0	6.0	n.a.	400	0
mozzarella:							
1 oz.	70	3.3	6.7	3.5	0	194	0
imitation *(Frigo)* . .	90	6.0	1.0	7.0	n.a.	240	0
imitation *(Sargento)*	80	7.0	<.5	6.0	2	310	0
Parmesan, Italian, grated *(Country Cottage Farms),* 1 tbsp.	14	1.0	2.0	0	0	60	0
sharp *(Smartbeat),* 1 slice	30	4.0	2.0	0	0	230	0
Swiss *(Smartbeat* Fat Free), 1 slice	30	4.0	2.0	0	0	180	0
Cheese dip, 1 oz., except as noted:							
(Chi-Chi's Fiesta) . .	41	1.0	3.0	3.0	9	296	0
blue *(Kraft* Premium), 2 tbsp.	50	1.0	2.0	4.0	10	210	0
cheddar *(Frito-Lay's)*	45	1.0	3.0	3.0	5	180	0
nacho *(Kraft* Premium), 2 tbsp.	55	2.0	2.0	4.0	10	200	0
nacho, jalapeño *(Price's)*	80	2.6	2.0	7.1	n.a.	m.q.	.1 d

Food and Measure	cal.	prot. (gms)	carbo. (gms)	fat (gms)	chol. (mgs)	sod. (mgs)	fiber (gms)
Cheese food, 1 oz.:							
(Heluva Good)	90	6.0	1.0	7.0	m.q.	360	0
(Land O'Lakes)	90	5.0	2.0	6.0	20	350	0
American:							
(Borden Singles) . .	90	5.0	3.0	7.0	20	360	0
(Kraft Singles) . . .	90	5.0	2.0	7.0	25	390	0
grated *(Kraft)* . . .	130	8.0	8.0	7.0	25	740	0
sharp *(Borden* Singles)	100	5.0	2.0	8.0	20	470	0
white *(Kraft* Singles)	90	5.0	2.0	7.0	20	400	0
w/bacon:							
(Cracker Barrel) . .	90	5.0	3.0	7.0	20	280	0
(Kraft Cheez'N Bacon)	90	6.0	2.0	7.0	25	400	0
cheddar:							
port wine *(Wispride Lite)*	77	4.0	4.0	4.0	16	195	0
port wine or sharp *(Cracker Barrel)*	100	4.0	4.0	7.0	20	230	0
extra sharp *(Cracker Barrel)*	90	5.0	3.0	7.0	20	240	0
w/garlic *(Kraft)*	90	5.0	2.0	7.0	20	370	(0)
Italian herb *(Land O'Lakes)*	90	6.0	2.0	7.0	20	430	(0)
w/jalapeños:							
(Kraft)	90	5.0	2.0	7.0	20	390	(0)
(Kraft Singles) . . .	90	5.0	2.0	7.0	25	450	(0)
(Land O'Lakes) . .	90	6.0	2.0	7.0	20	400	(0)
hot *(Velveeta* Mexican)*	100	6.0	3.0	7.0	25	430	(0)
mild *(Velveeta* Mexican)*	100	6.0	3.0	7.0	25	420	(0)
Monterey Jack *(Kraft* Singles)	90	5.0	2.0	7.0	25	390	0
(Nippy)	90	5.0	2.0	7.0	20	380	0
onion *(Land O'Lakes)*	90	6.0	2.0	7.0	20	410	(0)
pepperoni *(Land O'Lakes)*	90	6.0	1.0	7.0	20	430	0

Food and Measure	cal.	prot. (gms)	carbo. (gms)	fat (gms)	chol. (mgs)	sod. (mgs)	fiber (gms)
Cheese food (cont.)							
pimiento (Kraft Singles)	90	5.0	2.0	7.0	25	390	(0)
port wine, cold pack (Wispride)	100	5.0	3.0	7.0	25	210	0
salami (Land O'Lakes)	90	6.0	2.0	7.0	20	410	0
sharp (Kraft Singles)	100	6.0	1.0	8.0	25	400	0
shredded (Velveeta)	100	6.0	3.0	7.0	20	410	0
Swiss:							
(Borden Singles) . .	100	6.0	2.0	7.0	20	420	0
(Kraft Singles) . . .	90	6.0	2.0	7.0	25	440	0
Cheese nuggets, mozzarella, frozen (Banquet Hot Bites), 2.5 oz.	230	14.0	15.0	12.0	m.q.	510	m.q.
Cheese-nut ball or log, 1 oz., except as noted:							
ball, w/almonds:							
port wine cheddar (Wispride)	110	5.0	5.0	7.0	19	190	m.q.
sharp cheddar (Cracker Barrel)	100	5.0	4.0	7.0	20	250	m.q.
sharp cheddar (Wispride)	110	5.0	5.0	7.0	19	200	m.q.
sharp cheddar, mini (Wispride), 1 ball	80	2.0	5.0	6.0	13	130	m.q.
log:							
sharp or port wine cheddar (Sargento)	100	6.0	3.0	7.0	18	250	m.q.
sharp or smoky cheddar, w/almonds (Cracker Barrel)	90	5.0	4.0	6.0	15	250	m.q.
Swiss almond (Sargento)	90	6.0	2.0	7.0	21	350	m.q.

Food and Measure	cal.	prot. (gms)	carbo. (gms)	fat (gms)	chol. (mgs)	sod. (mgs)	fiber (gms)
Cheese product,							
1 oz., except as noted:							
(Kraft Free Singles)	45	7.0	4.0	0	5	420	0
(Lite-Line Low Sodium), 1 slice . . .	35	4.0	1.0	2.0	5	90	0
all varieties *(Borden* Fat Free Singles)	40	6.0	4.0	0	<5	380	0
American flavor:							
(Alpine Lace) . . .	90	6.0	2.0	7.0	20	200	0
(Borden Light) . . .	70	6.0	1.0	4.0	15	420	0
(Harvest Moon) . .	70	6.0	2.0	4.0	15	420	0
(Kraft Light)	70	6.0	2.0	4.0	15	420	0
(Light n' Lively) . .	70	6.0	2.0	4.0	15	420	0
(Lite-Line), 1 slice	35	4.0	1.0	2.0	5	280	0
white *(Kraft Light)*	70	6.0	2.0	4.0	15	410	0
white *(Light n' Lively)*	70	6.0	2.0	4.0	15	410	0
cheddar flavor:							
all varieties *(Lite-Line)*, 1 slice . .	35	4.0	1.0	2.0	5	300	0
medium *(Spreadery)*	70	5.0	3.0	4.0	15	250	0
sharp *(Borden* Light)	70	6.0	2.0	4.0	15	420	0
sharp *(Kraft Light)*	70	6.0	2.0	4.0	15	380	0
sharp *(Light n' Lively)*	70	6.0	2.0	4.0	15	380	0
sharp *(Spreadery)*	70	5.0	3.0	4.0	15	240	0
Vermont white *(Spreadery)* . . .	70	5.0	3.0	4.0	15	230	0
colby flavor *(Lite-Line)*, 1 slice	35	4.0	1.0	2.0	5	240	0
cream cheese, light *(Philadelphia Brand)*	60	3.0	2.0	5.0	10	160	0
Mexican, mild, w/ jalapeños *(Spreadery)*	70	5.0	3.0	4.0	15	260	0

Food and Measure	cal.	prot. (gms)	carbo. (gms)	fat (gms)	chol. (mgs)	sod. (mgs)	fiber (gms)
Cheese product *(cont.)*							
Monterey Jack or muenster flavor *(Lite-Line)*, 1 slice	35	4.0	1.0	2.0	5	245	0
mozzarella flavor *(Lite-Line)*, 1 slice	35	4.0	1.0	2.0	10	230	0
nacho *(Spreadery)* . .	70	5.0	3.0	4.0	15	240	0
Neufchâtel:							
French onion *(Spreadery)* . . .	70	2.0	2.0	6.0	20	135	(0)
garlic and herb *(Spreadery)* . . .	70	2.0	1.0	6.0	20	140	(0)
garlic and herb or garden vegetable *(Wispride* Cheese Snack)	60	3.0	2.0	5.0	15	170	.1 d
ranch *(Spreadery Classic)*	70	2.0	1.0	7.0	20	190	0
w/strawberries *(Spreadery)* . . .	70	2.0	m.q.	5.0	15	270	(0)
vegetables, garden *(Spreadery)* . . .	70	2.0	2.0	6.0	20	220	(0)
pizza topping *(Lunch Wagon)*	80	6.0	1.0	6.0	0	350	0
port wine *(Spreadery)*	70	5.0	3.0	4.0	15	250	0
sandwich slices *(Lunch Wagon)* . .	90	5.0	2.0	7.0	5	370	0
Swiss flavor:							
(Kraft Light)	70	6.0	2.0	3.0	15	350	0
(Lite-Line), 1 slice	35	4.0	1.0	2.0	10	260	0
(Light n' Lively) . .	70	6.0	2.0	3.0	15	350	0
(Velveeta Light) . . .	70	6.0	3.0	4.0	15	470	0
Cheese sauce mix, 1/4 pkg.:							
(French's)	35	1.0	4.0	1.0	5	430	n.a.
(McCormick/Schilling)	35	2.0	3.5	1.5	m.q.	477	n.a.

Food and Measure	cal.	prot. (gms)	carbo. (gms)	fat (gms)	chol. (mgs)	sod. (mgs)	fiber (gms)
nacho (McCormick/ Schilling)	42	2.4	4.5	1.5	m.q.	409	n.a.
Cheese spread (see also "Cheese"), 1 oz.:							
(Cheez Whiz)	80	4.0	2.0	6.0	20	470	0
(Heluva Good)	80	5.0	2.0	6.0	10	430	0
all varieties, except cheddar (Easy Cheese)	80	4.0	2.0	6.0	20	340	0
American, processed:							
(Borden Cheese Loaf).	90	5.0	3.0	6.0	20	360	0
(Kraft)	80	4.0	2.0	6.0	15	470	0
w/pimiento or sharp (Sargento Cracker Snacks)	110	6.0	<.5	9.0	27	410	(0)
w/bacon:							
(Kraft)	80	5.0	1.0	7.0	20	560	0
(Squeez-A-Snak) . .	80	5.0	1.0	7.0	20	500	0
blue (Roka)	70	3.0	2.0	6.0	20	270	0
brick (Sargento Cracker Snacks) . .	100	6.0	1.0	9.0	25	430	0
cheddar:							
regular or sharp (Easy Cheese) . .	80	4.0	2.0	6.0	20	360	0
sharp, cold pack (Wispride Lite) . .	80	3.0	4.0	5.0	15	180	0
garlic flavor (Squeez-A-Snak) . .	80	5.0	1.0	7.0	20	430	(0)
hickory smoke flavor (Squeez-A-Snak) . .	80	5.0	1.0	7.0	20	440	0
w/jalapeño peppers:							
(Cheez Whiz) . . .	80	4.0	2.0	6.0	20	430	(0)
(Kraft)	70	2.0	3.0	5.0	15	95	(0)
(Squeez-A-Snak) . .	80	5.0	1.0	6.0	20	510	(0)
loaf (Kraft)	80	5.0	2.0	6.0	20	470	(0)

Food and Measure	cal.	prot. (gms)	carbo. (gms)	fat (gms)	chol. (mgs)	sod. (mgs)	fiber (gms)
Cheese spread *(cont.)*							
(Land O'Lakes Golden							
Velvet)	80	5.0	2.0	6.0	20	370	0
limburger *(Mohawk*							
Valley)	70	4.0	0	6.0	20	420	0
Mexican:							
hot *(Velveeta)* . . .	80	5.0	3.0	6.0	20	520	(0)
mild *(Cheez Whiz)*	80	4.0	2.0	6.0	20	430	(0)
mild *(Velveeta)* . . .	80	5.0	3.0	6.0	20	440	(0)
olive and pimiento							
(Kraft)	60	2.0	2.0	5.0	15	160	(0)
pimiento *(Kraft)* . . .	70	2.0	3.0	5.0	15	120	(0)
pimiento *(Velveeta)* . .	80	5.0	3.0	6.0	20	400	(0)
pineapple *(Kraft)* . . .	70	2.0	4.0	5.0	15	75	(0)
port wine, cold pack							
(Wispride Lite) . . .	80	4.0	4.0	5.0	16	200	0
sharp:							
(Old English)	80	5.0	1.0	7.0	20	480	0
(Squeez-A-Snak) . .	80	5.0	1.0	7.0	20	440	0
Swiss *(Sargento*							
Cracker Snacks) . .	100	7.0	1.0	7.0	24	390	0
(Velveeta)	80	5.0	3.0	6.0	20	430	0
(Velveeta Slices) . . .	90	5.0	3.0	6.0	20	400	0
Cheese sticks, frozen							
(Stilwell), 1 piece:							
cheddar, breaded . .	50	3.0	5.0	2.5	5	180	1.0 d
mozzarella, battered	70	3.0	5.0	4.0	5	150	1.0 d
Cheesecake, see							
"Cake, frozen" and							
"Cake, snack, fro-							
zen"							
Cheeseburger, see							
"Beef entree, fro-							
zen"							
Cherimoya:							
1 medium, 1.9 lb. . . .	515	7.1	131.3	2.2	0	m.q.	13.1 d
(Frieda's), 1 oz.	27	.4	6.8	.1	0	m.q.	m.q.

Food and Measure	cal.	prot. (gms)	carbo. (gms)	fat (gms)	chol. (mgs)	sod. (mgs)	fiber (gms)
Cherry, 1/2 cup, except as noted:							
fresh, sour, red:							
w/pits, 1 oz.	14	.3	3.5	.1	0	1	1.2 d
w/pits	26	.5	6.3	.2	0	2	.6 d
pitted	39	.8	9.4	.2	0	3	.9 d
fresh, sweet:							
w/pits	52	.9	12.0	.7	0	1	1.5 d
10 medium, 2.6 oz.	49	.8	11.3	.7	0	tr.	1.6 d
canned, sour, pitted:							
in water *(Stokely)*	45	1.0	10.0	0	0	15	m.q.
in heavy syrup . . .	116	.9	29.8	.1	0	9	1.0 d
canned, sweet:							
in heavy syrup . . .	107	.8	27.4	.2	0	3	.9 d
dark, w/pits *(Del Monte)*	90	0	23.0	0	0	5	m.q.
dark or light, pitted *(Del Monte)* . . .	90	0	24.0	0	0	5	m.q.
light, w/pits *(Del Monte)*	100	0	26.0	0	0	0	m.q.
dried, bing *(Frieda's)*, 1 oz.	79	1.4	19.8	.3	0	2	m.q.
frozen, 4 oz.:							
sour, red, unsweetened . . .	52	1.0	12.5	.5	0	1	1.4 d
sweet, sweetened	101	1.3	25.4	.1	0	1	1.1 d
Cherry, maraschino, w/liquid, 1 oz. . . .	33	.1	8.3	.1	0	n.a.	.1 c
Cherry cider *(R.W. Knudsen)*, 8 fl. oz.	100	<1.0	24.0	<1.0	0	(0)	m.q.
Cherry drink:							
(Hi-C), 6 fl. oz.	100	0	24.0	0	0	25	(0)
(Kool-Aid Kool Bursts), 6.75 oz.	110	0	28.0	0	0	10	(0)
mix*, 8 fl. oz.:							
(Kool-Aid Presweetened)	70	0	18.0	0	0	0	(0)

Food and Measure	cal.	prot. (gms)	carbo. (gms)	fat (gms)	chol. (mgs)	sod. (mgs)	fiber (gms)
Cherry drink, mix *(cont.)*							
regular or black							
(Kool-Aid)	100	0	25.0	0	0	0	(0)
wild *(Wylers)*	80	(0)	21.0	(0)	0	0	(0)
Cherry fruit concen-							
trate, black *(Hain),*							
2 tbsp.	67	0	17.0	0	0	0	n.a.
Cherry fruit roll, see							
"Fruit snack"							
Cherry juice:							
(R.W. Knudsen Cherry							
Tart), 8 fl. oz. . . .	125	<1.0	30.0	<1.0	0	(0)	m.q.
black *(R.W. Knudsen),*							
8 fl. oz.	150	2.0	38.0	<1.0	0	(0)	m.q.
black *(Smucker's* Nat-							
urally 100%),							
8 fl. oz.	130	0	31.0	0	0	10	m.q.
blend *(Juicy Juice),*							
6 fl. oz.	90	1.0	23.0	0	0	10	m.q.
cocktail *(Welch's*							
Orchard), 6 fl. oz.	180	0	45.0	0	0	10	0
Cherry juice drink,							
8.45 fl. oz.:							
(Kool-Aid Koolers) . .	140	0	38.0	0	0	10	(0)
(Tang Fruit Box) . . .	130	0	34.0	0	0	10	(0)
Cherry-grape juice							
drink *(Boku),*							
8 fl. oz.	120	0	29.0	0	0	35	0
Chervil, dried, 1 tsp.	1	.1	.3	<.1	0	tr.	.1 d
Chestnut, California,							
(Frieda's), 1 oz. . .	55	.8	11.9	.4	0	2	m.q.
Chestnut, Chinese,							
shelled, 1 oz.:							
raw	64	1.2	13.9	.3	0	1	.5 c
dried	103	1.9	22.7	.5	0	2	.8 c
boiled or steamed . .	44	.8	9.6	.2	0	1	.3 c
roasted	68	1.3	14.9	.3	0	1	.5 c

Food and Measure	cal.	prot. (gms)	carbo. (gms)	fat (gms)	chol. (mgs)	sod. (mgs)	fiber (gms)
Chestnut, European:							
raw, in shell, 1 lb. . .	714	8.1	152.8	7.6	0	9	27.2 d
raw, shelled, w/peel,							
1 cup or 13 kernels	308	3.5	66.0	3.3	0	4	11.7 d
dried, peeled, 1 oz.	105	1.4	22.3	1.1	0	11	1.4 c
boiled, 1 oz.	37	.8	7.9	.4	0	8	.2 c
roasted, peeled:							
1 oz.	70	.9	15.0	.6	0	1	3.7 d
1 cup or 17 kernels	350	4.3	75.7	3.2	0	3	18.4 d
Chestnut, Japanese:							
raw, 1 oz.	44	.6	9.9	.2	0	4	.3 c
dried, 1 oz.	102	1.5	23.1	.4	0	10	.6 c
boiled or steamed,							
1 oz.	16	.2	3.6	.1	0	1	.1 c
roasted, 1 oz.	57	.8	12.8	.2	0	m.q.	.3 c
Chicken, fresh, 4 oz.,							
except as noted:							
broiler-fryer, roasted:							
w/skin, 1/2 chicken,							
10.5 oz. (15.8 oz.							
w/bone)	715	81.6	0	40.7	263	244	0
w/skin	271	31.0	0	15.4	100	93	0
meat only	215	32.8	0	8.4	101	98	0
meat only, chopped							
or diced, 1 cup	266	40.5	0	10.4	125	120	0
skin only, 1 oz. . .	129	5.8	0	11.5	24	18	0
dark meat only . .	232	31.0	0	11.0	105	105	0
light meat only . .	196	35.1	0	5.1	96	87	0
breast, w/skin,							
1/2 breast, 3.5 oz.							
(8.5 oz. w/bone)	193	29.2	0	7.6	83	69	0
drumstick, w/skin,							
1.8 oz. (2.9 oz.							
w/bone)	112	14.1	0	5.8	48	47	0
leg, w/skin (5.7 oz.							
w/bone)	265	29.6	0	15.4	105	99	0

Food and Measure	cal.	prot. (gms)	carbo. (gms)	fat (gms)	chol. (mgs)	sod. (mgs)	fiber (gms)
Chicken, broiler-fryer, roasted *(cont.)*							
thigh, w/skin, 2.2 oz. (2.9 oz. w/bone)	153	15.5	0	9.6	58	52	0
wing, w/skin, 1.2 oz. (2.3 oz. w/bone)	99	9.1	0	6.6	29	28	0
capon, roasted, w/skin:							
½ capon, 1.4 lbs. (2 lbs. w/bone)	1457	184.5	0	74.2	549	313	0
meat w/skin	260	32.8	0	13.2	98	56	0
roaster, roasted:							
w/skin, ½ chicken, 1 lb. (1.5 lbs. w/bone)	1071	115.0	0	64.3	365	349	0
meat w/skin	253	27.2	0	15.2	86	83	0
stewing, stewed:							
w/skin, ½ chicken, 9.2 oz. (13.5 oz. w/bone)	744	70.2	0	49.2	205	190	0
meat w/skin	323	30.5	0	21.4	90	83	0
meat only	269	34.5	0	13.5	94	88	0
meat only, chopped or diced, 1 cup	332	42.6	0	16.6	117	109	0
Chicken, boneless, and luncheon meat, 1 oz., except as noted:							
bologna, see "Chicken bologna"							
breast:							
(Longacre Gourmet)	34	5.3	.9	1.1	15	202	0
hickory smoked *(Louis Rich)* . . .	30	5.0	<1.0	1.0	15	360	0
hickory smoked *(Tyson)*, 1 slice . . .	25	4.0	.8	1.0	m.q.	195	0
honey flavored *(Tyson)*, 1 slice . . .	25	4.0	.8	1.0	m.q.	m.q.	0

Food and Measure	cal.	prot. (gms)	carbo. (gms)	fat (gms)	chol. (mgs)	sod. (mgs)	fiber (gms)
roast (Oscar Mayer Deli-Thin), 5 slices	60	11.0	2.0	1.5	35	790	0
breast, oven roasted:							
(Longacre Premium)	45	4.3	1.0	2.6	19	333	0
(Louis Rich Thin Sliced), 5 slices	60	10.0	1.0	1.5	25	650	0
(Louis Rich Deluxe)	30	5.0	<1.0	1.0	15	330	0
(Oscar Mayer), 1 slice	25	5.0	<1.0	0	10	290	0
(Oscar Mayer Healthy Favorites), 5 slices	60	12.0	1.0	.5	25	550	0
(Tyson), 1 slice . .	25	3.7	.8	.5	m.q.	185	0
(Weight Watchers)	30	5.0	1.0	1.0	15	230	0
mesquite (Tyson), 1 slice	25	4.0	.8	1.0	m.q.	m.q.	0
breast, smoked:							
(Hillshire Farm Deli Select)	31	6.0	<1.0	.2	m.q.	290	0
(Louis Rich Thin Sliced), 5 slices	60	10.0	1.0	1.5	30	700	0
(Oscar Mayer) . . .	25	5.0	<1.0	0	10	270	0
roll:							
(Tyson), 1 slice . .	26	3.2	1.4	.5	m.q.	153	0
breast (Longacre)	63	4.5	.6	4.5	27	235	0
light meat	45	5.5	.7	2.1	14	166	0
white, oven roasted (Louis Rich)	35	4.0	<1.0	2.0	15	340	0
Chicken, canned, chunk, 2.5 oz.:							
(Hormel)	100	15.0	0	4.0	40	250	0
(Hormel No Salt) . . .	90	16.0	0	3.0	35	25	0
(Swanson Premium)	90	15.0	0	3.0	m.q.	250	0
breast (Hormel) . . .	90	15.0	0	3.0	30	310	0
style (Swanson Mixin' Chicken)	130	13.0	1.0	8.0	m.q.	230	0
white (Swanson Premium)	100	15.0	0	4.0	m.q.	235	0

Food and Measure	cal.	prot. (gms)	carbo. (gms)	fat (gms)	chol. (mgs)	sod. (mgs)	fiber (gms)
Chicken, ground, 1 oz.:							
refrigerated, cooked *(Perdue)*	46	5.0	0	3.0	32	15	0
frozen *(Longacre)* . .	60	4.3	0	4.5	35	15	0
"Chicken," vegetar-ian:							
canned:							
(Worthington Fri-Chik), 2 pieces	180	11.0	4.0	13.0	0	610	m.q.
diced *(Worthington)*, 1/4 cup	90	4.0	2.0	8.0	0	330	m.q.
fried, w/gravy *(LaLoma)*, 2 pieces	140	9.0	4.0	10.0	0	340	m.q.
sliced *(Worthington)*, 2 slices	90	4.0	2.0	8.0	0	330	m.q.
frozen:							
(Worthington Chick-etts), 1/2 cup . .	160	19.0	6.0	7.0	0	640	m.q.
(Worthington Chik-Stiks), 1 stick . . .	110	9.0	4.0	7.0	0	390	m.q.
(Morningstar Farms), 1 patty	170	8.0	13.0	10.0	0	590	m.q.
(Morningstar Farms Country Crisps Patties), 1 patty	220	8.0	13.0	15.0	0	620	m.q.
diced *(Worthington Meatless)*, 1/2 cup	190	13.0	5.0	13.0	0	680	m.q.
fried *(LaLoma)*, 1 piece	180	11.0	2.0	14.0	0	570	m.q.
nuggets *(LaLoma)*, 5 pieces	270	15.0	8.0	20.0	0	530	m.q.
nuggets *(Worthing-ton Crispy Chik)*, 6 pieces	280	10.0	17.0	19.0	0	500	m.q.

Food and Measure	cal.	prot. (gms)	carbo. (gms)	fat (gms)	chol. (mgs)	sod. (mgs)	fiber (gms)
patties (Worthington Crispy Chik), 1 patty	220	8.0	13.0	15.0	0	620	m.q.
pie (Worthington), 1 pie	380	7.0	43.0	20.0	0	1200	m.q.
sliced (Worthington), 2 slices	130	9.0	3.0	9.0	0	460	m.q.
mix, supreme (LaLoma), 1/4 cup	50	9.0	4.0	0	0	450	m.q.
Chicken bologna:							
(Perdue), 1-oz. slice	64	4.0	2.0	5.0	31	290	0
(Tyson), 1 slice	44	2.2	3.7	.5	m.q.	185	0
Chicken dinner, frozen:							
à la king (Armour Classics Lite), 11.25 oz.	290	19.0	38.0	7.0	55	630	m.q.
baked (Swanson Hungry Man), 15 oz. . . .	740	42.0	57.0	38.0	m.q.	1340	m.q.
w/barbecue sauce (Healthy Choice), 12.75 oz.	380	24.0	57.0	6.0	60	560	m.q.
barbecue (Tyson Healthy Portion), 12.5 oz.	400	27.0	56.0	8.0	50	600	m.q.
boneless (Swanson Hungry Man), 17.25 oz.	670	36.0	71.0	27.0	m.q.	1260	m.q.
breast, 11 oz.: herbed, w/fettuccini (The Budget Gourmet Light and Healthy) . .	240	21.0	30.0	6.0	45	430	m.q.
mesquite (The Budget Gourmet Light and Healthy) . .	250	23.0	33.0	6.0	40	550	m.q.
Burgundy (Armour Classics Lite), 10 oz.	210	23.0	25.0	2.0	45	780	m.q.

Food and Measure	cal.	prot. (gms)	carbo. (gms)	fat (gms)	chol. (mgs)	sod. (mgs)	fiber (gms)
Chicken dinner, frozen *(cont.)*							
Cordon Bleu, grilled *(Le Menu New American Cuisine)*, 10.5 oz.	390	27.0	34.0	16.0	m.q.	960	m.q.
Dijon *(Healthy Choice)*, 11 oz.	250	21.0	40.0	3.0	40	470	m.q.
Français *(Tyson Premium)*, 9.5 oz. . . .	280	19.0	20.0	14.0	54	1130	m.q.
fried:							
(Banquet Extra Helping), 14.25 oz.	790	33.0	68.0	43.0	150	1490	m.q.
barbecue flavored *(Swanson)*, 10 oz.	550	25.0	61.0	23.0	m.q.	1170	m.q.
dark meat *(Swanson, 4 Compartment)*, 9.75 oz.	560	21.0	55.0	28.0	m.q.	1130	m.q.
dark meat *(Swanson Hungry Man)*, 14.25 oz.	860	36.0	77.0	45.0	m.q.	1660	m.q.
Southern *(Banquet Extra Helping)*, 13.25 oz.	790	35.0	75.0	39.0	135	2390	m.q.
thigh meat *(Freezer Queen)*, 10 oz.	400	21.0	39.0	17.0	65	790	m.q.
white meat *(Banquet Extra Helping)*, 14.25 oz.	760	36.0	69.0	38.0	120	1770	m.q.
white meat *(Freezer Queen)*, 10 oz.	400	13.0	47.0	13.0	60	1150	m.q.
white meat *(Swanson)*, 10.25 oz.	550	22.0	59.0	25.0	m.q.	1410	m.q.
white meat *(Swanson Hungry Man Mostly White)*, 14.25 oz.	870	35.0	80.0	46.0	m.q.	2150	m.q.

Food and Measure	cal.	prot. (gms)	carbo. (gms)	fat (gms)	chol. (mgs)	sod. (mgs)	fiber (gms)
garlic (Swanson Hungry Man), 16.5 oz.	500	27.0	55.0	19.0	m.q.	1450	m.q.
glazed:							
(Armour Classics), 10.75 oz.	300	15.0	24.0	16.0	60	960	m.q.
golden (Le Menu New American Cuisine Healthy), 11 oz.	330	23.0	52.0	3.0	30	420	m.q.
w/sauce (Tyson Premium), 9.25 oz.	240	22.0	29.0	4.0	44	930	m.q.
grilled:							
(Tyson Premium), 7.75 oz.	220	26.0	22.0	3.0	55	520	m.q.
(Swanson Hungry Man), 17 oz. . . .	660	33.0	78.0	24.0	m.q.	1760	m.q.
w/almonds (Swanson), 10 oz. . . .	310	17.0	39.0	9.0	30	630	m.q.
herb:							
(Tyson Healthy Portion), 13.75 oz.	340	32.0	43.0	4.0	50	550	m.q.
roasted (Healthy Choice), 11.5 oz.	380	26.0	56.0	7.0	60	470	m.q.
roasted (Le Menu New American Cuisine Healthy), 10 oz.	300	22.0	43.0	4.0	30	470	m.q.
honey mustard:							
(Tyson Healthy Portion), 13.75 oz.	390	31.0	52.0	6.0	50	520	m.q.
grilled (Le Menu New American Cuisine), 9 oz. . .	390	20.0	50.0	12.0	m.q.	670	m.q.
honey roasted (Tyson Premium), 9 oz. . .	220	26.0	23.0	4.0	48	500	m.q.
Italian:							
grilled (Tyson Premium), 9 oz.	210	28.0	19.0	3.0	40	420	m.q.

Food and Measure	cal.	prot. (gms)	carbo. (gms)	fat (gms)	chol. (mgs)	sod. (mgs)	fiber (gms)
Chicken dinner, frozen, Italian *(cont.)*							
style *(Tyson* Healthy Portion), 13.75 oz.	310	30.0	38.0	4.0	50	600	m.q.
Kiev *(Tyson* Premium), 9.25 oz.	450	18.0	39.0	25.0	78	950	m.q.
marinara *(Tyson* Healthy Portion), 13.75 oz.	340	31.0	37.0	7.0	45	590	m.q.
Marsala:							
(Armour Classics Lite), 10.5 oz. . .	250	20.0	27.0	7.0	80	930	m.q.
(Tyson Premium), 9 oz.	200	22.0	19.0	4.0	52	670	m.q.
mesquite:							
(Armour Classics), 9.5 oz.	370	15.0	42.0	16.0	55	660	m.q.
(Healthy Choice), 10.5 oz.	300	21.0	54.0	3.0	40	390	m.q.
(Le Menu New American Cuisine Healthy), 10.25 oz.	300	19.0	48.0	3.0	30	290	m.q.
(Tyson Healthy Portion), 13.25 oz.	330	34.0	38.0	5.0	45	600	m.q.
(Tyson Premium), 9 oz.	320	23.0	39.0	8.0	55	660	m.q.
and noodles *(Armour Classics)*, 11 oz. . .	230	19.0	23.0	7.0	50	660	m.q.
nuggets:							
(Freezer Queen), 6 oz.	310	12.0	33.0	15.0	15	830	m.q.
(Swanson), 8.75 oz.	470	19.0	48.0	23.0	m.q.	670	m.q.
w/barbecue or sweet and sour sauce *(Banquet Extra Helping)*, 10 oz.	540	32.0	68.0	19.0	80	2330	m.q.

Food and Measure	cal.	prot. (gms)	carbo. (gms)	fat (gms)	chol. (mgs)	sod. (mgs)	fiber (gms)
Oriental:							
(Armour Classics Lite), 10 oz. . . .	180	18.0	24.0	1.0	35	660	m.q.
(Healthy Choice), 11.25 oz.	200	19.0	32.0	1.0	35	440	m.q.
parmigiana:							
(Armour Classics), 11.5 oz.	370	22.0	27.0	19.0	75	1060	m.q.
(Healthy Choice), 11.5 oz.	290	23.0	41.0	6.0	55	340	m.q.
(Swanson 4 Compartment), 11.5 oz.	400	16.0	42.0	19.0	m.q.	1050	m.q.
(Tyson Premium), 11.25 oz.	380	19.0	37.0	17.0	36	1100	m.q.
breast (The Budget Gourmet Light and Healthy), 11 oz.	270	22.0	30.0	9.0	50	530	m.q.
breast (Le Menu New American Cuisine), 10.25 oz.	340	22.0	28.0	16.0	m.q.	870	m.q.
and pasta divan (Healthy Choice), 12.1 oz.	300	25.0	41.0	4.0	50	520	m.q.
pasta primavera (Le Menu New American Cuisine), 11.5 oz.	330	21.0	40.0	10.0	m.q.	830	m.q.
patty (Freezer Queen), 7.5 oz.	290	14.0	29.0	14.0	20	750	m.q.
picante (Tyson Premium), 9 oz.	250	28.0	26.0	4.0	50	390	m.q.
picatta (Tyson Premium), 9 oz.	200	24.0	18.0	4.0	60	550	m.q.
roast, homestyle gravy (The Budget Gourmet Light and Healthy), 11 oz. . .	280	20.0	36.0	8.0	35	560	m.q.

Food and Measure	cal.	prot. (gms)	carbo. (gms)	fat (gms)	chol. (mgs)	sod. (mgs)	fiber (gms)
Chicken dinner, frozen *(cont.)*							
roasted *(Tyson Premium)*, 9 oz.	200	21.0	21.0	2.0	42	430	m.q.
salsa:							
(Healthy Choice), 11.25 oz.	240	20.0	36.0	2.0	50	450	m.q.
(Le Menu New American Cuisine Healthy), 10.75 oz.	300	20.0	45.0	4.0	35	340	m.q.
(Tyson Healthy Portion), 13.75 oz.	370	34.0	52.0	6.0	45	470	m.q.
Santa Fe style, grilled *(Le Menu New American Cuisine)*, 10 oz.	320	20.0	37.0	10.0	m.q.	600	m.q.
sesame *(Tyson Healthy Portion)*, 13.5 oz.	400	27.0	59.0	6.0	45	400	m.q.
Southwestern style *(Healthy Choice)*, 12.5 oz.	340	25.0	51.0	5.0	60	550	m.q.
supreme *(Tyson Premium)*, 9 oz.	230	21.0	23.0	6.0	51	480	m.q.
sweet and sour:							
(Armour Classics Lite), 11 oz. . . .	240	18.0	39.0	2.0	35	820	m.q.
(Healthy Choice), 11.5 oz.	280	20.0	52.0	2.0	35	320	m.q.
(Le Menu New American Cuisine), 11.25 oz.	360	22.0	47.0	9.0	m.q.	720	m.q.
(Tyson Premium), 11 oz.	420	22.0	50.0	15.0	m.q.	850	m.q.
teriyaki:							
(The Budget Gourmet Light and Healthy), 11 oz.	300	18.0	41.0	8.0	30	480	m.q.

Food and Measure	cal.	prot. (gms)	carbo. (gms)	fat (gms)	chol. (mgs)	sod. (mgs)	fiber (gms)
(Healthy Choice),							
12.25 oz.	290	24.0	39.0	4.0	55	560	m.q.
tomato garden *(Le Menu New American Cuisine),* 10 oz.	240	22.0	24.0	6.0	m.q.	780	m.q.
w/wine and mushroom sauce *(Armour Classics),* 10.75 oz. . .	280	22.0	24.0	11.0	50	900	m.q.
Chicken entree, canned or packaged:							
à la king:							
(Hormel Top Shelf),							
10 oz.	360	18.0	49.0	10.0	37	890	m.q.
(Swanson), 5.25 oz.	190	10.0	9.0	12.0	m.q.	690	m.q.
breast, 10 oz.:							
glazed *(Hormel Top Shelf)*	170	19.0	19.0	2.0	35	780	m.q.
w/Spanish rice *(Hormel Top Shelf)* . .	400	27.0	38.0	15.0	75	810	m.q.
cacciatore *(Hormel Top Shelf),* 10 oz.	210	21.0	25.0	3.0	50	810	m.q.
chow mein:							
(La Choy), 3/4 cup	70	6.0	5.0	4.0	16	850	2.0 d
(La Choy Bi-Pack), 3/4 cup	80	7.0	8.0	3.0	18	970	1.0 d
(La Choy Dinner), 1/2 pkg.	300	12.0	29.0	17.0	16	1800	2.0 d
and dumplings:							
(Dinty Moore), 7.5 oz.	166	12.0	17.0	5.0	19	683	m.q.
(Swanson), 7.5 oz.	220	11.0	19.0	11.0	m.q.	980	m.q.
stew:							
(Dinty Moore), 7.5 oz.	260	11.0	15.0	18.0	80	850	m.q.
(Swanson), 7.6 oz.	160	9.0	15.0	7.0	m.q.	990	m.q.

Food and Measure	cal.	prot. (gms)	carbo. (gms)	fat (gms)	chol. (mgs)	sod. (mgs)	fiber (gms)
Chicken entree, canned or packaged (cont.)							
sweet and sour, 3/4 cup:							
(La Choy)	240	8.0	47.0	2.0	19	1420	1.0 d
(La Choy Bi-Pack)	120	7.0	18.0	2.0	13	440	2.0 d
teriyaki (La Choy Bi-Pack), 3/4 cup . . .	85	8.0	8.0	2.0	20	850	1.0 d
Chicken entree, freeze-dried (Mountain House), 1 cup*:							
à la king	300	18.0	33.0	10.0	m.q.	1350	m.q.
Polynesian	210	10.0	33.0	4.0	m.q.	810	m.q.
stew	230	9.0	30.0	8.0	m.q.	1200	m.q.
Chicken entree, frozen:							
à la king:							
(Dining Lite), 9 oz.	240	14.0	30.0	7.0	40	780	m.q.
(Freezer Queen Cook-in-Pouch), 4 oz.	60	7.0	7.0	1.0	10	420	n.a.
(Stouffer's Lunch Express), 97/8 oz.	350	21.0	41.0	11.0	m.q.	930	m.q.
w/rice (Stouffer's), 9.5 oz.	270	18.0	38.0	5.0	m.q.	800	m.q.
à l'orange:							
(Healthy Choice), 9 oz.	260	23.0	38.0	2.0	40	340	m.q.
w/almond rice (Lean Cuisine), 8 oz. . .	280	27.0	33.0	4.0	55	290	m.q.
au gratin (The Budget Gourmet Light and Healthy), 9.1 oz. . . .	230	18.0	23.0	8.0	40	820	m.q.
barbecue:							
(Banquet Meals), 9 oz.	310	18.0	37.0	12.0	60	810	m.q.
glazed (Weight Watchers Ultimate 200), 6.5 oz. . . .	180	17.0	16.0	5.0	25	300	n.a.

Food and Measure	cal.	prot. (gms)	carbo. (gms)	fat (gms)	chol. (mgs)	sod. (mgs)	fiber (gms)
sauce, w/pilaf (Lean Cuisine), 8.75 oz.	260	20.0	32.0	6.0	50	500	m.q.
breast:							
baked, nuggets, patties, or tenders (Banquet Healthy Balance), 2.25 oz.	120	12.0	8.0	4.0	30	310	n.a.
baked, whipped potatoes (Stouffer's Homestyle), 8⅞ oz.	250	22.0	18.0	10.0	m.q.	550	m.q.
batter dipped (Weaver), 4.4 oz.	310	20.0	13.0	20.0	m.q.	220	m.q.
breaded, Parmesan (Lean Cuisine), 10⅞ oz.	260	24.0	25.0	7.0	60	580	m.q.
chunks (Tyson), 3 oz.	240	13.0	10.0	17.0	30	430	m.q.
fillet (Tyson), 3 oz.	190	13.0	15.0	9.0	25	400	m.q.
fillet (Weaver), 4.5 oz.	270	20.0	18.0	13.0	m.q.	520	m.q.
fillet, barbecue (Tyson), 3 oz.	110	14.0	6.0	3.0	35	310	n.a.
fillet, grilled (Tyson), 2.75 oz.	100	15.0	4.0	3.0	45	410	n.a.
fillet, Mesquite (Tyson), 2.75 oz. . .	100	16.0	3.0	2.0	50	250	n.a.
fillet, Southern fried (Tyson), 3 oz. . .	220	14.0	15.0	11.0	25	630	m.q.
fillet strips (Tyson), 3.3 oz.	200	13.0	14.0	10.0	m.q.	500	m.q.
fried (Weaver Crispy Dutch Frye), 4.5 oz.	350	22.0	17.0	22.0	m.q.	520	m.q.
fried, whipped potato (Stouffer's Homestyle), 7⅛ oz.	350	17.0	30.0	18.0	m.q.	900	m.q.

Food and Measure	cal.	prot. (gms)	carbo. (gms)	fat (gms)	chol. (mgs)	sod. (mgs)	fiber (gms)
Chicken entree, frozen, breast *(cont.)*							
glazed *(Healthy Choice)*, 8.5 oz.	220	21.0	27.0	3.0	45	390	m.q.
grilled, barbecue sauce *(Stouffer's Homestyle)*, 7⅝ oz.	210	23.0	14.0	7.0	m.q.	550	m.q.
Marsala w/vegetables *(Lean Cuisine)*, 8⅛ oz.	180	22.0	13.0	4.0	55	430	m.q.
oven baked, breaded *(Lean Cuisine)*, 8 oz.	200	17.0	21.0	5.0	35	480	m.q.
patties *(Tyson)*, 2.6 oz.	220	10.0	11.0	15.0	35	640	m.q.
patties *(Weaver)*, 3 oz.	205	12.0	14.0	11.0	m.q.	640	m.q.
patties, Southern fried *(Tyson)*, 2.6 oz.	220	11.0	9.0	15.0	35	460	m.q.
portions, fried *(Banquet)*, 5.75 oz.	220	16.0	13.0	11.0	m.q.	710	m.q.
strips, Mesquite *(Tyson)*, 2.75 oz.	100	17.0	2.0	2.0	50	240	0
breast tenders:							
(Banquet Hot Bites), 2.25 oz.	150	11.0	12.0	6.0	m.q.	280	m.q.
(Tyson), 3 oz.	220	14.0	13.0	12.0	m.q.	500	m.q.
(Tyson Microwave), 3.5 oz.	230	16.0	19.0	11.0	m.q.	600	m.q.
(Weaver Premium), 3 oz.	170	12.0	11.0	9.0	m.q.	500	m.q.
breaded, O'Brien potatoes *(Stouffer's Homestyle)*, 8⅜ oz.	430	20.0	46.0	18.0	m.q.	950	m.q.
honey batter *(Weaver)*, 3 oz.	220	13.0	14.0	12.0	m.q.	500	m.q.

Food and Measure	cal.	prot. (gms)	carbo. (gms)	fat (gms)	chol. (mgs)	sod. (mgs)	fiber (gms)
hot barbecue (Tyson), 2.75 oz. . . .	110	16.0	4.0	3.0	45	580	n.a.
mesquite (Tyson), 2.75 oz.	110	17.0	4.0	3.0	45	420	n.a.
Southern fried (Banquet Hot Bites), 2.25 oz.	160	10.0	13.0	7.0	m.q.	340	m.q.
w/spaghetti swirls (On-Cor), 8 oz.	209	12.0	29.0	6.0	m.q.	1065	m.q.
cacciatore, w/vermicelli (Lean Cuisine), 10⅞ oz.	280	22.0	31.0	7.0	45	570	m.q.
cannelloni, see "Cannelloni entree"							
w/cheddar (Tyson Chick 'n Cheddar), 2.6 oz.	220	11.0	11.0	15.0	40	310	n.a.
chow mein:							
(Banquet Meals), 9 oz.	240	9.0	29.0	9.0	35	1070	m.q.
(Chun King), 13 oz.	370	25.0	53.0	6.0	85	1560	m.q.
(Dining Lite), 9 oz.	180	10.0	31.0	2.0	30	650	m.q.
(Healthy Choice), 9 oz.	240	20.0	29.0	5.0	45	530	m.q.
(Stouffer's Lunch Express), 10⅝ oz.	270	12.0	47.0	4.0	m.q.	790	m.q.
(Weight Watchers Smart Ones), 9 oz.	170	14.0	27.0	1.0	20	470	m.q.
w/rice (Stouffer's), 10.75 oz.	250	13.0	39.0	5.0	m.q.	720	m.q.
w/rice (Lean Cuisine), 9 oz. . . .	240	14.0	34.0	5.0	30	530	m.q.
chunks:							
(Country Skillet), 3 oz.	260	10.0	17.0	16.0	25	470	m.q.
(Tyson Chick'n Chunks), 2.6 oz.	220	10.0	11.0	15.0	35	500	n.a.

Food and Measure	cal.	prot. (gms)	carbo. (gms)	fat (gms)	chol. (mgs)	sod. (mgs)	fiber (gms)
Chicken entree, frozen, chunks (cont.)							
(*Tyson* Microwave), 3.5 oz.	220	10.0	11.0	15.0	m.q.	m.q.	n.a.
Southern fried (*Country Skillet*), 3 oz.	270	11.0	15.0	18.0	30	570	m.q.
Southern fried (*Tyson* Chick'n Chunks), 2.6 oz.	220	10.0	11.0	15.0	35	540	m.q.
Cordon Bleu (*Weight Watchers Ultimate 200*), 7.7 oz.	170	19.0	15.0	5.0	40	560	n.a.
creamed (*Stouffer's*), 6.5 oz.	300	19.0	8.0	21.0	m.q.	690	m.q.
croquettes:							
(*Freezer Queen* Family), 7 oz. . .	240	12.0	20.0	12.0	m.q.	1000	m.q.
w/gravy (*Weaver*), 2 croquettes, 1/2 gravy cup . .	306	15.0	26.0	18.0	m.q.	1040	m.q.
diced (*Tyson*), 3 oz.	130	24.0	1.0	3.0	70	40	0
divan (*Stouffer's*), 8 oz.	220	24.0	11.0	10.0	m.q.	610	m.q.
drumsticks:							
(*Banquet Drum-Snackers*), 2.5 oz.	210	9.0	12.0	14.0	m.q.	510	m.q.
crispy (*Weaver* Mini Drums), 3 oz. . .	210	13.0	13.0	12.0	m.q.	480	m.q.
herb and spice (*Weaver* Mini Drums), 3 oz. . .	200	13.0	13.0	11.0	m.q.	320	m.q.
drumsticks and thighs:							
batter dipped (*Weaver*), 3 oz.	210	11.0	11.0	14.0	m.q.	220	m.q.
fried (*Weaver* Crispy Dutch Frye), 3.5 oz.	290	16.0	14.0	19.0	m.q.	640	m.q.

Food and Measure	cal.	prot. (gms)	carbo. (gms)	fat (gms)	chol. (mgs)	sod. (mgs)	fiber (gms)
dumplings and *(Banquet* Family), 7 oz.	280	12.0	28.0	14.0	m.q.	m.q.	m.q.
and dumplings *(Banquet* Meals), 10 oz.	250	13.0	35.0	8.0	35	780	m.q.
enchilada, see "Enchilada entree"							
escalloped, w/noodles *(Stouffer's)*, 10 oz.	420	21.0	30.0	24.0	m.q.	840	m.q.
fajita, see "Fajita entree"							
fettuccine, see "Fettuccine entree"							
w/fettuccine *(The Budget Gourmet)*, 10 oz.	400	24.0	29.0	21.0	85	700	m.q.
fiesta:							
(Lean Cuisine), 8.5 oz.	240	19.0	30.0	5.0	40	560	m.q.
(Weight Watchers Smart Ones), 8 oz.	210	14.0	37.0	1.0	20	390	m.q.
Français *(Weight Watcher's Smart Ones)*, 8.5 oz. . . .	150	15.0	18.0	1.0	5	400	m.q.
French recipe *(The Budget Gourmet Light and Healthy)*, 10 oz.	220	17.0	21.0	9.0	40	870	m.q.
fried:							
(Banquet Meals), 9 oz.	520	22.0	41.0	29.0	90	1130	m.q.
(Swanson Plump & Juicy), 3.25 oz.	270	15.0	16.0	16.0	m.q.	650	m.q.
breast half *(Swanson Plump & Juicy)*, 4.5 oz. . .	360	23.0	21.0	20.0	m.q.	800	m.q.
hot'n spicy *(Banquet)*, 6.4 oz. . .	330	18.0	29.0	19.0	m.q.	1210	m.q.

Food and Measure	cal.	prot. (gms)	carbo. (gms)	fat (gms)	chol. (mgs)	sod. (mgs)	fiber (gms)
Chicken entree, frozen, fried *(cont.)*							
hot'n spicy *(Banquet Snack'n)*, 3.75 oz.	140	6.0	8.0	9.0	m.q.	480	n.a.
nibbles *(Swanson)*, 3.25 oz.	300	12.0	19.0	19.0	m.q.	690	m.q.
original or Southern *(Banquet)*, 5.6 oz.	290	15.0	26.0	17.0	m.q.	1060	m.q.
and whipped potatoes *(Swanson)*, 7 oz.	400	18.0	34.0	21.0	m.q.	1080	m.q.
spicy *(Swanson Take-Out)*, 3.25 oz.	270	14.0	17.0	16.0	m.q.	700	m.q.
thighs and drumsticks *(Banquet)*, 6.25 oz.	250	14.0	14.0	14.0	m.q.	790	m.q.
ginger, vegetable Hunan and *(Weight Watchers Stir-Fry)*, 9 oz.	160	15.0	21.0	2.0	15	430	m.q.
glazed, w/vegetable rice *(Lean Cuisine)*, 8.5 oz.	250	21.0	24.0	7.0	50	590	m.q.
grilled, glazed *(Weight Watchers Ultimate 200)*, 7.5 oz.	150	15.0	17.0	2.0	20	520	n.a.
honey mustard:							
(Healthy Choice), 9.5 oz.	250	24.0	37.0	3.0	40	480	n.a.
(Lean Cuisine), 7.5 oz.	230	18.0	30.0	4.0	40	540	n.a.
imperial:							
(Chun King), 13 oz.	300	17.0	54.0	1.0	30	1540	m.q.
(Weight Watchers Ultimate 200), 8.5 oz.	200	18.0	25.0	3.0	25	420	m.q.

Food and Measure	cal.	prot. (gms)	carbo. (gms)	fat (gms)	chol. (mgs)	sod. (mgs)	fiber (gms)
Italiano, w/fettuccine and vegetables (*Lean Cuisine*), 9 oz.	270	22.0	33.0	6.0	40	590	m.q.
Kiev (*Weight Watchers Ultimate 200*), 7 oz.	190	14.0	22.0	5.0	15	470	m.q.
mandarin:							
(*The Budget Gourmet Light and Healthy*), 10 oz.	240	15.0	38.0	5.0	40	710	m.q.
(*Healthy Choice*), 10 oz.	240	21.0	35.0	2.0	45	370	m.q.
Marsala (*The Budget Gourmet*), 9 oz.	260	17.0	31.0	8.0	90	730	m.q.
mesquite (*Banquet Healthy Balance*), 10.5 oz.	310	21.0	36.0	9.0	45	800	m.q.
mirabella (*Weight Watchers Smart Ones*), 9.2 oz.	160	13.0	26.0	1.0	10	420	m.q.
nibbles, w/french fries (*Swanson*), 4.25 oz.	330	10.0	30.0	19.0	m.q.	730	m.q.
and noodles:							
(*Banquet Entree Express*), 8.5 oz.	240	16.0	23.0	10.0	m.q.	1120	m.q.
(*Dining Lite*), 9 oz.	240	17.0	28.0	7.0	50	570	m.q.
(*Stouffer's Homestyle*), 10 oz.	290	22.0	21.0	13.0	m.q.	1040	m.q.
(*Swanson*), 9 oz.	310	14.0	30.0	15.0	m.q.	990	m.q.
(*Weight Watchers*), 9 oz.	240	19.0	25.0	7.0	30	450	m.q.
egg noodles (*The Budget Gourmet*), 10 oz.	440	24.0	28.0	26.0	90	880	m.q.
nuggets:							
(*Banquet Hot Bites*), 2.5 oz.	200	10.0	10.0	13.0	m.q.	530	m.q.
(*Banquet Meals*), 6.75 oz.	400	18.0	38.0	21.0	50	660	m.q.

Food and Measure	cal.	prot. (gms)	carbo. (gms)	fat (gms)	chol. (mgs)	sod. (mgs)	fiber (gms)
Chicken entree, frozen, nuggets *(cont.)*							
(Country Skillet),							
3 oz.	250	13.0	14.0	15.0	40	580	m.q.
(Freezer Queen							
Family), 7 oz. . .	290	15.0	16.0	18.0	m.q.	1180	m.q.
(Swanson), 3 oz. . .	230	13.0	14.0	14.0	m.q.	360	m.q.
(Weaver), 2.6 oz.	190	10.0	10.0	12.0	m.q.	450	m.q.
(Weight Watchers),							
5.9 oz.	220	16.0	23.0	7.0	40	500	m.q.
w/cheddar *(Banquet*							
Hot Bites), 2.5 oz.	240	10.0	10.0	17.0	m.q.	530	m.q.
w/french fries							
(Swanson),							
4.75 oz.	290	12.0	30.0	14.0	m.q.	550	m.q.
hot'n spicy *(Banquet*							
Hot Bites), 2.5 oz.	240	10.0	10.0	18.0	m.q.	360	m.q.
Southern fried *(Ban-*							
quet Hot Bites),							
2.5 oz.	210	10.0	12.0	14.0	m.q.	500	m.q.
orange glazed:							
(The Budget Gour-							
met Light and							
Healthy), 9 oz.	270	17.0	46.0	3.0	25	870	m.q.
w/rice *(Weight*							
Watchers Stir-Fry),							
9 oz.	170	14.0	25.0	2.0	10	360	m.q.
Oriental:							
(Banquet Meals),							
9 oz.	300	11.0	37.0	12.0	40	780	m.q.
(Freezer Queen),							
8.5 oz.	200	20.0	21.0	4.0	27	640	m.q.
w/peanut sauce							
(Healthy Choice),							
9.5 oz.	280	29.0	31.0	5.0	45	400	m.q.
w/vegetables *(The*							
Budget Gourmet),							
9 oz.	280	19.0	44.0	6.0	20	690	m.q.

Food and Measure	cal.	prot. (gms)	carbo. (gms)	fat (gms)	chol. (mgs)	sod. (mgs)	fiber (gms)
w/vegetables, vermicelli (Lean Cuisine), 9 oz. . . .	280	22.0	31.0	7.0	35	480	m.q.
Parmesan (Banquet Healthy Balance), 10.8 oz.	300	21.0	34.0	9.0	50	800	m.q.
parmigiana:							
(Banquet Meals), 9.5 oz.	280	14.0	27.0	14.0	50	900	m.q.
(Celentano), 9 oz.	380	33.0	17.0	22.0	100	550	4.0 d
(Freezer Queen), 8.5 oz.	370	12.0	42.0	17.0	20	1440	m.q.
(On-Cor), 8 oz. . .	343	18.0	26.0	19.0	m.q.	1450	m.q.
and pasta Alfredo (Stouffer's Homestyle), 10 5/8 oz.	310	28.0	31.0	8.0	m.q.	550	m.q.
patties:							
(Banquet Hot Bites), 2.5 oz.	190	11.0	11.0	12.0	m.q.	440	m.q.
(Country Skillet), 3 oz.	230	12.0	14.0	15.0	40	560	m.q.
(Tyson Thick & Crispy), 2.6 oz.	220	11.0	13.0	14.0	40	490	m.q.
Southern fried (Banquet Hot Bites), 2.5 oz.	200	10.0	12.0	12.0	m.q.	590	m.q.
Southern fried (Country Skillet), 3 oz.	240	11.0	14.0	15.0	35	540	m.q.
piccata, lemon herb (Weight Watchers Smart Ones), 7.5 oz.	160	13.0	25.0	1.0	5	500	m.q.
pie:							
(Freezer Queen Family), 7 oz. . .	220	9.0	25.0	9.0	m.q.	670	m.q.
(Stouffer's), 10 oz.	520	22.0	37.0	32.0	m.q.	950	m.q.
(Swanson), 7 oz. . .	390	10.0	35.0	23.0	m.q.	760	m.q.

Food and Measure	cal.	prot. (gms)	carbo. (gms)	fat (gms)	chol. (mgs)	sod. (mgs)	fiber (gms)
Chicken entree, frozen, pie *(cont.)*							
(Swanson Deluxe),							
9 oz.	410	15.0	39.0	22.0	m.q.	1020	m.q.
(Swanson Hungry							
Man), 16 oz. . . .	700	26.0	57.0	40.0	m.q.	1560	m.q.
Polynesian *(Weight*							
Watchers Stir-Fry),							
9 oz.	190	12.0	34.0	1.0	20	240	m.q.
primavera *(Celentano),*							
11.5 oz.	230	23.0	27.0	7.0	40	630	7.0 d
rondolet *(Weaver):*							
original, 3 oz. . . .	190	13.0	13.0	10.0	m.q.	610	m.q.
cheese, 2.6 oz. . .	190	11.0	12.0	11.0	m.q.	520	m.q.
Italian, 2.6 oz. . . .	190	11.0	11.0	11.0	m.q.	560	m.q.
sandwich, see							
"Chicken sandwich"							
sesame, w/lo mein							
noodles *(Weight*							
Watchers Stir-Fry),							
9 oz.	200	19.0	23.0	4.0	10	420	m.q.
skinless *(Weaver*							
Crispy Light), 2.9 oz.	170	14.0	9.0	9.0	m.q.	320	n.a.
sliced, gravy and							
(Freezer Queen							
Cook-in-Pouch),							
4 oz.	70	5.0	4.0	3.0	10	600	n.a.
Southern baked							
(Weight Watchers							
Ultimate 200),							
6.3 oz.	170	17.0	10.0	7.0	45	520	n.a.
sticks *(Banquet Hot*							
Bites), 2.5 oz. . . .	210	10.0	10.0	14.0	m.q.	340	m.q.
stir-fry, w/pasta							
(Healthy Choice Ex-							
tra Portion), 12 oz.	300	23.0	42.0	5.0	30	550	m.q.
sweet and sour:							
(Banquet Healthy							
Balance),							
10.25 oz.	270	11.0	47.0	4.0	35	590	m.q.

Food and Measure	cal.	prot. (gms)	carbo. (gms)	fat (gms)	chol. (mgs)	sod. (mgs)	fiber (gms)
(The Budget Gourmet), 10 oz. . . .	340	17.0	55.0	5.0	30	620	m.q.
(Freezer Queen), 9 oz.	240	11.0	46.0	1.0	15	640	m.q.
w/rice *(Lean Cuisine)*, 9 oz. . . .	280	17.0	39.0	6.0	50	490	m.q.
tenderloins:							
in herb cream sauce *(Lean Cuisine)*, 9.5 oz.	240	29.0	19.0	5.0	60	490	m.q.
in peanut sauce *(Lean Cuisine)*, 9 oz.	290	23.0	33.0	7.0	45	530	m.q.
teriyaki:							
(Weight Watchers Ultimate 200), 7.6 oz.	150	21.0	7.0	4.0	50	590	n.a.
spring vegetables *(Weight Watchers Stir-Fry)*, 9 oz. . . .	140	13.0	16.0	3.0	20	470	m.q.
thighs and drumsticks *(Swanson* Plump & Juicy), 3.25 oz. . .	290	15.0	17.0	18.0	m.q.	610	m.q.
and vegetables:							
(Freezer Queen), 9 oz.	200	16.0	30.0	2.5	35	510	m.q.
(Healthy Choice), 11.5 oz.	280	24.0	39.0	3.0	25	380	m.q.
primavera *(Banquet Cookin' Bag)*, 4 oz.	100	6.0	14.0	2.0	m.q.	m.q.	m.q.
primavera *(Banquet Family)*, 7 oz. . .	140	9.0	18.0	3.0	m.q.	m.q.	m.q.
w/vermicelli *(Lean Cuisine)*, 11.75 oz.	240	18.0	30.0	5.0	30	500	m.q.
walnut, crunchy *(Chun King)*, 13 oz.	310	16.0	49.0	5.0	45	1700	m.q.

Food and Measure	cal.	prot. (gms)	carbo. (gms)	fat (gms)	chol. (mgs)	sod. (mgs)	fiber (gms)
Chicken entree, frozen (cont.)							
wings:							
(Banquet Meals),							
8.75 oz.	390	33.0	37.0	13.0	80	1620	m.q.
all varieties (Tyson),							
3.5 oz.	218	23.0	0	14.0	m.q.	400	0
batter dipped							
(Weaver), 4 oz.	400	16.0	20.0	28.0	m.q.	520	m.q.
fried (Weaver Crispy							
Dutch Frye), 4 oz.	400	16.0	20.0	28.0	m.q.	520	m.q.
hot (Weaver), 2.7 oz.	170	17.0	1.0	11.0	m.q.	670	0
Chicken entree, mix*:							
broccoli, cheesy (Skil-							
let Chicken Helper),							
7 oz.	310	24.0	34.0	9.0	65	790	m.q.
creamy (Skillet							
Chicken Helper),							
8.25 oz.	330	26.0	29.0	13.0	100	820	m.q.
fettuccine Alfredo							
(Skillet Chicken							
Helper), 7.5 oz. . .	320	26.0	27.0	12.0	70	780	m.q.
mushroom, creamy							
(Skillet Chicken							
Helper), 8 oz. . . .	320	25.0	31.0	11.0	90	810	m.q.
stir-fried (Skillet							
Chicken Helper),							
7 oz.	370	25.0	36.0	14.0	145	950	m.q.
sweet and sour (La							
Choy Dinner Clas-							
sics), 3/4 cup . . .	310	32.0	30.0	6.0	50	860	<1.0 d
Chicken entree, re-							
frigerated:							
barbecue, 1 oz.:							
breast half (Perdue							
Done It!)	46	7.0	1.0	2.0	28	150	0
drumstick (Perdue							
Done It!)	53	6.0	2.0	2.0	34	106	0

Food and Measure	cal.	prot. (gms)	carbo. (gms)	fat (gms)	chol. (mgs)	sod. (mgs)	fiber (gms)
half, dark meat *(Perdue Done It!)* . .	57	5.0	1.0	4.0	31	108	0
half, white meat *(Perdue Done It!)*	40	7.0	1.0	1.0	22	110	0
thigh *(Perdue Done It!)*	59	6.0	1.0	3.0	37	98	0
wings *(Perdue Done It!)*	62	6.0	1.0	4.0	35	169	0
breast cutlet *(Perdue Done It!)*, 3.5 oz.	250	14.0	17.0	14.0	39	445	m.q.
breast nugget, 1 piece: *(Perdue Done It!)*	48	3.0	3.0	3.0	7	85	n.a.
chicken and cheese *(Perdue Done It!)*	54	3.0	3.0	3.0	8	108	n.a.
breast tenders *(Perdue Done It!)*, 1 oz. . .	62	5.0	4.0	3.0	10	116	n.a.
bleu cheese, Italian *(Chicken By George)*, 5 oz.	180	26.0	2.0	8.0	85	890	n.a.
Cajun *(Chicken By George)*, 5 oz.	180	25.0	4.0	8.0	80	890	n.a.
Caribbean grill *(Chicken By George)*, 5 oz.	200	25.0	10.0	6.0	80	610	n.a.
lemon herb *(Chicken By George)*, 5 oz.	170	24.0	6.0	6.0	70	870	n.a.
lemon oregano *(Chicken By George)*, 5 oz.	160	26.0	4.0	4.0	75	580	n.a.
mesquite barbecue *(Chicken By George)*, 5 oz.	170	25.0	6.0	6.0	70	790	n.a.
mustard dill *(Chicken By George)*, 5 oz.	180	26.0	3.0	7.0	80	640	n.a.
roasted, 1 oz.: breast half *(Perdue Done It!)*	45	7.0	1.0	2.0	22	116	0

Food and Measure	cal.	prot. (gms)	carbo. (gms)	fat (gms)	chol. (mgs)	sod. (mgs)	fiber (gms)
Chicken entree, refrigerated, roasted (cont.)							
drumstick (Perdue Done It!)	40	7.0	0	1.0	33	115	0
thigh (Perdue Done It!)	46	6.0	<1.0	2.0	32	114	0
whole or half, dark meat (Perdue Done It!)	51	6.0	<1.0	3.0	27	73	0
whole or half, white meat (Perdue Done It!)	37	7.0	<1.0	1.0	21	85	0
teriyaki (Chicken By George), 5 oz. . . .	180	25.0	9.0	5.0	70	740	n.a.
tomato herb w/basil (Chicken By George), 5 oz. . . .	190	25.0	7.0	7.0	80	800	n.a.
wings, hot and spicy (Perdue Done It!), 1 oz.	60	6.0	1.0	4.0	37	190	0
Chicken fat, 1 oz. . . .	178	1.1	0	19.3	16	9	0
Chicken frankfurter:							
(Longacre), 1 oz.	65	3.9	0	5.4	34	301	0
(Perdue), 2-oz. link . .	136	8.0	3.0	10.0	65	708	0
(Tyson), 1 link	115	6.0	1.0	10.0	m.q.	700	0
cheese (Tyson), 1 link	145	7.0	1.0	11.0	m.q.	680	0
Chicken giblets, simmered:							
4 oz.	178	29.3	1.1	5.4	446	66	0
chopped, 1 cup . . .	228	37.5	1.4	6.9	570	85	0
Chicken gravy:							
canned, 2 oz. or 1/4 cup:							
(Franco-American)	45	0	3.0	4.0	m.q.	240	n.a.
(Heinz HomeStyle)	35	1.0	3.0	2.0	1	350	.4 d
giblet (Franco-American)	30	1.0	3.0	2.0	m.q.	310	n.a.
golden (Pepperidge Farm)	25	1.0	3.0	1.0	m.q.	240	n.a.

Food and Measure	cal.	prot. (gms)	carbo. (gms)	fat (gms)	chol. (mgs)	sod. (mgs)	fiber (gms)
w/mushroom and onion (Heinz HomeStyle) . . .	35	1.0	3.0	2.0	1	330	0
mix:							
(Lawry's), 1/6 pkg. .	20	1.0	5.0	0	0	680	n.a.
(McCormick/Schilling), 1/4 cup* . .	22	.8	3.7	.4	n.a.	300	n.a.
(McCormick/Schilling Lite), 1/4 cup*	12	<1.0	.2	1.0	n.a.	450	n.a.
(Pillsbury), 1/4 cup*	25	<1.0	4.0	<1.0	0	170	n.a.
"Chicken" gravy, vegetarian, mix* (LaLoma Gravy Quik), 2 tbsp. . . .	45	<1.0	2.0	4.0	0	180	n.a.
Chicken luncheon meat, see "Chicken, boneless and luncheon meat"							
Chicken pie, see "Chicken entree, frozen"							
Chicken salad:							
(Longacre), 1 oz. . . .	63	2.6	3.0	4.6	15	142	m.q.
(Longacre Lite), 1 oz.	43	2.5	3.3	2.2	11	95	m.q.
spread (Libby's Spreadables), 1.9 oz.	90	5.0	5.0	6.0	15	230	1/0 d
Chicken sandwich, frozen, 1 piece:							
(Hormel Quick Meal)	320	16.0	40.0	11.0	65	640	m.q.
(MicroMagic), 4.5 oz.	390	13.0	42.0	16.0	35	650	m.q.
barbecue (Tyson Microwave), 4 oz. . .	230	16.0	27.0	6.0	50	600	m.q.
biscuit (Hormel Quick Meal)	310	13.0	36.0	13.0	50	900	m.q.
breast (Tyson Microwave), 4.25 oz. . .	328	16.0	33.0	14.0	m.q.	520	m.q.

Food and Measure	cal.	prot. (gms)	carbo. (gms)	fat (gms)	chol. (mgs)	sod. (mgs)	fiber (gms)
Chicken sandwich *(cont.)*							
breast, grilled *(Tyson)*,							
3.5 oz.	150	17.0	2.0	8.0	44	400	m.q.
grilled:							
(Hormel Quick Meal)	300	21.0	35.0	9.0	60	620	m.q.
(Tyson), 3.5 oz. . .	200	15.0	25.0	5.0	32	470	m.q.
(Weight Watchers							
Ultimate 200) . .	200	18.0	22.0	5.0	20	420	m.q.
pocket, 4.5 oz.:							
and cheddar w/ba-							
con *(Hot Pockets)*	300	13.0	35.0	12.0	50	700	m.q.
fajita *(Lean Pockets)*	270	11.0	33.0	10.0	30	840	m.q.
glazed *(Lean Pock-*							
ets Supreme) . .	250	11.0	32.0	8.0	35	640	m.q.
Oriental *(Lean Pock-*							
ets)	260	10.0	33.0	9.0	35	1040	m.q.
Parmesan *(Lean*							
Pockets)	270	12.0	31.0	11.0	30	670	m.q.
Chicken sauce,							
canned, see "En-							
tree sauce"							
Chicken sauce mix*							
(see also specific							
listings) *(McCor-*							
mick/Schilling Sauce							
Blends), 1 serving:							
cacciatore	575	46.0	17.0	35.0	n.a.	798	m.q.
Creole	229	30.0	16.0	5.0	n.a.	711	m.q.
curry, creamy	237	30.0	9.0	8.0	n.a.	429	m.q.
Dijon	238	30.0	8.0	8.0	n.a.	461	m.q.
Italian marinade . . .	324	48.0	3.0	12.0	n.a.	608	m.q.
mesquite	545	39.0	4.0	41.0	n.a.	488	m.q.
Parmesan	366	41.0	6.0	20.0	n.a.	671	m.q.
Southwest style . . .	359	40.0	4.0	20.0	n.a.	658	m.q.
stir fry	237	23.0	18.0	8.0	n.a.	928	m.q.
sweet and sour . . .	208	21.0	20.0	5.0	n.a.	262	m.q.
teriyaki	202	29.0	7.0	6.0	n.a.	421	m.q.

Food and Measure	cal.	prot. (gms)	carbo. (gms)	fat (gms)	chol. (mgs)	sod. (mgs)	fiber (gms)
Chicken seasoning:							
fried *(McCormick/ Schilling* Spice Blends), 1 tsp. . . .	5	.4	.6	.1	n.a.	526	n.a.
mix, Southwest *(Lawry's* Seasoning Blends), 1 pkg. . .	71	1.2	16.0	.3	n.a.	3947	m.q.
Chicken seasoning and coating mix:							
(French's Roasting Bag), 1/5 pkg. . . .	25	1.0	4.0	0	0	210	n.a.
(McCormick/Schilling Bag'n Season), 1 pkg.	122	4.0	22.0	2.0	0	2371	m.q.
(Shake'n Bake), 1/4 pkt.	80	2.0	14.0	2.0	0	450	m.q.
barbecue *(Shake'n Bake),* 1/4 pkt. . . .	90	1.0	18.0	2.0	0	840	m.q.
batter, Cajun *(Tone's),* 1 tsp.	12	.3	2.6	.1	0	75	.1 d
country *(McCormick/ Schilling* Bag'n Season), 1 pkg.	134	3.0	19.0	5.0	n.a.	4771	m.q.
extra crispy *(Oven Fry),* 1/4 pkt.	120	3.0	21.0	2.0	0	840	m.q.
frying *(Golden Dipt),* 1 oz.	90	2.0	20.0	0	0	1430	m.q.
homestyle *(Oven Fry),* 1/4 pkt.	90	1.0	15.0	2.0	0	980	m.q.
hot and spicy *(Shake'n Bake),* 1/4 pkt. . . .	80	2.0	15.0	2.0	0	380	m.q.
Chicken spread, chunky, canned:							
(Swanson), 1 oz. . . .	60	4.0	2.0	4.0	m.q.	140	n.a.
(Underwood), 2 1/8 oz.	150	10.0	2.0	9.0	40	440	n.a.
(Underwood Light), 2 1/8 oz.	100	11.0	2.0	5.0	30	330	n.a.

Food and Measure	cal.	prot. (gms)	carbo. (gms)	fat (gms)	chol. (mgs)	sod. (mgs)	fiber (gms)
Chicken and fish seasoning *(McCormick/Schilling Grillmates)*, 1 tsp.	8	0	2.0	0	n.a.	507	n.a.
Chick-fil-A, 1 serving:							
sandwiches:							
chicken	360	40.3	28.1	8.5	66	1174	.7 c
chicken, chargrilled	258	30.1	23.7	4.8	40	1121	.1 c
chicken, chargrilled, deluxe	266	30.5	25.5	4.9	40	1125	.1 c
chicken deluxe . .	368	40.7	29.8	8.6	66	1178	.7 c
chicken salad . . .	365	24.4	26.4	18.1	8	840	1.4 c
Chick-N-Q	409	28.4	40.9	14.7	10	1197	1.4 c
chicken dishes:							
garden salad, char-grilled	126	20.3	8.3	2.1	28	567	3.7 c
Grilled'n Lites, 2 skewers	97	20.0	.4	1.8	3	280	tr.c
Nuggets, 8-pack	287	28.2	12.5	15.1	61	1326	.6 c
salad plate	291	22.0	9.8	18.7	7	584	4.1 c
side dishes:							
carrot and raisin salad, cup	116	.8	17.9	4.8	6	8	1.0 c
chicken soup, breast of, hearty, cup	152	15.8	11.1	2.7	46	530	.7 c
coleslaw, cup . . .	175	1.4	11.2	14.2	13	158	1.1 c
potato salad, cup	198	2.5	13.9	15.0	6	337	.7 c
tossed salad	21	1.0	4.2	.3	0	19	2.1 c
w/dressing:							
blue cheese . . .	243	3.0	6.0	24.0	38	475	2.1 c
honey French . .	277	1.0	21.0	21.0	0	396	2.4 c
lite Italian	43	1.0	7.0	1.2	0	856	2.2 c
lite ranch	114	1.0	13.2	6.3	6	292	2.1 c
ranch	298	1.0	6.0	30.0	5	387	2.1 c
Thousand Island	250	1.0	12.0	22.0	25	396	2.2 c
Waffle Fries, small	270	3.0	33.0	13.5	8	45	m.q.

Food and Measure	cal.	prot. (gms)	carbo. (gms)	fat (gms)	chol. (mgs)	sod. (mgs)	fiber (gms)
desserts:							
fudge brownie,							
w/nuts	369	5.0	45.0	19.1	31	213	.3 c
cheesecake	299	6.6	24.7	19.1	13	272	.1 c
w/topping:							
blueberry	350	6.8	37.3	19.1	13	294	.4 c
strawberry	343	6.9	35.2	19.2	13	309	.5 c
Icedream, small cup	134	3.7	18.9	4.9	24	51	.3 c
lemon pie	329	7.5	63.8	5.1	7	300	.3 c
lemonade, small . . .	138	.3	34.2	tr.	tr.	tr.	.1 c
Chickpea flour (*Ar-*							
rowhead Mills), 2 oz.	200	12.0	35.0	3.0	0	9	7.4 d
Chickpeas, 1/2 cup,							
except as noted:							
dry (*Arrowhead Mills*),							
2 oz.	200	12.0	35.0	3.0	0	9	7.0 d
dry, boiled	134	7.3	22.5	2.1	0	6	2.9 d
canned:							
w/liquid	143	5.9	27.1	1.4	0	359	5.3 d
(*Allens*)	110	5.0	18.0	2.0	0	390	4.0 d
(*Eden*)	110	6.0	17.0	2.0	0	15	4.0 d
(*Eden* No Salt							
Added)	90	6.0	17.0	1.0	0	10	4.0 d
(*Green Giant/Joan*							
of Arc)	90	6.0	18.0	2.0	0	320	5.0 d
(*Green Giant/Joan*							
of Arc 50% Less							
Salt)	90	6.0	18.0	2.0	0	160	5.0 d
(*Hain*), 4 oz.	80	4.0	18.0	2.0	0	240	6.0 d
(*Old El Paso*) . . .	190	5.0	16.0	<1.0	0	250	m.q.
(*Progresso*), 4 oz.	110	9.0	22.0	1.0	0	200	6.0 d
Chicory, witloof:							
5–7″-long head,							
2.1 oz.	9	.5	2.1	.1	0	1	1.6 d
1/2 cup	8	.4	1.8	<.1	0	1	1.4 d
Chicory greens:							
trimmed, 1 oz.	7	.5	1.3	.1	0	13	1.1 d
chopped, 1/2 cup . .	21	1.5	4.2	.3	0	41	3.6 d

Food and Measure	cal.	prot. (gms)	carbo. (gms)	fat (gms)	chol. (mgs)	sod. (mgs)	fiber (gms)
Chicory root:							
1 medium, 2.6 oz. . . .	44	.8	10.5	.1	0	30	1.2 c
1″ pieces, 1/2 cup . .	33	.6	7.9	.1	0	23	.9 c
Chili, canned or packaged, 7.5 oz., except as noted:							
w/beans:							
(Gebhardt), 1 cup	495	20.0	47.0	28.0	92	1010	6.0 d
(Hormel)	300	15.0	27.0	15.0	55	1030	m.q.
(Hormel Micro Cup)	250	15.0	23.0	11.0	49	977	m.q.
(Just Rite), 4 oz. . .	200	10.0	16.0	11.0	33	500	1.0 d
(Libby's)	270	13.0	25.0	13.0	m.q.	810	m.q.
(Libby's Diner), 7.75 oz.	280	15.0	29.0	12.0	40	820	m.q.
(Old El Paso), 1 cup	217	15.0	17.0	10.0	32	480	6.0 d
chunky *(Hormel)* . .	290	15.0	25.0	14.0	50	780	m.q.
hot *(Gebhardt),* 1 cup	470	16.0	47.0	27.0	65	1000	6.0 d
hot *(Hormel)*	300	15.0	27.0	15.0	55	1030	m.q.
hot *(Hormel Micro Cup),* 7.4 oz. . .	250	15.0	24.0	11.0	49	977	m.q.
hot *(Just Rite),* 4 oz.	195	11.0	16.0	10.0	33	495	1.0 d
spicy, and turkey *(Healthy Choice)*	210	17.0	26.0	5.0	40	530	m.q.
w/out beans:							
(Gebhardt), 1 cup	530	21.0	20.0	43.0	150	990	1.0 d
(Hormel)	360	16.0	14.0	27.0	60	860	m.q.
(Hormel Micro Cup), 7.4 oz.	290	18.0	15.0	17.0	60	830	m.q.
(Just Rite), 4 oz. . .	180	13.0	9.0	11.0	41	515	<1.0 d
(Libby's)	390	18.0	11.0	30.0	m.q.	800	m.q.
hot *(Hormel)*	360	16.0	14.0	27.0	60	860	m.q.
w/chicken, spicy *(Hain)*	130	11.0	19.0	2.0	40	1030	m.q.
turkey, w/beans *(Healthy Choice)* . .	200	18.0	20.0	5.0	45	560	m.q.
vegetarian: *(Natural Touch),* 2/3 cup	230	12.0	19.0	12.0	0	890	m.q.

Food and Measure	cal.	prot. (gms)	carbo. (gms)	fat (gms)	chol. (mgs)	sod. (mgs)	fiber (gms)
(Worthington),							
2/3 cup	190	10.0	15.0	10.0	0	550	m.q.
mild, 3 bean *(Health Valley* Fat Free),							
5 oz.	90	10.0	12.0	<1.0	0	180	9.0 d
mild or spicy, w/black beans *(Health Valley* Fat Free), 5 oz. . . .	140	11.0	23.0	<1.0	0	290	12.2 d
spicy *(Hain)*	160	7.0	29.0	1.0	0	1060	m.q.
spicy *(Hain* Reduced Sodium)	170	7.0	31.0	1.0	0	200	m.q.
tempeh, spicy *(Hain)*	160	7.0	24.0	4.0	0	1350	m.q.
w/macaroni *(Hormel Micro Cup Chili Mac)*	192	10.0	18.0	9.0	22	977	m.q.
Chili, freeze-dried* *(Mountain House):*							
w/beans, 1 cup . . .	310	16.0	30.0	14.0	n.a.	950	m.q.
mac, w/beef, 1 cup	220	12.0	30.0	6.0	m.q.	540	m.q.
Chili, frozen (see also "Chili entree"):							
w/beans, meatless *(Bodin's),* 4 oz. . .	90	8.0	14.0	0	0	310	1.0 d
turkey *(Banquet Cookin' Bag),* 4 oz.	80	5.0	11.0	2.0	15	740	m.q.
Chili, mix*:							
(Fantastic Cha-Cha Chili), 10 oz.	240	20.0	38.0	1.0	0	490	13.0 d
(Hunt's Manwich Chili Fixin's),* 8 oz. . . .	290	20.0	20.0	14.0	65	980	5.0 d
black bean *(Aunt Patsy's* Souper Black Bean),* 8 oz.	152	9.0	30.0	1.0	n.a.	363	5.0 d
lentil *(Aunt Patsy's* Pantry),* 8 oz. . . .	150	11.0	27.0	1.0	n.a.	363	6.0 d
vegetarian *(Fantastic),* 4 oz.	106	7.0	18.0	.7	0	419	2.4 d

Food and Measure	cal.	prot. (gms)	carbo. (gms)	fat (gms)	chol. (mgs)	sod. (mgs)	fiber (gms)
Chili beans, canned:							
(Gebhardt), 4 oz. . . .	115	7.0	21.0	1.0	0	580	5.0 d
(Green Giant/Joan of Arc 50% Less Salt), 1/2 cup	100	7.0	21.0	1.0	0	310	7.0 d
(Hunt's), 4 oz.	100	6.0	18.0	<1.0	0	490	6.0 d
extra spicy *(Green Giant/Joan of Arc)*, 1/2 cup	100	7.0	21.0	1.0	0	580	6.0 d
hot *(Campbell's)*, 4 oz.	110	5.0	19.0	2.0	n.a.	440	5.0 d
spicy *(Green Giant/ Joan of Arc)*, 1/2 cup	100	7.0	21.0	1.0	0	620	7.0 d
Chili dip:							
(La Victoria), 2 tbsp.	10	0	2.0	0	0	180	m.q.
mix, caliente *(Knorr)*, 1 serving dry . . .	5	.2	.8	.1	<1	80	n.a.
Chili entree, frozen:							
con carne:							
(Swanson Homestyle)*, 8.25 oz.	270	20.0	26.0	10.0	m.q.	740	m.q.
w/beans *(Stouffer's)*, 8 3/4 oz.	280	20.0	28.0	10.0	m.q.	910	m.q.
vegetarian *(Right Course)*, 9 3/4 oz. . .	280	9.0	45.0	7.0	0	590	m.q.
Chili powder:							
1 tbsp.	24	.9	4.1	1.3	0	76	2.6 d
1 tsp.	8	.3	1.4	.4	0	26	.9 d
(Gebhardt), 1 tsp. . .	15	<1.0	3.0	<1.0	0	0	<1.0 d
Chili sauce:							
(Bennett's), 1 tbsp.	16	0	4.0	0	0	115	m.q.
(Heinz), 1 oz.	30	0	7.0	0	0	430	m.q.
(Tabasco 7 Spice)*, 1 oz.	11	.5	2.5	.2	0	137	.6 d
hot dog:							
(Gebhardt), 2 tbsp.	30	1.0	4.0	1.0	3	180	<1.0 d
(Just Rite), 2 oz. . . .	60	2.0	6.0	3.0	7	220	<1.0 d
red *(Las Palmas)*, 1/2 cup	25	1.0	3.0	1.0	0	670	0

Food and Measure	cal.	prot. (gms)	carbo. (gms)	fat (gms)	chol. (mgs)	sod. (mgs)	fiber (gms)
spicy *(Tabasco 7 Spice)*, 1 oz.	10	.5	2.4	.1	0	120	.6 d
Chili seasoning mix:							
(French's Chili O),							
1/6 pkg.	20	1.0	5.0	0	0	680	m.q.
(Gebhardt Chili Quik),							
1 tsp.	10	<1.0	2.0	<1.0	0	165	<1.0 d
(Lawry's Seasoning Blends), 1 pkg. . .	143	4.9	26.6	1.8	<1	2291	2.1 c
(McCormick/Schilling),							
1/4 pkg.	27	1.0	4.5	.5	0	290	m.q.
(Old El Paso), 1/5 pkg.	21	1.0	4.0	1.0	0	717	1.0 d
(Tio Sancho), 1.23 oz.	109	4.1	60.9	2.2	n.a.	832	4.2 c
medium *(Hain),*							
1/4 pkg.	30	<1.0	5.0	1.0	n.a.	300	m.q.
onion, real *(French's Chili O),* 1/6 pkg. . .	35	1.0	7.0	0	0	710	m.q.
Texas style *(French's Chili O),* 1/4 pkg. . .	35	1.0	<1.0	1.0	0	770	m.q.
Chimichanga, frozen, 1 piece:							
beef *(Old El Paso)* . .	410	10.0	35.0	25.0	m.q.	410	m.q.
chicken *(Old El Paso)*	370	13.0	34.0	20.0	m.q.	480	m.q.
Chimichanga entree, frozen beef and bean *(Banquet Meals),* 9.5 oz. . . .	480	13.0	60.0	21.0	15	1480	m.q.
Chitterlings, pork, simmered, 4 oz. . .	344	11.6	0	32.6	162	44	0
Chives:							
fresh:							
1 oz.	9	.9	1.2	.2	0	1	.9 d
chopped, 1 tbsp.	1	.1	.1	<.1	0	tr.	.1 d
freeze-dried:							
1/4 cup	2	.2	.5	<.1	0	24	.1 c
1 tbsp.	1	<.1	.1	<.1	0	6	<.1 c
Chocolate, see "Candy"							

Food and Measure	cal.	prot. (gms)	carbo. (gms)	fat (gms)	chol. (mgs)	sod. (mgs)	fiber (gms)
Chocolate, baking:							
bar, 1 oz.:							
semisweet *(Hershey's* Premium)	140	1.0	16.0	8.0	n.a.	0	m.q.
semisweet *(Nestlé)*	160	2.0	16.0	9.0	n.a.	0	m.q.
unsweetened *(Hershey's* Premium)	190	4.0	7.0	16.0	0	5	m.q.
unsweetened *(Nestlé)*	180	4.0	9.0	14.0	n.a.	0	m.q.
white *(Nestlé Premier)*	160	2.0	16.0	10.0	0	30	n.a.
chips, 1 oz., except as noted:							
milk *(Hershey's),* 1/4 cup	220	2.0	27.0	12.0	10	55	m.q.
milk *(Nestlé* Toll House Morsels)	150	1.0	19.0	7.0	n.a.	15	m.q.
milk, maxi *(Guittard)*	145	2.0	18.0	8.0	<5	20	<1.0 c
mint *(Hershey's),* 1/4 cup	230	2.0	28.0	12.0	n.a.	0	m.q.
rainbow *(Nestlé* Toll House Morsels)	140	2.0	20.0	6.0	0	0	m.q.
semisweet *(Guittard)*	130	1.0	19.0	8.0	0	0	<1.0 c
semisweet *(Nestlé* Merry Morsels)	140	1.0	21.0	5.0	n.a.	0	m.q.
semisweet or mint *(Nestlé* Toll House Morsels)	140	2.0	14.0	8.0	n.a.	0	4.0 d
semisweet, mini *(Nestlé* Toll House Morsels)	140	2.0	14.0	8.0	n.a.	0	4.0 d
semisweet, regular/ mini *(Hershey's),* 1/4 cup	220	2.0	27.0	12.0	0	0	m.q.
vanilla *(Hershey's),* 1/4 cup	220	1.0	25.0	13.0	n.a.	100	m.q.
chunks, 1 oz.:							
milk *(Hershey's)* . .	160	2.0	16.0	9.0	10	25	m.q.

Food and Measure	cal.	prot. (gms)	carbo. (gms)	fat (gms)	chol. (mgs)	sod. (mgs)	fiber (gms)
milk (Nestlé Treasures)	150	2.0	17.0	9.0	n.a.	n.a.	m.q.
semisweet (Hershey's)	140	1.0	15.0	8.0	n.a.	n.a.	m.q.
semisweet (Nestlé Treasures)	150	2.0	18.0	8.0	n.a.	0	m.q.
white (Nestlé Treasures)	160	2.0	15.0	10.0	n.a.	25	n.a.
premelted, un-sweetened, 1-oz. pkt.	134	3.4	9.6	13.5	0	3	.9 c
shreds (Tone's), 1 tsp.	21	.1	2.2	1.4	0	1	.1 d
Chocolate flavor drink, 1 cup:							
canned (Frostee) . . .	200	2.0	30.0	8.0	n.a.	160	(0)
chilled (Hershey's) . .	150	5.0	28.0	2.0	n.a.	85	(0)
Chocolate flavor drink mix, 1 pkt., except as noted:							
(Carnation Instant Breakfast)	130	4.0	27.0	1.0	2	105	m.q.
(Hershey's), 3 heaping tsp.	90	<1.0	22.0	<1.0	0	40	m.q.
(Nestlé Quik), 3/4 oz.	90	1.0	20.0	1.0	0	25	m.q.
(Pillsbury Instant Breakfast)	130	6.0	27.0	<1.0	0	100	m.q.
malt (Carnation Instant Breakfast)	130	4.0	27.0	2.0	3	125	m.q.
malt (Pillsbury Instant Breakfast)	130	6.0	25.0	0	0	135	m.q.
Chocolate milk, 1 cup:							
(Hershey's)	210	7.0	28.0	8.0	m.q.	120	(0)
(Nestlé Quik)	230	9.0	30.0	9.0	m.q.	120	(0)
lowfat (Nestlé Quik)	200	8.0	29.0	5.0	m.q.	150	(0)
lowfat (Hershey's) . .	190	8.0	29.0	5.0	20	130	(0)

Food and Measure	cal.	prot. (gms)	carbo. (gms)	fat (gms)	chol. (mgs)	sod. (mgs)	fiber (gms)
Chocolate mousse, see "Mousse"							
Chocolate soufflé mix (Knorr), 1 serving	40	3.9	5.4	.4	<1	190	n.a.
Chocolate syrup:							
(Hershey's), 2 tbsp.	110	1.0	25.0	<1.0	0	20	m.q.
(Nestlé Quik), 1²/₃ heaping tsp.	100	1.0	22.0	1.0	0	45	m.q.
(Smucker's), 2 tbsp.	130	1.0	27.0	2.0	0	35	m.q.
Chocolate topping, 2 tbsp., except as noted:							
(Kraft), 1 tbsp.	50	1.0	11.0	0	0	15	m.q.
(Smucker's Magic Shell)	190	1.0	16.0	15.0	n.a.	25	m.q.
dark (Smucker's Special)	130	1.0	31.0	1.0	n.a.	45	m.q.
fudge:							
(Hershey's)	120	2.0	17.0	5.0	5	40	m.q.
(Smucker's)	130	1.0	31.0	1.0	n.a.	50	m.q.
(Smucker's Magic Shell)	190	1.0	16.0	15.0	n.a.	50	m.q.
fudge, hot:							
(Kraft), 1 tbsp.	70	1.0	11.0	2.0	0	50	m.q.
(Smucker's)	110	1.0	18.0	4.0	n.a.	55	m.q.
(Smucker's Light)	70	2.0	19.0	0	n.a.	35	m.q.
(Smucker's Special)	150	2.0	23.0	5.0	n.a.	60	m.q.
Swiss milk chocolate (Smucker's)	140	3.0	31.0	1.0	n.a.	70	m.q.
toffee (Smucker's)	110	1.0	18.0	4.0	n.a.	55	m.q.
nut (Smucker's Magic Shell)	200	2.0	25.0	16.0	n.a.	40	m.q.
Chops, vegetarian, canned (Worthington Choplets), 2 slices	100	18.0	4.0	2.0	0	440	m.q.
Chow mein, see specific entree listings							

Food and Measure	cal.	prot. (gms)	carbo. (gms)	fat (gms)	chol. (mgs)	sod. (mgs)	fiber (gms)
Chow mein noodles, see "Noodles, Chinese"							
Chrysanthemum garland, 1/2 cup:							
raw, 1" pieces	2	.2	.5	<.1	0	7	.4 d
boiled, drained, 1" pieces	10	.8	2.2	.1	0	27	1.2 d
Churro, frozen (Tio Pepe's), 1 piece ..	130	2.0	16.0	7.0	1	120	m.q.
Cilantro, see "Coriander"							
Cinnamon, ground, (Tone's), 1 tsp. ...	6	.1	1.8	.1	0	1	.6 d
Cisco, meat only, raw, 4 oz.	112	21.5	0	2.2	m.q.	62	0
Citrus grill marinade (Lawry's), 2 tbsp.	34	3.8	3.4	.4	0	3350	.1 c
Citrus juice (Santa Cruz Natural), 8 fl. oz.	125	1.0	29.0	<1.0	0	(0)	m.q.
Citrus juice drink, 6 fl. oz:							
(Hi-C Citrus Cooler)	95	.1	23.3	<.1	0	17	(0)
chilled (Five Alive) ..	90	0	22.0	0	0	20	(0)
frozen (Five Alive) ..	90	0	22.0	0	0	0	(0)
berry, frozen (Five Alive)	90	0	22.0	0	0	5	(0)
tropical:							
chilled (Five Alive)	90	0	21.0	0	0	20	(0)
frozen (Five Alive)	90	0	21.0	0	0	0	(0)
Citrus punch (Minute Maid), 6 fl. oz.	90	0	23.0	0	0	20	(0)
Citrus-cranberry juice drink (Ocean Spray Refreshers), 6 fl. oz.	100	0	26.0	0	0	15	(0)

Food and Measure	cal.	prot. (gms)	carbo. (gms)	fat (gms)	chol. (mgs)	sod. (mgs)	fiber (gms)
Citrus-peach juice drink *(Ocean Spray Refreshers)*, 6 fl. oz.	90	0	23.0	0	0	15	(0)
Clam, meat only:							
raw:							
4 oz.	84	14.5	2.9	1.1	39	64	0
9 large or 20 small, 6.3 oz.	133	23.0	4.6	1.8	60	100	0
boiled, poached, or steamed, 4 oz. . .	168	29.0	5.8	2.2	76	127	0
Clam, canned, chopped or minced:							
(Gorton's), 1/2 can	70	12.0	4.0	1.0	m.q.	640	0
w/liquid *(Doxsee/ Snow's)*, 6.5 oz. . .	100	14.0	8.0	<1.0	35	1160	0
w/liquid *(Progresso)*, 1/2 cup	40	8.0	1.0	<1.0	15	500	0
drained *(Progresso)*, 1/2 cup	90	18.0	<1.0	1.0	45	410	0
Clam entree, frozen:							
fried *(Mrs. Paul's)*, 2.5 oz.	200	10.0	21.0	9.0	15	450	m.q.
strips, crunchy *(Gorton's* Microwave)*, 2.9 oz.	270	8.0	20.0	17.0	25	350	m.q.
Clam chowder, see "Soup"							
Clam dip, 2 tbsp.:							
(Breakstone's/Sealtest)	50	1.0	2.0	4.0	15	220	n.a.
(Breakstone's Gourmet Chesapeake) . . .	50	1.0	2.0	4.0	20	200	n.a.
(Kraft)	60	1.0	3.0	4.0	10	240	n.a.
(Kraft Premium) . . .	45	1.0	2.0	4.0	20	210	n.a.
Clam juice *(Doxsee/ Snow's)*, 3 fl. oz.	4	<1.0	0	0	n.a.	110	0
Clam sauce, canned:							
red *(Ferrara)*, 4 oz. . .	70	5.0	8.0	2.0	10	320	m.q.

Food and Measure	cal.	prot. (gms)	carbo. (gms)	fat (gms)	chol. (mgs)	sod. (mgs)	fiber (gms)
red (Progresso),							
1/2 cup	70	5.0	7.0	3.0	m.q.	560	n.a.
white (Ferrara), 4 oz.	80	5.0	4.0	5.0	10	570	m.q.
white (Progresso),							
1/2 cup	110	9.0	1.0	8.0	m.q.	280	n.a.
Clover seeds,							
sprouted, raw							
(Shaw's), 2 oz. . . .	7	1.0	0	<1.0	0	40	3.0 d
Cloves, ground:							
1 tbsp.	21	.4	4.0	1.3	0	16	2.1 d
1 tsp.	7	.1	1.3	.4	0	5	.7 d
Cobbler:							
apple, deep dish (Aw-							
rey's), 1/8 pie	320	2.0	48.0	14.0	0	300	1.0 d
blueberry, deep dish							
(Awrey's), 1/8 pie	310	2.0	45.0	14.0	0	360	2.0 d
frozen, 1/2 cup, except							
as noted:							
apple (Stilwell) . . .	250	3.0	55.0	2.5	0	350	3.0 d
apple or strawberry							
(Pet-Ritz), 1/6 pkg.	290	1.0	50.0	9.0	n.a.	m.q.	m.q.
apricot (Stilwell) . .	250	4.0	54.0	2.0	0	270	5.0 d
blackberry (Pet-Ritz),							
1/6 pkg.	250	2.0	39.0	10.0	n.a.	m.q.	m.q.
blackberry (Stilwell)	250	4.0	53.0	2.5	0	270	5.0 d
blueberry (Pet-Ritz),							
1/6 pkg.	370	3.0	50.0	12.0	n.a.	m.q.	m.q.
cherry (Pet-Ritz),							
1/6 pkg.	280	2.0	46.0	10.0	n.a.	m.q.	m.q.
cherry (Stilwell) . .	250	3.0	54.0	2.5	0	230	2.0 d
peach (Pet-Ritz),							
1/6 pkg.	260	2.0	46.0	10.0	n.a.	m.q.	m.q.
peach (Stilwell) . .	240	3.0	51.0	2.0	0	210	3.0 d
pecan (Stilwell) . .	440	6.0	88.0	7.0	45	290	4.0 d
strawberry (Stilwell)	240	3.0	53.0	2.0	0	174	4.0 d
mix* (Dromedary):							
apple crumb,							
1/8 cake	237	3.0	41.0	6.0	n.a.	49	m.q.

Food and Measure	cal.	prot. (gms)	carbo. (gms)	fat (gms)	chol. (mgs)	sod. (mgs)	fiber (gms)
Cobbler, mix *(cont.)*							
cherry crumb,							
1/8 cake	231	3.0	42.0	6.0	n.a.	16	m.q.
Cocktail sauce,							
1 tbsp., except as							
noted:							
(Bennett's)	20	0	4.0	<1.0	0	260	n.a.
(Sauceworks)	14	0	3.0	0	0	170	n.a.
seafood:							
(Heinz), 1/4 cup . .	60	1.0	13.0	0	0	680	0
hot *(Bennett's)* . . .	30	0	7.0	0	0	180	n.a.
regular or extra hot							
(Golden Dipt) . .	20	0	5.0	0	0	210	n.a.
Cocoa powder, 1 oz.:							
(Bensdorp)	130	6.0	8.0	7.0	<1.0	5	m.q.
(Hershey's)	110	8.0	12.0	3.0	0	25	m.q.
(Nestlé)	80	7.0	5.0	5.0	n.a.	<5	m.q.
European *(Hershey's)*	90	7.0	8.0	3.0	0	15	m.q.
Cocoa mix, 1 pkt.,							
except as noted:							
(Swiss Miss Lite) . . .	70	1.0	17.0	<1.0	1	160	0
all varieties *(Alba 66)*,							
.68 oz.	60	6.0	10.0	0	n.a.	160	m.q.
chocolate:							
Bavarian *(Swiss							
Miss)*	110	1.0	20.0	3.0	2	170	0
double rich *(Swiss							
Miss)*	110	2.0	22.0	1.0	0	150	0
milk or fudge *(Car-							
nation)*	110	2.0	24.0	1.0	0	130	(0)
milk *(Swiss Miss)*	110	2.0	24.0	1.0	5	125	0
rich or w/marshmal-							
low *(Carnation)*	110	1.0	24.0	1.0	0	120	(0)
rich *(Nestlé)*	110	2.0	23.0	1.0	n.a.	100	(0)
rich, w/marshmal-							
lows *(Nestlé)* . .	120	2.0	23.0	1.0	n.a.	115	(0)
w/mini marshmallows							
(Swiss Miss)	110	1.0	23.0	1.0	5	170	0

Food and Measure	cal.	prot. (gms)	carbo. (gms)	fat (gms)	chol. (mgs)	sod. (mgs)	fiber (gms)
Coconut:							
fresh, shelled:							
1 oz.	100	.9	4.3	9.5	0	6	2.6 d
shredded or grated,							
1 cup not packed	283	2.7	12.2	26.8	0	16	7.2 d
canned, 1/3 cup:							
sweetened, flaked	114	.9	10.5	8.1	0	5	1.2 d
(Baker's Angel Flake)	110	1.0	10.0	9.0	0	5	m.q.
dried, toasted, 1 oz.	168	1.5	12.6	13.4	0	11	.7 c
packaged, 1/3 cup:							
sweetened, flaked	117	.8	11.8	7.9	0	63	1.1 d
(Baker's Angel Flake)	120	1.0	10.0	8.0	0	75	m.q.
(Baker's Premium							
Shred)	140	1.0	12.0	9.0	0	85	m.q.
Coconut cream,							
canned, sweetened:							
1 tbsp.	36	.5	1.6	3.4	0	10	.4 d
(Coco Lopez), 2 tbsp.	120	0	20.0	5.0	0	10	m.q.
(Holland House),							
2 fl. oz.	144	<1.0	36.0	<1.0	0	42	m.q.
Coconut milk[1]:							
1 tbsp.	35	.3	.8	3.6	0	2	.3 d
canned, 1 tbsp. . . .	30	.3	.4	3.2	0	2	m.q.
Coconut nectar *(R.W.*							
Knudsen), 8 fl. oz.	150	<1.0	29.0	<1.0	0	(0)	m.q.
Coconut water[2],							
1 tbsp.	3	.1	.6	<.1	0	16	.2 d
Coconut-pineapple							
nectar *(Kern's),*							
6 fl. oz.	140	1.0	26.0	4.0	0	25	m.q.
Cod, meat only:							
fresh, Atlantic:							
raw, 4 oz.	93	20.2	0	.8	49	62	0
baked, broiled, or							
microwaved, 4 oz.	119	25.9	0	1.0	62	88	0

[1] Liquid expressed from mixture of grated coconut and water.
[2] Liquid from coconuts.

Food and Measure	cal.	prot. (gms)	carbo. (gms)	fat (gms)	chol. (mgs)	sod. (mgs)	fiber (gms)
Cod *(cont.)*							
fresh, Pacific:							
raw, 4 oz.	93	20.3	0	.7	42	81	0
baked, broiled, or							
microwaved, 4 oz.	119	26.0	0	.9	53	103	0
canned, Atlantic,							
w/liquid, 4 oz. . . .	119	25.8	0	1.0	62	247	0
dried, Atlantic, salted,							
1 oz.	81	17.6	0	.7	42	1968	0
frozen *(Van de Kamp's*							
Natural), 4 oz. . . .	90	20.0	0	1.0	25	90	0
Cod entree, frozen:							
breaded *(Van de*							
Kamp's Light),							
1 piece	250	17.0	20.0	11.0	35	510	m.q.
breaded *(Mrs. Paul's*							
Light), 4.25 oz. . .	240	15.0	22.0	11.0	50	430	m.q.
lemon thyme *(Gorton's*							
Select), 1 piece . .	90	13.0	5.0	2.0	40	260	n.a.
minced, nuggets,							
crunchy *(Frionor*							
Bunch O'Crunch),							
8 nuggets, 4 oz. . .	320	14.2	19.0	21.3	22	411	<.1 d
Cod liver oil, see							
"Oil"							
Coffee:							
brewed, 6 fl. oz. . . .	4	.1	.8	0	0	4	0
instant, regular,							
1 rounded tsp.* . .	4	.2	.7	tr.	0	1	0
freeze-dried, all vari-							
eties *(Taster's*							
Choice), 1 cup* . .	4	<1.0	1.0	<1.0	0	0	0

Food and Measure	cal.	prot. (gms)	carbo. (gms)	fat (gms)	chol. (mgs)	sod. (mgs)	fiber (gms)
Coffee, flavored (see also ''Cappuccino''), 6 fl. oz.*:							
café Amaretto (General Foods International)	50	0	7.0	3.0	0	90	(0)
café Français:							
(General Foods International) . . .	60	0	6.0	3.0	0	25	(0)
(Hills Bros.)	60	0	8.0	2.0	n.a.	35	(0)
café Vienna:							
(General Foods International) . . .	60	0	10.0	2.0	0	95	(0)
(Hills Bros.)	60	1.0	9.0	2.0	n.a.	35	(0)
chocolate, double Dutch (General Foods International)	50	0	8.0	2.0	0	30	(0)
chocolate, Viennese (General Foods International Café) . .	50	0	8.0	2.0	0	20	(0)
hazelnut, Belgian:							
(General Foods International) . . .	60	0	10.0	2.0	0	55	(0)
(Hills Bros.)	60	1.0	9.0	2.0	n.a.	30	(0)
mocha, Suisse:							
(General Foods International) . . .	50	0	7.0	3.0	0	40	(0)
(General Foods International Decaffeinated)	50	0	7.0	3.0	0	30	(0)
Swiss (Hills Bros.)	60	1.0	8.0	2.0	n.a.	10	(0)
orange cappuccino (General Foods International)	60	0	10.0	2.0	0	90	(0)
vanilla, French (General Foods International)	60	0	9.0	3.0	0	50	(0)

Food and Measure	cal.	prot. (gms)	carbo. (gms)	fat (gms)	chol. (mgs)	sod. (mgs)	fiber (gms)
Coffee creamer, see "Cream" and "Creamer, nondairy"							
Coffee flavored drink mix (*Carnation* Instant Breakfast), 1 pkt.	130	4.0	28.0	0	2	95	m.q.
Coffee liqueur, 1 fl. oz.:							
53 proof	117	tr.	16.3	.1	0	3	n.a.
w/cream, 34 proof . .	102	.9	6.5	4.9	n.a.	29	n.a.
Coffee substitute, cereal grain:							
powder, 1 tsp.	9	.1	1.9	.1	0	2	tr.c
(*Kaffree Roma*), 1 tsp.	6	0	1.0	0	0	n.a.	n.a.
all varieties (*Postum* Instant), 6 fl. oz.*	12	0	3.0	0	0	0	(0)
Cold cuts, see specific listings							
Collards:							
fresh:							
raw, 1 oz.	9	.4	2.0	.1	0	6	1.0 d
raw, chopped, 1/2 cup	6	.3	1.3	<.1	0	4	.7 d
boiled, drained, chopped, 1/2 cup	17	.9	3.9	.1	0	10	1.3 d
canned (*Allens/Sunshine*), 1/2 cup . . .	20	2.0	2.0	<1.0	0	15	m.q.
frozen, chopped:							
boiled, drained, 1/2 cup	31	2.5	6.1	.4	0	42	.9 c
(*Seabrook*), 3.3 oz.	25	3.0	4.0	0	0	45	1.0 c
(*Southern*), 3.5 oz.	30	2.7	4.6	.4	0	60	m.q.
Cookie, 1 piece, except as noted:							
almond:							
(*Frieda's*)	76	1.0	8.0	4.0	n.a.	43	m.q.

Food and Measure	cal.	prot. (gms)	carbo. (gms)	fat (gms)	chol. (mgs)	sod. (mgs)	fiber (gms)
(Stella D'Oro Breakfast Treats) . . .	100	2.0	15.0	4.0	<1	m.q.	m.q.
(Stella D'Oro Chinese Dessert) . .	170	2.0	19.0	9.0	<1	m.q.	m.q.
biscuit (Almondina)	30	1.0	5.5	1.3	0	3	.4 d
toast (Stella D'Oro Mandel)	60	1.0	10.0	1.0	<1	m.q.	m.q.
animal crackers: (Sunshine),							
13 pieces	130	2.0	21.0	4.0	0	160	m.q.
(Tom's), 2.5-oz. pkg.	300	5.0	54.0	7.0	n.a.	350	m.q.
candied (Grandma's),							
5 pieces	140	1.0	20.0	6.0	0	80	m.q.
anise: (Stella D'Oro Anisette Sponge) . .	50	1.0	10.0	1.0	<1	m.q.	m.q.
(Stella D'Oro Anisette Toast)	50	1.0	9.0	1.0	<1	m.q.	m.q.
(Stella D'Oro Anisette Toast Jumbo)	110	2.0	23.0	1.0	<1	m.q.	m.q.
apple: bar (Apple Newtons)	70	1.0	15.0	2.0	0	70	m.q.
bar, Dutch (Stella D'Oro)	110	1.0	19.0	3.0	<1	m.q.	m.q.
bar, fat free (Apple Newtons)	70	1.0	16.0	0	0	45	m.q.
pastry (Stella D'Oro Dietetic)	80	1.0	13.0	3.0	<1	10	m.q.
apple filled: (Archway)	110	1.0	20.0	4.0	5	115	0
(Little Debbie Apple Delights)	140	2.0	22.0	5.0	5	115	m.q.
apple-oatmeal tart (Pepperidge Farm Wholesome Choice)	70	1.0	12.0	2.0	0	45	m.q.
apple n'raisin (Archway)	130	2.0	20.0	5.0	5	105	1.0 d

Food and Measure	cal.	prot. (gms)	carbo. (gms)	fat (gms)	chol. (mgs)	sod. (mgs)	fiber (gms)
Cookie *(cont.)*							
apple-raisin filled *(Health Valley Fruit Centers)*	70	2.0	16.0	<1.0	0	35	3.5 d
apple or apricot filled *(Health Valley Fruit Centers)*	80	2.0	17.0	0	0	80	2.0 d
apricot filled *(Archway)*	110	1.0	19.0	5.0	5	85	1.0 d
apricot-raspberry:							
(Pepperidge Farm Fruit Cookies), 2 pieces	100	1.0	15.0	4.0	10	50	m.q.
(Pepperidge Farm Zurich)	60	1.0	10.0	2.0	0	30	m.q.
arrowroot biscuit:							
(National)	20	<1.0	3.0	<1.0	<2	15	m.q.
(Peek Freans), 5 pieces	181	2.9	30.5	5.3	0	91	m.q.
biscottini cashews *(Stella D'Oro)* . . .	110	1.5	13.5	5.5	n.a.	m.q.	m.q.
blueberry filled *(Archway)*	110	1.0	20.0	4.0	5	125	1.0 d
bourbon creme *(Peek Freans)*, 3 pieces	195	2.0	28.9	7.9	n.a.	31	m.q.
bran crunch *(Peek Freans)*, 4 pieces	177	2.5	26.0	7.0	n.a.	153	m.q.
brownie chocolate nut *(Pepperidge Farm)*, 2 pieces	110	1.0	11.0	7.0	0	45	m.q.
butter flavor:							
(Peek Freans Petit Beurre), 6 pieces	177	2.1	32.0	4.5	n.a.	148	m.q.
(Pepperidge Farm Chessmen) . . .	45	.5	6.0	2.0	5	30	m.q.
fudge creme filled *(Keebler E.L. Fudge)*	60	<1.0	8.0	3.0	0	35	m.q.

Food and Measure	cal.	prot. (gms)	carbo. (gms)	fat (gms)	chol. (mgs)	sod. (mgs)	fiber (gms)
butter pecan (Dare)	68	.6	7.5	4.0	7	41	.1 d
caramel:							
bar (Little Debbie)	150	1.0	22.0	7.0	5	85	m.q.
golden (Dare) . . .	64	.6	9.0	3.0	0	26	.1 d
carob chip (Health Valley Healthy Chip), 1.17 oz. or 3 pieces	80	2.0	18.0	0	0	80	3.0 d
carrot cake (Archway)	120	1.0	19.0	6.0	5	130	0 d
carrot walnut (Pepperidge Farm Wholesome Choice) . . .	60	1.0	11.0	1.0	0	45	m.q.
(Carr's Hob Nobs) . .	70	1.0	9.3	3.1	<1	76	.7 d
cherry filled (Archway)	110	1.0	20.0	4.0	10	105	1.0 d
chocolate:							
(Grandma's Grab), 8 pieces	140	2.0	19.0	6.0	0	180	m.q.
(Stella D'Oro Castelets)	60	1.0	9.0	3.0	<1	m.q.	m.q.
(Stella D'Oro Margherite) . . .	70	1.0	10.0	3.0	<1	m.q.	m.q.
dark (Peek Freans), 3 pieces	200	2.3	25.8	9.8	n.a.	113	m.q.
fudge (Dare)	93	.7	13.0	4.2	0	38	.3 d
milk (Peek Freans), 3 pieces	200	2.3	26.3	9.5	n.a.	120	m.q.
milk, fudge (Dare)	96	.9	13.0	4.6	0	32	.2 d
snaps (Nabisco), 4 pieces	60	1.0	10.0	2.0	<2	80	m.q.
chocolate chip/chunk:							
(Almost Home Real)	60	1.0	7.0	3.0	<2	45	m.q.
(Archway Mini), 12 pieces	150	1.0	20.0	7.0	5	95	0
(Archway Super Pak)	130	1.0	20.0	6.0	5	140	1.0 d
(Chips Ahoy!) . . .	50	1.0	7.0	2.0	0	40	m.q.
(Chips Ahoy! Rockers)	60	1.0	8.0	3.0	0	40	m.q.
(Dare)	73	1.0	9.7	3.3	11	42	.2 d

Food and Measure	cal.	prot. (gms)	carbo. (gms)	fat (gms)	chol. (mgs)	sod. (mgs)	fiber (gms)
Cookie, chocolate chip/chunk *(cont.)*							
(Dare Breaktime) . .	36	.4	5.0	1.7	0	37	.1 d
(Drake's), 2 pieces	140	1.0	18.0	6.0	0	110	m.q.
(Famous Amos), 3 pieces	140	2.0	20.0	6.0	n.a.	100	m.q.
(Grandma's), 2 pieces	370	4.0	50.0	17.0	5	270	m.q.
(Grandma's Rich'N Chewy), 3 pieces	140	1.0	20.0	6.0	5	80	m.q.
(Hostess), 5 pieces	250	2.0	33.0	13.0	35	110	2.0 d
(Keebler Chips Deluxe)	80	1.0	10.0	5.0	<5	55	m.q.
(Keebler Chips Deluxe Bakery Crisp)	60	1.0	7.0	3.0	0	45	m.q.
(Master Choice) . .	80	1.0	10.0	4.0	4	80	m.q.
(Mini Chips Ahoy!), 6 pieces	70	1.0	9.0	3.0	0	50	m.q.
(Pepperidge Farm Family Request), 2 pieces	90	1.0	15.0	5.0	0	55	1.0 d
(Pepperidge Farm Old Fashioned), 2 pieces	100	1.0	12.0	5.0	5	45	m.q.
(SnackWell's), 6 pieces	60	<1.0	11.0	1.0	0	85	m.q.
(Tom's), 2.25-oz. pkg.	320	4.0	43.0	14.0	n.a.	210	m.q.
bar *(Tastykake)* . . .	190	3.0	28.0	8.0	5	95	1.0 d
chewy *(Chips Ahoy!)*	60	1.0	8.0	3.0	<2	40	m.q.
chocolate *(Drake's)*, 2 pieces	130	2.0	19.0	10.0	0	85	m.q.
pecan *(Keebler Pecan Chips Deluxe)*	70	1.0	8.0	4.0	0	40	m.q.
toffee *(Pepperidge Farm)*, 2 pieces	100	1.0	12.0	5.0	5	75	m.q.

Food and Measure	cal.	prot. (gms)	carbo. (gms)	fat (gms)	chol. (mgs)	sod. (mgs)	fiber (gms)
chocolate walnut (Pepperidge Farm Beacon Hill) . . .	120	2.0	14.0	7.0	5	65	1.0 d
chocolate walnut (Pepperidge Farm Soft Baked) . . .	130	1.0	17.0	6.0	5	45	m.q.
chunk (Pepperidge Farm Nantucket)	120	1.0	15.0	6.0	5	60	1.0 d
chunk (Pepperidge Farm Soft Baked)	130	2.0	17.0	6.0	10	45	m.q.
chunk, macadamia (Tastykake) . . .	310	2.0	42.0	14.0	40	180	2.0 d
chunk, pecan (Chips Ahoy!)	100	1.0	10.0	6.0	10	65	m.q.
chunk, pecan (Pepperidge Farm Chesapeake) . .	120	1.0	14.0	7.0	5	60	1.0 d
chunky (Chips Ahoy!)	90	1.0	11.0	5.0	10	90	m.q.
coconut (Keebler Chocolate Drop)	80	1.0	10.0	5.0	0	60	m.q.
drop (Archway) . .	100	1.0	16.0	4.0	5	110	.5 d
Dutch, crunch or mint (Master Choice Patisserie)	80	<1.0	10.0	4.0	5	0	m.q.
fudge (Almost Home)	70	1.0	9.0	3.0	<2	50	m.q.
fudge (Grandma's), 2 pieces	350	4.0	54.0	13.0	5	380	m.q.
fudge, white, chunk (Chips Ahoy!) . .	90	1.0	10.0	5.0	<5	75	m.q.
Heath toffee chunk (Chips Ahoy!) . .	90	1.0	10.0	5.0	5	90	m.q.
milk (Dare Jersey Milk Chip)	64	1.0	8.0	3.5	3	36	.1 d
milk, macadamia (Pepperidge Farm Sausalito)	120	1.0	14.0	7.0	5	65	0

Food and Measure	cal.	prot. (gms)	carbo. (gms)	fat (gms)	chol. (mgs)	sod. (mgs)	fiber (gms)
Cookie, chocolate chip/chunk *(cont.)*							
milk, macadamia (Pepperidge Farm Soft Baked) . . .	130	1.0	16.0	7.0	10	45	m.q.
milk or regular (Duncan Hines), 2 pieces	110	1.0	15.0	5.0	n.a.	85	m.q.
pecan (Famous Amos), 3 pieces	150	2.0	18.0	8.0	n.a.	98	m.q.
snaps (Nabisco), 3 pieces	70	1.0	11.0	2.0	0	50	m.q.
sprinkled (Chips Ahoy!)	60	1.0	8.0	3.0	0	40	m.q.
striped (Chips Ahoy!)	90	1.0	10.0	5.0	0	45	m.q.
toffee (Archway) . .	140	1.0	19.0	7.0	5	125	1.0 d
chocolate sandwich:							
(Famous Amos), 3 pieces	150	1.0	21.0	8.0	0	105	1.0 d
(Little Debbie) . . .	250	3.0	35.0	12.0	<1	260	m.q.
(Mini Oreo), 5 pieces	70	1.0	10.0	3.0	0	90	m.q.
(Oreo)	50	1.0	8.0	2.0	<2	75	m.q.
(Oreo Double Stuf)	70	1.0	9.0	4.0	<2	75	m.q.
creme (Tom's), 1.6-oz. pkg. . . .	220	3.0	32.0	9.0	1	210	m.q.
fudge covered (Oreo)	110	1.0	13.0	6.0	0	75	m.q.
peanut butter creme (Dunkaroos), 1 tray	140	3.0	15.0	8.0	0	140	m.q.
vanilla creme filled (Keebler E.L. Fudge)	60	<1.0	8.0	3.0	0	35	m.q.
white fudge covered (Oreo)	110	1.0	14.0	6.0	0	70	m.q.
chocolate filled sandwich:							
(Nabisco Pure Chocolate Middles)	80	1.0	9.0	5.0	<5	35	m.q.

Food and Measure	cal.	prot. (gms)	carbo. (gms)	fat (gms)	chol. (mgs)	sod. (mgs)	fiber (gms)
(Pepperidge Farm Brussels), 2 pieces	110	1.0	13.0	5.0	0	65	m.q.
(Pepperidge Farm Lido)	90	1.0	10.0	5.0	0	30	m.q.
(Pepperidge Farm Milano), 2 pieces	120	1.0	15.0	6.0	5	45	m.q.
mint *(Pepperidge Farm Brussels Mint)*, 2 pieces	130	1.0	17.0	7.0	0	40	m.q.
mint or orange *(Pepperidge Farm Milano)*, 2 pieces	150	1.0	17.0	7.0	5	60	m.q.
chocolate peanut bar *(Ideal)*	90	1.0	10.0	5.0	0	80	m.q.
cinnamon:							
crisp *(Tom's)*, 2.5-oz. pkg.	340	4.0	49.0	14.0	0	360	m.q.
snap *(Archway)*, 6 pieces	150	1.0	20.0	7.0	0	115	0
sugar *(Pepperidge Farm Family Request)*, 2 pieces	80	1.0	12.0	4.0	15	40	0
cocoa, Dutch *(Archway)*	120	1.0	19.0	4.0	5	110	0
coconut:							
(Dare Breaktime) . .	34	.4	5.0	1.4	0	15	.1 d
(Drake's), 2 pieces	120	2.0	19.0	4.0	0	50	m.q.
(Stella D'Oro Dietetic)	50	1.0	6.0	2.0	<1	<10	m.q.
creme *(Dare)*	96	1.1	12.0	4.8	0	42	.2 d
macaroon *(Archway)*	110	1.0	19.0	6.0	0	60	3.0 d
macaroon *(Drake's)*	135	1.0	17.0	7.0	0	80	m.q.
macaroon *(Stella D'Oro)*	60	1.0	7.0	3.0	<1	m.q.	m.q.
coffee creme *(Peek Freans)*, 3 pieces	198	3.1	26.8	8.7	n.a.	85	m.q.

Food and Measure	cal.	prot. (gms)	carbo. (gms)	fat (gms)	chol. (mgs)	sod. (mgs)	fiber (gms)
Cookie *(cont.)*							
cranberry honey *(Pepperidge Farm Wholesome Choice)*	60	1.0	11.0	2.0	0	50	m.q.
creme sandwich, see specific listings							
Danish *(Imported Danish Cookies),* 2 pieces	70	1.0	9.0	4.0	0	15	m.q.
(Dare Harvest from the Rain Forest)	68	1.0	8.0	4.0	4	39	.2 d
date filled *(Health Valley Fruit Centers)*	70	2.0	16.0	<1.0	0	35	3.5 d
date walnut *(Pepperidge Farm Wholesome Choice)* . . .	60	1.0	10.0	2.0	0	45	m.q.
devil's food cakes:							
(Nabisco)	70	1.0	15.0	1.0	0	40	m.q.
(SnackWell's) . . .	50	1.0	12.0	0	0	25	m.q.
egg biscuit:							
(Stella D'Oro Dietetic)	45	1.5	6.5	1.0	<1	<10	m.q.
(Stella D'Oro Jumbo)	50	1.0	9.0	1.0	<1	m.q.	m.q.
Roman *(Stella D'Oro)*	140	3.0	20.0	5.0	<1	m.q.	m.q.
sugared *(Stella D'Oro)*	80	2.0	14.0	1.0	<1	m.q.	m.q.
fig bar:							
(Drake's)	380	6.0	50.0	18.0	9	220	m.q.
(Fig Newtons) . . .	60	1.0	11.0	1.0	0	60	m.q.
(Little Debbie Figaroo), 1.5 oz.	150	1.0	31.0	3.0	5	95	m.q.
(Tom's), 2-oz. pkg.	200	2.0	43.0	2.0	0	180	m.q.
fat free *(Fig Newtons)*	70	1.0	15.0	0	0	80	m.q.
fortune *(La Choy)* . .	15	<1.0	4.0	<1.0	0	1	<1.0 d

Food and Measure	cal.	prot. (gms)	carbo. (gms)	fat (gms)	chol. (mgs)	sod. (mgs)	fiber (gms)
French creme *(Dare)*	79	.9	8.4	4.7	0	21	.2 d
fruit (see also specific fruits):							
all varieties *(Health Valley Fat Free Jumbo Fruit Cookies)*	80	2.0	17.0	0	0	80	2.0 d
chunks, all varieties *(Health Valley Fat Free)*, 3 pieces	85	2.0	19.0	0	0	80	3.0 d
creme *(Peek Freans)*, 3 pieces . .	196	1.7	27.6	8.7	n.a.	36	m.q.
filled, all varieties *(Baker's Own)* . .	70	<1.0	12.0	2.0	0	80	m.q.
filled, all varieties *(Health Valley Mini Fruit Centers Fat Free)*, 3 pieces	75	2.0	17.0	0	0	60	3.0 d
slices *(Stella D'Oro)*	60	2.0	9.0	2.0	<1	m.q.	m.q.
tropical, filled *(Health Valley Fruit Centers)*	80	2.0	17.0	0	0	80	2.0 d
fruit cake *(Archway)*, 3 pieces	140	2.0	20.0	7.0	0	100	2.0 d
fruit and honey bar *(Archway)*	110	1.0	18.0	4.0	5	120	1.0 d
fudge (see also "chocolate," above):							
(Stella D'Oro Swiss)	70	1.0	9.0	3.0	<1	m.q.	m.q.
bar *(Tastykake)* . . .	200	2.0	35.0	7.0	5	160	1.0 d
bar, w/caramel and peanut *(Heyday)*	110	2.0	13.0	6.0	0	40	m.q.
deep night *(Stella D'Oro)*	65	1.0	8.0	4.0	<1	m.q.	m.q.
fudge creme filled *(Keebler E.L. Fudge)*	60	<1.0	7.0	3.0	0	40	m.q.

Food and Measure	cal.	prot. (gms)	carbo. (gms)	fat (gms)	chol. (mgs)	sod. (mgs)	fiber (gms)
Cookie, fudge *(cont.)*							
mint *(Keebler Grasshopper)*, 2 pieces	70	<1.0	10.0	3.0	0	35	m.q.
nut *(Tom's)*, 2.25-oz. pkg.	320	4.0	39.0	16.0	0	250	m.q.
nut bar *(Archway)*	110	2.0	17.0	4.0	5	120	1.0 d
wafer *(Nabisco Famous Wafers)*, 1/2 oz.	60	1.0	11.0	2.0	0	100	m.q.
garden creme *(Peek Freans)*, 3 pieces	197	2.7	26.9	8.7	n.a.	97	m.q.
ginger:							
(Little Debbie) . . .	80	1.0	14.0	3.0	5	55	m.q.
(Pepperidge Farm Gingerman), 2 pieces	70	1.0	10.0	3.0	5	50	m.q.
crisp *(Peek Freans)*, 5 pieces	178	2.1	31.7	4.6	0	85	m.q.
gingersnaps:							
(Archway), 6 pieces	130	1.0	23.0	5.0	0	105	1.0 d
(Nabisco Old Fashioned), 2 pieces	60	<1.0	11.0	1.0	0	80	m.q.
(Sunshine), 5 pieces	100	1.0	16.0	3.0	0	120	m.q.
golden bar *(Stella D'Oro)*	110	2.0	16.0	4.0	<1	m.q.	m.q.
graham cracker:							
(Carr's Home Wheat) . . : . .	74	1.0	10.0	3.3	<1	<1	.4 d
(Nabisco), 2 pieces	60	1.0	11.0	1.0	0	90	m.q.
(Regal), 2 pieces	140	1.0	19.0	7.0	n.a.	120	m.q.
carob chip, ginger or orange *(Mitchelhill)*	58	<1.0	8.0	3.0	n.a.	38	m.q.
chocolate, see "graham cracker, chocolate," below							
cinnamon *(Honey Maid)*, 2 pieces	60	1.0	12.0	1.0	0	85	m.q.

Food and Measure	cal.	prot. (gms)	carbo. (gms)	fat (gms)	chol. (mgs)	sod. (mgs)	fiber (gms)
cinnamon (Snack-Well's), 9 pieces	50	1.0	12.0	0	0	50	m.q.
cinnamon (Snoopy's), 11 pieces	60	1.0	11.0	2.0	0	80	m.q.
cinnamon (Sunshine), 4 scored sections	70	1.0	11.0	3.0	0	95	m.q.
cinnamon (Teddy Grahams), 11 pieces	60	1.0	11.0	2.0	0	80	m.q.
honey (Grahamy Bears), 9 pieces	130	2.0	21.0	5.0	0	160	m.q.
honey (Honey Maid), 2 pieces	60	1.0	11.0	1.0	0	90	m.q.
honey (Mitchelhill)	55	<1.0	9.0	2.0	n.a.	25	m.q.
honey (Snoopy's), 11 pieces	60	1.0	11.0	2.0	0	90	m.q.
honey (Sunshine), 4 scored sections	60	1.0	10.0	2.0	0	90	m.q.
honey (Teddy Grahams), 11 pieces	60	1.0	11.0	2.0	0	90	m.q.
muesli (Mitchelhill)	56	<1.0	9.0	2.0	n.a.	25	m.q.
vanilla (Teddy Grahams), 11 pieces	60	1.0	11.0	2.0	0	65	m.q.
vanilla frosted (Dunkaroos), 1 tray	130	<1.0	21.0	5.0	0	60	m.q.
wheat (Carr's Home Graham)	74	1.0	10.9	3.3	n.a.	<1	m.q.
wholemeal (Mitchelhill)	63	<1.0	8.0	3.0	n.a.	53	m.q.
graham cracker, chocolate: (Nabisco)	50	1.0	7.0	3.0	0	30	m.q.

Food and Measure	cal.	prot. (gms)	carbo. (gms)	fat (gms)	chol. (mgs)	sod. (mgs)	fiber (gms)
Cookie, graham cracker, chocolate (cont.)							
(Teddy Grahams),							
11 pieces	60	1.0	10.0	2.0	0	80	m.q.
(Snoopy's),							
11 pieces	60	1.0	10.0	2.0	0	90	m.q.
dark (Carr's Home							
Wheat)	64	.7	8.2	3.1	<1	49	.3 d
milk (Carr's Home							
Wheat)	65	.8	8.3	3.1	<1	53	.3 d
frosted (Dunkaroos),							
1 tray	130	1.0	19.0	5.0	0	70	m.q.
w/fudge (Cookies'N							
Fudge)	45	<1.0	6.0	2.0	0	35	m.q.
fudge covered (Kee-bler Deluxe),							
2 pieces	90	<1.0	12.0	5.0	0	80	m.q.
hazelnut (Pepperidge							
Farm), 2 pieces . .	110	1.0	15.0	6.0	0	75	m.q.
hazelnut crunch (Mas-ter Choice)	90	<1.0	9.0	4.0	10	0	m.q.
heart (Little Debbie)	100	1.0	12.0	5.0	5	50	m.q.
kichel (Stella D'Oro Di-etetic)	8	.2	.7	.5	0	<10	n.a.
lemon:							
butter finger (Master							
Choice)	70	<1.0	7.0	3.0	6	0	m.q.
creme (Dare)	93	1.1	13.0	4.1	0	36	.2 d
creme sandwich							
(Tom's), 1 pkg.	220	3.0	32.0	9.0	0	210	m.q.
frosty (Archway) . .	120	1.0	19.0	5.0	0	110	0
nut crunch (Pepper-idge Farm),							
2 pieces	110	1.0	13.0	7.0	0	50	m.q.
snaps (Archway),							
6 pieces	150	1.0	19.0	7.0	5	115	1.0 d
maple leaf creme							
(Dare)	82	.7	15.0	3.6	0	35	.3 d

Food and Measure	cal.	prot. (gms)	carbo. (gms)	fat (gms)	chol. (mgs)	sod. (mgs)	fiber (gms)
maple walnut fudge							
(Dare)	96	.9	12.0	4.6	0	36	.2 d
marshmallow cake:							
(Mallomars)	60	1.0	9.0	3.0	0	20	m.q.
(Nabisco Puffs) . .	90	1.0	14.0	4.0	0	40	m.q.
(Nabisco Twirls) . .	130	1.0	20.0	5.0	0	50	m.q.
(Pinwheels)	130	1.0	20.0	5.0	0	35	m.q.
all flavors (Dare Belmont Mallow) . .	69	.6	11.0	2.8	0	23	.1 d
mint (Dare Midnight Mint)	71	.5	9.0	4.0	0	28	.1 d
mint (Mystic Mint) . .	90	1.0	11.0	4.0	0	65	m.q.
molasses:							
(Archway)	110	1.0	20.0	4.0	5	140	1.0 d
(Archway Old Fashioned)	120	1.0	20.0	3.0	5	140	0
(Grandma's Old Time), 2 pieces	320	4.0	58.0	9.0	5	520	m.q.
crisps (Pepperidge Farm), 2 pieces	70	1.0	8.0	3.0	0	50	m.q.
iced (Archway) . . .	110	1.0	19.0	4.0	0	140	1.0 d
New Orleans cake (Archway)	110	1.0	18.0	4.0	0	105	1.0 d
nougat, nutty (Archway), 3 pieces . . .	160	1.0	18.0	10.0	0	60	0
oat bran raisin (Awrey's)	100	1.0	14.0	4.0	0	115	1.0 d
oatmeal:							
(Archway)	110	2.0	20.0	3.0	5	100	1.0 d
(Archway Mini), 12 pieces	150	2.0	19.0	8.0	5	130	1.0 d
(Baker's Bonus) . .	80	1.0	12.0	3.0	0	65	m.q.
(Dare Breaktime) . .	29	.5	5.0	1.3	0	27	.2 d
(Drake's), 2 pieces	120	2.0	19.0	4.0	0	50	m.q.
(Peek Freans Traditional), 4 pieces	183	1.9	30.3	6.0	0	231	m.q.

Food and Measure	cal.	prot. (gms)	carbo. (gms)	fat (gms)	chol. (mgs)	sod. (mgs)	fiber (gms)
Cookie, oatmeal *(cont.)*							
(Pepperidge Farm Family Request, 2 pieces	90	1.0	13.0	4.0	10	70	1.0 d
(Sunshine), 2 pieces	110	1.0	16.0	5.0	0	125	m.q.
apple spice *(Grandma's)*, 2 pieces	330	5.0	51.0	12.0	10	570	m.q.
chocolate *(Pepper- idge Farm* Dakota)	110	1.0	15.0	6.0	5	70	1.0 d
creme *(Drake's)* . .	240	3.0	38.0	9.0	2	250	m.q.
creme cakes *(Tom's)*, 1.8-oz. pkg.	230	3.0	33.0	10.0	2	190	m.q.
date filled *(Archway)*	90	1.0	19.0	2.0	5	110	1.0 d
golden *(Archway Ruth's)*	120	2.0	19.0	4.0	5	105	1.0 d
iced *(Archway)* . . .	120	1.0	19.0	5.0	5	85	1.0 d
Irish *(Pepperidge Farm)*, 2 pieces	90	1.0	13.0	5.0	5	80	m.q.
oatmeal raisin:							
(Almost Home) . .	70	1.0	10.0	3.0	<2	40	m.q.
(Archway)	110	2.0	19.0	4.0	5	115	1.0 d
(Dare)	58	.7	7.9	2.7	12	22	.5 d
(Duncan Hines), 2 pieces	110	1.0	15.0	5.0	n.a.	85	m.q.
(Pepperidge Farm Old Fashioned), 2 pieces	110	1.0	15.0	5.0	10	115	m.q.
(Pepperidge Farm Santa Fe)	100	1.0	16.0	4.0	0	70	1.0 d
(Pepperidge Farm Wholesome Choice)*	60	1.0	11.0	1.0	0	50	m.q.
(SnackWell's) . . .	60	1.0	10.0	1.0	0	65	m.q.
bar *(Tastykake)* . . .	210	3.0	32.0	8.0	15	250	1.0 d
bran *(Archway)* . .	110	2.0	19.0	4.0	5	100	1.0 d

Food and Measure	cal.	prot. (gms)	carbo. (gms)	fat (gms)	chol. (mgs)	sod. (mgs)	fiber (gms)
regular or chocolate coated raisins *(Keebler Raisin Ruckus)*	70	1.0	10.0	3.0	0	45	m.q.
cinnamon *(Famous Amos)*, 3 pieces	134	2.0	19.0	6.0	n.a.	137	m.q.
orange:							
butter fingers *(Master Choice)* . . .	70	<1.0	7.0	3.0	6	0	m.q.
chocolate tea *(Peek Freans)*, 5 pieces	200	2.2	28.0	8.8	n.a.	142	m.q.
frosty *(Archway)* . .	120	1.0	19.0	4.0	0	140	0
peach-apricot pastry *(Stella D'Oro)* . . .	90	1.0	13.0	4.0	<1	10	m.q.
peanut butter:							
(Archway)	140	3.0	16.0	7.0	10	125	1.0 d
(Dare Peanut Butter Delites)	72	1.0	8.0	4.0	0	50	.2 d
(Grandma's), 2 pieces	410	7.0	43.0	30.0	10	410	m.q.
(Grandma's Grab), 8 pieces	140	3.0	19.0	6.0	0	125	m.q.
(Pepperidge Farm Family Request), 2 pieces	80	2.0	10.0	5.0	0	65	1.0 d
bar *(Frito-Lay's)*, 1.75 oz.	270	2.0	30.0	16.0	0	65	m.q.
N' chips *(Archway)*	140	3.0	16.0	7.0	5	115	1.0 d
chip *(Dare)*	59	1.1	7.3	2.9	<1	35	.1 d
chocolate chip *(Pepperidge Farm Cheyenne)*	110	2.0	13.0	6.0	5	80	1.0 d
nougat *(Archway)*, 3 pieces	160	2.0	18.0	9.0	0	140	1.0 d
sandwich *(Nutter Butter)*	70	1.0	9.0	3.0	<2	50	m.q.

Food and Measure	cal.	prot. (gms)	carbo. (gms)	fat (gms)	chol. (mgs)	sod. (mgs)	fiber (gms)
Cookie, peanut butter *(cont.)*							
sandwich *(Nutter Butter* Bites),							
1/2 oz.	70	1.0	9.0	3.0	<2	55	m.q.
wafer *(Drake's)* . .	325	4.0	43.0	16.0	0	135	m.q.
peanut creme patties *(Nutter Butter),*							
2 pieces	80	2.0	8.0	4.0	0	45	m.q.
pecan:							
(Pecan Supremes)	80	1.0	9.0	5.0	<2	45	m.q.
crunch *(Archway)*	140	2.0	17.0	7.0	5	120	1.0 d
icebox *(Archway)*	140	1.0	18.0	7.0	10	80	0
nougat, malted *(Archway),*							
3 pieces	160	2.0	17.0	10.0	0	60	2.0 d
pineapple filled *(Archway)*	100	1.0	16.0	.4.0	5	75	1.0 d
prune pastry *(Stella D'Oro* Dietetic) . .	90	1.0	13.0	3.0	<1	<10	m.q.
raisin:							
bran *(Pepperidge Farm),* 2 pieces	110	1.0	13.0	5.0	0	55	m.q.
oatmeal *(Archway)*	130	2.0	19.0	5.0	5	40	1.0 d
oatmeal *(Dare Sun • Maid* Raisin Oatmeal)	52	1.0	7.5	2.5	5	30	.3 d
soft *(Grandma's),* 2 pieces	320	3.0	54.0	10.0	10	280	m.q.
raspberry filled:							
(Archway)	110	1.0	18.0	4.0	5	55	1.0 d
(Health Valley Fruit Centers)	80	2.0	17.0	0	0	80	2.0 d
(Health Valley Fruit Centers, 2-Pack)	85	2.0	19.0	0	0	80	2.0 d
(Pepperidge Farm Chantilly)	80	1.0	14.0	2.0	0	35	m.q.
(Pepperidge Farm Linzer)	120	2.0	20.0	4.0	0	55	m.q.

Food and Measure	cal.	prot. (gms)	carbo. (gms)	fat (gms)	chol. (mgs)	sod. (mgs)	fiber (gms)
(Raspberry Newtons)	70	1.0	15.0	2.0	0	70	m.q.
chocolate (Pepper-							
idge Farm Chan-							
tilly)	90	1.0	14.0	3.0	0	35	m.q.
raspberry tart (Pepper-							
idge Farm Whole-							
some Choice) . . .	60	1.0	11.0	1.0	0	35	m.q.
rocky road (Archway)	130	2.0	18.0	6.0	10	85	1.0 d
sesame (Stella D'Oro							
Regina)	50	1.0	6.0	2.0	<1	m.q.	m.q.
shortbread:							
(Lorna Doone),							
2 pieces	70	1.0	9.0	4.0	<5	65	m.q.
(Pepperidge Farm),							
2 pieces	150	1.0	17.0	8.0	0	85	m.q.
butter (Dare)	63	.7	7.0	3.7	6	45	.2 d
w/chocolate drop							
(Keebler Sweet							
Spots), 2 pieces	50	<1.0	8.0	3.0	<2	40	m.q.
fudge covered,							
w/toffee (Keebler							
Toffee Toppers),							
2 pieces	60	<1.0	10.0	4.0	0	50	m.q.
fudge striped (Kee-							
bler)	50	<1.0	7.0	3.0	0	55	m.q.
fudge striped (Cook-							
ies 'N Fudge) . .	60	1.0	7.0	3.0	0	50	m.q.
fudge-caramel cov-							
ered (Keebler							
Fudge'n Caramel)	60	1.0	8.0	3.0	0	30	m.q.
pecan (Pepperidge							
Farm)	70	1.0	7.0	5.0	0	15	m.q.
toffee chip (Keebler							
Toffee Sandies)	70	1.0	8.0	4.0	0	45	m.q.
shortcake (Peek Fre-							
ans), 3 pieces . . .	205	2.4	26.3	10.1	n.a.	96	m.q.
spice drops (Stella							
D'Oro Pfeffernusse)	40	.5	7.0	1.0	<1	m.q.	m.q.

Food and Measure	cal.	prot. (gms)	carbo. (gms)	fat (gms)	chol. (mgs)	sod. (mgs)	fiber (gms)
Cookie *(cont.)*							
(Stella D'Oro Angel Bars)	80	1.0	7.0	5.0	<1	m.q.	m.q.
(Stella D'Oro Angel Wings)	70	1.0	7.0	5.0	<1	m.q.	m.q.
(Stella D'Oro Angelica Goodies)	110	2.0	16.0	4.0	<1	m.q.	m.q.
(Stella D'Oro Como Delights)	150	2.0	18.0	7.0	1	m.q.	m.q.
(Stella D'Oro Love Cookies)	110	1.0	13.0	5.0	<1	m.q.	m.q.
strawberry:							
(Pepperidge Farm Fruit Cookies), 2 pieces	100	1.0	15.0	5.0	10	50	m.q.
bar *(Strawberry Newtons)*	70	1.0	15.0	2.0	0	70	m.q.
filled *(Archway)* . .	110	1.0	18.0	4.0	5	90	1.0 d
sugar:							
(Almost Home Old Fashioned) . . .	70	1.0	10.0	3.0	<2	80	m.q.
(Archway)	140	2.0	19.0	4.0	5	140	0
(Dare)	39	.4	6.0	1.4	0	13	m.q.
(Pepperidge Farm), 2 pieces	100	1.0	13.0	5.0	10	55	m.q.
drop, soft *(Archway)*	110	1.0	18.0	4.0	5	110	0
wafer *(Biscos),* 4 pieces	70	<1.0	10.0	3.0	0	20	m.q.
wafer, vanilla *(Tastykake)*	35	0	4.0	2.0	0	10	0
sweetmeal *(Peek Freans),* 4 pieces . . .	192	2.5	27.7	8.0	n.a.	161	m.q.
tea biscuit:							
(Dare Social Tea)	26	.3	4.1	1.0	0	23	.3 d
(Social Tea), 3 pieces	70	1.0	11.0	2.0	5	60	m.q.
rich *(Peek Freans),* 4 pieces	186	2.8	29.6	6.3	0	158	m.q.

Food and Measure	cal.	prot. (gms)	carbo. (gms)	fat (gms)	chol. (mgs)	sod. (mgs)	fiber (gms)
vanilla:							
(Grandma's Grab), 8 pieces	140	2.0	20.0	6.0	5	75	m.q.
(Pepperidge Farm Bordeaux), 2 pieces	70	1.0	11.0	3.0	0	40	m.q.
(Stella D'Oro Castelets)	70	1.0	10.0	3.0	<1	m.q.	m.q.
(Stella D'Oro Margherite) . . .	70	1.0	11.0	3.0	<1	m.q.	m.q.
chocolate laced (Pepperidge Farm Pirouettes), 2 pieces	70	1.0	8.0	4.0	0	20	m.q.
chocolate nut coated (Pepperidge Farm Geneva), 2 pieces	130	1.0	14.0	6.0	0	50	m.q.
creme sandwich:							
(Cameo)	70	1.0	10.0	3.0	0	50	m.q.
(Tom's), 1.6-oz. pkg.	220	2.0	32.0	9.0	0	210	m.q.
French (Peek Freans), 3 pieces	208	4.0	24.9	10.2	n.a.	92	m.q.
wafer:							
(Nilla Wafers), 1/2 oz.	60	1.0	11.0	2.0	<5	45	m.q.
(Tom's), 2.5-oz. pkg.	320	4.0	52.0	11.0	n.a.	280	m.q.
wafer (see also specific listings):							
brown edge (Nabisco), 1/2 oz.	70	1.0	10.0	3.0	<2	45	m.q.
creme, fudge covered (Keebler Fudge Sticks), 2 pieces	100	<1.0	13.0	5.0	0	35	m.q.

Food and Measure	cal.	prot. (gms)	carbo. (gms)	fat (gms)	chol. (mgs)	sod. (mgs)	fiber (gms)
Cookie, wafer (cont.)							
fudge striped (Cookies'N Fudge) . .	70	1.0	8.0	4.0	0	25	m.q.
waffle cremes (Biscos)	40	<1.0	6.0	2.0	0	10	m.q.
wedding cake (Archway), 3 pieces . . .	160	1.0	20.0	8.0	0	45	0
wheat (Carr's Wheatolo)	74	1.0	10.0	3.3	<1	<1	.4 d
wheatmeal:							
large (Carr's)	66	1.0	9.0	2.8	<1	80	.9 d
small (Carr's) . . .	40	.6	5.5	1.7	<1	48	.5 d
windmill (Archway Old Fashioned)	130	2.0	20.0	5.0	0	120	0
Cookie, frozen (Nestlé Toll House Ready To Bake), 1.2 oz., approx. 2 pieces:							
chocolate chip:							
double	150	1.0	20.0	7.0	n.a.	115	m.q.
w/nuts	150	2.0	19.0	7.0	n.a.	60	m.q.
oatmeal raisin	160	2.0	19.0	8.0	n.a.	90	m.q.
Cookie, mix, see "Dessert bar mix"							
Cookie crumbs, see "Pie crust"							
Cookie dough, refrigerated*, 1 piece:							
candy (Pillsbury Oven Lovin')	70	<1.0	10.0	3.0	0	40	m.q.
chocolate chip:							
(Pillsbury Oven Lovin')	70	<1.0	9.0	3.0	5	50	m.q.
(Pillsbury's Best) . .	70	1.0	9.0	3.0	5	55	m.q.
chocolate (Pillsbury's Best) . . .	70	1.0	9.0	3.0	0	35	m.q.
oatmeal raisin (Pillsbury's Best)	60	1.0	10.0	2.0	0	55	m.q.

Food and Measure	cal.	prot. (gms)	carbo. (gms)	fat (gms)	chol. (mgs)	sod. (mgs)	fiber (gms)
peanut butter *(Pillsbury's Best)*	70	1.0	9.0	3.0	5	75	m.q.
Reese's Pieces (Pillsbury Oven Lovin')	70	1.0	9.0	3.0	5	50	m.q.
sugar *(Pillsbury's Best)*	70	1.0	9.0	3.0 .	0	70	m.q.
Coquito nut, shelled, *(Frieda's),* 1 oz. . . .	180	2.3	5.0	17.0	0	n.a.	3.4 d
Coriander:							
fresh, 1/4 cup	1	.1	.1	<.1	0	1	.1 d
dried, leaf, 1 tsp. . . .	2	.1	.3	<.1	0	1	.1 d
seed, 1 tsp.	5	.2	1.0	.3	0	1	.5 c
Corn:							
fresh, kernels, boiled, drained, 1/2 cup . .	89	2.7	20.6	1.1	0	14	2.3 d
canned, kernel, 1/2 cup:							
drained	66	2.2	15.2	.8	0	m.q.	1.6 d
(Comstock)	100	3.0	21.0	.5	0	430	2.0 d
(Green Giant Delicorn)	80	2.0	19.0	<1.0	0	350	2.0 d
(Green Giant Niblets)	80	2.0	20.0	0	0	310	2.0 d
(Green Giant Niblets No Salt No Sugar)	80	2.0	18.0	<1.0	0	0	2.0 d
(Green Giant Sweet Select)	60	2.0	15.0	<1.0	0	280	3.0 d
golden *(Stokely)* . .	80	5.0	16.0	0	0	390	m.q.
golden, sweet *(Green Giant)* . .	70	2.0	18.0	0	0	360	2.0 d
golden, sweet *(Green Giant 50% Less Salt)*	70	2.0	16.0	<1.0	0	180	2.0 d
white *(Green Giant)*	80	2.0	20.0	0	0	310	2.0 d
w/peppers *(Green Giant Mexicorn)*	70	2.0	18.0	<1.0	0	580	3.0 d
cream-style *(Green Giant)*	100	2.0	24.0	<1.0	0	480	2.0 d
cream-style *(Stokely)*	100	2.0	23.0	0	0	380	m.q.

Food and Measure	cal.	prot. (gms)	carbo. (gms)	fat (gms)	chol. (mgs)	sod. (mgs)	fiber (gms)
Corn *(cont.)*							
freeze-dried *(Mountain House)*, 1/2 cup* . .	90	2.0	18.0	1.0	0	1	m.q.
frozen, on cob, 1 ear, except as noted:							
(Green Giant Nibblers), 2 ears . .	120	4.0	27.0	1.0	0	10	2.0 d
(Green Giant Nibblers One Serving), 2 half ears	120	4.0	26.0	1.0	0	10	2.0 d
(Green Giant Niblet Ears)	120	4.0	27.0	1.0	0	10	2.0 d
(Green Giant Sweet Select)	90	3.0	19.0	2.0	0	10	2.0 d
(Green Giant Sweet Select Half Ears), 2 ears	90	3.0	19.0	2.0	0	10	2.0 d
(Ore-Ida)	190	5.0	40.0	<1.0	0	10	m.q.
miniature *(Ore-Ida Mini-Gold)*	90	2.0	20.0	<1.0	0	5	m.q.
frozen, kernel, 3.3 oz., except as noted:							
(Green Giant Harvest Fresh Niblets), 1/2 cup	80	2.0	17.0	1.0	0	40	2.0 d
(Green Giant Niblets), 1/2 cup	90	2.0	19.0	<1.0	0	5	2.0 d
(Green Giant Sweet Select), 1/2 cup	60	2.0	13.0	1.0	0	5	2.0 d
cream-style *(Green Giant)*, 1/2 cup . .	110	3.0	25.0	1.0	0	370	2.5 d
cut *(Frosty Acres)*	80	3.0	20.0	1.0	0	3	1.0 c
white *(Seabrook)*	80	3.0	19.0	1.0	0	3	1.0 c
white shoepeg *(Green Giant Harvest Fresh)*, 1/2 cup	90	3.0	19.0	1.0	0	60	2.0 d

Food and Measure	cal.	prot. (gms)	carbo. (gms)	fat (gms)	chol. (mgs)	sod. (mgs)	fiber (gms)
white shoepeg *(Green Giant Select)*, 1/2 cup . . .	90	2.0	19.0	<1.0	0	5	2.0 d
frozen, in butter sauce:							
(Green Giant Niblets), 1/2 cup . . .	100	3.0	19.0	2.0	5	310	2.0 d
(Green Giant Niblets One Serving), 4.5 oz.	120	3.0	23.0	2.0	5	260	3.0 d
white shoepeg *(Green Giant)*, 1/2 cup	100	2.0	20.0	2.0	5	280	2.0 d
Corn, whole-grain:							
1 oz.	103	2.7	21.1	1.3	0	10	.8 c
1 cup	605	15.6	123.3	7.9	0	58	4.8 c
blue *(Arrowhead Mills)*, 2 oz.	210	6.0	41.0	3.0	0	tr.	5.6 d
yellow *(Arrowhead Mills)*, 2 oz.	210	4.0	43.0	2.0	0	tr.	6.8 d
Corn bran, crude:							
1 oz.	64	2.4	24.3	.3	0	2	24.0 d
1 cup	170	6.4	65.1	.7	0	5	64.3 d
Corn chips and similar snacks, 1 oz., except as noted:							
(Bugles)	150	2.0	18.0	8.0	n.a.	290	m.q.
(Fritos Original)	150	2.0	16.0	10.0	0	220	1.1 d
(Fritos Crisp'N Thin)	160	2.0	16.0	10.0	0	210	1.1 d
(Fritos Dip Size) . . .	150	1.0	16.0	10.0	0	190	1.1 d
(Santitas Cantina Style)	140	2.0	19.0	6.0	0	75	1.5 d
(Santitas Chips) . . .	140	2.0	19.0	7.0	0	50	1.5 d
(Santitas Strips) . . .	140	2.0	19.0	7.0	0	65	1.5 d
(Tom's), 13/4-oz. pkg.	270	3.0	29.0	16.0	0	420	m.q.
barbecue flavor:							
(Fritos Rowdy Rustlers Bar-B-Q) . .	150	2.0	17.0	9.0	0	300	1.1 d

Food and Measure	cal.	prot. (gms)	carbo. (gms)	fat (gms)	chol. (mgs)	sod. (mgs)	fiber (gms)
Corn chips and similar snacks, barbecue flavor *(cont.)*							
(Tom's), 15/8-oz. pkg.	250	3.0	26.0	15.0	0	420	m.q.
caramel corn puffs:							
(Health Valley) . . .	100	3.0	21.0	<1.0	0	45	m.q.
apple cinnamon *(Health Valley)* . .	100	3.0	21.0	<1.0	0	50	m.q.
peanut flavor *(Health Valley)*	100	3.0	21.0	<1.0	0	65	m.q.
cheese:							
(Cheddar Valley) . .	160	2.0	16.0	9.0	0	240	1.0 d
(Chee•tos Balls) . .	160	2.0	16.0	10.0	0	360	1.0 d
(Chee•tos Crunchy)	150	1.0	17.0	9.0	0	310	1.0 d
(Chee•tos Curls)	150	1.0	17.0	9.0	0	270	1.0 d
(Chee•tos Light)	140	2.0	19.0	6.0	0	280	1.0 d
(Chee•tos Paws)	160	1.0	15.0	10.0	0	310	1.0 d
(Chee•tos Puffs)	160	1.0	16.0	9.0	0	330	1.0 d
(Health Valley Cheese Puffs) . .	100	3.0	21.0	0	0	210	2.2 d
(Tom's Cheese Crunchies)	250	2.0	23.0	16.0	n.a.	340	m.q.
(Tom's Cheese Puffs), 7/8-oz. pkg.	200	2.0	20.0	12.0	n.a.	380	m.q.
chili, zesty or green onion *(Health Valley Cheese Puffs)*	100	3.0	21.0	<1.0	0	75	m.q.
hot *(Flamin' Hot)* . .	150	2.0	16.0	9.0	0	240	1.0 d
nacho *(Bugles)* . .	160	2.0	17.0	9.0	n.a.	250	m.q.
nacho *(Fritos Non-Stop)*	150	2.0	16.0	9.0	0	220	1.1 d
nacho, rings *(Tom's),* 7/8 oz.	140	2.0	10.0	10.0	n.a.	330	m.q.
puffs *(No Fries)* . .	120	3.0	22.0	2.0	n.a.	55	m.q.
chili cheese *(Fritos)*	160	2.0	15.0	10.0	0	300	1.1 d
fajita flavor *(Santitas Cantina Style)* . . .	140	2.0	18.0	7.0	0	95	1.5 d

Food and Measure	cal.	prot. (gms)	carbo. (gms)	fat (gms)	chol. (mgs)	sod. (mgs)	fiber (gms)
nuggets, toasted (Frito-Lay's), 1.38 oz.	170	3.0	29.0	5.0	0	265	m.q.
ranch:							
(Bugles)	150	2.0	16.0	9.0	n.a.	290	m.q.
(Fritos Wild'N Mild)	160	2.0	16.0	9.0	0	240	1.1 d
(No Fries Ranch-O's)	120	2.0	22.0	2.0	n.a.	55	m.q.
roasted, fresh (Pringles)	140	2.0	17.0	7.0	0	195	m.q.
tortilla, see "Tortilla chips"							
Corn combinations, packaged, 1/2 cup:							
w/carrots (Del Monte Vegetable Classics)	70	1.0	12.0	2.0	n.a.	330	m.q.
w/green beans, carrots, pasta (Green Giant Pantry Express)	80	2.0	17.0	2.0	0	330	3.0 d
Corn flake crumbs (Kellogg's), 1 oz.	100	2.0	24.0	0	0	290	1.0 d
Corn flour:							
whole-grain, 1 oz. . . .	102	2.0	21.8	1.1	0	1	3.8 d
whole-grain, 1 cup . .	422	8.1	89.9	4.5	0	6	15.7 d
masa, 1 oz.	103	2.6	21.6	1.1	0	1	2.7 d
masa, 1 cup	416	10.7	87.0	4.3	0	6	10.9 d
Corn fritter, frozen (Mrs. Paul's), 4 oz.	240	5.0	35.0	9.0	10	560	m.q.
Corn grits:							
dry:							
instant (Quaker Original), 1 oz.	100	2.0	22.0	0	0	340	1.5 d
instant, quick, dry (Albers Hominy), 1/4 cup	150	4.0	33.0	0	0	0	m.q.
white (Arrowhead Mills), 2 oz. . . .	200	5.0	43.0	1.0	0	1	1.5 d

Food and Measure	cal.	prot. (gms)	carbo. (gms)	fat (gms)	chol. (mgs)	sod. (mgs)	fiber (gms)
Corn grits, dry *(cont.)*							
yellow *(Arrowhead Mills),* 2 oz.	200	5.0	44.0	1.0	0	1	1.5 d
cooked, 1 cup	146	3.5	31.4	.5	0	tr.	.2 c
Corn soufflé, frozen *(Stouffer's),* 6 oz.	240	7.0	27.0	11.0	n.a.	760	m.q.
Corn syrup:							
dark *(Karo),* 1 tbsp.	60	0	15.0	0	0	40	0
light *(Karo),* 1 tbsp.	60	0	15.0	0	0	30	0
Cornbread, see "Bread, sweet, mix"							
Cornish game hen:							
fresh, roasted:							
dark meat w/skin *(Perdue),* 1 oz.	43	4.0	0	3.0	29	14	0
white meat w/skin *(Perdue),* 1 oz.	43	5.0	0	3.0	25	9	0
frozen, w/skin *(Tyson),* 3.5 oz.	250	27.0	1.0	15.0	155	80	0
refrigerated, roasted:							
dark meat *(Perdue Done It!),* 1 oz.	45	5.0	<1.0	3.0	26	72	0
white meat *(Perdue Done It!),* 1 oz.	39	6.0	<1.0	1.0	18	93	0
Cornmeal (see also "Corn flour" and "Polenta"):							
blue *(Arrowhead Mills),* 2 oz.	210	6.0	41.0	3.0	0	1	5.6 d
white or yellow *(Albers),* 1 oz.	100	2.0	22.0	1.0	0	0	1.5 d
white or yellow *(Quaker),* 1 oz. . . .	100	2.0	22.0	1.0	0	0	m.q.
yellow or hi-lysine *(Arrowhead Mills),* 2 oz.	210	4.0	43.0	2.0	0	1	6.8 d
Cornmeal mix, white *(Aunt Jemima),* 1 oz.	90	.2	18.0	1.0	0	380	3.0 d

Food and Measure	cal.	prot. (gms)	carbo. (gms)	fat (gms)	chol. (mgs)	sod. (mgs)	fiber (gms)
Cornstarch *(Argo/ Kingsford)*, 1 tbsp.	30	0	7.0	0	0	0	tr.d
Cottonseed kernels, roasted, 1 tbsp. . . .	51	3.3	2.2	3.6	0	3	.6 d
Cottonseed meal, partially defatted, 1 oz.	104	13.9	10.9	1.4	0	10	.7 c
Cough drop, see "Candy"							
Country coating mix, mild *(Shake'n Bake)*, 1/4 pouch	80	1.0	10.0	4.0	0	500	m.q.
Country gravy mix: *(McCormick/Schilling)*, 1/4 cup*	40	1.0	5.0	2.0	n.a.	289	n.a.
sausage *(McCormick/ Schilling)*, 1/4 cup*	41	1.0	5.0	2.0	n.a.	265	n.a.
vegetarian *(LaLoma Gravy Quik)*, 2 tbsp.	10	<1.0	2.0	<1.0	0	200	m.q.
Couscous:							
dry, 1 oz.	107	3.6	22.0	.2	0	3	1.4 d
cooked, 1/2 cup . . .	101	3.4	20.9	.1	0	4	1.3 d
Couscous mix*: *(Fantastic Foods)*, 1/2 cup	96	3.0	21.0	.1	0	5	2.6 d
almond chicken *(Casbah Couscous Cup)*, 6 oz.	140	7.0	22.0	3.0	m.q.	390	m.q.
asparagus au gratin *(Casbah Couscous Cup)*, 6 oz.	130	7.0	21.0	3.0	m.q.	390	m.q.
cheddar broccoli *(Casbah Couscous Cup)*, 6 oz.	125	6.0	22.0	1.0	m.q.	380	m.q.
lentil curry *(Marakesh Express)*, 1/2 cup	130	5.0	25.0	2.0	0	95	m.q.

Food and Measure	cal.	prot. (gms)	carbo. (gms)	fat (gms)	chol. (mgs)	sod. (mgs)	fiber (gms)
Couscous mix *(cont.)*							
mushroom tofu *(Casbah Couscous Cup)*,							
6 oz.	145	8.0	24.0	2.0	m.q.	380	m.q.
pilaf, savory:							
(Quick Pilaf), 1/2 cup	121	5.0	24.0	.5	0	237	3.0 d
w/butter *(Quick Pilaf)*, 1/2 cup . . .	124	4.0	19.0	3.0	m.q.	254	m.q.
shrimp paella *(Casbah Couscous Cup)*,							
6 oz.	130	8.0	21.0	2.0	m.q.	390	m.q.
spicy, w/raisins and almonds *(Knorr Pilafs)*, 1 serving . . .	150	5.7	29.4	1.0	0	340	1.4 d
tomato Parmesan *(Casbah Couscous Cup)*, 6 oz.	130	6.0	22.0	2.0	m.q.	380	m.q.
whole wheat *(Fantastic Foods)*, 1/2 cup . .	100	4.0	21.0	.2	0	3	3.0 d
Cowpeas, 1/2 cup, except as noted:							
fresh:							
raw, trimmed . . .	65	2.1	13.6	.3	0	3	3.6 d
boiled, drained . .	79	2.6	16.7	.3	0	3	4.1 d
fresh, leafy tips:							
raw, chopped . . .	5	.7	.9	<.1	0	1	.2 c
boiled, drained, 4 oz.	25	5.3	3.2	.1	0	7	3.0 c
fresh, pods, w/seeds:							
raw, trimmed . . .	21	1.6	4.5	.1	0	2	.8 c
boiled, drained . .	16	1.2	3.3	.1	0	1	.8 c
canned:							
(Allens/East Texas Fair)	100	7.0	18.0	<1.0	0	350	4.0 d
w/jalapeños *(Home-Folks)*	80	4.0	10.0	<1.0	0	560	4.0 d
w/snaps *(Allens/East Texas Fair)*	100	5.0	20.0	<1.0	0	370	m.q.

Food and Measure	cal.	prot. (gms)	carbo. (gms)	fat (gms)	chol. (mgs)	sod. (mgs)	fiber (gms)
frozen:							
boiled, drained . .	112	7.2	20.2	.6	0	5	4.3 d
(Frosty Acres),							
3.3 oz.	130	9.0	23.0	1.0	0	6	1.0 c
Cowpeas, mature:							
boiled, 1/2 cup	100	6.7	17.9	.5	0	3	5.6 d
canned, 1/2 cup:							
w/liquid	92	5.7	16.4	.7	0	359	4.0 d
(Allens/East Texas							
Fair)	110	5.0	20.0	<1.0	0	300	2.0 d
(Green Giant/Joan							
of Arc)	90	7.0	18.0	<1.0	0	300	4.0 d
w/bacon (Allens/							
Sunshine)	110	5.0	18.0	1.0	m.q.	300	2.0 d
w/pork	99	3.3	19.8	1.9	8	420	4.0 d
Cowpeas, catjang,							
see "Catjang"							
Crab, meat only:							
Alaska king:							
raw, 4 oz.	95	20.8	0	.7	47	948	0
boiled, poached, or							
steamed, 4 oz.	110	21.9	0	1.7	60	1216	0
blue:							
raw, 4 oz.	99	20.5	.1	1.2	89	332	0
boiled, poached, or							
steamed, 4 oz.	116	22.9	0	2.0	113	316	0
dungeness:							
raw, 4 oz.	98	19.8	.8	1.1	67	335	0
boiled, poached, or							
steamed, 4 oz.	125	25.3	1.1	1.4	86	429	0
queen:							
raw, 4 oz.	102	21.0	0	1.4	62	611	0
boiled, poached, or							
steamed, 4 oz.	130	26.9	0	1.7	81	784	0
Crab, canned, blue,							
4 oz.	112	23.3	0	1.4	101	378	0
"Crab," imitation:							
from surimi, 1 oz. . .	29	3.4	3.0	.4	6	238	0

Food and Measure	cal.	prot. (gms)	carbo. (gms)	fat (gms)	chol. (mgs)	sod. (mgs)	fiber (gms)
"Crab," imitation (cont.)							
(Louis Kemp Crab De-Lights), 2 oz. . . .	50	6.0	5.0	<1.0	m.q.	320	0
Crab cake, deviled, frozen:							
(Mrs. Paul's), 3 oz. . .	180	8.0	18.0	9.0	20	480	m.q.
miniature (Mrs. Paul's), 3.5 oz.	240	9.0	25.0	12.0	20	540	m.q.
Crab cake seasoning mix (Old Bay Crab Cake Classic), 1 pkg.	133	7.0	18.0	4.0	n.a.	1498	m.q.
Crabapple, fresh, w/ peel:							
1 oz.	22	.1	5.7	.1	0	<1	.2 c
sliced, 1/2 cup	42	.2	11.0	.2	0	1	.3 c
(Frieda's), 1 oz. . . .	19	.1	5.0	.1	0	<1	m.q.
Cracker, 1/2 oz., ex-cept as noted:							
all varieties (Mc-Cracken's Cracker Crisp), 1 oz.	140	2.0	18.0	8.0	0	170	m.q.
animal, see "Cookies"							
bacon flavor (Nabisco)	70	1.0	9.0	4.0	0	210	m.q.
w/bacon and cheese (Handi-Snacks), 1 pkg.	130	4.0	8.0	9.0	20	410	m.q.
butter flavor:							
(Carr's Butterpuff), 1 piece	52	.9	6.3	2.5	n.a.	58	.3 d
(Escort), 3 pieces	70	1.0	9.0	4.0	0	115	m.q.
(Keebler Club), 4 pieces	60	1.0	9.0	3.0	0	150	m.q.
(Keebler Club Low Salt), 4 pieces . .	60	1.0	9.0	3.0	0	75	m.q.
(Keebler Toasteds Complements), 4 pieces	60	1.0	8.0	3.0	0	180	m.q.

Food and Measure	cal.	prot. (gms)	carbo. (gms)	fat (gms)	chol. (mgs)	sod. (mgs)	fiber (gms)
(Keebler Town House), 4 pieces	70	1.0	8.0	4.0	0	200	m.q.
(Keebler Town House Low Salt), 4 pieces	70	1.0	8.0	4.0	0	120	m.q.
(Ritz/Ritz Bits) . . .	70	1.0	9.0	4.0	0	120	m.q.
(Ritz/Ritz Bits Low Salt)	70	1.0	9.0	4.0	0	60	m.q.
dairy *(American Classic)*, 4 pieces	70	1.0	9.0	3.0	<2	140	m.q.
thins *(Pepperidge Farm)*, 4 pieces	70	1.0	10.0	3.0	<5	115	0
cheddar:							
(Carr's), 1 piece . . .	21	.4	1.9	1.3	<1	32	.1 d
(Cheddar Wedges)	70	1.0	9.0	3.0	<2	150	m.q.
(Combos), 1.8 oz.	240	5.0	34.0	10.0	n.a.	580	m.q.
(Frito-Lay Cracker Snacks)	70	1.0	8.0	4.0	0	150	m.q.
(Munch'ems)	60	1.0	9.0	3.0	0	170	m.q.
(Pepperidge Farm Goldfish)	60	2.0	9.0	3.0	5	115	m.q.
(Pepperidge Farm Low Salt Goldfish)	60	2.0	9.0	2.0	<5	65	m.q.
(Snorkels)	60	2.0	9.0	2.0	0	130	m.q.
thins *(Better Cheddars)*	70	2.0	8.0	4.0	<2	130	m.q.
thins *(Better Cheddars Low Salt)* . .	70	2.0	8.0	4.0	<2	65	m.q.
cheese:							
(Cheese Nips) . . .	70	1.0	9.0	3.0	<2	130	m.q.
(Cheez-it), 12 pieces	70	2.0	7.0	4.0	<2	135	m.q.
(Cheez-it Low Salt), 12 pieces	70	2.0	7.0	4.0	<2	65	m.q.
(Hain), 6 pieces . .	70	2.0	9.0	3.0	0	100	m.q.
(Nips)	70	1.0	9.0	3.0	<2	150	m.q.
(Ritz Bits)	70	1.0	8.0	4.0	<2	130	m.q.
(SnackWell's) . . .	60	2.0	11.0	1.0	0	160	m.q.
(Tid Bits)	70	1.0	8.0	4.0	<2	200	m.q.

Food and Measure	cal.	prot. (gms)	carbo. (gms)	fat (gms)	chol. (mgs)	sod. (mgs)	fiber (gms)
Cracker, cheese *(cont.)*							
nacho *(Doritos Nacho Cheese)*, 1 oz.	140	2.0	18.0	7.0	0	150	m.q.
nacho *(Munch'ems)*	60	1.0	8.0	2.0	0	140	m.q.
Parmesan *(Pepperidge Farm* Goldfish)*	60	2.0	9.0	2.0	0	160	m.q.
Swiss *(Nabisco Swiss Cheese)*	70	1.0	9.0	3.0	<2	170	m.q.
three *(Pepperidge Farm* Snack Sticks), 8 pieces	130	4.0	19.0	5.0	0	400	1.0 d
cheese sandwich:							
(Tom's Cheese Crisp), 1 1/4 oz.	170	6.0	18.0	10.0	0	370	m.q.
(Tom's Cheezer), 1 1/4 oz.	160	3.0	21.0	8.0	2	560	m.q.
cheese filled *(Frito-Lay's)*, 1.5 oz. . . .	210	4.0	24.0	10.0	5	470	m.q.
cheese filled *(Ritz Bits Real Cheese)*	80	1.0	7.0	5.0	<2	135	m.q.
nacho or pizza *(Ritz Bits)*	80	1.0	8.0	5.0	<2	140	m.q.
peanut butter filled *(Frito-Lay's)*, 1.5 oz.	210	6.0	24.0	10.0	0	450	m.q.
and peanut butter *(Handi-Snacks)*, 1 pkg.	190	6.0	11.0	14.0	0	180	m.q.
and peanut butter *(Tom's Eat-A-Snax)*, 1.4 oz.	200	4.0	22.0	11.0	0	490	m.q.
and cheese *(Handi-Snacks)*, 1 pkg.	120	4.0	9.0	8.0	20	360	m.q.
(Chicken In A Biskit)	80	1.0	8.0	5.0	0	130	m.q.
chips:							
(Zings! Original) . .	70	1.0	10.0	3.0	0	115	m.q.

Food and Measure	cal.	prot. (gms)	carbo. (gms)	fat (gms)	chol. (mgs)	sod. (mgs)	fiber (gms)
cheddar (Zings!) . .	70	1.0	9.0	3.0	0	130	m.q.
club (Red Oval Farms), 6 pieces	121	1.9	16.7	5.2	0	160	m.q.
ranch (Zings!) . . .	70	1.0	9.0	3.0	0	135	m.q.
crispbread (see also specific cracker listings):							
(Wasa Breakfast), 1 piece	50	2.0	8.0	1.0	0	65	.7 d
(Wasa Extra Crisp), 1 piece	25	1.0	5.0	0	0	40	m.q.
(Wasa Fiber Plus), 1 piece	35	1.0	5.0	1.0	0	65	2.8 d
cinnamon sugar wheat (Pepperidge Farm)	60	1.0	11.0	1.0	0	100	1.0 d
dark, regular or w/caraway (Finn Crisp), 2 pieces . .	38	1.0	9.0	<1.0	0	130	1.6 d
high fiber:							
(Ryvita Crisp Bread), 1 piece	23	.9	4.0	<1.0	0	10	2.0 d
(Ryvita Snack- bread), 1 piece	14	.6	3.0	<1.0	0	25	1.0 d
croissant (Carr's), 1 piece	24	.4	3.2	1.0	<1	33	.1 d
(Dare Breton), 1 piece	21	.5	2.6	.9	0	40	.1 d
(Dare Breton 50% Less Salt), 1 piece	21	.5	2.6	1.0	0	15	.1 d
(Dare Cabaret), 1 piece	23	.4	3.0	1.1	0	45	.1 d
(Dare Vivant), 1 piece	20	.4	2.8	.8	0	32	.1 d
flatbread, 1 piece:							
(J.J. Flats Flavorall)	50	2.0	10.0	1.0	0	130	1.0 d
plain (J.J. Flats) . .	50	2.0	11.0	1.0	0	140	<1.0 d
garlic (J.J. Flats) . .	50	2.0	11.0	1.0	0	135	1.0 d
garlic (New York)	65	2.0	12.0	1.0	0	70	m.q.
Italian herb (J.J. Flats)	50	2.0	11.0	1.5	0	80	1.0 d

Food and Measure	cal.	prot. (gms)	carbo. (gms)	fat (gms)	chol. (mgs)	sod. (mgs)	fiber (gms)
Cracker, flatbread *(cont.)*							
multi grain *(J.J. Flats)*	50	1.0	11.0	1.5	0	120	1.0 d
oat bran *(J.J. Flats)*	50	2.0	11.0	.5	0	65	1.0 d
onion *(J.J. Flats)* . .	50	2.0	11.0	1.0	0	130	<1.0 d
poppy *(J.J. Flats)*	50	2.0	10.0	1.0	0	130	<1.0 d
sesame *(J.J. Flats)*	50	2.0	10.0	1.0	0	130	1.0 d
garlic *(Manischewitz Tams),* 10 pieces	153	2.0	19.0	8.0	0	165	m.q.
graham, see "Cookies"							
grain, mixed *(Harvest Crisps 5 Grain)* . .	60	1.0	10.0	2.0	0	135	m.q.
grain, multi *(Pepperidge Farm Wholesome),* 4 pieces . .	70	1.0	12.0	2.0	0	115	m.q.
Italian, zesty *(Frito-Lay Cracker Snacks)* . .	70	1.0	9.0	3.0	0	115	m.q.
(Manischewitz Tam Tams), 10 pieces	147	2.0	17.0	8.0	0	171	m.q.
(Manischewitz Tam Tams No Salt), 10 pieces	138	2.0	18.0	7.0	0	<10	m.q.
matzo, 1 board, except as noted:							
(Manischewitz Daily Unsalted)	110	3.0	24.0	.3	0	1	.1 d
(Manischewitz Miniatures), 10 pieces	80	2.0	20.0	<1.0	0	<10	m.q.
(Manischewitz Passover)	129	3.3	27.0	.4	0	<5	m.q.
American *(Manischewitz)*	115	2.9	22.0	1.9	0	m.q.	m.q.
egg *(Manischewitz Passover)*	132	4.0	27.0	2.0	25	<5	m.q.
egg *(Manischewitz Passover Crackers),* 10 pieces	108	3.0	20.0	2.0	20	<10	m.q.

Food and Measure	cal.	prot. (gms)	carbo. (gms)	fat (gms)	chol. (mgs)	sod. (mgs)	fiber (gms)
egg n' onion (Manischewitz)	112	3.1	23.0	1.0	15	180	m.q.
tea, thin (Manischewitz Daily)	103	3.0	22.0	.3	0	1	.1 d
thin (Manischewitz)	100	3.0	21.0	.3	0	m.q.	.1 d
thin, dietetic (Manischewitz)	91	2.6	19.0	.4	0	<1	.1 d
whole wheat w/bran (Manischewitz)	110	4.0	21.0	.6	0	1	.6 d
melba toast:							
(Devonsheer Rounds)	50	2.0	11.0	<1.0	0	85	m.q.
bacon (Old London Snacks)	60	2.0	9.0	2.0	0	130	m.q.
garlic (Devonsheer Rounds)	60	1.0	10.0	2.0	0	80	m.q.
garlic (Old London Snacks)	60	1.0	9.0	2.0	0	130	m.q.
honey bran (Devonsheer Rounds)	50	2.0	12.0	<1.0	0	85	m.q.
oat bran (Devonsheer Rounds)	50	2.0	11.0	<1.0	0	90	m.q.
onion (Devonsheer Rounds)	50	2.0	11.0	1.0	0	90	m.q.
onion or rye (Old London Snacks)	60	2.0	9.0	2.0	0	140	m.q.
sesame (Devonsheer Rounds)	60	2.0	9.0	2.0	0	130	m.q.
sesame (Old London Snacks)	60	2.0	8.0	2.0	0	160	m.q.
sesame (Old London Toast)	50	2.0	9.0	2.0	0	160	m.q.
sesame (Old London Unsalted Toast)	50	2.0	9.0	2.0	0	<5	m.q.
white or whole grain (Old London Snacks)	60	2.0	9.0	2.0	0	130	m.q.

Food and Measure	cal.	prot. (gms)	carbo. (gms)	fat (gms)	chol. (mgs)	sod. (mgs)	fiber (gms)
Cracker, melba toast *(cont.)*							
white or wheat *(Old London Toast)* . .	50	2.0	10.0	<1.0	0	130	m.q.
whole grain *(Old London Toast)* . .	50	2.0	10.0	<1.0	0	130	m.q.
milk *(Royal Lunch)* . .	60	1.0	10.0	2.0	<2	80	m.q.
oat *(Harvest Crisps)*	60	1.0	10.0	2.0	0	135	m.q.
oat *(Oat Thins)*	70	1.0	10.0	3.0	0	90	m.q.
oat bran *(Oat Bran Krisp)*	60	1.0	9.0	3.0	0	140	3.2 d
onion:							
(Hain), 6 pieces . .	70	1.0	9.0	3.0	0	80	m.q.
(Hain No Salt Added)*, 6 pieces	70	1.0	9.0	3.0	0	0	m.q.
(Manischewitz Tams), 10 pieces	150	2.0	18.0	8.0	0	157	m.q.
oyster, see "soup and oyster," below							
peanut butter:							
(Combos), 1.8 oz.	240	6.0	30.0	10.0	n.a.	360	m.q.
(Tom's Peanut Butter Malt), 1¼ oz.	180	4.0	20.0	8.0	0	280	m.q.
(Tom's Peanut Butter Squares), 1¾ oz.	230	5.0	31.0	11.0	0	340	m.q.
(Tom's Peanut Butter Toast), 1¼ oz.	180	4.0	19.0	10.0	0	390	m.q.
sandwich *(Little Debbie Toasty)*, 4 pieces	120	3.0	15.0	6.0	5	240	m.q.
sandwich *(Ritz Bits)*	70	1.0	8.0	4.0	0	110	m.q.
(Pepperidge Farm Original Goldfish)	60	1.0	9.0	3.0	0	95	m.q.
pizza flavor *(Pepperidge Farm Goldfish)*	60	2.0	9.0	3.0	0	110	1.0 d
pizza flavor *(Snorkels)*	60	1.0	10.0	2.0	0	110	m.q.
poppy, toasted *(American Classic)*	70	1.0	9.0	3.0	0	140	m.q.

Food and Measure	cal.	prot. (gms)	carbo. (gms)	fat (gms)	chol. (mgs)	sod. (mgs)	fiber (gms)
poppy and sesame seed *(Carr's)*, 1 piece	21	.4	2.1	1.2	<1	24	.1 d
pretzel:							
(Pepperidge Farm Goldfish)	60	1.0	10.0	2.0	0	80	m.q.
(Pepperidge Farm Snack Sticks), 8 pieces	120	3.0	23.0	3.0	0	430	1.0 d
pumpernickel *(Pepperidge Farm Snack Sticks)*, 8 pieces	140	3.0	20.0	6.0	0	330	1.0 d
ranch *(Munch'ems)*	90	1.0	17.0	3.0	<1	170	m.q.
ranch *(Snorkels)* . .	60	1.0	10.0	2.0	0	110	m.q.
rich, 4 pieces:							
(Hain)	70	2.0	9.0	3.0	0	55	m.q.
(Hain No Salt Added)	70	2.0	9.0	3.0	0	5	m.q.
rye:							
(Hain), 6 pieces . .	70	1.0	10.0	3.0	0	65	m.q.
(Hain No Salt Added)*, 6 pieces	60	1.0	10.0	2.0	0	0	m.q.
(Rykrisp)	40	1.0	11.0	0	0	75	3.6 d
(Triscuit Deli Style)	60	1.0	10.0	2.0	0	80	m.q.
dark *(Ryvita* Crisp Bread)*, 1 piece	26	.7	6.0	<1.0	0	35	1.3 d
light *(Ryvita* Crisp Bread)*, 1 piece	26	.7	6.0	<1.0	0	20	1.3 d
light *(Wasa* Crispbread)*, 1 piece	25	1.0	5.0	0	0	40	1.2 d
seasoned *(Rykrisp)*	45	1.0	11.0	1.0	0	105	3.0 d
sesame *(Rykrisp)*	50	1.0	10.0	2.0	0	105	3.0 d
sesame, toasted *(Ryvita* Crisp Bread)*, 1 piece	31	1.1	5.0	<1.0	0	10	1.4 d
stoned *(Red Oval Farms)*, 7 pieces	104	2.7	18.0	2.3	0	323	m.q.

Food and Measure	cal.	prot. (gms)	carbo. (gms)	fat (gms)	chol. (mgs)	sod. (mgs)	fiber (gms)
Cracker *(cont.)*							
saltine:							
(Premium)	60	1.0	10.0	2.0	0	180	m.q.
(Premium Bits) . . .	70	1.0	9.0	3.0	0	160	m.q.
(Premium Fat Free)	50	1.0	12.0	0	0	115	m.q.
(Premium Low Salt)	60	1.0	10.0	2.0	0	115	m.q.
(Premium Unsalted Tops)*	60	1.0	10.0	2.0	0.	135	m.q.
(Sunshine Krispy), 5 pieces	60	1.0	11.0	1.0	0	210	m.q.
(Sunshine Krispy Unsalted Tops),* 5 pieces	60	1.0	11.0	1.0	0	120	m.q.
multigrain *(Premium)*	60	1.0	10.0	2.0	0	170	m.q.
sandwich, see specific cracker listings							
seasoned *(Munch'ems Original)*	60	1.0	9.0	2.0	0	160	m.q.
sesame:							
(Dare Breton), 1 piece	22	.4	2.5	1.1	0	40	.1 d
(Hain), 6 pieces . .	70	1.0	9.0	3.0	0	80	m.q.
(Hain No Salt Added), 6 pieces	70	1.0	9.0	3.0	0	0	m.q.
(Keebler Toasteds Complements), 4 pieces	60	1.0	8.0	3.0	0	135	m.q.
(Pepperidge Farm), 4 pieces	80	2.0	12.0	4.0	0	140	2.0 d
(Pepperidge Farm Snack Sticks),* 8 pieces	140	4.0	19.0	5.0	0	280	1.0 d
golden *(American Classic)*	70	1.0	9.0	3.0	0	120	m.q.
thins *(Sesmark* Original), 4 pieces . .	71	2.0	8.0	3.0	0	170	m.q.
sesame and cheese *(Twigs* Snack Sticks)	70	1.0	8.0	4.0	<2	140	m.q.

Food and Measure	cal.	prot. (gms)	carbo. (gms)	fat (gms)	chol. (mgs)	sod. (mgs)	fiber (gms)
sesame and onion *(Red Oval Farms)*, 6 pieces	114	2.3	16.7	4.2	0	337	m.q.
soda or water:							
(Carr's Table Water, Bite Size), 1 piece	15	.3	2.7	.3	tr.	20	.1 d
(Carr's Table Water, King Size), 1 piece	33	.7	5.9	.6	tr.	44	.3 d
(Carr's Table Water Oblong), 1 piece	18	.4	3.1	.4	n.a.	24	.1 d
(Crown Pilot)	70	1.0	11.0	2.0	0	70	m.q.
(Pepperidge Farm English Water Biscuit), 4 pieces	70	2.0	13.0	1.0	0	100	0
w/cracked pepper *(Carr's* Table Water), 1 piece	15	.3	2.6	.3	tr.	20	.1 d
w/sesame seeds *(Carr's* Table Water), 1 piece	15	.3	2.6	.3	tr.	21	.1 d
soup and oyster:							
(Carr's Scalloped Round), 1 piece	16	.3	2.5	.5	n.a.	28	.1 d
(Oysterettes)	60	1.0	10.0	1.0	0	140	m.q.
(Premium)	60	1.0	10.0	1.0	0	210	m.q.
(Sunshine), 16 pieces	60	1.0	11.0	1.0	0	190	m.q.
sour cream and onion *(Munch'ems)*	60	1.0	9.0	3.0	0	150	m.q.
sourdough, 6 pieces:							
(Hain)	70	1.0	9.0	3.0	0	85	m.q.
(Hain Low Salt)	70	1.0	9.0	3.0	0	5	m.q.
toast *(Uneeda* Biscuits Unsalted Tops)	60	1.0	10.0	2.0	0	100	m.q.
vegetable:							
(Garden Crisps)	60	1.0	11.0	2.0	0	135	m.q.

Food and Measure	cal.	prot. (gms)	carbo. (gms)	fat (gms)	chol. (mgs)	sod. (mgs)	fiber (gms)
Cracker, vegetable *(cont.)*							
(Hain), 6 pieces . .	60	1.0	9.0	3.0	0	100	m.q.
(Hain No Salt Added), 6 pieces	70	1.0	9.0	3.0	0	25	m.q.
(Vegetable Thins)	70	1.0	8.0	4.0	0	140	m.q.
garden *(Pepperidge Farm Whole-some)*, 5 pieces	60	1.0	10.0	2.0	0	125	m.q.
wheat:							
(Keebler Toasteds Complements), 4 pieces	60	1.0	8.0	3.0	0	130	m.q.
(Manischewitz Tams), 10 pieces	150	2.0	18.0	8.0	0	180	m.q.
(Ryvita Original Snackbread), 1 piece	20	.5	4.0	<1.0	0	20	.2 d
(SnackWell's) . . .	50	1.0	12.0	0	0	160	m.q.
(Sociables)	70	1.0	9.0	4.0	0	135	m.q.
(Sunshine Wheats), 8 pieces	70	1.0	9.0	4.0	0	170	m.q.
(Triscuit)	60	1.0	10.0	2.0	0	75	m.q.
(Triscuit Low Salt)	60	1.0	10.0	2.0	0	35	m.q.
(Waverly), 4 pieces	70	1.0	10.0	3.0	0	160	m.q.
(Waverly Low Salt)	70	1.0	10.0	3.0	0	80	m.q.
(Wheat Thins) . . .	70	1.0	9.0	3.0	0	120	m.q.
(Wheat Thins Low Salt)	70	1.0	9.0	3.0	0	60	m.q.
(Wheatsworth Stone Ground)	70	1.0	9.0	3.0	0	135	m.q.
cracked *(American Classic)*	70	1.0	8.0	4.0	0	140	m.q.
cracked *(Pepperidge Farm)*, 3 pieces	100	2.0	14.0	4.0	0	180	1.0 d
grain *(Carr's)*, 1 piece	36	.8	6.1	.8	n.a.	67	.3 d
hearty *(Pepperidge Farm)*, 4 pieces	100	2.0	13.0	5.0	0	140	1.0 d

Food and Measure	cal.	prot. (gms)	carbo. (gms)	fat (gms)	chol. (mgs)	sod. (mgs)	fiber (gms)
multigrain (Wheat Thins)	60	1.0	10.0	2.0	0	135	m.q.
nutty (Wheat Thins)	70	1.0	9.0	4.0	0	170	m.q.
thins, stoned (Red Oval Farms), 7 pieces	105	2.8	18.0	2.4	0	340	m.q.
thins, stoned (Red Oval Farms Low Salt), 7 pieces . .	105	2.7	18.4	2.3	0	144	m.q.
toasted, w/onion (Pepperidge Farm), 4 pieces	80	2.0	12.0	3.0	0	140	1.0 d
wheat, whole:							
(Carr's Star), 1 piece	16	.4	2.5	.4	n.a.	30	.2 d
(Carr's Wheatmeal), 1 piece	40	.6	5.5	1.7	<1	48	.5 d
(Keebler Club), 4 pieces	70	1.0	9.0	3.0	0	55	m.q.
(Keebler Town House), 4 pieces	70	1.0	8.0	4.0	0	60	m.q.
(Keebler Wheatables)	70	1.0	8.0	3.0	0	150	m.q.
(Keebler Wheatables Low Salt)	70	1.0	8.0	3.0	0	75	m.q.
(Manischewitz), 10 pieces	80	3.0	18.0	1.0	0	<10	m.q.
(Ritz)	60	1.0	10.0	2.0	0	135	m.q.
wheat'n bran (Triscuit)	60	1.0	10.0	2.0	0	75	m.q.
wheat sandwich, cheese:							
(Tom's Wheat'N Cheese), 1.4 oz.	200	5.0	22.0	10.0	2	520	m.q.
cheddar (Little Debbie), 4 pieces	130	5.0	17.0	5.0	0	270	m.q.
wheat sandwich, peanut butter (Tom's Wheat'N Peanut Butter), 1.4 oz. . .	200	5.0	22.0	11.0	0	420	m.q.

Food and Measure	cal.	prot. (gms)	carbo. (gms)	fat (gms)	chol. (mgs)	sod. (mgs)	fiber (gms)
Cracker, *(cont.)*							
zwieback toast							
(Nabisco), 2 pieces	60	2.0	10.0	1.0	<2	20	m.q.
Cracker crumbs and							
meal:							
(Golden Dipt), 1 oz.	100	3.0	22.0	0	0	0	m.q.
matzo *(Manischewitz*							
Farfel), 1 cup . . .	180	6.8	60.0	.8	0	2	.2 d
matzo meal *(Mani-*							
schewitz Daily),							
1 cup	514	13.0	109.0	1.4	0	3	.5 d
meal *(Nabisco),*							
1/4 cup	100	3.0	23.0	<1.0	0	10	m.q.
saltine, fat free *(Pre-*							
mium, 2 tbsp.	50	1.0	11.0	0	0	0	m.q.
Cranberry fresh, raw:							
whole, 1/2 cup	23	.2	6.0	.1	0	1	2.0 d
chopped, 1/2 cup . .	27	.2	7.0	.1	0	1	2.3 d
Cranberry bean:							
boiled, 1/2 cup	120	8.2	21.5	.4	0	1	3.0 d
canned, w/liquid,							
1/2 cup	108	7.2	19.7	.4	0	431	1.2 c
Cranberry fruit							
blends, crushed, for							
chicken, 2 oz.:							
w/orange or raspberry							
(Ocean Spray							
Cran• Fruit)	90	0	23.0	0	0	10	m.q.
w/strawberry *(Ocean*							
Spray Cran• Fruit)	90	0	22.0	0	0	10	m.q.
Cranberry fruit con-							
centrate *(Hain),*							
2 tbsp.	45	0	12.0	0	0	9	<1.0 d
Cranberry juice:							
(R.W. Knudsen Just							
Cranberry), 8 fl. oz.	40	<1.0	10.0	<1.0	0	(0)	n.a.
(Master Choice),							
6 fl. oz.	100	0	25.0	0	0	10	n.a.

Food and Measure	cal.	prot. (gms)	carbo. (gms)	fat (gms)	chol. (mgs)	sod. (mgs)	fiber (gms)
(Smucker's Naturally 100%), 8 fl. oz. . . .	130	0	30.0	0	0	10	(0)
cocktail, 6 fl. oz.:							
(Ocean Spray) . . .	100	0	25.0	0	0	15	(0)
(Sunkist)	110	.1	28.2	.1	0	8	(0)
frozen* *(Sunkist)* . .	110	.1	28.2	.1	0	8	(0)
frozen* *(Welch's)* . .	100	0	26.0	0	0	0	0
frozen* *(Welch's* No Sugar Added) . .	40	0	10.0	0	0	5	(0)
sparkling *(Santa Cruz Natural)*, 8 fl. oz.	90	<1.0	22.0	<1.0	0	n.a.	n.a.
Cranberry juice drink, blend *(Ocean Spray CranTastic)*, 6 fl. oz.	100	0	26.0	0	0	15	(0)
Cranberry nectar, 8 fl. oz.:							
(R.W. Knudsen) . . .	110	<1.0	28.0	<1.0	0	(0)	m.q.
(Santa Cruz Natural)	110	<1.0	28.0	<1.0	0	(0)	m.q.
Cranberry sauce, canned:							
(R.W. Knudsen), 1 oz.	30	<1.0	8.0	<1.0	0	(0)	m.q.
whole or jellied, 1/2 cup	209	.3	53.7	.2	0	40	1.4 d
whole *(Ocean Spray)*, 2 oz.	80	0	21.0	0	0	10	m.q.
jellied *(Ocean Spray)*, 2 oz.	80	0	22.0	0	0	10	m.q.
Cranberry-apple drink *(Ocean Spray CranApple)*, 6 fl. oz.	120	0	31.0	0	0	15	(0)
Cranberry-apple juice cocktail, 6 fl. oz.:							
canned *(Minute Maid)*	120	0	30.0	0	0	20	(0)
frozen* *(Welch's)* . . .	120	0	30.0	0	0	0	0

Food and Measure	cal.	prot. (gms)	carbo. (gms)	fat (gms)	chol. (mgs)	sod. (mgs)	fiber (gms)
Cranberry-apricot juice drink (Ocean Spray Cranicot), 6 fl. oz.	120	0	29.0	0	0	15	(0)
Cranberry-blueberry juice:							
(R.W. Knudsen), 8 fl. oz.	115	<1.0	36.0	<1.0	0	(0)	m.q.
cocktail, frozen* (Welch's), 6 fl. oz.	110	0	27.0	0	0	0	0
Cranberry-cherry juice cocktail, frozen* (Welch's), 6 fl. oz.	110	0	28.0	0	0	0	(0)
Cranberry-grape drink (Ocean Spray Cran• Grape), 6 fl. oz.	120	0	31.0	0	0	15	(0)
Cranberry-grape juice cocktail, frozen* (Welch's), 6 fl. oz.	110	0	27.0	0	0	0	(0)
Cranberry-orange juice cocktail, frozen* (Welch's), 6 fl. oz.	110	0	28.0	0	0	0	(0)
Cranberry-orange relish, canned, 1/2 cup	246	.4	63.8	.1	0	44	.8 c
Cranberry-raspberry drink (Ocean Spray Cran• Raspberry), 6 fl. oz.	110	0	27.0	0	0	15	(0)
Cranberry-raspberry juice:							
(R.W. Knudsen), 8 fl. oz.	100	<1.0	25.0	<1.0	0	(0)	m.q.

Food and Measure	cal.	prot. (gms)	carbo. (gms)	fat (gms)	chol. (mgs)	sod. (mgs)	fiber (gms)
cocktail, frozen*:							
(Welch's), 6 fl. oz.	110	0	28.0	0	0	0	0
(Welch's No Sugar Added), 6 fl. oz.	40	0	10.0	0	0	0	(0)
Cranberry-raspberry-strawberry juice drink *(Tropicana Twister)*, 6 fl. oz. . . .	110	<1.0	27.0	<1.0	0	4	(0)
Cranberry-strawberry drink *(Ocean Spray Cran• Strawberry)*, 6 fl. oz.	110	0	27.0	0	0	15	(0)
Crayfish, meat only:							
mixed species, wild:							
raw, 4 oz.	87	18.1	0	1.1	130	66	0
raw, 8 medium, 1 oz.	22	4.5	0	.3	32	16	0
boiled or steamed, 4 oz.	100	19.0	0	1.4	151	107	0
mixed species, farmed, 4 oz.							
raw	82	16.9	0	1.1	122	70	0
boiled or steamed	99	19.9	0	1.5	155	110	0
Cream (see also "Creamer, nondairy"):							
half and half:							
1 cup	315	7.2	10.4	27.8	89	98	0
1 tbsp.	20	.4	.6	1.7	6	6	0
light, coffee or table:							
1 cup	469	6.5	8.8	46.3	159	95	0
1 tbsp.	29	.4	.6	2.9	10	6	0
medium (25% fat):							
1 cup	583	5.9	8.3	59.8	209	88	0
1 tbsp.	37	.4	.5	3.8	13	6	0
sour, see "Cream, sour"							

Food and Measure	cal.	prot. (gms)	carbo. (gms)	fat (gms)	chol. (mgs)	sod. (mgs)	fiber (gms)
Cream *(cont.)*							
whipping[1], light:							
1 cup	699	5.2	7.1	73.9	265	82	0
1 tbsp.	44	.3	.4	4.6	17	5	0
whipping[1], heavy:							
1 cup	821	4.9	6.6	88.1	326	89	0
1 tbsp.	52	.3	.4	5.6	21	6	0
whipped topping:							
frozen *(Kraft Real Cream)*, 1/4 cup	30	0	2.0	2.0	10	5	0
frozen *(La Creme)*, 1 tbsp.	16	0	1.0	1.0	<1	5	0
nondairy, see "Cream topping, non-dairy"							
pressurized, 1 tbsp.	8	.1	.4	.7	2	4	0
Cream, sour:							
1 cup	493	7.3	9.8	48.2	102	123	0
1 tbsp.	26	.4	.5	2.5	5	6	0
(Bison), 1 oz.	60	1.0	2.0	6.0	m.q.	20	0
(Breakstone's/Sealtest), 1 tbsp.	30	0	1.0	3.0	10	5	0
(Friendship), 1 oz. or 2 tbsp.	55	1.0	1.0	5.0	42	15	0
(Heluva Good), 1 tbsp.	26	1.0	1.0	3.0	m.q.	6	0
(Knudsen Hampshire), 1 oz.	60	1.0	1.0	6.0	20	10	0
half and half:							
1 tbsp.	20	.4	.6	1.8	6	6	0
(Breakstone's Light Choice/Sealtest Light), 1 tbsp.	25	1.0	1.0	2.0	5	10	0
light, 2 tbsp.:							
(Borden Lite-Line/ Viva Lite)	40	2.0	2.0	2.0	10	30	0
(Friendship)	35	1.0	2.0	2.0	8	25	0

[1] *Unwhipped; volume approximately doubled when whipped.*

Food and Measure	cal.	prot. (gms)	carbo. (gms)	fat (gms)	chol. (mgs)	sod. (mgs)	fiber (gms)
(Knudsen Light n' Lively)	40	1.0	2.0	3.0	10	20	0
(Land O'Lakes) . .	40	2.0	4.0	2.0	5	35	0
w/chives *(Land O'Lakes)*	40	2.0	4.0	2.0	5	150	(0)
no fat:							
(Land O'Lakes) . .	30	2.0	5.0	0	0	40	0
(Naturally Yours) . .	15	3.0	1.0	0	0	15	0
Cream, sour, nondairy:							
1 oz.	59	.7	1.9	5.5	0	29	0
(Friendship Sour Treat), 1 oz.	36	1.0	2.0	3.0	0	15	0
imitation *(Pet/Dairy-mate)*, 1 tbsp. . . .	25	<1.0	<1.0	2.0	0	25	0
Crème de menthe, 72 proof, 1 fl. oz.	125	0	14.0	.1	0	2	0
Cream gravy, canned *(Franco-American)*, 2 oz.	35	(0)	4.0	2.0	n.a.	220	n.a.
Cream puff, Bavarian, frozen *(Rich's)*, 1 piece	140	2.0	17.0	7.0	25	40	0
Cream of tartar *(Tone's)*, 1 tsp. . .	2	0	.6	0	0	n.a.	0
Cream topping, dairy, see "Cream"							
Cream topping, nondairy, 1 tbsp., except as noted:							
frozen:							
1 cup	239	.9	17.3	19.0	0	19	0
(Cool Whip Extra Creamy)	14	0	1.0	1.0	0	0	0
(Cool Whip Lite) . .	8	0	1.0	<1.0	0	0	0
(Kraft Whipped Topping), 1/4 cup . .	35	0	2.0	3.0	0	10	0
(Pet Whip)	14	0	1.0	1.0	0	0	0

Food and Measure	cal.	prot. (gms)	carbo. (gms)	fat (gms)	chol. (mgs)	sod. (mgs)	fiber (gms)
Cream topping, nondairy, frozen *(cont.)*							
(Richwhip)	12	<1.0	1.0	1.0	0	0	0
regular or chocolate							
(Cool Whip) . . .	12	0	1.0	1.0	0	0	0
mix*:							
1 cup	151	2.9	13.2	9.9	0	53	0
(D-Zerta)	8	0	0	1.0	0	5	0
(Dream Whip) . . .	10	0	1.0	0	0	0	0
pressurized *(Rich's)*,							
1/4 oz.	20	<1.0	1.0	2.0	0	5	0
Creamer, nondairy,							
1 tbsp., except as							
noted:							
(N.Rich), 1 tsp.	10	<1.0	1.0	<1.0	0	0	0
(Rich's Coffee Rich)	25	<1.0	2.0	2.0	0	10	0
(Rich's Coffee Rich							
Light)	12	<1.0	1.0	<1.0	0	5	0
(Rich's Farm Rich) . .	20	<1.0	1.0	2.0	0	5	0
(Rich's Farm Rich							
Light)	10	<1.0	<1.0	<1.0	0	5	0
liquid:							
(Coffee-mate) . . .	16	0	2.0	1.0	0	5	0
(Coffee-mate Lite)	10	0	1.0	<1.0	0	10	0
all flavors *(Carna-*							
tion)	40	0	5.0	2.0	0	5	0
Amaretto, cinna-							
mon-hazelnut or							
Irish creme *(Inter-*							
national Delight)	45	0	7.0	2.0	0	9	0
Suisse chocolate							
mocha *(Interna-*							
tional Delight) . .	45	0	7.0	2.0	0	11	0
powder, 1 tsp.:							
(Coffee-mate) . . .	10	<1.0	1.0	<1.0	0	5	0
(Coffee-mate Lite)	8	<1.0	2.0	<1.0	0	0	0
Creole sauce, Cajun							
(Enrico's Light),							
4 oz.	76	2.0	9.0	2.8	0	284	n.a.

Food and Measure	cal.	prot. (gms)	carbo. (gms)	fat (gms)	chol. (mgs)	sod. (mgs)	fiber (gms)
Crepe, fresh *(Frieda's),* 1 piece	45	1.0	7.0	1.0	m.q.	80	m.q.
Cress, garden, 1/2 cup:							
raw	8	.7	1.4	.2	0	4	.3 d
boiled, drained	16	1.3	2.6	.4	0	5	.5 d
Cress, water, see "Watercress"							
Croaker, meat only, raw, Atlantic, 4 oz.	119	20.2	0	3.6	69	63	0
Croissant, 1 piece:							
butter *(Awrey's),* 3 oz.	300	5.0	32.0	17.0	45	280	1.0 d
margarine *(Awrey's),* 2.5 oz.	250	4.0	26.0	14.0	5	360	1.0 d
wheat *(Awrey's)* . . .	240	4.0	24.0	14.0	5	390	1.0 d
frozen, butter *(Sara Lee Original)*	170	4.0	19.0	9.0	m.q.	240	m.q.
Crookneck squash:							
fresh, sliced, 1/2 cup:							
raw, ends trimmed	12	.6	2.6	.2	0	1	.7 d
boiled, drained . .	18	.8	3.9	.3	0	1	1.3 d
canned, cut, 1/2 cup:							
drained, no salt . .	14	.7	3.2	.1	0	5	1.1 d
yellow *(Allens/Sunshine)*	16	1.0	3.0	<1.0	0	230	m.q.
frozen, boiled, sliced, 1/2 cup	24	1.2	5.3	.2	0	6	1.2 d
Croquettes, vegetarian, frozen *(Worthington* Golden), 5 pieces	280	19.0	20.0	14.0	0	890	m.q.
Croutons, 1/2 oz.:							
Caesar *(Pepperidge Farm* Homestyle)	70	2.0	8.0	3.0	0	180	m.q.
Caesar salad *(Brownberry)*	60	2.0	7.0	3.0	0	170	<1.0 d
cheddar *(Brownberry)*	60	2.0	8.0	3.0	0	160	<1.0 d

Food and Measure	cal.	prot. (gms)	carbo. (gms)	fat (gms)	chol. (mgs)	sod. (mgs)	fiber (gms)
Croutons (cont.)							
cheddar and Romano							
(Pepperidge Farm)	60	2.0	10.0	2.0	0	200	m.q.
cheese and garlic:							
(Arnold Crispy) . .	60	2.0	9.0	2.0	0	130	<1.0 d
(Brownberry)	60	1.0	8.0	3.0	0	160	<1.0 d
(Pepperidge Farm)	70	2.0	9.0	3.0	0	180	m.q.
fine herb (Arnold							
Crispy)	50	2.0	10.0	1.0	0	150	1.0 d
Italian:							
(Arnold Crispy) . .	60	2.0	8.0	3.0	0	150	<1.0 d
(Pepperidge Farm							
Homestyle) . . .	70	2.0	9.0	3.0	0	170	m.q.
olive oil and garlic							
(Pepperidge Farm)	60	2.0	10.0	2.0	0	160	1.0 d
onion and garlic:							
(Arnold Crispy) . .	60	2.0	9.0	2.0	0	190	m.q.
(Brownberry)	60	2.0	9.0	2.0	0	190	1.0 d
(Pepperidge Farm)	70	2.0	9.0	3.0	0	160	m.q.
ranch (Brownberry)	60	2.0	9.0	2.0	0	180	m.q.
ranch (Pepperidge							
Farm)	70	2.0	9.0	3.0	5	130	1.0 d
seasoned:							
(Arnold)	60	2.0	8.0	3.0	0	160	<1.0 d
(Brownberry)	60	2.0	8.0	2.0	0	160	<1.0 d
(Pepperidge Farm)	70	2.0	9.0	3.0	0	180	m.q.
wheat (Brownberry)	60	1.0	9.0	3.0	0	170	1.0 d
sourdough cheese							
(Pepperidge Farm							
Homestyle) . . .	70	2.0	9.0	2.0	5	160	m.q.
toasted (Brownberry)	60	2.0	9.0	1.0	0	150	<1.0 d
Cucumber, w/peel:							
1 medium, 8¼" long	38	2.1	8.3	.4	0	6	2.4 d
sliced, ½ cup	7	.4	1.4	.1	0	1	.4 d
hot house, unpeeled							
(Frieda's), 1 oz. . .	4	.2	.8	<.1	0	1	m.q.

Food and Measure	cal.	prot. (gms)	carbo. (gms)	fat (gms)	chol. (mgs)	sod. (mgs)	fiber (gms)
Cucumber dip, 2 tbsp.:							
creamy (Kraft Premium)	50	1.0	2.0	4.0	10	130	n.a.
and onion (Breakstone's/Sealtest) . .	50	1.0	2.0	4.0	15	160	n.a.
Cumin seed, 1 tsp.	8	.4	.9	.5	0	4	.2 d
Cupcake, see "Cake, snack"							
Cupuassu punch (R.W. Knudsen Rain Forest), 8 fl. oz. . . .	110	<1.0	25.0	<1.0	0	(0)	m.q.
Currant, trimmed, 1/2 cup:							
black, European . . .	36	.8	8.6	.2	0	1	3.0 d
red or white	31	.8	7.7	.1	0	1	2.4 d
zante, dried	204	2.9	53.3	.2	0	6	4.9 d
Curry powder:							
1 tbsp.	20	.8	3.7	.9	0	3	2.2 d
1 tsp.	6	.3	1.2	.3	0	1	.7 d
Curry sauce mix, 1.25-oz. pkt.	151	3.3	17.9	8.2	tr.	1444	.5 c
Cusk, meat only:							
raw, 4 oz.	99	21.6	0	.8	47	36	0
baked, broiled, or microwaved, 4 oz. . .	127	27.6	0	1.0	60	45	0
Custard, see "Pudding mix"							
Custard apple, trimmed, 1 oz. . . .	29	.5	7.1	.2	0	1	1.0 c
Cutlets, vegetarian: canned, 2 pieces:							
(LaLoma Dinner Cuts)	110	22.0	2.0	1.0	0	340	m.q.
(Worthington) . . .	100	16.0	4.0	2.0	0	270	m.q.
multigrain (Worthington)	90	14.0	5.0	2.0	0	550	m.q.

Food and Measure	cal.	prot. (gms)	carbo. (gms)	fat (gms)	chol. (mgs)	sod. (mgs)	fiber (gms)
Cutlets, vegetarian *(cont.)*							
frozen, breaded							
(Morningstar Farms),							
1 piece	230	14.0	12.0	14.0	0	390	m.q.
Cuttlefish, meat only:							
raw, 4 oz.	90	18.4	.9	.8	127	422	0
boiled or steamed,							
4 oz.	179	36.8	1.9	1.6	254	844	0

D

Food and Measure	cal.	prot. (gms)	carbo. (gms)	fat (gms)	chol. (mgs)	sod. (mgs)	fiber (gms)
Daikon, see "Radish, Oriental"							
Daiquiri mixer:							
bottled, 3 fl. oz.:							
(Holland House) . .	108	<1.0	27.0	<1.0	0	333	(0)
raspberry *(Holland House)*	84	<1.0	21.0	<1.0	0	12	(0)
strawberry *(Holland House)*	98	<1.0	24.0	<1.0	0	10	(0)
instant *(Holland House)*, .56 oz. dry	64	<1.0	16.0	<1.0	0	21	(0)
frozen*, w/rum, 7 fl. oz.:							
banana *(Bacardi)*	210	0	35.0	1.0	0	0	n.a.
lime *(Bacardi)* . . .	210	0	33.0	0	0	10	n.a.
peach *(Bacardi)* . .	200	0	33.0	0	0	5	n.a.
strawberry *(Bacardi)*	200	0	34.0	0	0	5	n.a.
Dairy Queen/Brazier,							
1 serving:							
burgers and sandwiches:							
BBQ beef	225	12.0	34.0	4.0	20	700	m.q.
chicken fillet, breaded	430	24.0	37.0	20.0	55	760	m.q.
chicken fillet, breaded, w/ cheese	480	27.0	38.0	25.0	70	980	m.q.
chicken fillet, grilled	300	25.0	33.0	8.0	50	800	m.q.
DQ Homestyle Ultimate burger . . .	700	43.0	30.0	47.0	140	1110	m.q.

Food and Measure	cal.	prot. (gms)	carbo. (gms)	fat (gms)	chol. (mgs)	sod. (mgs)	fiber (gms)
Dairy Queen/Brazier, burgers and sandwiches _(cont.)_							
fish fillet	370	16.0	39.0	16.0	45	630	m.q.
fish fillet w/cheese	420	19.0	40.0	21.0	60	850	m.q.
hamburger, single	310	17.0	29.0	13.0	45	580	m.q.
hamburger, double	460	31.0	29.0	25.0	95	630	m.q.
cheeseburger, single	365	20.0	30.0	18.0	60	800	m.q.
cheeseburger, double	570	37.0	31.0	34.0	120	1070	m.q.
hot dog	280	9.0	23.0	16.0	25	700	m.q.
hot dog, w/cheese	330	12.0	24.0	21.0	35	920	m.q.
hot dog, w/chili . .	320	11.0	26.0	19.0	30	720	m.q.
hot dog, 1/4# _Super Dog_	590	20.0	41.0	38.0	60	1360	m.q.
side dishes:							
french fries, large	390	5.0	52.0	18.0	0	200	m.q.
french fries, regular	300	4.0	40.0	14.0	0	160	m.q.
french fries, small	210	3.0	29.0	10.0	0	115	m.q.
onion rings, regular	240	4.0	29.0	12.0	0	135	m.q.
salad, no dressing:							
garden	200	13.0	7.0	13.0	185	240	m.q.
side	25	1.0	4.0	0	0	15	m.q.
salad dressing, 2 oz.:							
French, reduced cal.	90	<1.0	11.0	5.0	0	450	n.a.
Thousand Island . .	225	<1.0	10.0	21.0	25	570	n.a.
desserts and shakes, regular size:							
banana split	510	9.0	93.0	11.0	30	250	m.q.
Blizzard, Heath . .	820	16.0	114.0	36.0	60	410	n.a.
Blizzard, strawberry	570	13.0	92.0	16.0	50	230	n.a.
Breeze, Heath . . .	680	15.0	113.0	21.0	15	360	n.a.
Breeze, strawberry	420	12.0	90.0	1.0	5	170	n.a.
Buster Bar	450	11.0	40.0	29.0	15	220	n.a.
cone, chocolate . .	230	6.0	36.0	7.0	20	115	m.q.
cone, vanilla	230	6.0	36.0	7.0	20	95	m.q.
cone, chocolate dip	330	6.0	40.0	16.0	20	100	m.q.
Dilly Bar	210	3.0	21.0	13.0	10	50	n.a.
DQ cake slice, un-decorated	380	6.0	50.0	18.0	20	210	m.q.

Food and Measure	cal.	prot. (gms)	carbo. (gms)	fat (gms)	chol. (mgs)	sod. (mgs)	fiber (gms)
DQ Sandwich . . .	140	3.0	24.0	4.0	5	135	m.q.
Hot Fudge Brownie							
Delight	710	11.0	102.0	29.0	35	340	m.q.
malt, vanilla	610	13.0	106.0	14.0	45	230	n.a.
Mr. Misty	250	0	63.0	0	0	0	n.a.
Nutty Double Fudge	580	10.0	85.0	22.0	35	170	m.q.
Peanut Buster Par-							
fait	710	16.0	94.0	32.0	30	410	m.q.
QC Big Scoop:							
chocolate	310	5.0	40.0	14.0	35	100	n.a.
vanilla	300	5.0	39.0	14.0	35	100	n.a.
shake, chocolate	540	12.0	94.0	14.0	45	290	(0)
shake, vanilla . . .	520	12.0	88.0	14.0	45	230	0
Strawberry Waffle							
Cone Sundae . .	350	8.0	56.0	12.0	20	220	m.q.
sundae, chocolate	300	6.0	54.0	7.0	20	140	(0)
yogurt:							
cone	180	6.0	38.0	<1.0	<5	80	m.q.
cup	170	6.0	35.0	<1.0	<5	70	n.a.
strawberry sundae	200	6.0	43.0	<1.0	<5	80	n.a.
Dandelion greens:							
raw, 1 oz. or 1/2 cup							
chopped	13	.8	2.6	.2	0	22	1.0 d
boiled, drained,							
chopped, 1/2 cup	17	1.0	3.3	.3	0	23	1.5 d
Danish, 1 piece:							
packaged (Awrey's):							
apple, round	390	4.0	50.0	20.0	10	390	1.0 d
apple, square . . .	220	3.0	34.0	8.0	10	230	1.0 d
apple, miniature . .	160	2.0	21.0	8.0	5	170	0
cheese, round . . .	420	5.0	52.0	22.0	15	530	1.0 d
cheese, square . .	210	4.0	25.0	11.0	15	300	1.0 d
cheese, miniature	170	2.0	21.0	9.0	5	200	m.q.
cinnamon raisin							
square	290	3.0	41.0	12.0	15	280	1.0 d
cinnamon raisin,							
miniature	160	2.0	21.0	8.0	5	150	1.0 d

Food and Measure	cal.	prot. (gms)	carbo. (gms)	fat (gms)	chol. (mgs)	sod. (mgs)	fiber (gms)
Danish, packaged (Awrey's) (cont.)							
cinnamon walnut, round	300	4.0	31.0	18.0	5	290	1.0 d
pineapple, miniature	157	2.0	21.0	8.0	5	180	1.0 d
raspberry, square	260	3.0	45.0	8.0	10	210	1.0 d
strawberry, round	400	4.0	53.0	20.0	10	410	1.0 d
frozen (Pepperidge Farm):							
apple	220	2.0	35.0	8.0	n.a.	130	m.q.
cheese	240	3.0	25.0	14.0	m.q.	230	m.q.
cinnamon raisin . .	250	3.0	35.0	11.0	n.a.	170	m.q.
raspberry	220	3.0	31.0	9.0	n.a.	140	m.q.
refrigerated, iced (Pillsbury):							
cinnamon raisin . .	150	2.0	20.0	7.0	0	230	m.q.
orange	150	2.0	19.0	7.0	0	250	m.q.
Dasheen, see "Taro"							
Date, pitted:							
(Bordo), 2 oz.	204	1.2	47.2	1.2	0	5	1.5 c
(Dole), 1/2 cup	280	5.0	62.0	0	0	0	m.q.
(Dromedary), 1 oz. or 5 dates	100	1.0	23.0	0	0	0	m.q.
chopped (Dole), 1/2 cup	230	1.0	56.0	0	0	5	m.q.
chopped (Dromedary), 1/4 cup	130	1.0	31.0	0	0	0	m.q.
diced (Bordo), 2 oz.	203	1.0	47.5	1.1	0	5	1.2 c
domestic, natural, dry, 10 dates, 2.9 oz.	228	1.6	61.0	.4	0	2	6.2 d
Date bar, see "Dessert bar, mix"							
Denny's, 1 serving:							
breakfast:							
bacon, 1 slice . . .	48	3.0	.5	4.0	m.q.	142	0
bagel	240	9.0	47.0	1.0	n.a.	450	m.q.
biscuit	217	4.0	35.0	7.0	n.a.	800	m.q.
blueberry muffin . .	309	4.0	42.0	14.0	n.a.	190	m.q.
cinnamon roll . . .	450	9.0	73.0	14.0	n.a.	750	m.q.

Food and Measure	cal.	prot. (gms)	carbo. (gms)	fat (gms)	chol. (mgs)	sod. (mgs)	fiber (gms)
country gravy, 1 oz.	140	8.0	14.0	8.0	n.a.	712	n.a.
eggs	80	6.0	0	6.0	m.q.	0	0
eggs Benedict . . .	658	32.9	20.2	35.6	m.q.	2197	m.q.
English muffin . . .	137	6.0	25.8	1.2	n.a.	186	m.q.
French toast, 2 slices	729	12.0	46.0	56.0	m.q.	275	m.q.
ham slice	156	14.0	.9	6.8	m.q.	1303	0
hashed browns, 4 oz.	164	4.4	32.1	2.0	n.a.	310	m.q.
omelette:							
chili cheese . . .	490	28.0	17.0	32.0	230	1130	2.0 d
Denver	580	15.0	4.0	56.0	m.q.	806	n.a.
ham 'N' cheddar	480	28.0	7.0	33.0	235	1120	n.a.
Mexican	540	29.0	14.0	40.0	245	1060	1.0 d
ultimate	577	24.9	7.7	41.0	m.q.	649	n.a.
pancakes	136	4.0	26.0	2.0	n.a.	656	m.q.
sausage, 1 link . .	113	2.5	0	10.0	m.q.	250	0
waffles	261	6.3	35.0	10.4	n.a.	62	m.q.
sandwiches/burgers:							
BLT	492	17.0	42.0	34.0	m.q.	662	m.q.
bacon Swiss burger[1]	819	53.0	38.0	52.0	m.q.	1127	m.q.
cheese, grilled . . .	454	17.0	29.0	29.0	m.q.	1519	m.q.
chicken, grilled[1] . .	439	27.0	40.0	12.0	m.q.	413	m.q.
club sandwich . . .	590	29.0	40.0	35.0	m.q.	1383	m.q.
Dennyburger	629	34.8	36.7	37.4	m.q.	427	m.q.
patty melt	761	40.0	27.0	47.0	n.a.	887	m.q.
roast beef deluxe	840	45.0	44.0	55.0	145	1720	4.0 d
San Fran burger[2]	872	58.0	51.0	48.0	m.q.	1335	m.q.
Superbird	625	37.0	81.0	24.0	n.a.	1750	n.a.
veggie cheese . . .	350	21.0	29.0	20.0	n.a.	909	m.q.
works burger[1] . . .	944	49.0	48.0	60.9	m.q.	1306	m.q.
finger food:							
chicken strips, 4 pieces	290	23.0	21.0	12.0	50	670	n.a.

[1] *Without lettuce and tomato.*
[2] *Without lettuce, tomatoes, and guacamole.*

Food and Measure	cal.	prot. (gms)	carbo. (gms)	fat (gms)	chol. (mgs)	sod. (mgs)	fiber (gms)
Denny's, finger food *(cont.)*							
mozzarella strips,							
1 piece	88	4.2	7.3	6.7	m.q.	206	n.a.
entree (entree only):							
catfish, seasoned	317	14.4	1.0	28.8	m.q.	59	0
chicken, fried,							
4 pieces	463	61.7	7.5	29.6	m.q.	1304	n.a.
chicken, grilled . .	192	34.5	2.5	3.9	m.q.	71	0
chicken fried steak,							
w/out gravy . . .	252	14.2	16.0	14.6	m.q.	422	n.a.
fried shrimp, 1 piece	46	3.0	7.3	.3	m.q.	393	n.a.
hamburger steak	669	37.6	8.6	53.8	m.q.	201	n.a.
liver w/bacon and							
onions, 2 slices	334	39.8	10.0	14.5	m.q.	516	m.q.
New York steak . .	582	65.0	0	36.0	m.q.	100	0
roast beef	965	60.0	41.0	32.0	180	820	2.0 d
spaghetti w/meat-							
balls	1000	37.0	119.0	38.0	110	170	5.0 d
stir-fry	328	36.0	5.0	10.9	m.q.	109	n.a.
top sirloin steak . .	223	36.0	.7	6.3	m.q.	62	0
turkey, no gravy,							
6 slices	505	56.0	40.0	14.4	m.q.	895	n.a.
side dishes:							
carrots, 3 oz. . . .	17	.4	3.8	<.1	0	31	m.q.
chili, 4 oz.	169	9.5	15.0	7.5	n.a.	677	m.q.
coleslaw, 1 cup . .	119	1.4	8.5	9.5	n.a.	149	m.q.
corn, 3 oz.	63	1.8	15.0	.8	n.a.	37	m.q.
french fries, 4 oz.	303	2.2	38.0	15.8	n.a.	74	m.q.
green beans, 3 oz.	13	.8	2.6	<.1	0	22	m.q.
onion rings, 1 piece	86	1.0	9.0	5.0	n.a.	198	m.q.
peas, 3 oz.	40	3.1	7.0	.2	n.a.	54	m.q.
potato, baked . . .	90	3.0	21.0	0	0	7	m.q.
potato, mashed,							
4 oz.	74	2.0	15.0	.4	n.a.	302	m.q.
rice pilaf, 1/3 cup .	89	1.8	15.5	2.3	n.a.	320	m.q.
stuffing, 1/2 cup . .	180	4.0	20.0	9.0	n.a.	400	m.q.
soups, 1 bowl:							
beef barley	79	4.7	10.9	2.1	m.q.	847	m.q.

Food and Measure	cal.	prot. (gms)	carbo. (gms)	fat (gms)	chol. (mgs)	sod. (mgs)	fiber (gms)
cheese	309	5.6	19.0	22.0	m.q.	898	n.a.
chicken noodle . .	105	3.9	14.8	3.3	m.q.	1118	m.q.
clam chowder . . .	235	5.3	21.0	14.2	m.q.	856	m.q.
potato . . , ...	248	5.0	38.0	8.6	n.a.	1560	m.q.
split pea	231	14.0	33.0	4.9	n.a.	1519	m.q.
salad:							
chef	492	36.1	12.9	20.3	m.q.	3418	m.q.
chicken, no shell	207	36.0	4.0	4.0	m.q.	93	m.q.
taco, no shell . . .	514	31.0	35.0	20.0	n.a.	2022	m.q.
tuna	340	29.6	13.2	17.8	m.q.	652	m.q.
salad condiments:							
cheese:							
American, 1 slice	55	3.0	.5	4.5	m.q.	230	0
cheddar, 1 oz.	114	5.6	0	10.0	m.q.	369	0
Jack, 1 slice . .	52	5.5	.2	4.3	m.q.	195	0
Swiss, 1 slice . .	47	6.0	.3	3.5	m.q.	195	0
guacamole, 1 oz.	60	1.4	2.3	6.2	n.a.	130	m.q.
ranch dressing,							
1 tbsp.	52	.4	.6	5.5	n.a.	117	n.a.
tortilla shell, fried	439	6.0	37.0	30.0	n.a.	606	m.q.
Dessert bar mix,							
1 bar*, except as							
noted:							
caramel oatmeal (Betty							
Crocker Supreme)	110	1.0	15.0	5.0	0	65	m.q.
chocolate peanut but-							
ter (Betty Crocker							
Supreme)	110	1.0	14.0	5.0	10	100	m.q.
chocolate and toffee							
(Betty Crocker Su-							
preme)	110	1.0	17.0	4.0	10	55	m.q.
date (Betty Crocker							
Classic), 1/32 pkg.	60	1.0	9.0	2.0	0	35	m.q.
Sunkist lemon (Betty							
Crocker Supreme)	110	1.0	17.0	4.0	30	65	m.q.
Diable sauce (Escof-							
fier), 1 tbsp.	20	0	4.0	0	0	160	n.a.

Food and Measure	cal.	prot. (gms)	carbo. (gms)	fat (gms)	chol. (mgs)	sod. (mgs)	fiber (gms)
Dill dip:							
(Nasoya Vegi-Dip),							
1 oz.	100	1.0	4.0	9.0	0	135	n.a.
mix, garden *(Knorr),*							
1 serving dry . . .	2	.1	.5	0	0	110	n.a.
Dill seasoning *(Mc-*							
Cormick/Schilling							
Parsley Patch It's a							
Dilly), 1/2 tsp. . . .	4	.2	1.0	0	0	2	(0)
Dill seed:							
1 tsp.	6	.3	1.2	.3	0	tr.	.4 d
sprouted, raw							
(Shaw's), 2 oz. . . .	8	2.0	<1.0	<1.0	0	55	3.0 d
Dill weed:							
fresh:							
5 sprigs	<1	<1.0	.1	<.1	0	1	m.q.
1/2 cup loosely							
packed	2	.2	.3	.1	0	3	m.q.
dried, 1 tsp.	3	.2	.6	<.1	0	2	.1 d
Dock, boiled, drained,							
4 oz.	23	2.1	3.3	.7	0	3	.8 c
Dolphin fish, meat							
only:							
raw, 4 oz.	97	21.0	0	.8	83	99	0
baked, broiled, or mi-							
crowaved, 4 oz. . .	124	26.9	0	1.0	107	128	0
Donut, 1 piece, ex-							
cept as noted:							
plain:							
(Awrey's)	490	6.0	48.0	30.0	35	650	1.0 d
(Hostess Breakfast							
Bake Shop Pan-							
try)	190	3.0	21.0	11.0	10	270	.9 d
(Tastykake Assorted)	190	3.0	22.0	10.0	10	170	1.0 d
cinnamon:							
(Hostess Breakfast							
Bake Shop							
Donette Gems)	60	1.0	7.0	3.0	5	70	.3 d

Food and Measure	cal.	prot. (gms)	carbo. (gms)	fat (gms)	chol. (mgs)	sod. (mgs)	fiber (gms)
(Hostess Breakfast Bake Shop Pantry)	190	3.0	24.0	10.0	10	240	.9 d
(Tastykake Assorted)	180	3.0	25.0	8.0	10	210	1.0 d
(Tastykake Mini) . .	50	1.0	6.0	2.0	5	55	0
apple filled *(Hostess Breakfast Bake Shop Donette Gems)*	70	1.0	10.0	3.0	5	70	.3 d
crumb:							
(Hostess Breakfast Bake Shop) . . .	160	1.0	16.0	10.0	10	140	.9 d
(Hostess Breakfast Bake Shop Donette Gems)	80	1.0	8.0	5.0	5	70	.4 d
crunch *(Awrey's)* . .	600	7.0	65.0	34.0	40	730	2.0 d
frosted:							
(Hostess Breakfast Bake Shop), 1.5 oz.	190	2.0	20.0	12.0	5	180	1.1 d
(Hostess Breakfast Bake Shop Donette Gems)	80	1.0	8.0	5.0	<5	70	.4 d
(Hostess Breakfast Bake Shop O's)	260	3.0	32.0	14.0	5	240	1.7 d
rich *(Tastykake)* . .	260	4.0	28.0	16.0	10	200	3.0 d
rich *(Tastykake* Mini)	60	1.0	8.0	3.0	5	60	1.0 d
strawberry filled *(Hostess Breakfast Bake Shop Donette Gems)*	80	1.0	10.0	4.0	<5	70	.5 d
glazed:							
(Hostess Breakfast Bake Shop Old Fashioned) . . .	250	3.0	33.0	12.0	15	230	1.4 d
whirl *(Hostess Breakfast Bake Shop)*	190	3.0	27.0	7.0	5	230	.9 d

Food and Measure	cal.	prot. (gms)	carbo. (gms)	fat (gms)	chol. (mgs)	sod. (mgs)	fiber (gms)
Donut *(cont.)*							
honey wheat:							
(Hostess Breakfast Bake Shop) . . .	250	3.0	32.0	12.0	25	280	1.2 d
(Tastykake)	210	3.0	32.0	8.0	10	200	1.0 d
(Tastykake Mini) . .	40	1.0	7.0	1.0	5	50	0
(Hostess Breakfast Bake Shop O's)	230	3.0	34.0	10.0	5	230	1.0 d
(Hostess Breakfast Bake Shop Old Fashioned) . . .	170	3.0	21.0	9.0	10	230	.9 d
orange glazed *(Tastykake)*	220	3.0	32.0	9.0	10	180	1.0 d
powdered sugar:							
(Awrey's)	610	7.0	68.0	35.0	40	735	2.0 d
(Hostess Breakfast Bake Shop Assorted)	190	2.0	24.0	10.0	10	230	.8 d
(Hostess Breakfast Bake Shop Donette Gems)	60	1.0	7.0	3.0	5	70	.2 d
(Tastykake Assorted)	180	3.0	24.0	9.0	10	220	1.0 d
(Tastykake Mini) . .	40	1.0	7.0	1.0	5	70	0
strawberry filled *(Hostess Breakfast Bake Shop Donette Gems)*	70	1.0	10.0	3.0	5	70	.3 d
frozen:							
glazed *(Rich's Ever Fresh)*	140	2.0	14.0	8.0	0	30	m.q.
sugar and spice *(Rich's Ever Fresh* Mini), 3 pieces	200	2.0	24.0	11.0	10	290	m.q.
Drum, freshwater, meat only:							
raw, 4 oz.	135	19.9	0	5.6	73	85	0
baked, broiled, or microwaved, 4 oz. . .	173	25.5	0	7.2	93	109	0

Food and Measure	cal.	prot. (gms)	carbo. (gms)	fat (gms)	chol. (mgs)	sod. (mgs)	fiber (gms)
Duck, domesticated, roasted:							
meat w/skin, 4 oz...	382	21.5	0	32.1	95	67	0
meat only, 4 oz. . . .	228	26.6	0	12.7	101	74	0
Duck, wild, raw:							
meat w/skin, 4 oz. . .	239	19.8	0	17.2	91	64	0
breast meat only, 4 oz.	139	22.5	0	4.8	m.q.	65	0
Duck sauce, see "Sweet and sour sauce"							
Dunkin' Donuts, 1 piece:							
apple filled, cinnamon sugar	250	5.0	33.0	11.0	0	280	1.0 d
Bavarian filled, choco- late frosting	240	5.0	32.0	11.0	0	260	2.0 d
blueberry filled	210	4.0	29.0	8.0	0	240	2.0 d
buttermilk ring, glazed	290	4.0	37.0	14.0	10	370	1.0 d
cake ring, plain . . .	270	4.0	25.0	17.0	0	330	1.0 d
chocolate ring, glazed	324	3.5	34.0	21.0	0	383	1.9 d
coffee roll, glazed . .	280	5.0	37.0	12.0	0	310	2.0 d
cookie:							
chocolate chunk . .	200	3.0	25.0	10.0	30	110	1.0 d
chocolate chunk, nuts	210	3.0	23.0	11.0	30	100	2.0 d
oatmeal pecan raisin	200	3.0	28.0	9.0	25	100	1.0 d
croissant:							
plain	310	7.0	27.0	19.0	0	240	2.0 d
almond	420	8.0	38.0	27.0	0	280	3.0 d
chocolate	440	7.0	38.0	29.0	0	220	3.0 d
French cruller, glazed	140	2.0	16.0	8.0	30	130	0
jelly filled	220	4.0	31.0	9.0	0	230	1.0 d
lemon filled	260	4.0	33.0	12.0	0	280	1.0 d
muffin:							
apple N'spice . . .	300	6.0	52.0	8.0	25	360	2.0 d
banana nut	310	7.0	49.0	10.0	30	410	3.0 d
blueberry	280	6.0	46.0	8.0	30	340	2.0 d

Food and Measure	cal.	prot. (gms)	carbo. (gms)	fat (gms)	chol. (mgs)	sod. (mgs)	fiber (gms)
Dunkin' Donuts, muffin (cont.)							
bran w/raisins . . .	310	6.0	51.0	9.0	15	560	4.0 d
corn	340	7.0	51.0	12.0	40	560	1.0 d
cranberry nut . . .	290	6.0	44.0	9.0	25	360	2.0 d
oat bran muffin . .	330	7.0	50.0	11.0	0	450	3.0 d
whole wheat ring, glazed	330	4.0	39.0	18.0	0	380	2.0 d
yeast ring:							
chocolate frosted	200	4.0	25.0	10.0	0	190	1.0 d
glazed	200	4.0	26.0	9.0	0	230	1.0 d
Dutch brand loaf (Kahn's), 1 slice . .	80	3.0	1.0	7.0	m.q.	280	(0)

E

Food and Measure	cal.	prot. (gms)	carbo. (gms)	fat (gms)	chol. (mgs)	sod. (mgs)	fiber (gms)
Eclair, chocolate, frozen, 1 piece:							
(Rich's)	190	2.0	25.0	9.0	35	80	m.q.
(Weight Watchers Sweet Celebrations)	150	3.0	26.0	4.0	15	110	m.q.
Eel, meat only:							
raw, 4 oz.	209	20.9	0	13.2	143	58	0
baked, broiled, or microwaved, 4 oz. . .	268	26.8	0	17.0	183	74	0
Egg, chicken:							
raw, 1 large egg:							
whole	75	6.3	.6	5.0	213	63	0
white only	17	3.5	.3	0	0	55	0
yolk only[1]	59	2.8	.3	5.1	213	7	0
cooked:							
hard-boiled, chopped, 1 cup	210	17.1	1.5	14.4	578	169	0
poached, 1 large	74	6.2	.6	5.0	212	140	0
dried, 1 oz.:							
whole	168	13.0	1.4	11.9	544	148	0
whole, stabilized . .	174	13.7	.7	12.5	572	155	0
white, stabilized, flakes	100	21.8	1.2	<.1	0	328	0
yolk	195	8.7	.1	17.4	830	26	0

---

[1] Includes a small portion of white.

Food and Measure	cal.	prot. (gms)	carbo. (gms)	fat (gms)	chol. (mgs)	sod. (mgs)	fiber (gms)
Egg, substitute or imitation:							
frozen, 1/4 cup, except as noted:							
(Fleischmann's Egg Beaters)	25	5.0	1.0	0	0	80	0
(Healthy Choice) . .	30	5.0	1.0	<1.0	0	90	0
(Morningstar Farms Better'n Eggs) . .	30	6.0	1.0	0	0	100	0
(Morningstar Farms Scramblers) . . .	35	6.0	2.0	0	0	95	0
w/cheez (Fleischmann's Egg Beaters), 1/2 cup . . .	130	14.0	3.0	6.0	5	440	0
mix*, 1/2 cup:							
(Tofu Scrambler)[1]	117	9.0	9.0	5.0	0	263	2.3 d
(Tofu Scrambler)[2]	171	9.0	9.0	11.0	m.q.	333	2.3 d
refrigerated, 2 oz., except as noted:							
(Morningstar Farms Better'n Eggs), 1/4 cup	25	5.0	1.0	0	0	100	0
(Second Nature) . .	60	6.0	3.0	2.0	0	90	0
(Second Nature No Fat)	40	6.0	3.0	0	0	100	0
w/garden vegetables (Second Nature)	60	6.0	4.0	2.0	0	150	m.q.
w/garden vegetables (Second Nature No Fat)	40	6.0	4.0	0	0	100	m.q.
Egg, duck, 1 egg . .	130	9.0	1.0	9.6	619	102	0
Egg, goose, 1 egg	267	20.0	1.9	19.1	m.q.	n.a.	0
Egg, pickled (Penrose), 1 egg	80	8.0	1.0	5.0	m.q.	230	0
Egg, quail, 1 egg . .	14	1.2	<.1	1.0	76	n.a.	0

[1] Prepared with tofu; does not include fat or oil used in frying.
[2] Prepared with tofu and butter; does not include fat or oil used in frying.

Food and Measure	cal.	prot. (gms)	carbo. (gms)	fat (gms)	chol. (mgs)	sod. (mgs)	fiber (gms)
Egg, turkey, 1 egg	135	10.8	.9	9.4	737	n.a.	0
Egg breakfast, freeze-dried *(Mountain House),* 1/2 pkg.:							
w/bacon	160	10.0	6.0	11.0	m.q.	750	n.a.
w/bacon, precooked	190	12.0	6.0	13.0	m.q.	920	n.a.
omelet, cheese . . .	180	13.0	8.0	9.0	m.q.	600	n.a.
Egg breakfast, frozen:							
omelet, ham and cheese *(Weight Watchers Handy),* 4 oz.	180	14.0	18.0	5.0	10	420	m.q.
scrambled:							
w/bacon, home fries *(Swanson Great Starts),* 5.25 oz.	350	11.0	16.0	27.0	m.q.	700	m.q.
w/Canadian bacon, cheese, jalapeños, home fries *(Swanson Fiesta),* 6.5 oz.	390	12.0	18.0	29.0	m.q.	690	m.q.
w/home fries *(Swanson Budget),* 4.35 oz.	260	7.0	15.0	19.0	m.q.	390	m.q.
w/pancakes, silver dollar *(Swanson Budget),* 4.25 oz.	180	8.0	20.0	20.0	m.q.	550	m.q.
w/sausages, hash browns *(Swanson Great Starts),* 6.25 oz.	430	13.0	19.0	34.0	m.q.	750	m.q.
"Egg" breakfast, vegetarian *(Morningstar Farms Scramblers),* frozen:							
w/cheese and home fries, 5 oz.	210	11.0	20.0	9.0	0	310	m.q.

Food and Measure	cal.	prot. (gms)	carbo. (gms)	fat (gms)	chol. (mgs)	sod. (mgs)	fiber (gms)
"Egg" breakfast, vegetarian (cont.)							
w/hash browns and links, 5 oz.	240	11.0	20.0	13.0	0	580	m.q.
w/links and muffins, 4 oz.	220	11.0	22.0	10.0	0	400	m.q.
Egg breakfast biscuit, frozen:							
cheese and bacon (Swanson Great Starts), 4.2 oz. . . .	360	12.0	36.0	19.0	m.q.	960	m.q.
sausage and (Hormel Quick Meal), 4.5 oz.	350	11.0	30.0	21.0	110	780	m.q.
sausage and cheese (Swanson Great Starts), 5.5 oz. . . .	470	17.0	35.0	29.0	m.q.	1260	m.q.
Egg breakfast muffin, frozen:							
Canadian bacon, cheese:							
(Hormel Quick Meal), 4.5 oz. . .	250	16.0	29.0	8.0	115	680	m.q.
(Swanson Great Starts), 4.1 oz.	290	15.0	25.0	15.0	m.q.	750	m.q.
green chili pepper (Swanson Fiesta), 4.75 oz.	280	14.0	26.0	14.0	m.q.	680	m.q.
English (Healthy Choice), 4.25 oz.	200	16.0	30.0	3.0	20	510	m.q.
English (Weight Watchers), 4 oz. . .	240	14.0	29.0	8.0	15	540	m.q.
omelet:							
classic (Weight Watchers), 3.84 oz.	210	14.0	22.0	7.0	30	410	m.q.
garden (Weight Watchers), 3.6 oz.	210	9.0	28.0	6.0	15	480	m.q.

Food and Measure	cal.	prot. (gms)	carbo. (gms)	fat (gms)	chol. (mgs)	sod. (mgs)	fiber (gms)
turkey sausage (Healthy Choice), 4.75 oz.	210	16.0	30.0	4.0	20	470	m.q.
western (Healthy Choice), 4.75 oz.	200	16.0	29.0	3.0	15	480	m.q.
sausage and cheese (Hormel Quick Meal), 5.1 oz. . .	76	3.0	5.0	4.0	26	143	m.q.
"Egg" breakfast sandwich, vegetarian (Morningstar Farms Scramblers), frozen:							
w/cheese, 3.5 oz. . .	220	11.0	29.0	7.0	0	420	m.q.
w/pattie, 4.5 oz. . . .	300	18.0	29.0	12.0	0	590	m.q.
w/pattie, cheese, 5 oz.	350	20.0	33.0	15.0	0	780	m.q.
Egg foo young, mix* (La Choy Dinner Classics), 2 patties and 3 oz. sauce . .	170	8.0	20.0	7.0	275	1390	1.0 d
Egg roll, frozen:							
chicken:							
(Chun King), 3.6 oz.	220	5.0	32.0	8.0	20	600	m.q.
(La Choy Snack), 1.45 oz.	90	3.0	12.0	3.0	<1	140	m.q.
almond (La Choy), 3 oz.	120	5.0	19.0	3.0	5	290	m.q.
sweet and sour (La Choy), 3 oz. . . .	150	4.0	24.0	4.0	5	280	m.q.
lobster (La Choy Snack), 1.45 oz.	75	2.0	12.0	2.0	<1	150	m.q.
meat and shrimp:							
(Chun King), 3.6 oz.	220	6.0	31.0	8.0	20	680	m.q.
(La Choy Snack), 1.45 oz.	80	3.0	11.0	3.0	4	115	m.q.
pork:							
(Chun King Restaurant Style), 3 oz.	180	6.0	23.0	6.0	25	450	m.q.

Food and Measure	cal.	prot. (gms)	carbo. (gms)	fat (gms)	chol. (mgs)	sod. (mgs)	fiber (gms)
Egg roll, frozen, pork *(cont.)*							
(La Choy Restaurant Style), 3 oz. . . .	150	7.0	20.0	5.0	7	480	m.q.
shrimp:							
(Chun King), 3.6 oz.	220	4.0	31.0	6.0	20	480	m.q.
(La Choy Restaurant Style), 3 oz. . . .	130	5.0	19.0	4.0	5	260	m.q.
(La Choy Snack), 1.45 oz.	75	2.0	12.0	2.0	4	120	m.q.
vegetarian *(Worthington),* 3 oz. . . .	160	6.0	20.0	6.0	0	530	m.q.
Egg roll wrapper:							
(Azumaya), 1 oz. . . .	78	2.8	15.9	.3	0	126	m.q.
(Frieda's), 1 piece . .	32	1.0	1.0	n.a.	m.q.	61	m.q.
(Nasoya), 1 piece . .	90	3.0	20.0	0	0	35	m.q.
Eggless salad dip *(Nasoya Vegi-Dressing),* 1 oz.	80	2.0	4.0	7.0	0	160	n.a.
Eggnog, canned *(Borden),* 1/2 cup	160	3.0	16.0	9.0	90	80	0
Eggplant:							
raw, trimmed, 1" pieces, 1/2 cup	11	.4	2.5	.1	0	1	1.0 d
boiled, drained, 1" cubes, 1/2 cup	13	.4	3.2	.1	0	2	1.2 d
Japanese, raw, unpeeled *(Frieda's),* 1 oz.	7	.3	1.6	.1	0	1	m.q.
Eggplant appetizer:							
(Progresso Caponata), 1/4 cup	70	2.0	4.0	4.0	0	260	m.q.
baby, stuffed *(Krinos),* 1.1 oz.	20	0	0	2.0	0	550	1.0 d
Eggplant entree, frozen:							
parmigiana:							
(Celentano), 6.25 oz.	260	9.0	36.0	10.0	m.q.	220	m.q.
(Celentano), 10 oz.	490	14.0	30.0	35.0	45	800	m.q.

Food and Measure	cal.	prot. (gms)	carbo. (gms)	fat (gms)	chol. (mgs)	sod. (mgs)	fiber (gms)
(Mrs. Paul's), 5 oz.	240	6.0	18.0	16.0	15	600	m.q.
rollettes *(Celentano)*, 11 oz.	450	15.0	32.0	29.0	80	750	m.q.
El Pollo Loco, 1 serving:							
meals[1]:							
chicken fajita . . .	780	41.0	120.0	18.0	58	1060	17.0 d
steak fajita	1040	61.0	120.0	38.0	100	1550	17.0 d
chicken:							
breast	160	26.0	0	6.0	110	390	0
leg	90	11.0	0	5.0	75	150	0
thigh	180	16.0	0	12.0	130	230	0
wing	110	12.0	0	6.0	80	220	0
burritos and tacos:							
chicken burrito . .	310	23.0	30.0	11.0	65	510	4.0 d
chicken taco	180	13.0	18.0	7.0	35	300	2.0 d
steak burrito	450	31.0	31.0	22.0	70	740	4.0 d
steak taco	250	18.0	18.0	12.0	40	410	2.0 d
vegetarian burrito	340	14.0	54.0	7.0	20	360	7.0 d
salads and side dishes:							
beans	100	5.0	16.0	2.5	0	460	8.0 d
chicken salad . . .	160	22.0	11.0	4.0	45	440	4.0 d
cole slaw	90	1.0	7.0	8.0	0	35	1.0 d
corn	110	3.0	20.0	2.0	0	110	1.0 d
corn tortilla	60	1.0	13.0	.5	0	25	<1.0 d
flour tortilla	90	3.0	15.0	2.5	0	150	<1.0 d
guacamole, 1 oz.	60	1.0	2.0	6.0	0	130	0
potato salad	180	2.0	21.0	10.0	10	340	1.0 d
salsa, 2 oz.	10	1.0	3.0	0	0	180	1.0 d
side salad	50	3.0	10.0	1.0	0	30	4.0 d
salad dressing, 1 oz.:							
blue cheese	80	1.0	4.0	6.0	5	150	0
French, deluxe . .	60	<1.0	7.0	4.0	0	160	0
Italian, low calorie	25	0	2.0	2.0	0	170	0
ranch	75	<1.0	4.0	6.0	0	190	0

[1] Including guacamole, cheese, and sour cream.

Food and Measure	cal.	prot. (gms)	carbo. (gms)	fat (gms)	chol. (mgs)	sod. (mgs)	fiber (gms)
El Pollo Loco, salad dressing *(cont.)*							
Thousand Island . .	110	<1.0	4.0	10.0	5	240	0
dessert:							
cheesecake	310	8.0	30.0	18.0	60	230	0
churros	140	2.0	14.0	9.0	4	180	0
Orange or Piña Colada Bang	110	0	26.0	0	0	24	0
Elderberry, 1/2 cup	53	.5	13.3	.4	0	n.a.	5.1 d
Enchilada entree, frozen:							
beef and bean *(Lean Cuisine),* 91/4 oz.	240	15.0	32.0	6.0	45	480	m.q.
chicken *(Lean Cuisine),* 97/8 oz.	290	17.0	34.0	9.0	55	500	m.q.
Enchilada dinner, frozen:							
beef:							
(Healthy Choice), 13.4 oz.	370	15.0	66.0	5.0	30	450	m.q.
(Patio), 13.25 oz.	520	16.0	59.0	24.0	40	1810	m.q.
cheese *(Patio),* 12 oz.	370	14.0	58.0	10.0	20	1970	m.q.
chicken:							
(Banquet Healthy Balance), 11 oz.	300	8.0	58.0	4.0	15	630	m.q.
(Healthy Choice), 13.4 oz.	320	13.0	58.0	6.0	30	550	m.q.
Enchilada dinner mix:							
(Tio Sancho Dinner Kit):*							
sauce mix, 3 oz. . .	278	4.5	62.0	1.5	n.a.	4058	1.8 c
1 shell	80	1.3	10.8	3.5	n.a	2	.6 c
Enchilada entree, frozen:							
beef:							
(Banquet Meals), 11 oz.	390	14.0	57.0	12.0	15	1260	m.q.

Food and Measure	cal.	prot. (gms)	carbo. (gms)	fat (gms)	chol. (mgs)	sod. (mgs)	fiber (gms)
w/chili sauce *(Banquet* Family), 7 oz.	270	10.0	28.0	13.0	m.q.	m.q.	m.q.
Ranchero *(Weight Watchers Ultimate 200)*, 9.12 oz. . . .	190	18.0	18.0	5.0	20	500	m.q.
cheese:							
(Banquet Meals), 11 oz.	340	15.0	56.0	7.0	15	1500	m.q.
(Stouffer's), 9.75 oz.	490	23.0	33.0	29.0	m.q.	550	m.q.
nacho *(Weight Watchers)*, 8.87 oz.	230	10.0	33.0	6.0	25	520	m.q.
chicken:							
(Banquet Meals), 11 oz.	360	15.0	54.0	10.0	20	1580	m.q.
(Healthy Choice), 9.5 oz.	310	14.0	44.0	9.0	35	480	m.q.
(Stouffer's), 10 oz.	490	21.0	31.0	31.0	m.q.	860	m.q.
Suiza *(Weight Watchers)*, 9 oz.	230	16.0	25.0	7.0	40	530	m.q.
Enchilada sauce:							
(Gebhardt), 3 tbsp.	25	<1.0	3.0	1.0	<1	170	<1.0 d
green *(Old El Paso)*, 2 tbsp.	11	<1.0	3.0	0	0	200	0
hot:							
(Las Palmas), 1/2 cup	25	1.0	3.0	1.0	0	670	0
(Old El Paso), 1/4 cup	30	<1.0	4.0	1.0	0	250	(0)
or mild *(Ortega)*, 1 oz.	12	0	3.0	0	0	280	(0)
mild *(Old El Paso)*, 1/4 cup	25	<1.0	4.0	1.0	0	250	(0)
mild *(Rosarita)*, 2.5 oz.	25	<1.0	3.0	<1.0	0	230	<1.0 d
Enchilada seasoning mix:							
(Lawry's Seasoning Blends), 1 pkg. . .	152	5.3	29.9	1.2	0	1723	1.4 c

Food and Measure	cal.	prot. (gms)	carbo. (gms)	fat (gms)	chol. (mgs)	sod. (mgs)	fiber (gms)
Enchilada seasoning mix *(cont.)*							
(French's), 1/5 pkg. . . .	20	1.0	4.0	0	0	580	n.a.
(Old El Paso), 1/18 pkg.	6	0	1.0	0	0	80	0
Endive, chopped,							
1/2 cup	4	.3	.8	.1	0	6	.8 d
Endive, Belgian, see "Chickory, witloof"							
Energy shake, see "Protein shake mix"							
Entree sauce (see also specific listings):							
Alfredo *(Betty Crocker Recipe Sauces),* 4 oz.	190	1.0	8.0	17.0	20	650	n.a.
barbecue *(Beef Tonight),* 4 oz.	70	2.0	15.0	<1.0	0	580	n.a.
cacciatore *(Betty Crocker Recipe Sauces),* 3.9 oz. . .	40	1.0	9.0	<1.0	0	570	m.q.
cacciatore *(Chicken Tonight),* 4 oz. . . .	70	1.0	12.0	2.0	0	490	m.q.
country French *(Chicken Tonight),* 4 oz.	140	1.0	6.0	12.0	5	730	n.a.
herbed, w/wine *(Chicken Tonight),* 4 oz.	100	2.0	13.0	4.0	5	610	m.q.
honey mustard *(Chicken Tonight Light),* 4 oz.	50	1.0	12.0	<1.0	0	420	n.a.
lasagna, skillet *(Beef Tonight),* 4 oz. . . .	60	3.0	9.0	1.0	5	630	m.q.
Oriental *(Chicken Tonight),* 4 oz.	70	1.0	14.0	1.0	0	580	m.q.
parmigiana *(Betty Crocker Recipe Sauces),* 3.9 oz. . .	50	2.0	9.0	1.0	0	430	n.a.

Food and Measure	cal.	prot. (gms)	carbo. (gms)	fat (gms)	chol. (mgs)	sod. (mgs)	fiber (gms)
pepper steak *(Betty Crocker* Recipe Sauces), 3.8 oz. . .	45	1.0	8.0	1.0	0	520	m.q.
primavera, Italian *(Chicken Tonight Light)*, 4 oz.	50	2.0	9.0	<1.0	0	540	m.q.
Spanish *(Chicken Tonight)*, 4 oz.	70	2.0	10.0	2.0	0	640	m.q.
Stroganoff *(Beef Tonight)*, 4 oz.	130	1.0	6.0	12.0	10	770	n.a.
Stroganoff *(Betty Crocker* Recipe Sauces), 3.8 oz. . .	60	1.0	6.0	4.0	10	540	n.a.
sweet and sour *(Betty Crocker* Recipe Sauces), 4.1 oz. . .	130	<1.0	32.0	0	0	360	m.q.
sweet and sour *(Chicken Tonight)*, 4 oz.	80	0	19.0	0	0	280	m.q.
sweet and spicy *(Chicken Tonight Light)*, 4 oz.	50	2.0	10.0	<1.0	0	390	m.q.
teriyaki *(Betty Crocker* Recipe Sauces), 3.9 oz.	60	2.0	13.0	<1.0	0	820	n.a.
Eppaw, 1/2 cup . . .	75	2.3	15.8	.9	0	6	m.q.
Escarole, see "Endive"							
Etouffée dinner mix *(Luzianne)*, 1/4 pkg.	200	5.0	42.0	1.0	0	1030	<1.0 d

F

Food and Measure	cal.	prot. (gms)	carbo. (gms)	fat (gms)	chol. (mgs)	sod. (mgs)	fiber (gms)
Fajita entree, frozen:							
chicken *(Healthy Choice),* 7 oz.	200	17.0	25.0	3.0	35	310	m.q.
chicken *(Weight Watchers),* 6.75 oz.	210	17.0	24.0	5.0	25	490	m.q.
Fajita mix:							
(Tio Sancho Dinner Kit)							
fajita sauce, 1 oz.	14	.5	1.8	.5	<1	590	.1 c
tortilla, 1 piece	125	3.3	24.0	1.9	n.a.	569	m.q.
(Tyson), 4 oz.	80	7.0	2.0	2.0	n.a.	240	m.q.
Fajita sauce *(Lawry's Skillet Sauce),* 1 oz.	14	.5	1.8	.5	<1	590	.1 c
Fajita seasoning mix:							
(French's), 1/5 pkg. . .	16	0	3.0	0	0	450	n.a.
(Lawry's Seasoning Blends), 1 pkg. . .	63	2.0	14.0	.4	<1	2118	.5 c
(McCormick/Schilling), 1/4 pkg.	28	1.0	5.0	.5	n.a.	417	n.a.
Falafel mix:							
(Casbah), 11/4 oz. . .	100	5.0	20.0	1.0	0	240	m.q.
(Fantastic Falafel), 3 oz.	134	8.0	21.0	2.0	0	296	7.0 d
(Near East), 3 patties*	270	13.0	22.0	15.0	n.a.	680	m.q.
Farina, whole-grain (see also "Cereal"):							
dry, 1 oz.	105	3.0	22.1	.1	0	1	.8 d
cooked, 1 cup	116	3.4	24.6	.2	0	1	3.3 d
Fat, see specific listings							

Food and Measure	cal.	prot. (gms)	carbo. (gms)	fat (gms)	chol. (mgs)	sod. (mgs)	fiber (gms)
Fat, imitation							
(Rokeach Nyafat),							
1 tbsp.	99	0	0	11.0	0	0	0
Fava beans, see "Broad beans, mature"							
Feijoa, raw:							
w/skin, 1 medium,							
2.3 oz.	25	.6	5.3	.4	0	2	m.q.
pureed, 1/2 cup . . .	60	1.5	12.9	1.0	0	4	m.q.
(Frieda's), 1 oz. . . .	17	.3	4.0	.3	0	1	m.q.
Fennel, bulb, raw, trimmed:							
1 oz.	9	.4	2.1	.1	0	15	m.q.
1 bulb, 8.3 oz.	72	2.9	17.1	.5	0	122	m.q.
sliced, 1/2 cup	27	1.1	6.3	.2	0	45	m.q.
Fennel seed, 1 tsp.	7	.3	1.1	.3	0	2	.3 c
Fenugreek seed, 1 tsp.	12	.9	2.2	.2	0	2	.4 c
Fettuccine Alfredo, frozen *(Stouffer's),*							
5 oz.	245	8.0	22.0	14.0	n.a.	400	m.q.
Fettuccine Alfredo mix*, 1/2 cup:							
(Hain Pasta & Sauce)	190	6.0	21.0	10.0	10	440	1.5 d
(Kraft Pasta & Cheese)	180	7.0	19.0	9.0	30	590	m.q.
Fettuccine entree, frozen:							
Alfredo:							
(Healthy Choice Quick Meal), 8 oz.	240	10.0	36.0	7.0	45	460	m.q.
(Lean Cuisine), 9 oz.	280	14.0	41.0	7.0	15	570	m.q.
(Stouffer's Lunch Express), 10 oz.	490	16.0	45.0	27.0	n.a.	800	m.q.
(Weight Watchers), 8 oz.	230	15.0	28.0	7.0	25	550	m.q.

Food and Measure	cal.	prot. (gms)	carbo. (gms)	fat (gms)	chol. (mgs)	sod. (mgs)	fiber (gms)
Fettuccine entree, Alfredo *(cont.)*							
chicken *(Stouffer's Lunch Express),*							
9⅝ oz.	370	20.0	29.0	19.0	m.q.	700	m.q.
w/beef and broccoli *(Healthy Choice Extra Portion),* 12 oz.	290	19.0	46.0	3.0	20	520	m.q.
chicken:							
(Armour Classics),							
11 oz.	260	17.0	28.0	9.0	50	660	m.q.
(Healthy Choice),							
8.5 oz.	240	22.0	29.0	4.0	45	370	m.q.
(Lean Cuisine), 9 oz.	280	23.0	33.0	6.0	35	500	m.q.
(Weight Watchers),							
8.25 oz.	280	22.0	25.0	9.0	40	590	m.q.
w/vegetable medley *(Stouffer's* Homestyle), 9.5 oz. . .	340	22.0	28.0	16.0	m.q.	760	m.q.
primavera:							
(Green Giant),							
1 pkg.	230	13.0	26.0	8.0	25	610	6.0 d
(Green Giant Garden Gourmet Right for Lunch), 9.5 oz.	230	13.0	26.0	8.0	25	610	6.0 d
(Lean Cuisine),							
10 oz.	260	14.0	35.0	7.0	20	580	m.q.
Fettuccine entree mix, Alfredo *(Hain Pasta & Sauce),*							
¼ pkg.	180	5.0	27.0	4.0	n.a.	420	m.q.
Fiber supplement *(FiberSonic),*							
1.35-oz. pouch . .	120	2.0	24.0	2.0	0	0	11.0 d
Fig:							
fresh:							
1 large, 2.3 oz. . .	47	.5	12.3	.2	0	1	2.1 d
1 medium, 1.8 oz.	37	.4	9.6	.2	0	1	1.7 d

Food and Measure	cal.	prot. (gms)	carbo. (gms)	fat (gms)	chol. (mgs)	sod. (mgs)	fiber (gms)
California, 4 figs, 2 oz.	143	2.4	38.8	.7	0	6	9.5 d
Calimyrna (Frieda's), 1 oz.	23	.3	5.8	.1	0	<1	m.q.
canned in heavy syrup, 1/2 cup . . .	114	.5	29.7	.1	0	2	2.8 d
dried, 10 figs, 6.6 oz.	477	5.7	122.2	2.2	0	20	17.4 d
dried, Calamata string (Agora), 1/2 cup . .	250	3.0	58.0	2.0	0	<10	17.0 d
Filberts:							
dried:							
1 oz.	179	3.7	4.4	17.8	0	1	1.7 d
chopped, 1 cup . .	727	15.0	17.6	72.0	0	3	7.0 d
blanched, 1 oz. . .	191	3.6	4.5	19.1	0	1	.5 c
dry-roasted:							
1 oz.	188	2.8	5.1	18.8	0	1	1.1 c
salted, 1 oz.	188	2.8	5.1	18.8	0	221	1.1 c
oil-roasted:							
1 oz.	187	4.1	5.4	18.1	0	1	1.8 d
salted, 1 oz.	187	4.1	5.4	18.1	0	223	1.8 d
Fillo pastry, frozen:							
(Apollo), 1 oz.	80	3.0	18.0	.4	0	100	m.q.
(Athens Foods), 1 oz.	80	3.0	18.0	.4	0	100	m.q.
Finnan haddie, see "Haddock, smoked"							
Fish, see specific listings							
"Fish," vegetarian:							
frozen (Worthington Fillets), 2 pieces . .	180	15.0	9.0	9.0	0	910	m.q.
mix (LaLoma Ocean Platter), 1/4 cup . .	50	8.0	5.0	0	0	260	m.q.
Fish batter mix, see "Fish seasoning and coating mix"							
Fish cakes, see "Fish Entree"							

Food and Measure	cal.	prot. (gms)	carbo. (gms)	fat (gms)	chol. (mgs)	sod. (mgs)	fiber (gms)
Fish dinner, frozen (see also specific fish listings):							
'n' chips (Swanson), 10 oz.	500	20.0	59.0	21.0	m.q.	980	m.q.
lemon pepper (Healthy Choice), 10.7 oz.	300	13.0	52.0	5.0	40	470	m.q.
w/mashed potatoes and carrots (Morton), 9.25 oz. . . .	350	17.0	44.0	12.0	65	860	m.q.
sticks (Swanson), 7.5 oz.	270	8.0	32.0	12.0	m.q.	620	m.q.
Fish entree, frozen (see also specific fish listings):							
cakes (Mrs. Paul's), 4 oz.	190	9.0	24.0	7.0	20	690	m.q.
fillets:							
divan (Lean Cuisine), 10³/8 oz.	210	27.0	13.0	5.0	65	490	m.q.
Florentine (Lean Cuisine), 9⁵/8 oz. . . .	220	26.0	13.0	7.0	65	590	m.q.
w/macaroni and cheese (Stouffer's Homestyle), 9 oz.	440	24.0	40.0	20.0	m.q.	990	m.q.
fillets, battered, 2 pieces, except as noted:							
(Gorton's Crispy)	290	11.0	18.0	19.0	35	550	m.q.
(Gorton's Crunchy)	230	13.0	19.0	11.0	40	440	m.q.
(Gorton's Crunchy Microwave Portions)	300	11.0	19.0	20.0	30	510	m.q.
(Gorton's Potato Crisp)	300	12.0	18.0	20.0	30	360	m.q.
(Gorton's Value Pack Portions), 1 piece	180	7.0	15.0	10.0	25	450	m.q.

Food and Measure	cal.	prot. (gms)	carbo. (gms)	fat (gms)	chol. (mgs)	sod. (mgs)	fiber (gms)
(Mrs. Paul's), 6 oz.	400	14.0	35.0	23.0	40	750	m.q.
(Mrs. Paul's Crunchy), 4.5 oz.	280	12.0	26.0	14.0	25	730	m.q.
(Van de Kamp's), 1 piece	170	7.0	13.0	10.0	20	350	m.q.
minced *(Mrs. Paul's)*, 3 oz. . .	140	6.0	14.0	7.0	15	280	m.q.
fillets, breaded, 2 pieces, except as noted:							
(Healthy Choice) . .	160	12.0	16.0	5.0	30	350	m.q.
(Mrs. Paul's Crispy Crunchy), 4 oz.	230	14.0	23.0	10.0	35	520	m.q.
(Mrs. Paul's Healthy Treasures), 3 oz.	130	11.0	14.0	3.0	20	210	m.q.
(Van de Kamp's) . .	280	11.0	18.0	18.0	35	280	m.q.
(Van de Kamp's Crisp & Healthy)	150	12.0	18.0	3.0	25	350	m.q.
(Van de Kamp's Crispy Large Microwave), 1 piece	290	12.0	21.0	17.0	25	640	m.q.
(Van de Kamp's Crispy Microwave), 1 piece	140	6.0	9.0	9.0	15	210	m.q.
(Van de Kamp's Snack Pack) . .	220	8.0	13.0	10.0	20	280	m.q.
fillets, in sauce *(Mrs. Paul's Light)*, 4.1 oz.	110	16.0	5.0	3.0	25	410	n.a.
'n' chips *(Swanson)*, 5.5 oz.	300	12.0	39.0	11.0	m.q.	620	m.q.
nuggets, battered *(Van de Kamp's)*, 4 pieces	130	5.0	8.0	9.0	10	310	m.q.
oven baked *(Weight Watchers Ultimate 200)*, 6.64 oz. . . .	120	16.0	10.0	2.0	m.q.	390	n.a.

Food and Measure	cal.	prot. (gms)	carbo. (gms)	fat (gms)	chol. (mgs)	sod. (mgs)	fiber (gms)
Fish entree *(cont.)*							
portions, minced, battered *(Mrs. Paul's)*, 3.5 oz.	300	11.0	21.0	19.0	35	540	m.q.
sandwich, see "Fish sandwich"							
sticks, battered, 4 pieces, except as noted:							
(Gorton's Crispy)	260	9.0	16.0	18.0	25	480	m.q.
(Gorton's Crunchy)	200	8.0	15.0	12.0	30	240	m.q.
(Gorton's Crunchy Microwave), 6 pieces	360	13.0	27.0	22.0	30	690	m.q.
(Gorton's Potato Crisp)	220	7.0	16.0	14.0	25	330	m.q.
(Gorton's Value Pack)	190	7.0	13.0	12.0	20	330	m.q.
(Van de Kamp's) . .	160	8.0	12.0	9.0	20	380	m.q.
minced *(Mrs. Paul's)*, 3.5 oz.	210	7.0	20.0	12.0	25	590	m.q.
sticks, breaded, 4 pieces, except as noted:							
(Frionor Bunch O' Crunch)	210	9.2	13.0	14.1	22	267	<.1 d
(Healthy Choice), 8 pieces	120	8.0	14.0	4.0	20	250	m.q.
(Mrs. Paul's Crispy Crunchy), 2.7 oz.	170	9.0	16.0	8.0	20	460	m.q.
(Mrs. Paul's Healthy Treasures), 2.25 oz.	110	8.0	14.0	3.0	15	270	m.q.
(Mrs. Paul's Sea Pals), 3 oz. . . .	190	9.0	18.0	9.0	15	320	m.q.
(Van de Kamp's) . .	200	9.0	15.0	12.0	20	290	m.q.
(Van de Kamp's Crisp & Healthy)	120	9.0	17.0	2.0	15	330	m.q.

Food and Measure	cal.	prot. (gms)	carbo. (gms)	fat (gms)	chol. (mgs)	sod. (mgs)	fiber (gms)
(Van de Kamp's Crispy Micro- wave), 3 pieces	130	7.0	11.0	7.0	15	280	m.q.
(Van de Kamp's Snack/Value Pack)	170	8.0	13.0	10.0	20	270	m.q.
minced *(Mrs. Paul's),* 3 oz. . .	140	6.0	14.0	7.0	15	280	m.q.
Fish sandwich, fro- zen, fillet *(Hormel Quick Meal),* 5.2 oz.	430	16.0	56.0	16.0	68	910	m.q.
Fish seasoning and coating mix:							
(Shake'n Bake), 1/4 pkt.	70	1.0	14.0	1.0	0	410	m.q.
batter:							
Cajun *(Tone's),* 1 tsp.	12	.3	2.6	.1	0	49	.1 d
fish & chips *(Golden Dipt),* 1 1/4 oz. . .	120	2.0	27.0	0	0	910	m.q.
blackened Redfish *(Golden Dipt),* 1/4 tsp.	2	0	0	0	0	140	n.a.
broiled *(Golden Dipt),* 1/4 tsp. . .	2	0	0	0	0	125	n.a.
fish fry, 2/3 oz.:							
(Golden Dipt) . . .	60	2.0	14.0	0	0	430	m.q.
Cajun style *(Golden Dipt)*	60	2.0	14.0	0	0	470	m.q.
herb, Italian *(McCor- mick/Schilling* Bag'n Season), 1 pkg. . .	94	2.0	21.0	.2	0	1367	m.q.
lemon butter *(French's* Roasting Bag), 1/4 pkg.	25	0	6.0	0	0	390	n.a.
lemon and dill *(McCor- mick/Schilling* Bag'n Season), 1 pkg. . .	161	3.0	15.0	11.0	0	2035	m.q.
seafood:							
(Old Bay), 1 tsp. . . .	5	.2	.8	.3	0	577	m.q.

Food and Measure	cal.	prot. (gms)	carbo. (gms)	fat (gms)	chol. (mgs)	sod. (mgs)	fiber (gms)
Fish seasoning and coating mix, seafood *(cont.)*							
(Tone's), 1 tsp.	10	.5	.9	.7	0	1	.3 d
all purpose *(Golden Dipt)*, 1/4 tsp.	2	0	0	0	0	85	n.a.
Chesapeake Bay *(McCormick/ Schilling Spice Blends)*, 1 tsp.	7	.3	.8	.3	n.a.	806	n.a.
frying *(Golden Dipt)*, 2/3 oz.	60	1.0	14.0	0	0	600	m.q.
lemon pepper *(Golden Dipt)*, 1/4 tsp.	8	1.0	1.0	0	0	115	n.a.
shrimp and crab, Cajun style *(Golden Dipt)*, 1/4 tsp.	2	0	0	0	0	200	n.a.
Flatfish, meat only:							
raw, 4 oz.	104	21.4	0	1.4	54	92	0
baked, broiled, or microwaved, 4 oz.	133	27.4	0	1.7	77	119	0
Flavor enhancer							
(Ac'cent), 1/2 tsp.	5	0	0	0	0	300	0
Flax seeds *(Arrowhead Mills)*, 1 oz.	140	5.0	11.0	10.0	0	<1	6.0 d
Flounder:							
fresh, see "Flatfish"							
frozen:							
(Gorton's Fishmarket Fillets), 5 oz.	110	23.0	1.0	1.0	m.q.	170	0
(Van de Kamp's Natural), 4 oz.	100	22.0	0	2.0	35	100	0
Flounder entree, frozen:							
battered, 2 pieces:							
(Gorton's Crispy)	280	11.0	16.0	19.0	35	550	m.q.
(Mrs. Paul's Crunchy Batter)	220	12.0	23.0	9.0	40	560	m.q.

Food and Measure	cal.	prot. (gms)	carbo. (gms)	fat (gms)	chol. (mgs)	sod. (mgs)	fiber (gms)
breaded, 1 piece:							
(Mrs. Paul's Light)	240	16.0	20.0	10.0	50	450	m.q.
(Van de Kamp's Light)	260	18.0	21.0	12.0	45	480	m.q.
crunchy *(Gorton's Select)*	190	10.0	17.0	9.0	30	420	m.q.
Flour, see "Wheat flour" and specific listings							
Frankfurter, 1 link, except as noted:							
(Healthy Deli), 1 oz.	42	4.0	1.3	1.9	9	200	0
(Hillshire Farm Bun Size Wieners) . . .	180	7.0	2.0	16.0	m.q.	550	0
(Hormel Light & Lean)	45	6.0	2.0	1.0	15	390	0
(Hormel Wranglers)	180	7.0	1.0	16.0	40	500	0
(Jesse Jones, 1 lb.)	150	6.0	2.0	13.0	m.q.	540	0
(Kahn's Bun Size) . .	190	6.0	2.0	17.0	m.q.	600	0
(Kahn's Jumbo) . . .	190	6.0	2.0	17.0	m.q.	560	0
(Oscar Mayer Healthy Favorites)	50	8.0	2.0	1.5	20	520	0
(Oscar Mayer Light Wieners)	110	7.0	2.0	8.0	30	580	0
(Oscar Mayer Little Wieners), 6 links . .	170	6.0	1.0	16.0	35	580	0
(Oscar Mayer Wieners, 10/lb.)	150	5.0	1.0	13.0	30	450	0
(Oscar Mayer Wieners, 8/lb.)	180	6.0	1.0	17.0	35	570	0
beef:							
(Healthy Deli), 1 oz.	41	4.3	1.5	2.0	10	200	0
(Hebrew National)	149	5.8	<1.0	14.0	15	497	0
(Hillshire Farm Bun Size Wieners) . .	180	7.0	2.0	16.0	m.q.	560	0
(Hormel Wranglers)	170	7.0	1.0	15.0	40	530	0
(Jesse Jones) . . .	180	7.0	3.0	15.0	m.q.	620	0
(Kahn's)	140	5.0	2.0	13.0	m.q.	500	0
(Kahn's Bun Size)	190	6.0	3.0	17.0	m.q.	560	0

Food and Measure	cal.	prot. (gms)	carbo. (gms)	fat (gms)	chol. (mgs)	sod. (mgs)	fiber (gms)
Frankfurter, beef *(cont.)*							
(Kahn's Jumbo) . .	190	6.0	3.0	18.0	m.q.	560	0
(King Kold), 2 oz.	173	9.0	1.0	16.3	m.q.	815	0
(Oscar Mayer) . . .	150	5.0	1.0	13.0	25	450	0
(Oscar Mayer Big & Juicy), 4-oz. link	360	13.0	2.0	34.0	65	1150	0
(Oscar Mayer Big & Juicy Brooklyn)	240	9.0	0	23.0	45	690	0
(Oscar Mayer Bun Length)	180	6.0	1.0	17.0	35	570	0
(Oscar Mayer Light)	130	7.0	1.0	11.0	25	600	0
w/cheddar *(Kahn's)*	180	7.0	2.0	16.0	m.q.	640	0
hot *(Hillshire Farm Links)*, 2 oz. . . .	190	8.0	1.0	17.0	m.q.	560	0
cheese (cheesefurter or cheese smokie):							
(Hillshire Farm Bun Size Wieners) . .	180	7.0	2.0	16.0	m.q.	530	0
(Kahn's Wiener) . .	150	6.0	1.0	13.0	m.q.	490	0
(Oscar Mayer) . . .	150	5.0	<1.0	14.0	35	450	0
chicken, see "Chicken frankfurter"							
chili, frozen, w/cheese *(Hormel Quick Meal)*, 4.5 oz. . . .	340	14.0	25.0	20.0	80	540	m.q.
corn dog:							
(Jesse Jones) . . .	210	6.0	22.0	11.0	m.q.	870	m.q.
frozen *(Hormel)*, 2.75 oz.	210	6.0	24.0	10.0	35	510	m.q.
hot *(Hillshire Farm)*, 2 oz.	190	8.0	2.0	16.0	m.q.	530	0
hot and spicy *(Oscar Mayer)*	220	10.0	<1.0	20.0	45	770	0
natural casing *(Hillshire Farm* Wieners), 2 oz.	180	6.0	2.0	17.0	m.q.	470	0

Food and Measure	cal.	prot. (gms)	carbo. (gms)	fat (gms)	chol. (mgs)	sod. (mgs)	fiber (gms)
red hots *(Jesse Jones)*	180	9.0	3.0	15.0	m.q.	710	0
smoked:							
(Kahn's Big Red Smokey)	170	8.0	2.0	14.0	m.q.	550	0
(Kahn's Bun Size Smokey)	180	8.0	2.0	15.0	m.q.	550	0
beef *(Kahn's* Bun Size Beef Smokey)	190	7.0	2.0	17.0	m.q.	530	0
turkey, see "Turkey frankfurter"							
"Frankfurter," vege-tarian:							
canned:							
(LaLoma), 1 link . .	110	11.0	2.0	6.0	0	190	m.q.
(LaLoma Linketts), 2 links	140	15.0	2.0	8.0	0	320	m.q.
(LaLoma Sizzle Franks), 2 links	170	10.0	3.0	13.0	0	340	m.q.
(Worthington Veja-Links), 2 links . .	140	8.0	4.0	10.0	0	330	m.q.
(Worthington Super-Links), 1 link . . .	100	7.0	3.0	7.0	0	440	m.q.
frozen, 1 link:							
(Morningstar Farms Deli Franks) . . .	120	10.0	4.0	7.0	0	480	m.q.
(Worthington Leanies)	100	8.0	2.0	6.0	0	440	m.q.
corn battered *(LaLoma* Corn Dogs)	190	13.0	15.0	8.0	0	400	m.q.
Frankfurter wrap *(Weiner Wrap)*, 1 piece	60	1.0	10.0	2.0	n.a.	430	m.q.
French toast, frozen:							
(Aunt Jemima Origi-nal), 2 pieces . . .	240	9.0	36.0	7.0	m.q.	320	m.q.
(Downyflake), 1 piece	130	4.0	22.0	3.0	25	270	m.q.

Food and Measure	cal.	prot. (gms)	carbo. (gms)	fat (gms)	chol. (mgs)	sod. (mgs)	fiber (gms)
French toast, frozen (cont.)							
cinnamon (Aunt Jemima), 2 pieces . .	240	10.0	36.0	7.0	m.q.	310	m.q.
mini (Swanson Breakfast Blast), 3 oz. . . .	180	4.0	30.0	5.0	m.q.	190	m.q.
sticks (Qwik-Krisp), 4 pieces	450	7.0	52.0	24.0	45	420	1.0 d
sticks (Swanson Breakfast Blast), 3.75 oz.	280	6.0	44.0	9.0	m.q.	220	m.q.
French toast breakfast, frozen:							
(Aunt Jemima Homestyle), 5.9 oz. . . .	470	8.0	53.0	26.0	m.q.	330	m.q.
cinnamon swirl, w/sausage (Swanson Great Starts), 5.5 oz.	440	14.0	38.0	27.0	m.q.	580	m.q.
w/sausages (Aunt Jemima Homestyle), 5.3 oz.	390	13.0	35.0	22.0	m.q.	840	m.q.
w/sausages (Swanson Great Starts), 5.5 oz.	410	14.0	36.0	23.0	m.q.	600	m.q.
vegetarian, cinnamon swirl, w/patty (Morningstar Farms), 6.5 oz.	380	24.0	37.0	15.0	0	1220	4.0 d
Frog's legs, meat only, raw, 4 oz. . .	83	18.6	0	.3	m.q.	m.q.	0
Frosting, ready-to-use, 1/12 can, except as noted:							
butter fudge (Pillsbury Frosting Supreme)	140	1.0	22.0	6.0	0	50	(0)
butter pecan (Betty Crocker Creamy Deluxe)	170	0	26.0	7.0	0	50	(0)

Food and Measure	cal.	prot. (gms)	carbo. (gms)	fat (gms)	chol. (mgs)	sod. (mgs)	fiber (gms)
caramel pecan (Pillsbury Frosting Supreme)	150	0	20.0	8.0	0	70	0
cherry (Betty Crocker Creamy Deluxe) . .	160	0	27.0	6.0	0	50	(0)
chocolate:							
(Betty Crocker Creamy Deluxe)	160	<1.0	24.0	7.0	0	60	(0)
(Betty Crocker Creamy Deluxe Light)	130	<1.0	28.0	2.0	0	60	(0)
(Duncan Hines) . .	160	0	24.0	7.0	n.a.	90	(0)
double Dutch (Pillsbury Frosting Supreme)	140	1.0	22.0	6.0	0	50	(0)
chocolate, milk:							
(Betty Crocker Creamy Deluxe)	160	<1.0	25.0	6.0	0	55	(0)
(Betty Crocker Creamy Deluxe Light)	140	<1.0	29.0	2.0	0	60	(0)
(Duncan Hines) . .	160	0	24.0	7.0	n.a.	85	(0)
(Pillsbury Frosting Supreme)	150	0	23.0	6.0	0	65	(0)
w/fudge swirl (Pillsbury Frosting Supreme)	150	0	23.0	6.0	0	65	(0)
chocolate chip:							
(Betty Crocker Creamy Deluxe)	170	<1.0	27.0	7.0	0	30	(0)
(Pillsbury Frosting Supreme)	150	0	27.0	4.0	0	70	(0)
chocolate fudge:							
(Pillsbury Frosting Supreme)	150	0	22.0	6.0	0	88	(0)
Funfetti (Pillsbury Frosting Supreme)	140	0	23.0	6.0	0	80	(0)

Food and Measure	cal.	prot. (gms)	carbo. (gms)	fat (gms)	chol. (mgs)	sod. (mgs)	fiber (gms)
Frosting, ready-to-use, chocolate fudge *(cont.)*							
dark Dutch *(Betty Crocker Creamy Deluxe)*	160	1.0	22.0	7.0	0	70	(0)
Dutch *(Duncan Hines)*	160	0	24.0	7.0	n.a.	95	(0)
or milk *(Pillsbury Lovin' Lites)* . . .	130	<1.0	28.0	2.0	0	95	1.0 d
coconut almond *(Pillsbury Frosting Supreme)*	150	1.0	17.0	9.0	0	60	0
coconut pecan:							
(Betty Crocker Creamy Deluxe)	160	<1.0	20.0	9.0	0	60	(0)
(Pillsbury Frosting Supreme)	160	0	17.0	10.0	0	60	0
cream cheese:							
(Betty Crocker Creamy Deluxe)	170	0	26.0	7.0	0	70	n.a.
(Duncan Hines) . .	160	0	24.0	8.0	n.a.	120	n.a.
(Pillsbury Frosting Supreme)	160	0	26.0	6.0	0	75	0
decorator, all flavors *(Pillsbury)*, 1 tbsp.	60	0	12.0	2.0	0	0	(0)
lemon:							
(Betty Crocker Creamy Deluxe)	170	0	28.0	6.0	0	70	n.a.
(Duncan Hines) . .	120	0	18.0	6.0	n.a.	60	n.a.
(Pillsbury Frosting Supreme)	160	0	25.0	6.0	0	80	0
rainbow chip *(Betty Crocker Creamy Deluxe)*	170	<1.0	27.0	7.0	0	30	n.a.
sour cream:							
chocolate *(Betty Crocker Creamy Deluxe)*	160	<1.0	23.0	7.0	0	100	n.a.
white *(Betty Crocker Creamy Deluxe)*	160	0	27.0	6.0	0	50	n.a.

Food and Measure	cal.	prot. (gms)	carbo. (gms)	fat (gms)	chol. (mgs)	sod. (mgs)	fiber (gms)
strawberry (Pillsbury Frosting Supreme)	160	0	25.0	6.0	0	80	0
vanilla:							
(Betty Crocker Creamy Deluxe)	160	0	27.0	6.0	0	25	n.a.
(Betty Crocker Creamy Deluxe Light)	140	0	30.0	2.0	0	30	n.a.
(Duncan Hines) . .	160	0	24.0	7.0	n.a.	80	n.a.
(Pillsbury Frosting Supreme)	160	0	25.0	6.0	0	75	0
(Pillsbury Lovin' Lites)	130	0	29.0	2.0	0	70	0
w/fudge swirl (Pillsbury Frosting Supreme)	150	0	25.0	6.0	0	75	0
pink, Funfetti (Pillsbury Frosting Supreme)	150	0	25.0	6.0	0	70	0
plain or sunshine, Funfetti (Pillsbury Frosting Supreme)	150	0	25.0	6.0	0	75	0
Frosting mix*, 1/12 mix, except as noted:							
chocolate fudge (Betty Crocker)	180	<1.0	30.0	6.0	0	70	(0)
coconut pecan (Betty Crocker)	150	<1.0	19.0	8.0	0	50	(0)
vanilla, creamy (Betty Crocker)	170	0	32.0	5.0	0	50	(0)
white, fluffy (Betty Crocker)	70	<1.0	16.0	0	0	40	(0)
Fructose:							
(Estee), 1 tsp.	16	0	4.0	0	0	0	0
(Estee), 1 pkt.	12	0	3.0	0	0	0	0
Fruit, see specific listings							

Food and Measure	cal.	prot. (gms)	carbo. (gms)	fat (gms)	chol. (mgs)	sod. (mgs)	fiber (gms)
Fruit, mixed:							
canned (see also "Fruit cocktail" and "Fruit salad"), 1/2 cup:							
in juice (*Del Monte Fruit Naturals*) . .	60	0	16.0	0	0	10	1.0 d
in juice, chunky (*Libby's Lite*) . .	50	1.0	13.0	0	0	5	m.q.
in extra light syrup (*Del Monte Lite*)	60	0	16.0	0	0	10	1.0 d
in heavy syrup (*Del Monte*)	100	0	24.0	0	0	10	1.0 d
in heavy syrup, w/ berry flavor, chunky (*Libby's*)	90	0	24.0	0	0	15	m.q.
dried, 2 oz.:							
(*Del Monte*)	130	1.0	34.0	0	0	10	m.q.
(*Sun-Maid/Sunsweet*)	150	1.0	39.0	0	0	<20	m.q.
bits (*Sun-Maid/Sunsweet*)	150	2.0	40.0	<1.0	0	<50	m.q.
freeze-dried (*Mountain House Fruit Crisps*), 1/4 cup	60	0	15.0	0	0	5	m.q.
frozen:							
(*Stilwell*), 1 1/4 cup	60	0	14.0	0	0	30	1.0 d
in syrup (*Birds Eye*), 5 oz.	120	1.0	31.0	0	0	5	1.0 d
Fruit bar, see "Fruit snack" and "Snack bar"							
Fruit bar, frozen (see also "Ice bar" and "Yogurt bar"), 1 bar:							
all flavors (*Welch's Fruit Juice Bar*), 1.75 fl. oz.	45	0	11.0	0	0	0	n.a.

Food and Measure	cal.	prot. (gms)	carbo. (gms)	fat (gms)	chol. (mgs)	sod. (mgs)	fiber (gms)
all flavors (Welch's Fruit Juice Bar No Sugar Added), 1.75 fl. oz.	25	0	6.0	0	0	0	n.a.
banana (Frozfruit) . .	120	1.0	19.0	4.0	m.q.	n.a.	m.q.
berry, wild (Sunkist Fruit & Juice Bar)	103	.1	24.6	.5	0	11	n.a.
cantaloupe or cherry (Frozfruit)	70	0	16.0	0	0	n.a.	m.q.
coconut (Frozfruit) . .	120	1.0	18.0	5.0	m.q.	n.a.	m.q.
coconut (Sunkist) . .	137	2.7	12.8	8.4	0	58	1.4 c
lemon, lime, or orange (Frozfruit)	70	0	16.0	0	0	n.a.	m.q.
lemonade (Sunkist)	68	.1	17.6	.1	0	3	n.a.
orange (Sunkist Juice Bar)	72	.7	17.6	.1	0	1	n.a.
peach-passion fruit (Dole Fruit'n Juice)	70	<1.0	15.0	<1.0	0	10	n.a.
piña colada (Frozfruit)	120	1.0	16.0	6.0	m.q.	n.a.	m.q.
pineapple (Frozfruit)	70	0	16.0	0	0	n.a.	m.q.
raspberry (Dole Fruit'n Juice)	70	<1.0	15.0	<1.0	0	15	n.a.
raspberry, strawberry, or watermelon (Frozfruit)	70	0	16.0	0	0	n.a.	m.q.
strawberry cream (Frozfruit)	120	1.0	18.0	4.0	m.q.	n.a.	m.q.
strawberry-banana (Frozfruit)	120	1.0	20.0	5.0	m.q.	n.a.	m.q.
and cream: all flavors (Welch's No Sugar Added), 1.75 fl. oz.	45	1.0	6.0	2.0	0	12	n.a.
orange (Sunkist) . .	84	.9	16.6	1.5	n.a.	15	n.a.
Fruit cocktail, canned, 1/2 cup, except as noted:							
(Hunt's), 4 oz.	90	<1.0	23.0	<1.0	0	7	<1.0 d

Food and Measure	cal.	prot. (gms)	carbo. (gms)	fat (gms)	chol. (mgs)	sod. (mgs)	fiber (gms)
Fruit cocktail *(cont.)*							
(Stokely)	90	0	24.0	0	0	15	m.q.
in water	40	.5	10.4	.1	0	5	1.3 d
in water *(Libby's)* . .	40	0	10.0	0	0	5	m.q.
in juice *(Del Monte* Fruit Naturals*)* . . .	60	0	15.0	0	0	5	m.q.
in extra light syrup *(Del Monte* Lite Fruits*)*	50	0	13.0	0	0	5	m.q.
in light syrup	72	.5	18.8	.1	0	7	1.4 d
in heavy syrup *(Libby's)*	90	0	24.0	0	0	15	m.q.
Fruit juice blends (see also specific listings), 6 fl. oz.:							
(Chiquita Calypso Breeze)	100	0	24.0	0	0	30	(0)
(Chiquita Caribbean Splash)	90	0	23.0	0	0	15	(0)
(Chiquita Hawaiian Sunrise)	110	<1.0	26.0	<1.0	0	0	(0)
(Chiquita Tropical Squeeze)	90	0	23.0	0	0	15	(0)
cocktail, frozen* *(Welch's Orchard* Harvest Blend*)* . .	110	0	27.0	0	0	0	0
Fruit juice drink:							
(Boku Seven Fruit Blend*)*, 8 fl. oz. . .	120	0	29.0	0	0	5	0
mixed *(Tang Fruit Box)*, 8.45 fl. oz. . .	140	0	36.0	0	0	10	(0)
Fruit punch (see also specific fruit listings), 6 fl. oz., except as noted:							
canned or bottled:							
(Juicy Juice)	100	1.0	23.0	0	0	10	(0)
(Mott's 100%) . . .	188	<1.0	47.0	<1.0	0	5	(0)

Food and Measure	cal.	prot. (gms)	carbo. (gms)	fat (gms)	chol. (mgs)	sod. (mgs)	fiber (gms)
rainbow *(Kool-Aid Koolers),*							
8.45 fl. oz.	130	0	36.0	0	· 0	10	(0)
tropical *(Crush),*							
11.5 fl. oz.	188	0	47.0	0	0	5	(0)
tropical *(Juicy Juice)*	110	1.0	26.0	0	0	10	(0)
tropical *(R.W. Knud-*							
sen), 8 fl. oz. . .	105	<1.0	33.0	<1.0	0	(0)	m.q.
tropical *(Santa Cruz*							
Natural), 8 fl. oz.	110	<1.0	26.0	<1.0	0	(0)	m.q.
canned or chilled							
(Minute Maid) . . .	90	0	22.0	0	0	20	(0)
chilled *(Tropicana)* . .	90	<1.0	21.0	<1.0	0	15	(0)
cocktail, frozen*							
(Welch's Orchard							
Harvest Punch) . .	110	0	28.0	0	0	0	0
Fruit punch drink,							
6 fl. oz., except as							
noted:							
canned:							
(Hi-C)	90	0	23.0	0	0	20	(0)
(Hi-C Hula Cooler)	100	0	23.0	0	0	20	(0)
(Hi-C Hula Punch)	90	0	21.0	0	0	20	(0)
(Shasta), 12 fl. oz.	196	0	49.0	0	0	70	0
(Shasta Plus),							
12 fl. oz.	168	0	42.0	0	0	58	0
(Wylers), 8 fl. oz.	130	0	32.0	0	0	5	(0)
tropical *(Kool-Aid*							
Kool Bursts),							
6.75 oz.	110	0	28.0	0	⁻0	10	(0)
tropical *(Kool-Aid*							
Koolers),							
8.45 fl. oz.	130	0	35.0	0	0	10	(0)
tropical *(Wylers)* . .	80	(0)	21.0	(0)	0	10	(0)
frozen* *(Bright &*							
Early)	90	0	22.0	0	0	5	(0)
mix*, 8 fl. oz.:							
tropical *(Kool-Aid)*	100	0	25.0	0	0	0	0

Food and Measure	cal.	prot. (gms)	carbo. (gms)	fat (gms)	chol. (mgs)	sod. (mgs)	fiber (gms)
Fruit punch drink, mix *(cont.)*							
tropical *(Kool-Aid Presweetened)*	70	0	18.0	0	0	0	0
tropical *(Wylers Crystals)*	80	(0)	21.0	(0)	0	0	(0)
Fruit roll, see "Fruit snack"							
Fruit salad, canned:							
in heavy syrup, 1/2 cup	94	.4	24.5	.1	0	7	1.4 d
tropical, in heavy syrup, 1/2 cup . . .	110	.5	28.6	.1	0	3	1.7 d
Fruit snack (see also specific fruit listings):							
all varieties:							
(Fruit by the Foot), 1 roll	80	<1.0	17.0	2.0	0	45	m.q.
(Fruit Roll-Ups), 1/2 oz.	50	<1.0	12.0	<1.0	0	40	m.q.
(Gushers), 1 pouch	90	<1.0	21.0	1.0	0	45	m.q.
(Sunkist Fun Fruits), .9-oz. pouch . .	100	(0)	22.0	1.0	0	10	m.q.
bar *(Stretch Island Fruit Leather),* 1 oz. or 2 pieces:							
apple	90	0	25.0	0	0	0	3.0 d
apple, organic . . .	90	0	24.0	0	0	10	2.0 d
apricot	90	0	23.0	0	0	0	2.0 d
blackberry	90	0	24.0	0	0	0	3.0 d
cherry or grape . .	90	0	24.0	0	0	0	2.0 d
grape, organic . . .	90	0	24.0	0	0	5	2.0 d
raspberry	90	0	24.0	0	0	0	2.0 d
raspberry, organic	90	0	25.0	0	0	10	2.0 d
roll, *(Sunkist),* 1 piece:							
apple	80	(0)	19.0	(0)	0	15	m.q.
apricot	80	(0)	18.0	(0)	0	15	m.q.
cherry	80	(0)	18.0	(0)	0	20	m.q.
fruit punch	70	(0)	18.0	(0)	0	10	m.q.

Food and Measure	cal.	prot. (gms)	carbo. (gms)	fat (gms)	chol. (mgs)	sod. (mgs)	fiber (gms)
grape	80	(0)	18.0	(0)	0	35	m.q.
raspberry	80	(0)	18.0	(0)	0	20	m.q.
strawberry	70	(0)	18.0	(0)	0	10	m.q.
Fruit spreads (see also "Jam and preserves"):							
all flavors, 1 tsp., except as noted:							
(Knott's Berry Farm Light)	8	0	2.0	0	0	0	m.q.
(Master Choice), 2 tsp.	20	0	5.0	0	0	5	m.q.
(Polaner All Fruit)	14	0	4.0	0	0	0	m.q.
(Smucker's Extra Fruit)	15	0	3.0	0	0	0	m.q.
(Smucker's Simply Fruit)	16	0	4.0	0	0	0	m.q.
(Smucker's Light)	7	0	2.0	0	0	0	m.q.
(Smucker's Low Sugar)	8	0	2.0	0	0	0	m.q.
(Smucker's Slenderella)	7	0	2.0	0	0	0	m.q.
(Welch's), 2 tsp. . .	35	0	9.0	0	0	5	m.q.
except grape *(Welch's* Totally Fruit)*	14	0	4.0	0	0	5	m.q.
grape *(Welch's* Totally Fruit), 2 tsp.	28	0	8.0	0	0	5	m.q.
strawberry *(Master Choice),* 2 tsp. . . .	20	0	5.0	0	0	5	m.q.
Fruit syrup, 2 tbsp.:							
all flavors:							
(Knott's Berry Farm Light)	50	0	12.0	0	0	0	n.a.
(Knott's Berry Farm Light Microwave)	45	0	11.0	0	0	70	n.a.
(Knott's Berry Farm Microwave) . . .	110	0	28.0	0	0	90	n.a.

Food and Measure	cal.	prot. (gms)	carbo. (gms)	fat (gms)	chol. (mgs)	sod. (mgs)	fiber (gms)
Fruit syrup, all flavors *(cont.)*							
(Smucker's)	100	0	26.0	0	0	0	n.a.
except apricot							
(Knott's Berry							
Farm)	120	0	30.0	0	0	0	n.a.
apple *(R.W. Knudsen)*	75	<1.0	15.0	<1.0	0	(0)	n.a.
apricot *(Knott's Berry*							
Farm)	100	0	25.0	0	0	0	n.a.
blueberry *(R.W. Knud-*							
sen)	75	<1.0	19.0	<1.0	0	(0)	n.a.
w/maple *(R.W. Knud-*							
sen Fruit 'N Maple)	105	<1.0	26.0	<1.0	0	(0)	n.a.
raspberry or straw-							
berry *(R.W. Knud-*							
sen)	75	<1.0	18.0	<1.0	0	(0)	n.a.
Fruit topping, see							
"Fruit syrup" and							
specific listings							
Fudge, see "Candy"							
Fudge topping, see							
"Chocolate topping"							

G

Food and Measure	cal.	prot. (gms)	carbo. (gms)	fat (gms)	chol. (mgs)	sod. (mgs)	fiber (gms)
Garbanzo, see "Chickpea"							
Garlic:							
trimmed, 1 oz.	42	1.8	9.4	.1	0	5	.6 d
1 clove, approx. .1 oz.	4	.2	1.0	<.1	0	1	.1 d
crushed (Frieda's), 1 oz.	39	1.8	8.7	.1	0	5	m.q.
crushed (Gilroy), 1 tsp.	8	.3	2.0	0	0	4	m.q.
minced (Gilroy), 1 tsp.	23	.3	2.0	1.0	0	4	m.q.
Garlic and herb dip (Nasoya Vegi-Dip), 1 oz.	100	1.0	4.0	9.0	0	140	m.q.
Garlic pepper, 1 tsp.:							
(McCormick/Schilling California Style) . .	8	.2	2.0	.1	0	257	n.a.
(Lawry's Spice Blends)	11	.2	2.0	.1	0	292	.1 c
Garlic powder, 1 tsp.:							
(McCormick/Schilling California Style) . .	12	.5	2.0	0	0	3	n.a.
w/parsley (Lawry's Spice Blends) . . .	12	.5	2.3	.1	0	5	.1 c
Garlic puree (Progresso), 1 tsp.	4	<1.0	<1.0	<1.0	0	30	0
Garlic salt, 1 tsp.:							
(Lawry's Spice Blends)	4	.1	.8	<.1	0	968	<.1 c
(McCormick/Schilling California Style) . .	5	.1	1.0	0	0	833	n.a.

Food and Measure	cal.	prot. (gms)	carbo. (gms)	fat (gms)	chol. (mgs)	sod. (mgs)	fiber (gms)
Garlic seasoning:							
(McCormick/Schilling Garlic saltless), 1/2 tsp.	5	.2	1.1	0	0	1	n.a.
(McCormick/Schilling Season All), 1 tsp.	6	.1	.5	n.a.	0	652	n.a.
bread sprinkle *(Mc-Cormick/Schilling Spice Blends),* 1 tsp.	18	.2	.4	1.8	n.a.	100	n.a.
spread *(Lawry's),* 1/2 tbsp.	47	.2	1.0	4.6	<1	15	<.1 c
spread, concentrate *(Lawry's),* 1/2 tbsp.	15	0	.2	4.0	0	21	0
Gefilte fish, 1 piece:							
(Mothers Low Sodium)	60	6.0	2.0	3.0	25	45	<1.0 d
(Rokeach), 4 pieces	110	12.0	3.0	6.0	74	583	1.0 d
(Rokeach), 8 pieces	50	6.0	1.0	2.0	33	281	0
(Rokeach Low Sodium)	60	7.0	2.0	2.5	25	20	1.0 d
(Rokeach No Sugar)	50	6.0	1.0	3.0	34	250	1.0 d
(Rokeach Old Vienna)	60	6.0	2.0	3.0	29	240	1.0 d
jelled broth:							
(Mothers Old Fashioned), 4 pieces	45	5.0	1.0	2.0	18	196	1.0 d
(Mothers Old Fashioned), 6 pieces	60	7.0	1.0	3.0	22	237	2.0 d
(Rokeach)	45	5.0	1.0	2.0	34	265	0
liquid broth *(Mothers Old Fashioned)*	50	6.0	1.0	2.0	22	159	1.0 d
sweet:							
(Rokeach Gold Label Old Vienna)	50	5.0	2.0	1.0	32	236	1.0 d
(Rokeach Old Vienna)	110	11.0	4.0	5.0	55	463	1.0 d
jelled broth *(Mothers Old World)*	45	5.0	2.0	2.0	18	193	1.0 d

Food and Measure	cal.	prot. (gms)	carbo. (gms)	fat (gms)	chol. (mgs)	sod. (mgs)	fiber (gms)
whitefish, jelled broth							
(Rokeach No Sugar)	40	6.0	0	2.0	33	244	1.0 d
whitefish/pike, jelled broth:							
(Mothers), 4 pieces	45	6.0	2.0	1.0	18	203	1.0 d
(Rokeach)	80	11.0	1.0	4.0	64	478	3.0 d
(Rokeach Old Vienna), 6 oz. . . .	50	6.0	3.0	2.0	30	248	1.0 d
(Rokeach Old Vienna), 27 oz. . .	50	5.0	3.0	2.0	28	234	1.0 d
Gelatin, unflavored (Knox), 1 pkt. . . .	25	6.0	0	0	0	10	0
Gelatin bar, frozen, all flavors (Jell-O Gelatin Pops), 1 bar	35	1.0	8.0	0	0	25	0
Gelatin dessert, 1/2 cup, except as noted:							
(Jell-O Snacks), 3.5-oz. cup	80	1.0	18.0	0	0	40	0
mix*, all flavors:							
(D-Zerta)	8	2.0	0	0	0	0	0
(Jell-O)	80	2.0	19.0	0	0	—[1]	0
(Jell-O 1-2-3), 2/3 cup	130	2.0	27.0	2.0	0	55	0
Gelatin drink mix, orange flavor, w/Nutrasweet (Knox), 1 pkt.	40	6.0	4.0	(0)	0	15	(0)
Ginger, trimmed root:							
1 oz.	20	.5	4.3	.2	0	4	.6 d
sliced, 1/4 cup	17	.4	3.6	.2	0	3	.5 d
Ginger, crystallized (Frieda's), 1 oz. . .	96	.1	24.7	.1	0	m.q.	m.q.

[1] *Sodium values vary according to flavor: black raspberry, 35 mg.; lemon and pink lemonade, 75 mg.; lime, 55 mg.; orange-pineapple, 65 mg.; cherry, 70 mg.; all other flavors, 50 mg.*

Food and Measure	cal.	prot. (gms)	carbo. (gms)	fat (gms)	chol. (mgs)	sod. (mgs)	fiber (gms)
Ginger, ground, 1 tsp.	6	.2	1.3	.1	0	1	.2 d
Ginger, pickled,							
Japanese, 1 oz. . . .	10	.1	2.1	<.1	0	105	m.q.
Ginkgo nut, shelled:							
raw, 1 oz.	52	1.2	10.7	.5	0	2	.1 c
canned, drained, 1 oz.	32	.6	6.3	.5	0	87	2.6 d
dried, 1 oz.	99	2.9	20.6	.8	0	4	.3 c
Glaze *(Marie's):*							
blueberry, 2.35 oz. . . .	90	0	22.0	0	0	65	(0)
creamy, for bananas,							
2.2 oz.	120	0	18.0	5.0	n.a.	100	(0)
peach, 2.35 oz.	90	0	21.0	0	0	110	(0)
strawberry, 2.35 oz.	90	0	21.0	0	0	70	(0)
Goat, meat only,							
roasted, 4 oz.	162	30.7	0	3.4	85	98	0
Godfather's Pizza:							
original crust cheese:							
mini, 1/4 pie	138	6.0	20.0	4.0	13	159	m.q.
small, 1/6 pie . . .	239	10.0	32.0	7.0	25	289	m.q.
medium, 1/8 pie . .	242	10.0	35.0	7.0	22	285	m.q.
large, 1/10 pie . . .	271	12.0	37.0	8.0	28	329	m.q.
jumbo, 1/10 pie . .	402	17.5	54.6	12.2	42	479	.7 d
original crust combo:							
mini, 1/4 pie	164	8.0	21.0	5.0	17	287	m.q.
small, 1/6 pie . . .	299	15.0	34.0	11.0	37	573	m.q.
medium, 1/8 pie . .	318	16.0	37.0	12.0	38	569	m.q.
large, 1/10 pie . . .	332	16.0	39.0	12.0	39	617	m.q.
jumbo, 1/10 pie . .	508	26.2	58.5	18.8	63	984	2.5 d
original crust							
pepperoni:							
mini, 1/4 pie	149	6.3	19.9	4.8	15	207	.2 d
small, 1/6 pie . . .	256	10.8	32.3	9.0	26	398	.5 d
medium, 1/8 pie . .	277	11.6	35.1	9.7	28	430	.5 d
large, 1/10 pie . . .	309	13.4	37.3	11.5	34	483	.5 d
jumbo, 1/10 pie . .	458	19.9	54.9	17.2	51	710	.7 d
golden crust cheese:							
small, 1/6 pie . . .	207	8.1	25.7	7.9	19	253	.4 d
medium, 1/8 pie . .	223	8.3	26.9	9.1	19	265	.4 d

Food and Measure	cal.	prot. (gms)	carbo. (gms)	fat (gms)	chol. (mgs)	sod. (mgs)	fiber (gms)
large, 1/10 pie . . .	254	9.5	29.5	10.9	23	309	.5 d
golden crust combo:							
small, 1/6 pie . . .	273	13.0	29.0	12.0	31	542	m.q.
medium, 1/8 pie . .	283	13.0	30.0	13.0	29	526	m.q.
large, 1/10 pie . . .	322	14.0	33.0	15.0	34	602	m.q.
golden crust pepper-							
oni:							
small, 1/6 pie . . .	238	9.4	25.9	10.7	24	382	.4 d
medium, 1/8 pie . .	258	9.7	27.1	12.3	25	410	.4 d
large, 1/10 pie . . .	291	11.1	29.7	14.3	29	463	.5 d
Goose, roasted:							
meat w/skin, 4 oz. . .	346	28.5	0	24.9	103	79	0
meat only, 4 oz. . . .	270	32.9	0	14.4	109	86	0
Goose fat, 1 oz. . . .	255	0	0	28.3	28	0	0
Goose liver, see							
"Liver" and "Pâté"							
Gooseberry:							
fresh, 1/2 cup	34	.7	7.6	.4	0	1	3.2 d
fresh, green *(Frieda's)*,							
1 oz.	11	.2	2.7	.1	0	<1	m.q.
canned, in light syrup,							
1/2 cup	93	.8	23.6	.3	0	3	3.0 d
Gourd, 1/2 cup:							
dishcloth, boiled,							
drained, 1″ slices	50	.6	12.8	.3	0	18	.4 d
white-flower, boiled,							
drained, 1″ cubes	11	.4	2.7	<.1	0	1	.5 c
Grain dishes, mix*,							
3-grain, w/herbs,							
1/2 cup:							
(Quick Pilaf)	121	4.0	24.0	1.0	0	267	1.3 d
w/butter *(Quick Pilaf)*	157	4.0	24.0	5.0	m.q.	306	1.3 d
Granola, see "Cereal"							

Food and Measure	cal.	prot. (gms)	carbo. (gms)	fat (gms)	chol. (mgs)	sod. (mgs)	fiber (gms)
Granola and cereal bars, (see also "Snack bars"), 1 bar, except as noted:							
all varieties:							
(Kellogg's Nutri-Grain)	150	2.0	25.0	5.0	0	65	1.0 d
(Sunbelt Fruit Boosters)	130	1.0	28.0	2.0	0	130	m.q.
except raisin (Health Valley Fat Free)	140	3.0	33.0	<1.0	0	10	3.7 d
w/almonds, chewy (Sunbelt)	120	3.0	18.0	6.0	0	65	m.q.
apple berry (Quaker Chewy)	120	2.0	20.0	4.0	0	95	m.q.
apple cinnamon (Nature Valley Granola Bites), 1 pouch	170	3.0	25.0	7.0	0	100	2.0 d
butter almond (Kudos)	180	3.0	20.0	10.0	n.a.	80	m.q.
chocolate chip:							
(Carnation Breakfast)	200	6.0	20.0	11.0	0	80	.2 d
(Kudos)	180	3.0	20.0	10.0	n.a.	60	m.q.
(Quaker Chewy) . .	130	2.0	20.0	5.0	0	70	m.q.
chewy (Sunbelt), 1.25 oz.	150	3.0	23.0	7.0	0	75	m.q.
fudge dipped, chewy (Sunbelt)	210	2.0	26.0	10.0	0	55	m.q.
chocolate crunch (Carnation Breakfast)	190	6.0	20.0	10.0	0	150	.2 d
cinnamon (Nature Valley)	120	2.0	17.0	5.0	0	70	1.0 d
w/coconut, fudge dipped (Sunbelt Macaroo), 1.4 oz. . . .	200	2.0	23.0	11.0	0	50	m.q.

Food and Measure	cal.	prot. (gms)	carbo. (gms)	fat (gms)	chol. (mgs)	sod. (mgs)	fiber (gms)
cookies and creme (Kudos)	180	3.0	20.0	10.0	n.a.	70	m.q.
fudge, nutty (Kudos)	200	3.0	20.0	12.0	n.a.	60	m.q.
honey nut (Nature Valley Granola Bites), 1 pouch	170	3.0	25.0	7.0	0	120	2.0 d
oat bran-honey graham (Nature Valley)	110	2.0	16.0	4.0	0	90	1.0 d
oats 'n honey (Nature Valley)	120	2.0	17.0	5.0	0	65	1.0 d
oats and honey, chewy (Sunbelt) . .	130	2.0	18.0	5.0	0	35	m.q.
peanut butter:							
(Kudos)	190	4.0	18.0	12.0	n.a.	70	m.q.
(Nature Valley) . . .	120	2.0	15.0	6.0	0	70	1.0 d
chocolate chip (Carnation Breakfast)	200	6.0	20.0	11.0	0	170	.1 d
crunch (Carnation Breakfast)	190	6.0	20.0	10.0	0	180	0
w/peanuts, fudge dipped, chewy (Sunbelt), 1.5 oz.	200	4.0	24.0	12.0	0	60	m.q.
raisin (Health Valley Fat Free)	140	3.0	33.0	0	0	10	3.0 d
w/raisins, chewy (Sunbelt)	150	2.0	24.0	6.0	0	65	m.q.
trail mix (Quaker Chewy)	130	2.0	18.0	5.0	0	105	m.q.
Grape:							
fresh, American type (slipskin): 10 medium	15	.2	4.1	.1	0	tr.	.3 d
peeled and seeded, 1/2 cup	29	.3	7.9	.2	0	1	.6 d
fresh, European type (adherent skin): seeded, 1 lb. . . .	287	2.7	72.0	2.3	0	7	2.7 d

Food and Measure	cal.	prot. (gms)	carbo. (gms)	fat (gms)	chol. (mgs)	sod. (mgs)	fiber (gms)
Grape, fresh, European type *(cont.)*							
seedless, 10 medium	36	.3	8.9	.3	0	1	.3 d
seedless or seeded, 1/2 cup	57	.5	14.2	.5	0	2	.5 d
canned, Thompson seedless, 1/2 cup:							
in water	48	.6	12.6	.1	0	7	1.2 d
in heavy syrup . . .	94	.6	25.2	.1	0	7	.5 d
Grape drink:							
canned, bottled, chilled or frozen*:							
(Crush), 11.5 fl. oz.	176	0	44.0	0	0	1	0
(Hi-C), 6 fl. oz. . . .	90	0	23.0	0	0	25	0
(Kool-Aid Kool Bursts), 6.75 fl. oz.	110	0	30.0	0	0	10	0
(Mott's), 10 fl. oz.	160	<1.0	39.0	<1.0	0	10	0
(Tropicana), 6 fl. oz.	90	<1.0	22.0	<1.0	0	10	0
mix*, 8 fl. oz.:							
(Kool-Aid)	100	0	25.0	0	0	0	0
(Kool-Aid Presweetened)* . . .	70	0	18.0	0	0	0	0
wild *(Wyler's)* . . .	80	(0)	21.0	(0)	0	0	(0)
Grape fruit roll, see "Fruit snack"							
Grape juice, 6 fl. oz., except as noted:							
canned or bottled:							
(R.W. Knudsen), 8 fl. oz.	130	1.0	32.0	<1.0	0	(0)	n.a.
(Tree Top)	120	1.0	30.0	0	0	10	(0)
blend *(Juicy Juice)*	90	1.0	22.0	0	0	5	(0)
Concord *(R.W. Knudsen)*, 8 fl. oz.	130	1.0	32.0	<1.0	0	(0)	n.a.
purple *(Welch's)* . .	120	0	30.0	0	0	10	(0)
red or white *(Welch's)*	120	0	30.0	0	0	15	0

Food and Measure	cal.	prot. (gms)	carbo. (gms)	fat (gms)	chol. (mgs)	sod. (mgs)	fiber (gms)
canned, sparkling:							
red *(Welch's)* . . .	130	0	32.0	0	0	30	0
white *(Welch's)* . .	110	0	28.0	0	0	30	0
chilled or frozen*							
(Minute Maid) . . .	90	0	24.0	0	0	0	(0)
frozen*:							
(Sunkist)	69	.3	17.1	.1	0	3	- 0
(Welch's 100%) . .	120	0	30.0	0	0	5	(0)
sweetened *(Welch's)*	100	0	25.0	0	0	0	(0)
white, sweetened							
(Welch's)	100	0	25.0	0	0	5	(0)
cocktail:							
(Welch's)	100	0	26.0	0	0	20	(0)
(Welch's Orchard)	110	0	27.0	0	0	20	(0)
frozen*, no sugar							
added *(Welch's)*	40	0	10.0	0	0	0	(0)
Grape juice drink:							
canned or bottled:							
(Kool-Aid Koolers),							
8.45 fl. oz.	140	0	36.0	0	0	10	(0)
(Shasta Plus),							
12 fl. oz.	176	0	44.0	0	0	58	0
(Tang Fruit Box),							
8.45 fl. oz.	130	0	34.0	0	0	10	(0)
frozen*, 6 fl. oz.:							
(Bright & Early) . .	100	0	24.0	0	0	0	(0)
(Sunkist)	69	.3	17.0	.1	0	3	0
Grape leaf, in jars,							
imported *(Krinos),*							
1 oz.	10	1.0	0	.5	0	450	2.0 d
Grape punch, regular							
or Concord *(Minute*							
Maid), 6 fl. oz. . . .	90	0	23.0	0	0	20	(0)
Grape-apple drink							
(Mott's), 11.5 fl. oz.	176	<1.0	44.0	<1.0	0	1	(0)
Grape-apple juice							
(Welch's), 6 fl. oz.	100	0	26.0	0	0	10	(0)

Food and Measure	cal.	prot. (gms)	carbo. (gms)	fat (gms)	chol. (mgs)	sod. (mgs)	fiber (gms)
Grape-cranberry juice *(Welch's)*, 6 fl. oz.	110	0	28.0	0	0	10	(0)
Grape-peach juice, white grape *(Welch's)*, 6 fl. oz.	120	0	30.0	0	0	10	(0)
Grape-raspberry juice drink *(Boku)*, 8 fl. oz.	120	0	29.0	0	0	75	0
Grapefruit:							
fresh, pink or red, California or Arizona:							
1/2 medium, 33/4″ diam. . . .	46	.6	11.9	.1	0	<1	1.4 d
sections w/juice, 1/2 cup	43	.6	11.1	.1	0	<1	1.3 d
fresh, pink or red, Florida:							
1/2 medium, 33/4″ diam. . . .	37	.7	9.2	.1	0	<1	1.4 d
sections w/juice, 1/2 cup	34	.6	8.6	.1	0	<1	1.3 d
fresh, white, California:							
1/2 medium, 33/4″ diam.	43	1.0	10.7	.1	0	tr.	1.3 d
sections w/juice, 1/2 cup	42	1.0	10.5	.1	0	tr.	1.3 d
fresh, white, Florida:							
1/2 medium, 33/4″ diam.	38	.7	9.7	.1	0	tr.	.2 d
sections w/juice, 1/2 cup	38	.7	9.4	.1	0	tr.	.2 d
canned or chilled:							
in water, 1/2 cup . .	44	.7	11.2	.1	0	2	.5 d
in juice, 1/2 cup . .	46	.9	11.4	.1	0	9	.5 d

Food and Measure	cal.	prot. (gms)	carbo. (gms)	fat (gms)	chol. (mgs)	sod. (mgs)	fiber (gms)
Grapefruit juice,							
6 fl. oz., except as noted:							
fresh	72	.9	17.0	.2	0	2	.2 d
canned or bottled:							
unsweetened . . .	70	1.0	16.6	.2	0	2	.2 d
(R.W. Knudsen),							
8 fl. oz.	70	1.0	17.0	<1.0	0	(0)	m.q.
(Minute Maid) . . .	70	1.0	17.0	0	0	20	m.q.
(Mott's), 11.5 oz.	148	<1.0	37.0	<1.0	0	6	m.q.
pink (R.W. Knud-							
sen), 8 fl. oz. . .	80	1.0	18.0	<1.0	0	n.a.	m.q.
canned or chilled:							
(Libby's)	70	1.0	17.0	0	0	0	m.q.
(Ocean Spray 100%)	60	1.0	18.0	0	0	15	m.q.
(Tree Top)	80	1.0	19.0	0	0	0	m.q.
(Welch's)	70	0	17.0	0	0	20	m.q.
chilled (Minute Maid)	70	1.0	17.0	0	0	20	m.q.
chilled, regular or							
ruby red (Tropi-							
cana)	70	1.0	14.0	<1.0	0	20	m.q.
frozen* (Minute							
Maid)	80	1.0	18.0	0	0	0	m.q.
cocktail, pink:							
(Minute Maid) . . .	80	0	20.0	0	0	20	(0)
(Ocean Spray) . . .	80	0	20.0	0	0	15	(0)
(Tropicana Twister)	80	<1.0	19.0	<1.0	0	30	(0)
(Tropicana Twister							
Light)	30	<1.0	6.0	<1.0	0	25	(0)
(Welch's)	90	0	22.0	0	0	20	(0)
chilled or frozen							
(Minute Maid) . .	80	0	20.0	0	0	0	(0)
Grapefruit juice							
drink, 6 fl. oz.:							
(Citrus Hill Plus Cal-							
cium)	70	<1.0	19.0	<1.0	0	10	(0)
(Ocean Spray Ruby							
Red)	100	0	24.0	0	0	15	(0)

Food and Measure	cal.	prot. (gms)	carbo. (gms)	fat (gms)	chol. (mgs)	sod. (mgs)	fiber (gms)
Gravy, see specific listings							
Great northern beans:							
boiled, 1/2 cup	104	7.3	18.6	.4	0	2	6.2 d
canned:							
w/liquid, 1/2 cup . .	150	9.7	27.6	.5	0	6	6.4 d
(Allens), 1/2 cup . .	110	5.0	17.0	<1.0	0	350	5.0 d
(Eden), 1/2 cup . . .	110	6.0	20.0	<1.0	0	15	6.4 d
(Green Giant/Joan of Arc), 1/2 cup	80	6.0	18.0	<1.0	0	290	5.0 d
(Hain), 4 oz.	80	6.0	18.0	1.0	0	220	7.0 d
Green bean:							
fresh:							
raw, 1/2 cup	17	1.0	3.9	.1	0	3	1.9 d
boiled, drained, 1/2 cup	22	1.2	4.9	.2	0	2	2.0 d
canned or packaged, 1/2 cup:							
(Green Giant Kitchen Sliced)	16	<1.0	4.0	0	0	390	1.0 d
(Stokely)	20	1.0	4.0	0	0	360	m.q.
whole (Allens/Sunshine)	25	1.0	4.0	<1.0	0	470	m.q.
cut (Green Giant)	16	<1.0	4.0	0	0	390	1.0 d
cut (Green Giant 50% Less Salt)	16	<1.0	4.0	0	0	195	1.0 d
cut (Green Giant Pantry Express)	12	<1.0	3.0	0	0	260	1.0 d
cut (Allens/Sunshine)	23	1.0	4.0	<1.0	0	350	m.q.
cut (Allens No Salt Added)	23	1.0	4.0	<1.0	0	10	m.q.
Almondine (Green Giant)	45	2.0	5.0	3.0	0	350	2.0 d
French (Allens) . . .	20	1.0	4.0	<1.0	0	290	m.q.
French (Green Giant)	16	<1.0	4.0	0	0	390	1.0 d
Italian (Allens/Sunshine)	18	1.0	3.0	<1.0	0	260	m.q.

Food and Measure	cal.	prot. (gms)	carbo. (gms)	fat (gms)	chol. (mgs)	sod. (mgs)	fiber (gms)
and potatoes (Allen/ Sunshine)	30	2.0	5.0	<1.0	0	260	m.q.
shell outs (Allens)	35	2.0	6.0	<1.0	0	395	m.q.
freeze-dried (Mountain House), 1/2 cup* . .	35	1.0	6.0	0	0	1	m.q.
frozen, 3 oz., except as noted: (Green Giant), 1/2 cup	14	1.0	4.0	0	0	10	1.0 d
whole (Seabrook)	25	1.0	5.0	0	0	1	1.0 c
whole (Southern), 3.5 oz.	33	1.6	6.8	.1	0	20	m.q.
cut (Frosty Acres)	25	1.0	6.0	0	0	3	1.0 c
cut (Green Giant Harvest Fresh), 1/2 cup	16	1.0	4.0	0	0	95	1.0 d
cut (Seabrook) . . .	25	1.0	6.0	0	0	3	1.0 c
French (Frosty Acres)	25	1.0	6.0	0	0	3	1.0 c
in butter sauce (Green Giant One Serving), 5.5 oz.	60	2.0	8.0	2.0	5	370	3.0 d
in butter sauce, cut (Green Giant), 1/2 cup	30	1.0	4.0	1.0	5	230	1.5 d
Green bean combinations, frozen or packaged:							
French, w/toasted almonds (Birds Eye), 3 oz.	50	3.0	8.0	2.0	0	340	2.0 d
mushroom, creamy (Green Giant Garden Gourmet Right for Lunch), 9.5 oz. . .	220	6.0	29.0	11.0	25	860	4.0 d
mushroom casserole (Stouffer's), 4.75 oz.	160	5.0	13.0	10.0	n.a.	550	m.q.

Food and Measure	cal.	prot. (gms)	carbo. (gms)	fat (gms)	chol. (mgs)	sod. (mgs)	fiber (gms)
Green bean combinations *(cont.)*							
potatoes and mushrooms, in sauce *(Green Giant Pantry Express)*, 1/2 cup	60	1.0	8.0	3	0	440	2.5 d
Grenadine syrup							
(Rose's), 1 tbsp. . . .	32	<1.0	8.0	<1.0	0	14	0
Grits, see "Corn grits"							
Ground cherry, trimmed, 1/2 cup	37	1.3	7.8	.5	0	m.q.	2.0 c
Grouper, meat only:							
raw, 4 oz.	104	22.0	0	1.2	42	60	0
baked, broiled, or microwaved, 4 oz. . . .	134	28.2	0	1.5	53	60	0
Guacamole, see "Avocado dip"							
Guacamole seasoning:							
(Lawry's Seasoning Blends), 1 pkg. . .	60	1.7	12.6	.4	0	1495	.8 c
mix *(Old El Paso)*, 1/7 pkg.	7	0	2.0	0	0	240	0
Guanabana nectar							
(Libby's), 6 fl. oz. . .	110	0	26.0	0	0	15	m.q.
Guanabana punch							
(R.W. Knudsen Rain Forest), 8 fl. oz. . .	125	<1.0	29.0	<1.0	0	(0)	m.q.
Guava:							
1 medium, 4 oz. . . .	45	.7	10.7	.5	0	2	4.9 d
1/2 cup	42	.7	9.8	.5	0	2	4.5 d
strawberry, 1/2 cup	85	.7	21.2	.7	0	45	7.8 c
Guava fruit drink *(Ocean Spray Mauna La'I)*, 6 fl. oz.	100	0	24.0	0	0	15	(0)

Food and Measure	cal.	prot. (gms)	carbo. (gms)	fat (gms)	chol. (mgs)	sod. (mgs)	fiber (gms)
Guava juice cocktail, frozen* *(Welch's Orchard Tropicals),* 6 fl. oz.	100	0	25.0	0	0	20	0
Guava nectar, canned:							
(Kern's), 6 fl. oz. . . .	110	0	28.0	0	0	0	m.q.
(Libby's), 6 fl. oz. . .	110	0	26.0	0	0	15	m.q.
(Libby's Ripe), 8 fl. oz.	140	0	35.0	0	0	20	m.q.
Guava sauce, cooked, 1/2 cup . .	43	.4	11.3	.2	0	4	4.3 d
Guava-passion fruit drink *(Ocean Spray Mauna La'l),* 6 fl. oz.	100	0	25.0	0	0	10	(0)
Guinea hen, raw:							
meat w/skin, 4 oz. . . .	179	26.5	0	7.3	m.q.	m.q.	0
meat only, 4 oz.	125	23.4	0	2.8	71	m.q.	0
Gumbo dinner mix *(Luzianne),* 1/5 pkg.	160	4.0	33.0	1.0	0	760	1.0 d

H

Food and Measure	cal.	prot. (gms)	carbo. (gms)	fat (gms)	chol. (mgs)	sod. (mgs)	fiber (gms)
Häagen-Dazs Ice Cream Shop, 4 fl. oz.:							
ice cream:							
cappuccino	270	5.0	22.0	18.0	120	85	0
cherry, brandied . .	250	4.0	24.0	15.0	100	80	(0)
chocolate, Belgian	330	5.0	29.0	18.0	90	80	(0)
chocolate Swiss almond	300	6.0	24.0	21.0	105	75	m.q.
coffee chip	300	5.0	26.0	20.0	105	80	n.a.
macadamia nut . .	330	5.0	24.0	24.0	m.q.	m.q.	m.q.
maple walnut . . .	330	6.0	18.0	26.0	125	75	m.q.
pralines and cream	290	5.0	27.0	18.0	100	180	n.a.
vanilla chip	300	5.0	26.0	20.0	105	80	n.a.
sorbet:							
lemon	140	0	35.0	0	0	20	(0)
orange	140	0	36.0	0	0	20	(0)
raspberry	110	0	27.0	0	0	15	(0)
yogurt, soft-serve:							
chocolate	120	4.0	26.0	0	0	65	(0)
coffee	140	5.0	22.0	4.0	35	75	0
raspberry	140	4.0	21.0	4.0	35	70	(0)
strawberry	120	4.0	26.0	0	5	70	(0)
vanilla	110	5.0	22.0	0	5	75	0
Haddock, meat only:							
raw, 4 oz.	99	21.5	0	.8	65	78	0
baked, broiled, or microwaved, 4 oz. . .	127	27.5	0	1.1	84	99	0
frozen (Van de Kamp's), 4 oz.	90	21.0	0	1.0	20	125	0

Food and Measure	cal.	prot. (gms)	carbo. (gms)	fat (gms)	chol. (mgs)	sod. (mgs)	fiber (gms)
smoked, 4 oz.	132	28.6	0	1.1	87	865	0
Haddock entree, frozen:							
battered, 2 pieces:							
(Gorton's Crispy)	300	11.0	16.0	21.0	35	560	m.q.
(Mrs. Paul's Crunchy Batter)	190	14.0	22.0	5.0	25	580	m.q.
(Van de Kamp's) . .	250	12.0	19.0	15.0	30	580	m.q.
breaded:							
(Mrs. Paul's Light), 1 piece	220	17.0	15.0	9.0	45	350	m.q.
(Van de Kamp's), 2 pieces	270	12.0	19.0	16.0	25	290	m.q.
(Van de Kamp's Light), 1 piece . .	240	15.0	21.0	11.0	35	590	m.q.
Hake, see "Whiting"							
Halibut, meat only:							
Atlantic and Pacific:							
raw, 4 oz.	124	23.6	0	2.6	37	61	0
baked, broiled, or microwaved, 4 oz.	159	30.3	0	3.3	46	78	0
Greenland:							
raw, 4 oz.	211	16.3	0	15.7	52	91	0
baked, broiled, or microwaved, 4 oz.	271	20.9	0	20.1	67	117	0
Halibut entree, frozen, battered (Van de Kamp's), 2 pieces	150	8.0	16.0	6.0	10	400	m.q.
Halvah:							
(Fantastic Foods), 1 bar	232	8.0	17.0	10.0	0	0	m.q.
(Joyva), 1 oz.	160	4.0	12.0	11.0	0	55	m.q.
Ham, fresh, meat only:							
whole leg, roasted:							
lean w/fat, 4 oz. . . .	333	28.4	0	23.5	105	67	0
lean w/fat, chopped or diced, 1 cup	411	35.0	0	29.0	131	83	0

Food and Measure	cal.	prot. (gms)	carbo. (gms)	fat (gms)	chol. (mgs)	sod. (mgs)	fiber (gms)
Ham, whole leg, roasted *(cont.)*							
lean only, 4 oz. . .	249	32.1	0	12.5	107	73	0
lean only, chopped or diced, 1 cup	309	39.7	0	15.4	131	90	0
rump half, roasted:							
lean w/fat, 4 oz. . .	311	30.2	0	20.2	108	69	0
lean only, 4 oz. . .	251	33.0	0	12.1	109	74	0
shank half, roasted:							
lean w/fat, 4 oz. . .	344	27.6	0	25.1	104	66	0
lean only, 4 oz. . .	244	32.0	0	11.9	104	73	0
Ham, cured:							
whole leg, lean w/fat:							
unheated, 4 oz. . .	279	21.0	.1	21.0	64	1456	0
roasted, 4 oz. . . .	276	24.5	0	19.0	70	1346	0
roasted, chopped or diced, 1 cup . .	341	30.2	0	23.5	86	1661	0
whole leg, lean only:							
unheated, 4 oz. . .	167	25.3	.1	6.5	59	1719	0
roasted, 4 oz. . . .	178	28.4	0	6.2	62	1505	0
roasted, chopped or diced, 1 cup . .	219	35.1	0	7.7	78	1858	0
boneless (11% fat):							
unheated, 4 oz. . .	206	19.9	3.5	12.0	65	1493	0
roasted, 4 oz. . . .	202	25.7	0	10.2	67	1701	0
roasted, chopped or diced, 1 cup . .	249	31.7	0	12.6	83	2100	0
boneless, extra lean (5% fat):							
unheated, 4 oz. . .	149	21.9	1.1	5.6	53	1620	0
roasted, 4 oz. . . .	164	23.7	1.7	6.3	60	1364	0
roasted, chopped or diced, 1 cup . .	203	29.3	2.1	7.7	74	1684	0
Ham, canned:							
(Black Label), 1 oz. .	37	5.0	<2.0	1.0	15	303	0
(Cure 81 Half Ham), 1 oz.	31	5.0	<2.0	1.0	15	291	0
(Hormel Curemaster Half Ham), 2 oz. . .	60	10.0	1.0	2.0	26	627	0

Food and Measure	cal.	prot. (gms)	carbo. (gms)	fat (gms)	chol. (mgs)	sod. (mgs)	fiber (gms)
(Hormel Light & Lean Half Ham), 2 oz. . .	60	10.0	1.0	2.0	26	450	0
(Oscar Mayer Jubilee), 3 oz.	90	16.0	0	3.0	40	870	0
w/natural juices *(Oscar Mayer Jubilee),* 3 oz.	110	15.0	0	6.0	45	940	0
"Ham," vegetarian, frozen *(Worthington Wham),* 3 slices . .	120	12.0	3.0	7.0	0	940	m.q.
Ham bologna *(Kahn's),* 1 slice . .	90	3.0	1.0	8.0	m.q.	330	0
Ham entree, frozen or packaged:							
and asparagus:							
au gratin *(The Budget Gourmet Light and Healthy),* 8.7 oz.	300	17.0	26.0	14.0	50	860	m.q.
bake *(Stouffer's),* 9.5 oz.	520	18.0	32.0	35.0	m.q.	1100	m.q.
scalloped potatoes:							
(Hormel Micro Cup), 7.5 oz.	260	8.0	21.0	16.0	33	768	m.q.
(Swanson), 9 oz. . .	300	18.0	25.0	14.0	m.q.	1030	m.q.
Ham luncheon meat, 1 oz., except as noted:							
(Healthy Deli Deluxe)	31	4.7	1.0	.9	11	290	0
(Healthy Deli Lessalt)	31	4.7	1.2	.8	13	200	0
(Healthy Deli Light AM)	27	3.9	1.4	.6	11	200	0
(Healthy Deli Old Tyme Taverne)	31	5.2	.3	.8	14	290	0
(Jones Dairy Farm Slices),* .8-oz. slice	30	4.5	tr.	1.0	14	210	0
(Jones Dairy Farm Family Ham)	40	6.0	tr.	1.5	14	310	0
(Kahn's Low Salt), 1 slice	30	5.0	1.0	1.0	m.q.	290	0

Food and Measure	cal.	prot. (gms)	carbo. (gms)	fat (gms)	chol. (mgs)	sod. (mgs)	fiber (gms)
Ham luncheon meat *(cont.)*							
(Oscar Mayer Jubilee),							
3 oz.	130	16.0	0	7.0	45	1100	0
baked:							
(Weight Watchers)	35	5.0	1.0	2.0	15	290	0
(Oscar Mayer),							
3 slices	60	12.0	1.0	1.5	35	710	0
Black Forest *(Healthy*							
Deli)	32	5.2	.7	.8	15	290	0
Virginia *(Healthy Deli)*	34	4.8	1.6	.9	11	290	0
boiled:							
(Oscar Mayer),							
3 slices	70	12.0	<1.0	2.0	35	840	0
(Oscar Mayer Deli-							
Thin), 5 slices . .	60	11.0	<1.0	2.0	35	800	0
(Oscar Mayer							
Healthy Favorites),							
5 slices	60	11.0	<1.0	2.0	35	570	0
breakfast *(Oscar*							
Mayer Healthy Fa-							
vorites), 3 slices . .	90	14.0	2.0	3.0	40	1050	0
Cajun *(Hillshire Farm*							
Deli Select)	31	6.0	<1.0	.9	m.q.	350	0
chopped:							
(Black Label)	70	4.0	1.0	6.0	16	326	0
(Kahn's), 1 slice . .	50	5.0	1.0	3.0	m.q.	360	0
(Oscar Mayer) . . .	50	4.0	<1.0	3.0	15	320	0
cooked:							
(Hormel Bread							
Ready)	33	5.0	1.0	1.0	14	442	0
(Hormel Deli) . . .	29	4.0	1.0	1.0	11	344	0
(Kahn's), 1 slice . .	30	5.0	1.0	1.0	m.q.	360	0
fresh *(Healthy Deli)*	33	5.9	.2	.8	13	120	0
cooked or honey							
roasted *(Weight*							
Watchers)	30	5.0	1.0	1.0	15	290	0

Food and Measure	cal.	prot. (gms)	carbo. (gms)	fat (gms)	chol. (mgs)	sod. (mgs)	fiber (gms)
honey:							
(Healthy Deli Honey							
Valley)	31	4.8	1.7	.8	10	260	0
(Hillshire Farm Deli							
Select)	31	6.0	<1.0	.9	m.q.	270	0
(Oscar Mayer),							
3 slices	70	12.0	2.0	2.0	35	800	0
(Oscar Mayer Deli-							
Thin), 5 slices . .	70	11.0	2.0	2.0	35	760	0
(Oscar Mayer							
Healthy Favorites),							
5 slices	70	11.0	2.0	2.0	35	570	0
minced	75	4.6	.5	5.9	20	353	0
slice (Oscar Mayer Ju-							
bilee), 3 oz.	90	14.0	0	3.0	45	1030	0
smoked:							
(Hillshire Farm Deli							
Select)	31	6.0	<1.0	.9	m.q.	300	0
(Oscar Mayer),							
3 slices	70	11.0	0	2.5	30	780	0
(Oscar Mayer Deli-							
Thin), 5 slices . .	60	11.0	0	2.5	30	750	0
(Oscar Mayer							
Healthy Favorites),							
5 slices	70	11.0	<1.0	2.0	35	580	0
steak (Oscar Mayer							
Jubilee), 2-oz. steak	60	10.0	0	2.0	30	750	0
Ham salad spread							
(Libby's Spread-							
ables), 1.9 oz. . . .	70	5.0	6.0	3.0	10	380	.6 d
Ham spread, deviled:							
(Hormel), 1 oz.	76	4.0	1.0	6.0	19	214	0
(Underwood), 2 1/8 oz.	220	8.0	<1.0	19.0	50	430	0
(Underwood Light),							
2 1/8 oz.	120	11.0	1.0	8.0	35	250	0

Food and Measure	cal.	prot. (gms)	carbo. (gms)	fat (gms)	chol. (mgs)	sod. (mgs)	fiber (gms)
Ham and cheese breakfast bagel *(Weight Watchers),* 3 oz.	210	13.0	28.0	6.0	15	460	m.q.
Ham and cheese loaf, 1 slice:							
(Kahn's)	70	4.0	1.0	6.0	m.q.	310	0
(Oscar Mayer)	70	4.0	1.0	5.0	20	350	0
Ham and cheese pocket sandwich, frozen:							
(Hot Pockets), 4.5 oz.	350	16.0	36.0	16.0	55	790	m.q.
(Weight Watchers Ultimate 200), 4 oz. . .	200	14.0	24.0	6.0	5	490	m.q.
Hamburger, see "Beef Entree, frozen"							
"Hamburger," vegetarian:							
mix:							
(LaLoma Patty Mix), 1/4 cup	50	9.0	4.0	0	0	200	m.q.
(Nature's Burger), 3 oz.[1]	155	6.0	26.0	3.0	0	287	4.0 d
burger *(Tofu Classics),* 3.4 oz.[2] . .	137	9.0	14.0	5.0	0	337	2.6 d
(Worthington Granburger), 6 tbsp.	110	19.0	7.0	1.0	0	730	m.q.
BBQ *(Nature's Burger),* 3 oz.[1]	133	5.0	26.0	1.0	0	430	3.0 d
chunk *(LaLoma Vita-Burger),* 1/4 cup	70	11.0	6.0	0	0	150	m.q.

[1] *Does not include fat or oil used in frying.*

[2] *Prepared with tofu; does not include fat or oil used in frying.*

Food and Measure	cal.	prot. (gms)	carbo. (gms)	fat (gms)	chol. (mgs)	sod. (mgs)	fiber (gms)
granules *(LaLoma Vita-Burger)*, 3 tbsp.	70	11.0	6.0	0	0	150	m.q.
pizza flavor *(Nature's Burger)*, 3 oz.[1]	133	5.0	26.0	1.0	1	431	3.0 d
canned:							
(LaLoma Redi-Burger), 1/2" slice	130	14.0	5.0	6.0	0	340	m.q.
(LaLoma Vege-Burger), 1/2 cup	110	21.0	3.0	2.0	0	190	m.q.
(Worthington Vegetarian Burger), 1/2 cup	150	19.0	9.0	4.0	0	780	m.q.
(Worthington Vegetarian Burger No Salt), 1/2 cup . .	150	22.0	7.0	4.0	0	170	m.q.
frozen, patties:							
(Ken & Robert's), 1 patty	110	5.0	19.0	2.0	0	370	m.q.
(LaLoma Sizzle Burger), 1 patty	220	17.0	10.0	12.0	0	420	m.q.
(Morningstar Farms Grillers), 1 patty	150	14.0	5.0	7.0	0	300	m.q.
(Morningstar Farms Prime), 1 patty	130	17.0	4.0	5.0	0	250	m.q.
(Worthington FriPats), 1 patty	180	13.0	5.0	12.0	0	360	m.q.
garden vegetable *(Morningstar Farms)*, 1 patty	120	12.0	9.0	4.0	0	380	m.q.
sandwich, w/cheese *(Morningstar Farms)*, 4.75 oz.	370	21.0	32.0	17.0	0	700	m.q.

[1] *Does not include fat or oil used in frying.*

Food and Measure	cal.	prot. (gms)	carbo. (gms)	fat (gms)	chol. (mgs)	sod. (mgs)	fiber (gms)
Hamburger entree mix* *(Hamburger Helper),* 1 cup, except as noted:							
beef:							
noodle	330	20.0	29.0	15.0	m.q.	970	m.q.
Romanoff	350	22.0	31.0	15.0	m.q.	1080	m.q.
teriyaki	360	20.0	38.0	14.0	m.q.	1160	m.q.
cheddar'n bacon . .	400	24.0	30.0	20.0	m.q.	1020	m.q.
cheeseburger macaroni	370	21.0	28.0	19.0	m.q.	1030	m.q.
chili macaroni	330	19.0	32.0	14.0	m.q.	960	m.q.
hamburger hash . . .	320	18.0	27.0	15.0	m.q.	1020	m.q.
hamburger stew . . .	300	19.0	26.0	13.0	m.q.	1030	m.q.
Italian, cheesy	360	21.0	31.0	17.0	m.q.	970	m.q.
Italian, zesty	350	20.0	36.0	14.0	m.q.	870	m.q.
lasagne	340	20.0	33.0	14.0	m.q.	940	m.q.
meatloaf	360	27.0	14.0	22.0	m.q.	740	m.q.
mushroom and wild rice	380	21.0	37.0	16.0	m.q.	950	m.q.
nacho cheese	360	21.0	35.0	15.0	m.q.	1050	m.q.
pizza, dish	360	21.0	37.0	14.0	m.q.	1010	m.q.
Pizzabake, 4.5 oz. . .	320	19.0	29.0	14.0	m.q.	840	m.q.
potato au gratin . . .	350	20.0	28.0	18.0	m.q.	900	m.q.
potato Stroganoff . .	330	20.0	27.0	16.0	m.q.	990	m.q.
rice Oriental	340	19.0	38.0	14.0	m.q.	1120	m.q.
Sloppy Joe Bake, 5 oz.	340	18.0	33.0	15.0	m.q.	1100	m.q.
spaghetti	330	20.0	32.0	14.0	m.q.	1020	m.q.
Stroganoff	390	22.0	33.0	19.0	m.q.	870	m.q.
taco, beef	330	19.0	33.0	14.0	m.q.	970	m.q.
Tacobake, 6 oz. . . .	320	17.0	31.0	15.0	m.q.	940	m.q.
Hardee's, 1 serving:							
Big Country Breakfast:							
bacon	660	24.0	51.0	40.0	305	1540	m.q.
country ham	670	29.0	52.0	38.0	345	2870	m.q.
ham	620	28.0	51.0	33.0	325	1780	m.q.
sausage	850	33.0	51.0	57.0	340	1980	m.q.

Food and Measure	cal.	prot. (gms)	carbo. (gms)	fat (gms)	chol. (mgs)	sod. (mgs)	fiber (gms)
Biscuit 'N' Gravy . . .	440	9.0	45.0	24.0	15	1250	m.q.
blueberry muffin . .	400	7.0	56.0	17.0	65	310	m.q.
breakfast bagel:							
plain	200	7.0	38.0	3.0	10	350	m.q.
w/bacon	280	12.0	38.0	9.0	20	590	m.q.
w/bacon and egg	330	17.0	38.0	12.0	165	635	m.q.
w/bacon, egg, and							
cheese	375	19.0	39.0	16.0	175	865	m.q.
w/egg	250	12.0	38.0	6.0	155	395	m.q.
w/egg and cheese	295	14.0	39.0	10.0	165	625	m.q.
w/sausage	350	15.0	38.0	16.0	35	750	m.q.
w/sausage and egg	400	20.0	38.0	19.0	180	795	m.q.
w/sausage, egg,							
and cheese . . .	445	22.0	39.0	23.0	190	1025	m.q.
breakfast biscuit:							
bacon	360	10.0	34.0	21.0	10	950	m.q.
bacon and egg . .	410	15.0	35.0	24.0	155	990	m.q.
bacon, egg, and							
cheese	460	17.0	35.0	28.0	165	1220	m.q.
country ham	350	11.0	35.0	18.0	25	1550	m.q.
country ham and							
egg	400	16.0	35.0	22.0	175	1600	m.q.
ham	320	10.0	34.0	16.0	15	1000	m.q.
ham and egg . . .	370	15.0	35.0	19.0	160	1050	m.q.
ham, egg, and							
cheese	420	18.0	35.0	23.0	170	1270	m.q.
Canadian Rise 'N'							
Shine	470	22.0	35.0	27.0	180	1550	m.q.
chicken	430	17.0	42.0	22.0	45	1330	m.q.
Cinnamon 'N' Raisin	320	4.0	37.0	17.0	0	510	m.q.
omelet, Ultimate . .	540	16.0	36.0	36.0	80	1120	m.q.
Rise 'N' Shine . . .	320	5.0	34.0	18.0	0	740	m.q.
sausage	440	13.0	34.0	28.0	25	1100	m.q.
sausage and egg	490	18.0	35.0	31.0	170	1150	m.q.
steak	500	15.0	46.0	29.0	30	1320	m.q.
steak and egg . . .	550	20.0	47.0	32.0	175	1370	m.q.
Western omelet . .	400	14.0	35.0	27.0	150	1050	m.q.

Food and Measure	cal.	prot. (gms)	carbo. (gms)	fat (gms)	chol. (mgs)	sod. (mgs)	fiber (gms)
Hardee's *(cont.)*							
breakfast sandwich:							
Frisco Ham	460	20.0	46.0	22.0	175	1320	m.q.
Frisco Sausage . .	720	33.0	43.0	47.0	205	1740	m.q.
Hash Rounds	230	3.0	24.0	14.0	0	560	m.q.
oat bran raisin muffin	410	8.0	59.0	16.0	50	380	m.q.
pancakes, three:							
regular	280	8.0	56.0	2.0	15	890	m.q.
w/2 bacon strips	350	13.0	56.0	9.0	25	1110	m.q.
w/1 sausage patty	430	16.0	56.0	16.0	40	1290	m.q.
sandwiches/burgers:							
Big Deluxe burger	500	27.0	32.0	30.0	70	760	m.q.
Big Roast Beef . .	380	26.0	29.0	18.0	60	1230	m.q.
Big Twin	450	23.0	34.0	25.0	55	580	m.q.
cheeseburger . . .	300	12.0	34.0	14.0	40	740	m.q.
cheeseburger,							
bacon	610	34.0	31.0	39.0	80	1030	m.q.
cheeseburger, 1/4 lb.	500	29.0	34.0	29.0	70	1060	m.q.
chicken breast							
sandwich, grilled	310	24.0	34.0	9.0	60	890	m.q.
Chicken Fillet . . .	370	19.0	44.0	13.0	55	1060	m.q.
combo sub	380	28.0	52.0	6.0	45	1440	m.q.
Fisherman's Fillet,							
bakery bun . . .	480	23.0	50.0	21.0	70	1210	m.q.
Frisco Burger . . .	760	36.0	43.0	50.0	70	1280	m.q.
Frisco Chicken . .	620	35.0	44.0	34.0	95	1730	m.q.
Frisco Club	620	30.0	46.0	35.0	75	1930	m.q.
ham sub	370	25.0	52.0	7.0	45	1400	m.q.
hamburger	260	10.0	33.0	10.0	30	510	m.q.
hot dog	290	11.0	26.0	16.0	30	760	m.q.
Hot Ham 'N' Cheese	330	23.0	32.0	12.0	65	1420	m.q.
Mushroom 'N' Swiss							
burger	490	30.0	33.0	27.0	70	940	m.q.
New York Patty Melt	780	35.0	45.0	51.0	80	990	m.q.
Real West bacon							
cheeseburger . .	560	33.0	38.0	31.0	45	1130	m.q.
Real West BBQ beef	350	18.0	48.0	9.0	36	1290	m.q.
Reuben	540	35.0	48.0	22.0	80	1610	m.q.

Food and Measure	cal.	prot. (gms)	carbo. (gms)	fat (gms)	chol. (mgs)	sod. (mgs)	fiber (gms)
roast beef, regular	280	18.0	29.0	11.0	40	870	m.q.
roast beef sub . . .	370	23.0	57.0	5.0	45	1400	m.q.
Turkey Club	390	29.0	32.0	16.0	70	1280	m.q.
turkey sub	390	29.0	53.0	7.0	65	1420	m.q.
chicken, fried:							
breast, 4 oz.	340	27.0	15.0	19.0	104	659	n.a.
leg, 2 oz.	152	12.0	6.0	8.0	80	207	n.a.
thigh, 3.8 oz. . . .	370	20.0	13.0	26.0	128	489	n.a.
wing, 1.9 oz. . . .	205	12.0	9.0	13.0	48	374	n.a.
Chicken Stix, 9 piece	310	28.0	20.0	14.0	55	1020	m.q.
Chicken Stix, 6 piece	210	19.0	13.0	9.0	35	680	m.q.
side dishes:							
breadstick, 1.6 oz.	150	5.0	24.0	4.0	0	190	m.q.
coleslaw, 4 oz. . .	240	2.0	13.0	20.0	10	340	m.q.
coleslaw, 12 oz. . .	710	5.0	38.0	60.0	35	1020	m.q.
Crispy Curls, 3 oz.	300	4.0	36.0	16.0	0	840	m.q.
fries, Big Fry	500	6.0	66.0	23.0	0	180	m.q.
fries, large	360	4.0	48.0	17.0	0	135	m.q.
fries, regular	230	3.0	30.0	11.0	0	85	m.q.
gravy, 1.5 oz. . . .	20	1.0	3.0	<1.0	0	260	n.a.
gravy, 5 oz.	60	3.0	11.0	1.0	5	850	n.a.
mashed potato, 4 oz.	70	2.0	16.0	<1.0	0	260	m.q.
mashed potato, 12 oz.	220	6.0	48.0	<1.0	0	760	m.q.
potato salad, 5 oz.	260	3.0	18.0	19.0	20	500	m.q.
Fixin's Cup	10	0	0	0	0	80	n.a.
salads:							
chef	214	20.0	5.0	13.0	44	910	m.q.
chicken, grilled . .	120	18.0	2.0	4.0	60	520	m.q.
garden	184	12.0	3.0	12.0	34	250	m.q.
side	20	2.0	1.0	<1.0	0	15	m.q.
desserts and shakes:							
apple turnover . . .	270	3.0	38.0	12.0	0	250	m.q.
Big Cookie	250	3.0	31.0	13.0	5	240	m.q.

Food and Measure	cal.	prot. (gms)	carbo. (gms)	fat (gms)	chol. (mgs)	sod. (mgs)	fiber (gms)
***Hardee's,* desserts and shakes** *(cont.)*							
Cool Twist cone, 4.2 oz.:							
chocolate	180	4.0	29.0	4.0	15	85	m.q.
vanilla	180	5.0	29.0	4.0	15	80	m.q.
vanilla/chocolate	170	5.0	29.0	4.0	15	85	m.q.
Cool Twist sundae:							
caramel, 6 oz. . . .	330	6.0	59.0	8.0	20	280	(0)
hot fudge, 5.9 oz.	320	8.0	50.0	10.0	25	260	(0)
strawberry, 5.9 oz.	260	6.0	48.0	6.0	15	100	(0)
shake:							
Butterfinger . . .	370	12.0	55.0	9.0	32	180	n.a.
chocolate	390	15.0	61.0	10.0	31	220	(0)
strawberry	390	13.0	65.0	8.0	30	200	(0)
vanilla	370	14.0	59.0	9.0	25	210	0
strudel, strawberry cream cheese . .	320	5.0	34.0	19.0	5	260	m.q.
Hazelnut butter *(Roaster Fresh),* 1 oz.	188	4.0	5.0	18.9	0	1	m.q.
Hazelnuts, see "Filberts"							
Head cheese *(Oscar Mayer),* 1 slice . . .	50	5.0	0	4.0	25	360	0
Heart, braised or simmered, 4 oz.:							
beef	199	32.6	.5	6.4	219	71	0
chicken, broiler-fryer	210	30.0	.1	9.0	274	54	0
lamb	210	28.3	2.2	9.0	282	71	0
pork	168	26.8	.5	5.7	251	40	0
turkey	201	30.3	2.3	6.9	256	62	0
veal	211	33.0	.1	7.7	200	66	0
Herb garlic marinade, w/lemon juice *(Lawry's),* 2 tbsp.	36	3.6	3.8	n.a.	0	3688	.4 c

Food and Measure	cal.	prot. (gms)	carbo. (gms)	fat (gms)	chol. (mgs)	sod. (mgs)	fiber (gms)
Herb gravy mix* *(McCormick/Schilling),* 1/4 cup	20	.5	3.0	.5	n.a.	312	n.a.
Herb seasoning and coating mix, Italian:							
(McCormick/Schilling Bag'n Season), 1 pkg.	94	2.0	21.0	.2	n.a.	1367	m.q.
(Shake'n Bake), 1/4 pkg.	80	2.0	14.0	1.0	0	620	m.q.
Herbs, see specific listings							
Herbs, mixed *(Lawry's* Pinch of Herbs), 1 tsp. . .	9	.3	.9	.5	0	259	.2 c
Herring, fresh:							
Atlantic, meat only:							
raw, 4 oz.	180	20.4	0	10.3	68	102	0
baked, broiled, or microwaved, 4 oz.	230	26.1	0	13.1	87	130	0
kippered, 4 oz. . .	246	27.9	0	14.0	93	1041	0
pickled, 4 oz. . . .	297	16.1	10.9	20.4	15	987	0
lake, see "Cisco"							
Pacific, meat only:							
raw, 4 oz.	224	18.6	0	15.8	87	84	0
baked, broiled, or microwaved, 4 oz.	284	23.8	0	20.2	112	108	0
Herring, canned, see "Sardine"							
Herring, in jars *(Elf),* 3 oz.:							
Cajun	167	12.0	7.0	10.0	42	798	0
cocktail sauce	121	9.0	16.0	3.0	27	1596	0
cream sauce, regular or black pepper . .	167	12.0	7.0	10.0	42	798	0
dill sauce	152	10.0	10.0	8.0	38	832	0
horseradish sauce . .	218	8.0	11.0	16.0	40	1512	0

Food and Measure	cal.	prot. (gms)	carbo. (gms)	fat (gms)	chol. (mgs)	sod. (mgs)	fiber (gms)
Herring, in jars *(cont.)*							
lunch, sliced	181	11.0	8.0	12.0	30	1680	0
rollmops, wine sauce	145	10.0	13.0	6.0	31	790	0
wine sauce	155	12.0	12.0	8.0	38	554	0
Hibiscus cooler *(R.W. Knudsen)*, 8 fl. oz.	95	<1.0	24.0	<1.0	0	(0)	n.a.
Hibiscus-cranberry juice *(R.W. Knudsen)*, 8 fl. oz. . . .	110	<1.0	28.0	<1.0	0	(0)	n.a.
Hickory nuts, dried, shelled, 1 oz. . . .	187	3.6	5.2	18.3	0	tr.	1.8 d
Hollandaise sauce mix:							
(French's), 1/5 pkg. . .	25	1.0	4.0	1.0	20	240	n.a.
(Knorr), 1 serving dry	16	.5	2.6	.3	<1	140	n.a.
(McCormick/Schilling), 1/4 pkg.	51	1.0	3.5	3.8	n.a.	170	n.a.
(McCormick/Schilling McCormick Collection), 1/4 cup* . . .	137	2.0	4.0	13.0	n.a.	418	n.a.
Homestyle gravy mix:							
(French's), 1/4 pkg. . .	18	0	3.0	0	0	210	n.a.
(McCormick/Schilling), 1/4 cup*	24	.5	3.8	.8	n.a.	295	n.a.
(Pillsbury), 1/4 cup* . .	16	0	3.0	0	0	240	n.a.
Hominy, canned *(Allens)*, 1/2 cup:							
golden	80	2.0	16.0	<1.0	0	350	m.q.
Mexican	80	2.0	16.0	<1.0	0	330	m.q.
white	70	2.0	16.0	<1.0	0	430	m.q.
Hominy grits, see "Corn grits"							
Honey *(Sue Bee)*, 1 tbsp.	60	0	16.0	0	0	1	(0)
Honey butter *(Honey Butter)*, 1 tbsp. . .	50	<1.0	11.0	1.0	m.q.	5	0
Honey loaf:							
(Kahn's), 1 slice . . .	40	4.0	1.0	2.0	m.q.	320	0

Food and Measure	cal.	prot. (gms)	carbo. (gms)	fat (gms)	chol. (mgs)	sod. (mgs)	fiber (gms)
(Oscar Mayer), 1 slice	35	5.0	1.0	1.0	15	380	0
Honey roll sausage,							
beef, 1 oz.	52	5.3	.6	3.0	14	375	0
Honeycomb, strained							
(Frieda's), 1 oz. . .	86	.1	23.3	0	0	1	0
Honeydew:							
1/10 melon, 7″ × 2″ . .	46	.6	11.8	.1	0	13	.8 d
pulp, cubed, 1/2 cup	30	.4	7.8	.1	0	9	.5 d
Horseradish:							
fresh, 1/2 cup:							
leafy tips, raw,							
chopped	6	.9	.8	.1	0	1	.2 d
leafy tips, boiled,							
drained, chopped	13	1.1	2.3	.2	0	2	.4 d
pods, raw, sliced	19	1.1	4.3	.1	0	21	1.6 d
pods, boiled,							
drained, sliced	21	1.2	4.8	.1	0	25	2.5 d
prepared:							
(Kraft), 1 tbsp.	10	0	1.0	0	0	140	m.q.
cream style *(Kraft)*,							
1 tbsp.	12	0	1.0	1.0	0	85	m.q.
hot *(Gold's)*, 1 tsp.	4	<1.0	<1.0	<1.0	0	60	m.q.
red *(Gold's)*, 1 tsp.	4	<1.0	<1.0	0	0	75	m.q.
white *(Gold's)*, 1 tsp.	4	<1.0	<1.0	<1.0	0	55	m.q.
Horseradish sauce:							
(Bennett's), 1 tbsp.	60	0	3.0	5.0	10	130	m.q.
(Heinz), 1 tbsp. . . .	80	0	1.0	8.0	5	110	m.q.
(Sauceworks), 1 tbsp.	50	0	2.0	5.0	5	105	m.q.
Hot dog, see "Frank-furter"							
Hot dog sauce, see "Chili sauce"							
Hot sauce, see "Pep-per sauce, hot" and specific listings							
Hubbard squash:							
raw *(Frieda's)*, 1 oz.	14	.5	3.3	.1	0	<1	m.q.
baked, cubed, 1/2 cup	51	2.5	11.0	.6	0	8	2.9 d

Food and Measure	cal.	prot. (gms)	carbo. (gms)	fat (gms)	chol. (mgs)	sod. (mgs)	fiber (gms)
Hubbard squash *(cont.)*							
boiled, drained,							
mashed, 1/2 cup . .	35	1.8	7.6	.4	0	6	3.4 d
Hummus mix:							
(Casbah), 1 oz.	120	5.0	12.0	5.0	0	200	m.q.
(Fantastic Foods),							
1/4 cup*	114	4.0	11.0	6.0	0	266	3.5 d
Hunter sauce mix*							
*(McCormick/Schilling							
McCormick Collec-*							
tion), 1/4 cup	104	1.0	5.0	9.0	n.a.	391	n.a.
Hushpuppies:							
frozen, 3 pieces:							
(Stilwell)	140	2.0	19.0	6.0	0	310	2.0 d
jalapeño *(Stilwell)*	70	2.0	4.0	5.0	0	360	2.0 d
mix, 1.25 oz.:							
deluxe *(Golden Dipt)*	120	3.0	26.0	0	0	520	m.q.
jalapeño *(Golden							
Dipt)*	120	3.0	27.0	0	0	570	m.q.
w/onion *(Golden							
Dipt)*	120	3.0	27.0	0	0	520	m.q.
Hyacinth beans,							
1/2 cup:							
fresh, raw, trimmed	19	.8	3.7	.1	0	1	.5 c
fresh, boiled, drained	22	1.3	4.1	.1	0	1	.8 c
dry, boiled	114	7.9	20.1	.6	0	7	2.4 c

I

Food and Measure	cal.	prot. (gms)	carbo. (gms)	fat (gms)	chol. (mgs)	sod. (mgs)	fiber (gms)
Ice, Italian (see also "Sorbet"), 4 fl. oz., except as noted:							
all flavors (Luigi's), 6 fl. oz.	95	0	24.0	0	0	0	(0)
chocolate (Mama-Tish's)	140	0	36.0	0	0	190	2.0 d
lemon (MamaTish's)	125	0	30.0	0	0	8	0
lemon-lime (Mama-Tish's)	104	0	26.0	0	0	3	n.a.
orange-pineapple-banana (MamaTish's)	105	0	26.0	0	0	6	n.a.
raspberry (Mama-Tish's)	140	0	34.0	0	0	10	0
strawberry (Mama-Tish's)	110	0	28.0	0	0	10	0
Ice bar (see also "Fruit bar, frozen"):							
(Blue Bell Rainbow Freeze), 3.75 fl. oz.	90	0	23.0	0	0	0	(0)
(Blue Bell Twin Pop), 3 fl. oz.	70	0	18.0	0	0	5	(0)
Ice cream, 1/2 cup, except as noted:							
almond praline (Dove Bite Size), .75 oz.	80	1.0	8.0	5.0	7	20	m.q.
almond praline (Edy's Grand)	150	3.0	19.0	7.0	26	91	m.q.
banana pudding (Blue Bell Supreme) . . .	180	3.0	25.0	8.0	30	65	n.a.

Food and Measure	cal.	prot. (gms)	carbo. (gms)	fat (gms)	chol. (mgs)	sod. (mgs)	fiber (gms)
Ice cream *(cont.)*							
banana split *(Edy's Grand)*	170	3.0	19.0	10.0	23	52	n.a.
brownie, double fudge *(Edy's Grand)* . . .	170	2.0	20.0	9.0	31	50	(0)
Brownie Overload, Triple (Häagen-Dazs Exträas)	330	5.0	28.0	22.0	m.q.	75	n.a.
butter almond *(Breyers)*	170	4.0	15.0	10.0	25	125	m.q.
butter crunch *(Sealtest)*	150	2.0	18.0	7.0	25	90	n.a.
butter pecan:							
(Blue Bell Supreme)	190	3.0	17.0	12.0	35	80	m.q.
(Breyers)	180	3.0	15.0	12.0	25	125	m.q.
(Chambord French)	325	4.0	19.0	26.0	102	104	m.q.
(Edy's Grand) . . .	160	3.0	17.0	9.0	27	50	m.q.
(Frusen Glädjé) . .	280	5.0	16.0	21.0	60	160	m.q.
(Häagen-Dazs) . . .	290	5.0	29.0	17.0	110	100	m.q.
(Sealtest)	160	3.0	16.0	9.0	15	125	m.q.
Cappuccino Commotion (Häagen-Dazs Exträas)	340	5.0	29.0	22.0	100	85	n.a.
Caramel Cone Explosion (Häagen-Dazs Exträas)	330	5.0	31.0	21.0	100	110	n.a.
caramel nut sundae *(Häagen-Dazs)* . . .	310	5.0	26.0	21.0	m.q.	100	m.q.
caramel pecan fudge *(Blue Bell* Supreme)	200	3.0	21.0	11.0	30	80	m.q.
caramel toasted almond *(Chambord* French)	335	4.0	21.0	21.0	47	92	m.q.
caramel toffee crunch *(Chambord* Lite)	225	5.0	30.0	9.0	45	60	(0)

Food and Measure	cal.	prot. (gms)	carbo. (gms)	fat (gms)	chol. (mgs)	sod. (mgs)	fiber (gms)
Carrot Cake Passion (Häagen-Dazs Exträas)	310	5.0	26.0	21.0	m.q.	90	n.a.
cherry chocolate chip *(Edy's Grand)* . . .	150	3.0	18.0	9.0	22	45	m.q.
cherry royale, chocolate coated *(Dove Bite Size)*, .75 oz.	60	1.0	6.0	4.0	7	10	n.a.
cherry vanilla:							
(Breyers)	150	3.0	17.0	7.0	20	45	(0)
brandied *(Chambord French)*	300	4.0	26.0	19.0	56	61	(0)
chocolate:							
(Breyers)	160	3.0	20.0	8.0	20	30	(0)
(Chambord French)	330	3.0	24.0	20.0	63	50	(0)
(Edy's Grand) . . .	160	2.0	16.0	9.0	31	30	(0)
(Frusen Glädjé) . .	240	5.0	17.0	17.0	75	65	(0)
(Häagen-Dazs) . . .	270	5.0	24.0	17.0	120	50	(0)
(Sealtest)	140	2.0	18.0	6.0	20	50	(0)
decadence *(Blue Bell Supreme)* . .	190	3.0	20.0	11.0	20	55	(0)
deep *(Häagen-Dazs)*	310	5.0	30.0	20.0	100	70	(0)
double *(Chambord Lite)*	230	5.0	30.0	9.0	40	50	(0)
Dutch *(Blue Bell Supreme)*	160	3.0	17.0	9.0	35	65	(0)
fudge mousse *(Edy's Grand)* . .	160	2.0	16.0	9.0	31	30	(0)
fudge sundae *(Edy's Grand)*	180	2.0	20.0	10.0	23	56	(0)
milk *(Blue Bell Supreme)*	180	4.0	21.0	9.0	40	80	(0)
sundae *(Blue Bell Supreme)*	170	3.0	20.0	8.0	35	55	(0)
swirl *(Borden)* . . .	130	2.0	18.0	6.0	m.q.	65	(0)
triple *(Blue Bell Supreme)*	170	3.0	21.0	8.0	30	60	(0)

Food and Measure	cal.	prot. (gms)	carbo. (gms)	fat (gms)	chol. (mgs)	sod. (mgs)	fiber (gms)
Ice cream, chocolate *(cont.)*							
triple stripes *(Sealtest)*	140	2.0	17.0	7.0	20	50	(0)
chocolate almond, Swiss *(Frusen Glädjé)*	270	6.0	18.0	19.0	55	60	m.q.
chocolate almond marshmallow *(Blue Bell* Supreme)	190	4.0	22.0	10.0	30	75	m.q.
chocolate chip:							
(Blue Bell Supreme)	170	3.0	18.0	9.0	35	60	(0)
(Edy's Grand Chocolate Chips!) . .	160	3.0	18.0	9.0	24	45	(0)
(Sealtest)	150	2.0	17.0	8.0	15	50	(0)
mint *(Chambord Lite)*	210	5.0	29.0	9.0	45	65	(0)
mint *(Edy's Grand* Chocolate Chips!)	160	3.0	18.0	9.0	29	42	(0)
mint supreme *(Blue Bell)*	170	3.0	18.0	9.0	60	35	(0)
chocolate chocolate chip:							
(Chambord French)	315	4.0	26.0	22.0	61	74	(0)
(Edy's Grand) . . .	160	2.0	17.0	10.0	30	29	(0)
(Frusen Glädjé) . .	270	5.0	21.0	18.0	55	60	(0)
(Häagen-Dazs) . . .	290	5.0	28.0	20.0	105	40	(0)
chocolate chocolate mint *(Häagen-Dazs)*	300	5.0	26.0	20.0	m.q.	50	(0)
chocolate fudge, deep *(Häagen-Dazs)* . . .	300	5.0	28.0	15.0	100	100	(0)
chocolate marshmallow sundae *(Sealtest)*	150	2.0	21.0	6.0	20	40	(0)
chocolate mint *(Breyers)*	170	3.0	18.0	10.0	25	45	(0)

Food and Measure	cal.	prot. (gms)	carbo. (gms)	fat (gms)	chol. (mgs)	sod. (mgs)	fiber (gms)
chocolate, deep, and peanut butter *(Häagen-Dazs)* . . .	330	7.0	25.0	19.0	m.q.	90	(0)
chocolate raspberry truffle *(Chambord French)*	285	6.0	26.0	17.0	48	65	(0)
chocolate Swiss almond *(Chambord Lite)*	230	5.0	30.0	9.0	35	55	m.q.
coconut almond fudge *(Chambord Lite)* . .	220	5.0	30.0	9.0	41	65	m.q.
coffee:							
(Breyers)	150	3.0	16.0	8.0	30	50	0
(Chambord French)	275	6.0	21.0	18.0	64	67	0
(Edy's Grand) . . .	140	3.0	15.0	8.0	30	41	0
(Häagen-Dazs) . . .	270	5.0	23.0	17.0	120	55	0
(Sealtest)	140	2.0	16.0	7.0	15	50	0
coffee-toffee crunch *(Häagen-Dazs)* . . .	300	4.0	27.0	19.0	145	110	0
cookie dough:							
(Edy's Grand) . . .	170	3.0	21.0	9.0	19	78	(0)
dynamo *(Häagen-Dazs)*	300	4.0	31.0	18.0	100	110	(0)
cookies n' cream:							
(Blue Bell Supreme)	180	3.0	20.0	9.0	35	95	(0)
(Breyers)	170	3.0	19.0	9.0	20	60	(0)
(Edy's Grand) . . .	160	2.0	18.0	9.0	28	80	(0)
(Häagen-Dazs) . . .	280	5.0	26.0	18.0	110	140	(0)
fruit special *(Blue Bell Supreme)*	150	3.0	17.0	8.0	35	50	n.a.
fudge:							
brownie nut *(Blue Bell Supreme)* . .	180	3.0	21.0	9.0	25	90	m.q.
marble *(Edy's Grand)*	150	3.0	18.0	8.0	28	50	(0)
royale *(Sealtest)* . .	140	3.0	19.0	7.0	15	55	(0)

Food and Measure	cal.	prot. (gms)	carbo. (gms)	fat (gms)	chol. (mgs)	sod. (mgs)	fiber (gms)
Ice cream *(cont.)*							
Heath candy crunch							
(Edy's Grand) . . .	160	3.0	18.0	9.0	25	70	n.a.
heavenly hash *(Seal-test)*	150	2.0	19.0	7.0	15	50	(0)
macadamia brittle							
(Häagen-Dazs) . . .	280	4.0	25.0	18.0	m.q.	60	m.q.
malt ball'n fudge							
(Edy's Grand) . . .	150	3.0	18.0	8.0	25	46	(0)
maple walnut *(Seal-test)*	150	3.0	17.0	9.0	20	40	m.q.
mint supreme *(Dove Bite Size)*, .75 oz.	70	1.0	8.0	4.0	8	10	n.a.
mocha almond fudge							
(Edy's Grand) . . .	160	3.0	17.0	9.0	27	46	m.q.
mud pie *(Edy's Grand)*	150	3.0	18.0	8.0	23	56	n.a.
Neapolitan *(Blue Bell Supreme)*	160	3.0	17.0	8.0	35	55	n.a.
peach *(Breyers)* . . .	130	2.0	18.0	6.0	15	35	(0)
peaches & cream *(Chambord French)*	265	4.0	24.0	17.0	47	68	(0)
peaches and vanilla *(Blue Bell* Home-made)	170	3.0	24.0	7.0	30	30	(0)
Peanut Butter Burst (Häagen-Dazs Ex-träas)	340	6.0	29.0	22.0	95	130	(0)
peanut butter cup *(Edy's Grand)* . . .	170	4.0	16.0	10.0	22	72	n.a.
peanut fudge sundae *(Sealtest)*	140	3.0	17.0	7.0	20	50	m.q.
pecan pralines 'n cream *(Blue Bell* Su-preme)	200	3.0	23.0	10.0	35	80	m.q.
rocky road *(Edy's Grand)*	170	3.0	18.0	10.0	30	30	(0)

Food and Measure	cal.	prot. (gms)	carbo. (gms)	fat (gms)	chol. (mgs)	sod. (mgs)	fiber (gms)
rum raisin *(Häagen-Dazs)*	250	4.0	21.0	17.0	110	45	m.q.
strawberry:							
(Blue Bell Supreme)	150	3.0	19.0	6.0	30	40	(0)
(Borden)	130	2.0	18.0	6.0	m.q.	55	(0)
(Breyers)	130	2.0	16.0	6.0	20	40	(0)
(Chambord French)	260	3.0	22.0	18.0	46	43	(0)
(Frusen Glädjé) . .	230	4.0	20.0	15.0	65	60	(0)
(Häagen-Dazs) . . .	250	4.0	23.0	15.0	95	40	(0)
(Sealtest)	130	2.0	18.0	5.0	15	40	(0)
real *(Edy's Grand)*	130	3.0	16.0	6.0	20	35	(0)
tin roof *(Blue Bell* Supreme)	190	4.0	21.0	10.0	30	55	n.a.
vanilla:							
(Breyers)	150	3.0	15.0	8.0	25	50	0
(Chambord French)	275	4.0	22.0	19.0	81	58	0
(Edy's Grand) . . .	160	2.0	14.0	10.0	40	30	0
(Frusen Glädjé) . .	230	5.0	16.0	17.0	65	70	0
(Häagen-Dazs) . . .	260	5.0	23.0	17.0	120	55	0
(Sealtest)	140	2.0	16.0	7.0	20	50	0
bean *(Chambord* Lite)	190	5.0	26.0	7.0	46	55	0
bean *(Edy's Grand)*	150	2.0	15.0	9.0	30	35	0
bean, natural *(Blue Bell* Supreme) . .	180	4.0	20.0	9.0	40	55	0
classic, chocolate coated *(Dove* Bite Size), .75 oz. . .	60	1.0	6.0	4.0	7	10	n.a.
French *(Blue Bell* Supreme)	160	3.0	18.0	8.0	75	50	0
French *(Edy's Grand)*	160	2.0	16.0	10.0	69	29	0
French *(Sealtest)*	140	2.0	16.0	7.0	35	50	0
French, chocolate coated *(Dove* Bite Size), .75 oz. . .	60	1.0	6.0	4.0	13	10	n.a.
French, soft-serve	185	3.5	19.1	11.2	78	52	0

Food and Measure	cal.	prot. (gms)	carbo. (gms)	fat (gms)	chol. (mgs)	sod. (mgs)	fiber (gms)
Ice cream, vanilla *(cont.)*							
homemade *(Blue Bell Supreme)* . .	180	4.0	20.0	9.0	40	70	0
honey *(Häagen-Dazs)*	250	5.0	22.0	16.0	135	55	0
vanilla and chocolate *(Breyers)*	160	3.0	17.0	8.0	25	40	(0)
vanilla-chocolate-strawberry:							
(Breyers)	150	3.0	17.0	8.0	20	40	(0)
(Edy's Grand) . . .	160	3.0	17.0	9.0	31	39	(0)
(Sealtest)	140	2.0	18.0	6.0	20	50	(0)
(Sealtest Cubic Scoops)	130	2.0	17.0	6.0	20	50	(0)
vanilla fudge:							
(Häagen-Dazs) . . .	270	5.0	26.0	17.0	m.q.	100	n.a.
pecan *(Chambord Grand Indulgence)*	320	3.0	24.0	23.0	90	70	m.q.
twirl *(Breyers)* . . .	160	3.0	19.0	8.0	20	55	(0)
vanilla-orange *(Sealtest Cubic Scoops)*	130	2.0	22.0	4.0	15	40	(0)
vanilla-peanut butter swirl *(Häagen-Dazs)*	280	5.0	19.0	20.0	110	120	(0)
vanilla-red raspberry *(Sealtest Cubic Scoops)*	130	2.0	22.0	4.0	15	40	(0)
vanilla Swiss almond:							
(Chambord French)	320	4.0	24.0	23.0	87	68	m.q.
(Frusen Glädjé) . .	270	6.0	18.0	19.0	60	65	m.q.
(Häagen-Dazs) . . .	290	5.0	24.0	19.0	110	55	m.q.
"Ice cream," substitute or imitation (see also "Ice milk"), 1/2 cup:							
almond praline *(Edy's Grand Light)*	110	3.0	16.0	4.0	18	70	m.q.

Food and Measure	cal.	prot. (gms)	carbo. (gms)	fat (gms)	chol. (mgs)	sod. (mgs)	fiber (gms)
brownie chunk fudge swirl *(Simple Pleasures* Light)	110	6.0	24.0	1.0	10	110	1.0 d
butter *Brickle (Edy's Grand Light)*	110	3.0	18.0	4.0	20	80	n.a.
butter pecan *(Edy's Grand Light)*	120	3.0	16.0	5.0	18	70	m.q.
butter pecan crunch *(Healthy Choice)* . .	140	3.0	26.0	2.0	5	80	m.q.
café au lait *(Edy's Grand Light)*	110	3.0	14.0	4.0	25	50	0
cappuccino *(Rice Dream)*	130	1.0	17.0	5.0	0	80	n.a.
caramel *Brickle (Simple Pleasures* Light)	100	5.0	22.0	1.0	10	105	0
caramel cream, dreamy *(Edy's Grand Light)*	110	3.0	15.0	4.0	24	60	n.a.
carob:							
(Rice Dream) . . .	130	1.0	20.0	5.0	0	80	n.a.
almond *(Rice Dream)*	140	1.0	20.0	6.0	0	80	n.a.
chip, plain or mint *(Rice Dream)* . .	140	1.0	20.0	6.0	0	80	n.a.
cherry:							
black *(Borden/ Meadow Gold* Fat Free)	90	2.0	21.0	<1.0	0	40	n.a.
black *(Sealtest Free)*	100	2.0	25.0	0	0	45	n.a.
chocolate:							
(Borden/Meadow Gold Fat Free) . .	100	3.0	21.0	<1.0	0	50	(0)
(Edy's Sugar Free)	90	3.0	13.0	4.0	15	70	(0)
(Healthy Choice) . .	130	3.0	24.0	2.0	5	70	(0)
(Sealtest Free) . . .	100	3.0	23.0	0	0	50	(0)
Dutch *(Simple Pleasures* Light) . . .	100	6.0	18.0	2.5	15	90	1.0 d

Food and Measure	cal.	prot. (gms)	carbo. (gms)	fat (gms)	chol. (mgs)	sod. (mgs)	fiber (gms)
"Ice cream," substitute or imitation (cont.)							
chocolate almond fudge (Edy's Grand Light)	120	4.0	15.0	5.0	23	60	m.q.
chocolate caramel:							
(C'est Bon Chocolat)	120	1.0	30.0	0	0	45	2.0 d
sundae (Simple Pleasures Light)	90	6.0	19.0	1.0	10	100	1.0 d
chocolate cherry/ brandy (C'est Bon Chocolat)	140	1.0	53.0	0	0	35	2.0 d
chocolate chip:							
(Edy's Grand Light)	110	3.0	15.0	5.0	24	50	(0)
(Edy's Sugar Free)	100	3.0	14.0	5.0	15	60	(0)
(Healthy Choice) . .	130	3.0	24.0	2.0	5	70	(0)
cherry, Bordeaux (Healthy Choice)	130	3.0	24.0	2.0	5	80	(0)
cookie dough (Simple Pleasures Light)	110	6.0	20.0	2.5	10	100	0
mint (Healthy Choice)	140	3.0	25.0	2.0	5	80	(0)
chocolate fudge mousse (Edy's Grand Light)	120	3.0	17.0	5.0	24	60	(0)
chocolate raspberry (C'est Bon Chocolat)	220	1.0	54.0	0	0	30	2.0 d
coffee toffee (Healthy Choice)	130	3.0	25.0	2.0	5	80	0
cookies n' cream:							
(Edy's Grand Light)	120	3.0	15.0	5.0	24	70	n.a.
(Healthy Choice) . .	130	4.0	24.0	2.0	5	80	n.a.
cookies N' dream (Rice Dream) . . .	160	1.0	23.0	7.0	0	90	n.a.
French silk (Edy's Grand Light)	120	3.0	18.0	5.0	20	60	n.a.
fudge:							
(Edy's Grand Light)	110	3.0	15.0	4.0	24	50	(0)

Food and Measure	cal.	prot. (gms)	carbo. (gms)	fat (gms)	chol. (mgs)	sod. (mgs)	fiber (gms)
brownie *(Healthy Choice)*	140	3.0	27.0	2.0	5	70	n.a.
chocolate or marble *(Edy's Fat Free)*	100	3.0	22.0	<1.0	0	80	(0)
cocoa marble *(Rice Dream)*	140	1.0	19.0	6.0	0	80	n.a.
marble, mint, or mocha *(Edy's Sugar Free)* . . .	110	3.0	17.0	4.0	15	80	(0)
mint *(Edy's Grand Light)*	110	3.0	16.0	4.0	25	55	(0)
mocha almond *(Edy's Grand Light)*	110	3.0	15.0	5.0	25	50	m.q.
peanut butter *(Rice Dream)*	160	3.0	19.0	7.0	0	100	n.a.
fudge, double, swirl *(Healthy Choice)* . .	130	3.0	24.0	2.0	5	70	(0)
fudgescotch swirl *(Edy's Grand Light)*	110	3.0	16.0	4.0	24	50	n.a.
lemon *(Rice Dream)*	130	1.0	17.0	5.0	0	80	n.a.
malt ball 'n fudge *(Edy's Grand Light)*	110	3.0	15.0	5.0	25	50	n.a.
Neapolitan:							
(Healthy Choice) . .	120	3.0	22.0	2.0	5	60	n.a.
(Rice Dream) . . .	130	1.0	21.0	5.0	0	80	n.a.
peach *(Sealtest Free)*	100	2.0	23.0	0	0	45	n.a.
peach or strawberry *(Borden/Meadow Gold Fat Free)* . . .	90	2.0	21.0	<1.0	0	40	n.a.
peanut butter cookie dough'n fudge *(Healthy Choice)* . .	130	4.0	24.0	2.0	5	80	n.a.
praline and caramel *(Healthy Choice)* . .	130	3.0	26.0	2.0	5	70	n.a.
rocky road: *(Edy's Grand Light)*	110	3.0	17.0	5.0	23	60	n.a.

Food and Measure	cal.	prot. (gms)	carbo. (gms)	fat (gms)	chol. (mgs)	sod. (mgs)	fiber (gms)
"Ice cream," substitute or imitation, rocky road *(cont.)*							
(Healthy Choice) . .	160	3.0	32.0	2.0	5	70	n.a.
(Simple Pleasures Light)	110	6.0	20.0	2.5	10	95	1.0 d
S'mores *(Edy's Grand Light)*	120	3.0	17.0	5.0	22	70	m.q.
strawberry:							
(Edy's Fat Free) . .	90	2.0	20.0	<1.0	0	60	n.a.
(Edy's Sugar Free)	90	3.0	13.0	4.0	15	55	n.a.
(Sealtest Free) . . .	100	2.0	23.0	0	0	40	n.a.
swirl *(Earle Swensen's Gourmet Sugar Free)* . . .	110	3.0	17.0	4.0	10	90	n.a.
strawberry or wildberry *(Rice Dream)*	130	1.0	17.0	5.0	0	80	n.a.
tin roof sundae *(Earle Swensen's Gourmet Sugar Free)*	140	4.0	18.0	6.0	10	100	n.a.
toffee crunch *(Simple Pleasures Light)* . .	100	5.0	21.0	1.0	15	120	0
vanilla:							
(Blue Bell Diet) . .	90	3.0	12.0	4.0	15	60	0
(Blue Bell Free) . .	80	4.0	16.0	0	0	65	0
(Borden/Meadow Gold Fat Free) . .	90	3.0	20.0	<1.0	0	50	0
(Edy's Fat Free) . .	90	3.0	20.0	<1.0	0	70	0
(Edy's Grand Light)	100	3.0	15.0	5.0	25	50	0
(Edy's Sugar Free)	100	3.0	13.0	4.0	15	60	0
(Rice Dream) . . .	130	1.0	17.0	5.0	0	80	n.a.
(Sealtest Free) . . .	100	3.0	24.0	0	0	45	0
(Simple Pleasures Light)	100	5.0	17.0	2.0	15	90	0
(Healthy Choice) . .	120	4.0	21.0	2.0	5	60	0
vanilla 'n caramel *(Edy's Sugar Free)*	100	3.0	16.0	4.0	15	70	0
vanilla fudge:							
(Rice Dream) . . .	140	1.0	21.0	6.0	0	80	n.a.

Food and Measure	cal.	prot. (gms)	carbo. (gms)	fat (gms)	chol. (mgs)	sod. (mgs)	fiber (gms)
royale *(Sealtest Free)*	100	3.0	24.0	0	0	50	(0)
swirl *(Simple Pleasures* Light) . . .	100	5.0	21.0	1.0	10	105	0
vanilla-chocolate-strawberry *(Sealtest Free)*	100	3.0	23.0	0	0	40	(0)
vanilla-strawberry royale *(Sealtest Free)*	100	3.0	25.0	0	0	35	(0)
vanilla Swiss almond: *(Earle Swensen's* Gourmet-Sugar Free)	140	4.0	15.0	7.0	10	100	m.q.
(Rice Dream) . . .	140	1.0	20.0	6.0	0	80	m.q.
Ice cream, mix*, 1 cup:							
chocolate *(Salada)* . .	310	4.0	31.0	19.0	m.q.	75	n.a.
strawberry or vanilla *(Salada)*	310	4.0	32.0	19.0	m.q.	60	n.a.
Ice cream bar, 1 bar:							
(Heath)	170	3.0	16.0	13.0	m.q.	155	n.a.
(Kool-Aid Pops) . . .	50	1.0	9.0	2.0	5	20	n.a.
(Snickers), 2 fl. oz. . .	220	5.0	20.0	14.0	15	65	n.a.
(Snickers), 1 fl. oz. . .	110	2.0	10.0	7.0	7	35	n.a.
almond *(Dove)*	350	5.0	32.0	23.0	41	70	m.q.
almond *(Mars)*	210	4.0	19.0	14.0	14	45	m.q.
chocolate, chocolate coated:							
(Klondike)	270	4.0	23.0	19.0	m.q.	60	n.a.
(3 Musketeers) . . .	170	2.0	16.0	10.0	18	40	n.a.
(3 Musketeers Snack)	60	1.0	6.0	4.0	7	15	n.a.
chocolate, dark chocolate coated:							
(Dove)	350	4.0	34.0	22.0	41	40	n.a.
(Häagen-Dazs) . . .	380	5.0	38.0	27.0	85	60	n.a.

Food and Measure	cal.	prot. (gms)	carbo. (gms)	fat (gms)	chol. (mgs)	sod. (mgs)	fiber (gms)
Ice cream bar *(cont.)*							
chocolate, milk chocolate coated:							
(Dove)	340	4.0	35.0	21.0	42	60	n.a.
(Milky Way)	190	2.0	21.0	11.0	16	60	n.a.
(Milky Way Snack)	70	1.0	8.0	4.0	6	20	n.a.
coconut, milk or dark chocolate coated							
(Bounty), .84 fl. oz.	70	1.0	7.0	5.0	7	20	m.q.
coconut, cherry, dark chocolate coated							
(Bounty), .84 fl. oz.	70	1.0	8.0	5.0	6	20	m.q.
crunch:							
caramel almond							
(Häagen-Dazs) . .	240	3.0	17.0	18.0	40	65	m.q.
chocolate-peanut butter *(Häagen-Dazs)*	270	6.0	16.0	21.0	35	55	m.q.
coffee almond							
(Häagen-Dazs) . .	360	5.0	28.0	26.0	100	90	m.q.
vanilla crisp							
(Häagen-Dazs) . .	220	3.0	16.0	16.0	40	55	m.q.
crunchy cookies							
(Dove)	330	4.0	34.0	20.0	43	70	n.a.
fudge *(Häagen-Dazs)*	210	4.0	19.0	14.0	75	50	n.a.
fudge, double *(Blue Bell)*	220	3.0	24.0	13.0	75	50	n.a.
peanut *(Dove)* . . .	350	6.0	32.0	23.0	40	95	m.q.
peanut butter-chocolate crisp							
(Häagen-Dazs) . .	390	7.0	29.0	28.0	m.q.	140	m.q.
vanilla, caramel brittle							
(Häagen-Dazs) . . .	370	5.0	32.0	25.0	85	170	n.a.
vanilla, chocolate coated:							
(Blue Bell)	310	4.0	27.0	21.0	170	30	n.a.
(Klondike)	280	4.0	23.0	19.0	m.q.	65	n.a.
(3 Musketeers) . . .	170	2.0	16.0	10.0	19	40	n.a.

Food and Measure	cal.	prot. (gms)	carbo. (gms)	fat (gms)	chol. (mgs)	sod. (mgs)	fiber (gms)
(3 Musketeers Snack)	60	1.0	6.0	4.0	7	15	n.a.
w/popcorn *(Klondike Krispy)*	290	4.0	26.0	19.0	m.q.	70	m.q.
vanilla, w/almonds *(Häagen-Dazs)* . . .	370	6.0	26.0	27.0	90	85	m.q.
vanilla, dark chocolate coated:							
(Dove)	340	4.0	33.0	22.0	40	45	n.a.
(Häagen-Dazs) . . .	380	5.0	38.0	27.0	90	65	n.a.
(Klondike)	280	4.0	23.0	19.0	m.q.	20	n.a.
(Milky Way)	190	2.0	22.0	11.0	17	50	n.a.
(Milky Way Snack)	70	1.0	8.0	4.0	7	20	n.a.
vanilla, milk chocolate coated:							
(Dove)	340	5.0	33.0	21.0	43	65	n.a.
(Häagen-Dazs) . . .	330	5.0	25.0	24.0	90	75	n.a.
"Ice cream" bar, substitute or imitation, 1 bar:							
(Blue Bell Bullet) . . .	40	0	11.0	0	0	5	n.a.
chocolate:							
(Rice Dream) . . .	270	1.0	33.0	16.0	0	115	n.a.
fudge *(Blue Bell)* . .	140	3.0	20.0	5.0	0	80	n.a.
fudge *(Blue Bell Sugar Free)* . . .	40	2.0	5.0	1.0	5	35	n.a.
fudge, double *(Light n' Lively)*	50	2.0	11.0	0	0	45	n.a.
fudge swirl *(Sealtest Free)*	90	3.0	19.0	0	0	30	n.a.
malt, chocolate crisp coated *(Blue Bell Grizzly Bar)*	160	2.0	20.0	8.0	n.a.	40	m.q.
mousse *(Light n' Lively)* . . . . . . :	50	2.0	12.0	0	0	45	n.a.
orange vanilla *(Blue Bell Dream Bar)* . .	100	1.0	16.0	4.0	0	30	n.a.

Food and Measure	cal.	prot. (gms)	carbo. (gms)	fat (gms)	chol. (mgs)	sod. (mgs)	fiber (gms)
"Ice cream" bar, substitute or imitation *(cont.)*							
orange vanilla *(Light n' Lively)*	40	1.0	10.0	0	0	15	n.a.
strawberry:							
(Light n' Lively) . .	80	2.0	12.0	0	0	25	n.a.
(Rice Dream) . . .	260	1.0	31.0	14.8	0	110	n.a.
vanilla *(Rice Dream)*	275	1.0	33.0	15.8	0	120	n.a.
vanilla, chocolate coated:							
(Blue Bell Mooo Bar)	140	1.0	17.0	8.0	n.a.	30	n.a.
(Klondike Lite) . . .	110	3.0	13.0	7.0	5	70	n.a.
(Light n' Lively) . .	110	2.0	14.0	6.0	0	35	n.a.
vanilla fudge swirl *(Sealtest Free)* . . .	80	3.0	18.0	0	0	30	n.a.
vanilla strawberry swirl *(Sealtest Free)* . . .	80	2.0	17.0	0	0	40	n.a.
Ice cream cone or cup, 1 piece:							
(Comet)	18	<1.0	4.0	<1.0	0	5	m.q.
rainbow *(Comet)* . . .	16	<1.0	4.0	<1.0	0	10	m.q.
sugar *(Comet)*	50	1.0	11.0	<1.0	0	40	m.q.
waffle *(Comet)*	70	1.0	15.0	<1.0	0	30	m.q.
filled, 3 fl. oz.:							
chocolate or vanilla *(Blue Bell)*	100	2.0	12.0	5.0	20	45	n.a.
strawberry *(Blue Bell)*	100	1.0	12.0	5.0	20	40	(0)
vanilla *(Blue Bell Homemade)* . . .	160	4.0	19.0	8.0	40	65	0
Ice cream sandwich, 1 piece:							
(Blue Bell)	170	3.0	27.0	6.0	m.q.	200	m.q.
(Klondike Lite)	100	2.0	17.0	2.0	5	110	m.q.
chocolate chip *(Klondike)*	200	5.0	35.0	9.0	m.q.	100	m.q.
vanilla *(Klondike)* . . .	230	5.0	33.0	9.0	m.q.	220	m.q.

Food and Measure	cal.	prot. (gms)	carbo. (gms)	fat (gms)	chol. (mgs)	sod. (mgs)	fiber (gms)
"Ice cream" sandwich, imitation, all varieties (Rice Dream Pie), 1 piece	380	3.0	47.0	19.0	0	225	m.q.
Ice cream and sorbet, see "Sorbet"							
Ice milk, 1/2 cup:							
almond praline:							
(Edy's Low Fat) . .	110	3.0	22.0	2.0	5	80	m.q.
delight (Swensen's)	130	3.0	20.0	4.0	10	60	m.q.
caramel nut (Light n' Lively)	120	3.0	18.0	4.0	10	85	m.q.
caramel turtle fudge (Swensen's)	120	3.0	18.0	4.0	10	50	n.a.
chocolate:							
(Borden)	100	3.0	18.0	2.0	n.a.	80	0
(Breyers Light) . . .	120	3.0	18.0	4.0	15	55	(0)
chocolate chip:							
(Light n' Lively) . .	120	3.0	18.0	4.0	10	35	0
(Weight Watchers Grand Collection)	120	3.0	19.0	4.0	10	75	n.a.
chocolate fudge twirl (Breyers Light) . . .	130	4.0	21.0	4.0	10	60	(0)
coffee (Light n' Lively)	100	3.0	16.0	3.0	10	40	0
cookies n' cream:							
(Edy's Low Fat) . .	110	3.0	20.0	2.0	5	85	n.a.
(Light n' Lively) . .	110	3.0	18.0	3.0	10	65	0
(Swensen's)	130	3.0	20.0	4.0	10	60	n.a.
heavenly hash:							
(Breyers Light) . . .	150	3.0	21.0	5.0	10	55	(0)
(Light n' Lively) . .	120	3.0	20.0	4.0	10	35	0
mocha almond fudge (Edy's Low Fat) . .	110	3.0	20.0	2.0	5	70	n.a.
peaches 'n cream (Blue Bell Light) . .	120	3.0	21.0	2.0	25	45	(0)

Food and Measure	cal.	prot. (gms)	carbo. (gms)	fat (gms)	chol. (mgs)	sod. (mgs)	fiber (gms)
Ice milk *(cont.)*							
pecan pralines 'n creme *(Weight Watchers Grand Collection)*	120	3.0	20.0	4.0	10	80	n.a.
praline almond *(Breyers Light)* . . .	130	3.0	19.0	5.0	10	70	m.q.
rocky road *(Edy's Low Fat)*	110	3.0	20.0	2.0	5	60	n.a.
strawberry:							
(Borden)	90	2.0	17.0	2.0	n.a.	65	0
(Breyers Light) . . .	110	3.0	18.0	3.0	15	50	n.a.
toffee fudge parfait *(Breyers Light)* . . .	140	3.0	22.0	5.0	10	90	(0)
vanilla:							
(Blue Bell Light) . .	100	3.0	17.0	2.0	10	65	0
(Borden)	90	2.0	17.0	2.0	n.a.	65	0
(Breyers Light) . . .	120	3.0	18.0	4.0	10	60	0
(Edy's Low Fat) . .	100	3.0	18.0	2.0	10	60	0
(Light n' Lively) . .	100	3.0	16.0	3.0	10	40	0
soft serve	111	4.3	19.2	2.3	10	62	0
vanilla-chocolate-almond *(Light n' Lively)*	120	3.0	17.0	4.0	10	45	0
vanilla-chocolate-strawberry:							
(Breyers Light) . . .	120	3.0	18.0	4.0	15	55	(0)
(Light n' Lively) . .	100	2.0	17.0	3.0	10	35	0
vanilla fudge twirl *(Light n' Lively)* . .	110	3.0	18.0	3.0	10	45	0
vanilla–red raspberry: parfait *(Breyers Light)*	130	3.0	23.0	3.0	15	50	(0)
swirl *(Light n' Lively)*	110	3.0	19.0	3.0	10	35	0
Icing, cake, see "Frosting"							
Italian sausage, see "Sausage"							

Food and Measure	cal.	prot. (gms)	carbo. (gms)	fat (gms)	chol. (mgs)	sod. (mgs)	fiber (gms)
Italian seasoning:							
(McCormick/Schilling Spice Blends),							
1 tsp.	4	.1	.6	n.a.	0	1	m.q.
(Tone's), 1 tsp.	3	.1	.7	.1	0	<1	.2 d

J

Food and Measure	cal.	prot. (gms)	carbo. (gms)	fat (gms)	chol. (mgs)	sod. (mgs)	fiber (gms)
Jack-in-the-Box,							
1 serving:							
breakfast:							
Breakfast Jack . . .	307	18.0	30.0	13.0	203	871	m.q.
crescent, sausage	584	22.0	28.0	43.0	187	1012	m.q.
crescent, supreme	547	20.0	27.0	40.0	178	1053	m.q.
hash browns	156	1.0	14.0	11.0	0	312	m.q.
pancake platter . .	612	15.0	87.0	22.0	99	888	m.q.
pancake syrup,							
1.5 oz.	121	0	30.0	0	0	6	0
scrambled egg:							
platter	559	18.0	50.0	32.0	378	1060	m.q.
pocket	431	29.0	31.0	21.0	354	1060	m.q.
sourdough sandwich	381	21.0	31.0	20.0	236	1120	m.q.
sandwiches:							
bacon bacon							
cheeseburger . .	705	35.0	41.0	45.0	113	1240	m.q.
cheeseburger:							
regular	315	15.0	33.0	14.0	41	746	m.q.
double	467	21.0	33.0	27.0	72	842	m.q.
ultimate	942	47.0	33.0	69.0	127	1176	m.q.
chicken, spicy							
crispy	556	24.0	55.0	27.0	49	1020	m.q.
chicken fajita pita	292	24.0	29.0	8.0	34	703	m.q.
chicken fillet, grilled	431	29.0	36.0	19.0	65	1070	m.q.
chicken supreme	641	27.0	47.0	39.0	85	1470	m.q.
chicken and mush-							
room	438	28.0	40.0	18.0	61	1340	m.q.
fish supreme . . .	510	24.0	44.0	27.0	55	1040	m.q.
gyro, beef	618	27.0	55.0	32.0	63	1310	m.q.

Food and Measure	cal.	prot. (gms)	carbo. (gms)	fat (gms)	chol. (mgs)	sod. (mgs)	fiber (gms)
hamburger	267	13.0	28.0	11.0	26	556	m.q.
Jumbo Jack	584	26.0	42.0	34.0	73	733	m.q.
Jumbo Jack, w/cheese	677	32.0	46.0	40.0	102	1090	m.q.
sirloin steak	517	29.0	49.0	23.0	66	1050	m.q.
sourdough burger, grilled	712	32.0	34.0	50.0	109	1140	m.q.
steak, country fried	450	14.0	42.0	25.0	36	891	m.q.
Mexican food:							
chimichangas, mini:							
4 pieces	571	22.0	57.0	28.0	64	633	m.q.
6 pieces	856	34.0	85.0	42.0	95	949	m.q.
guacamole, .9 oz.	30	1.0	2.0	3.0	0	128	m.q.
salsa, 1 oz.	8	<1.0	2.0	<1.0	0	27	m.q.
taco	187	7.0	15.0	11.0	18	414	m.q.
taco, super	281	12.0	22.0	17.0	29	718	m.q.
salads:							
chef	325	30.0	10.0	18.0	142	900	m.q.
side	51	7.0	<1.0	3.0	<1	84	m.q.
taco	503	34.0	28.0	31.0	92	1600	m.q.
finger foods:							
chicken strips:							
4 pieces	285	25.0	18.0	13.0	52	695	m.q.
6 pieces	451	39.0	28.0	20.0	82	1100	m.q.
chicken wings:							
6 pieces	846	34.0	78.0	44.0	181	1710	n.a.
9 pieces	1270	51.0	117.0	66.0	272	2560	n.a.
egg rolls:							
3 pieces	437	3.0	54.0	24.0	29	957	m.q.
5 pieces	753	5.0	92.0	41.0	49	1640	m.q.
ravioli, toasted:							
7 pieces	537	15.0	57.0	28.0	36	639	m.q.
10 pieces	768	22.0	81.0	40.0	52	913	m.q.
side dishes:							
fries:							
small	219	3.0	28.0	11.0	0	121	m.q.
regular	351	4.0	45.0	17.0	0	194	m.q.
jumbo	396	5.0	51.0	19.0	0	219	m.q.

Food and Measure	cal.	prot. (gms)	carbo. (gms)	fat (gms)	chol. (mgs)	sod. (mgs)	fiber (gms)
Jack-in-the-Box, side dishes, fries *(cont.)*							
seasoned, curly	358	5.0	39.0	20.0	0	1030	m.q.
onion rings	380	5.0	38.0	23.0	0	451	m.q.
sesame breadsticks	70	2.0	12.0	2.0	<1	110	m.q.
tortilla chips, 1 oz.	139	2.0	18.0	6.0	<1	134	m.q.
sauces:							
BBQ, 1 oz.	44	1.0	11.0	<1.0	0	300	n.a.
hot, .5 oz.	4	<1.0	1.0	0	0	112	n.a.
Italian, 1.5 oz. . . .	28	<1.0	6.0	<1.0	<1	176	n.a.
sweet and sour, 1 oz.	40	<1.0	11.0	<1.0	<1	160	n.a.
dressings, 2.5 oz.:							
bleu cheese	262	<1.0	14.0	22.0	18	918	n.a.
buttermilk, house	362	<1.0	8.0	36.0	21	694	n.a.
Italian, low calorie	25	<1.0	2.0	2.0	0	810	n.a.
Thousand Island . .	312	<1.0	12.0	30.0	23	700	n.a.
desserts:							
apple turnover . . .	354	3.0	48.0	19.0	0	479	m.q.
cheesecake	309	8.0	29.0	18.0	63	208	n.a.
double fudge cake	288	4.0	49.0	9.0	20	259	m.q.
shakes:							
chocolate	330	11.0	55.0	7.0	25	270	(0)
strawberry	320	10.0	55.0	7.0	25	240	(0)
vanilla	320	10.0	57.0	6.0	25	230	0
Jackfruit, trimmed, 1 oz.	27	.4	6.8	.1	0	1	.5 d
Jalapeño dip:							
(Kraft), 2 tbsp.	50	1.0	3.0	4.0	0	160	n.a.
cheddar *(Breakstone's Gourmet),* 2 tbsp.	70	2.0	2.0	6.0	15	90	n.a.
cheese *(Kraft Premium),* 2 tbsp. . . .	50	1.0	3.0	4.0	15	160	n.a.
nacho *(Price's),* 1 oz.	80	2.6	2.0	7.1	n.a.	m.q.	n.a.
Jalapeño loaf:							
(Kahn's), 1 slice . . .	70	3.0	2.0	6.0	m.q.	340	n.a.
(Oscar Mayer), 1 oz.	72	3.1	2.4	5.5	10	464	n.a.

Food and Measure	cal.	prot. (gms)	carbo. (gms)	fat (gms)	chol. (mgs)	sod. (mgs)	fiber (gms)
Jam and preserves							
(see also "Fruit							
spreads"), 1 tbsp.,							
except as noted:							
all varieties:							
(Knott's Berry Farm),							
1 tsp.	18	0	4.0	0	0	0	m.q.
(R.W. Knudsen Or-							
ganic), 2 tsp. . .	25	<1.0	7.0	<1.0	0	(0)	m.q.
(Kraft), 1 tsp. . . .	17	0	4.0	0	0	0	m.q.
(Polaner), 2 tsp. . .	35	0	9.0	0	0	0	m.q.
(Smucker's), 1 tsp. .	18	0	4.0	0	0	0	m.q.
except organic							
(R.W. Knudsen),							
2 tsp.	35	<1.0	8.0	<1.0	0	(0)	m.q.
apricot *(Chambord)*	44	.1	11.0	<.1	<1	2	.2 d
black currant							
(Chambord)	46	.2	12.0	<.1	<1	1	.7 d
blueberry *(Chambord)*	50	.1	13.0	<.1	<1	2	.4 d
cherry, black							
(Chambord)	45	.2	11.0	<.1	<1	3	.2 d
four fruit *(Chambord)*	43	.1	11.0	<.1	<1	2	.5 d
grape *(Welch's),* 2 tsp.	35	0	9.0	0	0	5	m.q.
orange:							
(Chambord)	45	<.1	11.6	<.1	<1	2	.4 d
marmalade *(R.W.*							
Knudsen), 2 tsp.	35	<1.0	8.0	<1.0	0	(0)	m.q.
marmalade							
(Smucker's),							
1 tsp.	18	0	4.0	0	0	0	m.q.
peach *(Chambord)* . .	50	.1	13.0	<.1	<1	3	.2 d
plum *(Chambord*							
Fancy)	47	.1	12.0	<.1	<1	2	.3 d
raspberry:							
black *(Chambord)*	46	.2	12.0	<.1	<1	2	.7 d
red *(Chambord)* . .	45	.2	12.0	<.1	<1	1	.5 d
strawberry:							
(Chambord)	48	.1	12.0	<.1	<1	2	.3 d

Food and Measure	cal.	prot. (gms)	carbo. (gms)	fat (gms)	chol. (mgs)	sod. (mgs)	fiber (gms)
Jam and preserves, strawberry *(cont.)*							
(Kraft Reduced Calorie), 1 tsp. . . .	6	0	2.0	0	0	5	0
(Smucker's Imitation), 1 tsp. . . .	2	0	1.0	0	0	2	n.a.
Jamaican jerk:							
dipping sauce *(Helen's Tropical Exotics),* 2 tbsp.	45	1.0	10.0	0	0	640	1.0 d
seasoning and marinade *(Helen's Tropical Exotics),* 1 tbsp. dry	30	1.0	7.0	0	0	210	1.0 d
Jambalaya dinner mix *(Luzianne),* 1/4 pkg.	200	5.0	43.0	1.0	0	690	1.0 d
Java plum:							
3 medium, .4 oz. . . .	5	.1	1.4	<.1	0	1	<.1 c
seeded, 1/2 cup . . .	41	.5	10.5	.2	0	9	.2 c
Jelly:							
all flavors:							
(Knott's Berry Farm), 1 tsp.	18	0	4.0	0	0	0	m.q.
(Kraft), 1 tsp. . . .	17	0	4.0	0	0	0	0
(Polaner), 2 tsp. . . .	35	0	9.0	0	0	n.a.	0
(Smucker's), 1 tsp. .	18	0	4.0	0	0	0	0
(Welch's), 2 tsp. . . .	35	0	9.0	0	0	5	0
grape:							
(Kraft Reduced Calorie), 1 tsp. . . .	6	0	2.0	0	0	5	0
(Smucker's Imitation), 1 tsp. . . .	2	0	1.0	0	0	2	0
(Welch's), 2 tsp. . . .	35	0	9.0	0	0	5	0
Jelly and peanut butter *(Smucker's Goober Grape/Strawberry),* 2 tbsp.	180	5.0	18.0	10.0	0	120	m.q.

Food and Measure	cal.	prot. (gms)	carbo. (gms)	fat (gms)	chol. (mgs)	sod. (mgs)	fiber (gms)
Jerusalem artichoke:							
sliced, 1/2 cup	57	1.5	13.1	<.1	0	n.a.	1.2 d
stored (Frieda's Sun-choke), 1 oz. . . .	75	2.3	16.7	.1	0	n.a.	m.q.
Jicama, see "Yam bean tuber"							
Jujube:							
raw, seeded, 1 oz. . .	22	.3	5.7	.1	0	1	.4 c
dried, 1 oz.	81	1.0	20.1	.3	0	3	.9 c
Jute, potherb:							
raw, 1/2 cup	5	.7	.8	<.1	0	1	.2 c
boiled, drained, 1/2 cup	16	1.6	3.1	.1	0	5	.9 d

K

Food and Measure	cal.	prot. (gms)	carbo. (gms)	fat (gms)	chol. (mgs)	sod. (mgs)	fiber (gms)
Kale:							
fresh, 1/2 cup:							
raw, chopped . . .	17	1.1	3.4	.2	0	15	.7 d
boiled, drained,							
chopped	21	1.2	3.7	.3	0	15	1.3 d
canned (Allens/Sun-							
shine), 1/2 cup	25	2.0	3.0	<1.0	0	15	2.0 d
frozen, chopped:							
(Frosty Acres),							
3.3 oz.	25	3.0	5.0	0	0	15	1.0 c
(Seabrook), 3.3 oz.	25	3.0	5.0	0	0	14	1.0 c
(Southern), 3.5 oz.	30	2.6	4.8	.5	0	30	m.q.
Kale, Scotch:							
raw, chopped, 1/2 cup	14	1.0	2.8	.2	0	24	.4 c
boiled, drained,							
chopped, 1/2 cup	18	1.2	3.7	.3	0	29	.6 c
Kamut:							
flakes (Arrowhead							
Mills), 1 oz.	110	4.0	22.0	1.0	0	60	3.0 d
grain, rolled, or flour							
(Arrowhead Mills),							
2 oz.	170	7.0	41.0	1.0	0	0	4.0 d
Kasha, see "Buck-							
wheat groats"							
Kauai punch (Santa							
Cruz Natural),							
8 fl. oz.	120	<1.0	28.0	1.0	0	(0)	m.q.
Kelp, see "Seaweed"							

Food and Measure	cal.	prot. (gms)	carbo. (gms)	fat (gms)	chol. (mgs)	sod. (mgs)	fiber (gms)
KFC, 1 serving:							
Original Recipe							
chicken:							
breast, center . . .	260	25.3	8.0	14.0	92	609	m.q.
breast, side	245	18.4	9.0	15.0	78	604	m.q.
drumstick	152	13.5	3.0	9.0	75	269	m.q.
thigh	287	17.9	8.0	21.0	112	591	m.q.
wing	172	11.8	5.0	11.0	59	383	m.q.
Extra Tasty Crispy							
chicken:							
breast, center . . .	330	26.0	14.0	19.0	75	740	m.q.
breast, side	400	21.0	19.0	27.0	75	710	m.q.
drumstick	190	14.0	6.0	12.0	65	310	m.q.
thigh	380	23.0	7.0	29.0	90	520	m.q.
wing	240	13.0	8.0	17.0	65	320	m.q.
Hot & Spicy chicken:							
breast, center . . .	360	28.0	13.0	22.0	80	750	m.q.
breast, side	400	22.0	16.0	28.0	80	850	m.q.
drumstick	180	14.0	6.0	12.0	55	320	m.q.
thigh	370	24.0	10.0	27.0	100	670	m.q.
wing	220	14.0	5.0	16.0	65	440	m.q.
Hot Wings, 6 pieces	471	26.5	18.0	33.0	150	1230	m.q.
Kentucky Nuggets,							
6 pieces	284	15.5	15.0	18.0	66	865	m.q.
Kentucky Nuggets							
sauce:							
barbeque, 1 oz. . .	35	.3	7.0	1.0	<5	450	n.a.
honey, .5 oz. . . .	49	0	12.0	0	<5	15	n.a.
Chicken Littles sand-							
wich	169	5.7	14.0	10.0	18	331	m.q.
Colonel's chicken							
sandwich	482	20.8	39.0	27.0	47	1060	m.q.
side dishes:							
biscuit	220	5.0	26.0	12.0	<5	530	m.q.
coleslaw	114	.9	13.0	6.0	4	177	m.q.
corn-on-the-cob . .	176	5.0	32.0	3.0	<5	21	m.q.
fries, crispy	294	3.6	33.0	17.0	<5	761	m.q.

Food and Measure	cal.	prot. (gms)	carbo. (gms)	fat (gms)	chol. (mgs)	sod. (mgs)	fiber (gms)
KFC, side dishes (cont.)							
mashed potatoes w/ gravy	70	3.0	15.0	1.0	<5	370	m.q.
Kidney beans,							
1/2 cup, except as noted:							
dry, boiled	112	7.6	20.1	.4	0	2	6.5 d
dry (Arrowhead Mills), 2 oz.	190	13.0	35.0	1.0	0	3	11.7 d
canned, red:							
w/liquid	108	6.7	20.0	.4	0	437	8.2 d
(Hunt's), 4 oz. . . .	100	6.0	20.0	<1.0	0	400	5.0 d
(Progresso), 4 oz.	100	9.0	21.0	<1.0	0	210	7.0 d
(Stokely)	110	7.0	20.0	1.0	0	360	m.q.
dark (Allens/East Texas Fair)	110	5.0	20.0	<1.0	0	280	6.0 d
dark (Hain), 4 oz.	60	7.0	16.0	0	0	260	7.0 d
dark or light (Green Giant/Joan of Arc)	90	7.0	20.0	<1.0	0	330	5.0 d
dark or light (Green Giant/Joan of Arc) 50% Less Salt)	90	7.0	20.0	<1.0	0	165	5.0 d
light (Allens)	110	5.0	20.0	1.0	0	290	6.0 d
canned, white (Progresso Cannellini), 4 oz.	80	8.0	19.0	<1.0	0	220	6.5 d
Kidney beans, sprouted:							
raw, 1/2 cup	27	3.9	3.8	.5	0	m.q.	m.q.
boiled, drained, 4 oz.	37	5.5	5.4	.7	0	m.q.	m.q.
Kidneys, braised:							
beef, 4 oz.	163	28.9	1.1	3.9	439	152	0
lamb, 4 oz.	155	26.8	1.1	4.1	641	171	0
pork, 4 oz.	171	28.8	0	5.3	544	91	0
pork, chopped, 1 cup	211	35.6	0	6.6	673	111	0
veal, 4 oz.	185	29.8	0	6.4	897	125	0

Food and Measure	cal.	prot. (gms)	carbo. (gms)	fat (gms)	chol. (mgs)	sod. (mgs)	fiber (gms)
Kielbasa (see also "Polish sausage"), 2 oz.:							
(Hillshire Farm Bun Size)	180	8.0	2.0	16.0	m.q.	570	0
(Hillshire Farm Polska Flavorseal)	190	8.0	2.0	17.0	m.q.	540	0
(Hillshire Farm Polska Flavorseal Lite)	130	8.0	1.0	11.0	m.q.	m.q.	0
(Hillshire Farm Polska Links)	190	7.0	2.0	17.0	m.q.	530	0
(Kahn's Bun Size Polska), 1 link	190	7.0	2.0	17.0	m.q.	530	0
beef (Hillshire Farm Polska Flavorseal)	190	7.0	1.0	17.0	m.q.	550	0
mild (Hillshire Farm Polska Flavorseal)	190	7.0	2.0	17.0	m.q.	530	0
Kiwi nectar (R.W. Knudsen), 8 fl. oz.	60	<1.0	14.0	<1.0	0	(0)	m.q.
Kiwifruit:							
1 large, 3.7 oz.	55	.9	13.5	.4	0	4	3.1 d
1 medium, 3.1 oz.	46	.8	11.3	.3	0	4	2.6 d
fuzzless (Frieda's), 1 oz.	10	.2	2.1	<.1	0	m.q.	m.q.
Knockwurst:							
(Hillshire Farm), 2 oz.	180	7.0	1.0	16.0	m.q.	460	0
beef (Hebrew National), 1 link	263	10.2	<1.0	25.0	26	877	0
Kohlrabi:							
raw, sliced, 1/2 cup	19	1.2	4.3	.1	0	14	2.5 d
boiled, drained, sliced, 1/2 cup	24	1.5	5.5	.1	0	17	.9 d
Kumquat:							
1 medium, .7 oz.	12	.2	3.1	<.1	0	1	1.3 d
seeded, 1 oz.	18	.3	4.7	<.1	0	2	1.9 d

L

Food and Measure	cal.	prot. (gms)	carbo. (gms)	fat (gms)	chol. (mgs)	sod. (mgs)	fiber (gms)
Lamb, choice, meat only, 4 oz., except as noted:							
cubed, leg/shoulder:							
braised or stewed	253	38.2	0	10.0	122	79	0
broiled	211	31.8	0	8.3	102	86	0
foreshank, braised:							
lean w/fat	276	32.2	0	15.3	120	82	0
lean only	212	35.2	0	6.8	118	84	0
ground:							
raw	320	18.8	0	26.5	83	67	0
broiled	321	28.1	0	22.3	110	92	0
broiled, 1 cup . . .	328	28.7	0	23.1	113	94	0
leg, whole, roasted:							
lean w/fat	293	29.0	0	18.7	105	75	0
lean w/fat, 1 slice, 3″ diam. × 1/4″ . .	73	7.2	0	4.7	26	19	0
lean only	217	32.1	0	8.8	101	77	0
lean only, 3″ slice	54	8.0	0	2.2	25	19	0
leg, shank, roasted:							
lean w/fat	255	29.9	0	14.1	102	74	0
lean w/fat, 1 slice, 3″ diam. × 1/4″ . .	64	7.5	0	3.5	26	18	0
lean only	204	31.9	0	7.6	99	75	0
lean only, 3″ slice	51	8.0	0	1.9	25	19	0
leg, sirloin, roasted:							
lean w/fat	331	27.9	0	23.4	110	77	0
lean w/fat, 1 slice, 3″ diam. × 1/4″ . .	83	7.0	0	5.9	27	19	0
lean only	231	32.1	0	10.4	104	81	0

Food and Measure	cal.	prot. (gms)	carbo. (gms)	fat (gms)	chol. (mgs)	sod. (mgs)	fiber (gms)
lean only, 3″ slice	58	8.0	0	2.6	26	20	0
loin chop, broiled:							
lean w/fat, 2.25 oz.							
(4.2 oz. raw							
w/bone)	201	16.1	0	14.7	64	49	0
lean w/fat	358	28.5	0	26.2	113	87	0
lean only, 1.6 oz.							
(4.2 oz. raw							
w/bone and fat)	100	13.9	0	4.5	44	39	0
lean only	245	34.0	0	11.0	108	95	0
loin, roasted:							
lean w/fat	350	25.6	0	26.8	108	73	0
lean only	229	30.2	0	11.1	99	75	0
rib:							
broiled, lean w/fat	409	25.1	0	33.6	112	86	0
broiled, lean only	266	31.5	0	14.7	103	96	0
roasted, lean w/fat	407	24.0	0	33.8	110	83	0
roasted, lean only	263	29.7	0	15.1	100	92	0
shoulder, whole:							
braised, lean w/fat	390	32.5	0	27.8	132	85	0
braised, lean only	321	37.2	0	10.0	133	90	0
roasted, lean w/fat	313	25.5	0	22.6	104	75	0
roasted, lean only	231	28.3	0	12.2	99	77	0
Lamb, New Zealand,							
frozen, meat only,							
4 oz.:							
foreshank:							
braised, lean w/fat	293	30.6	0	18.0	116	53	0
braised, lean only	211	34.9	0	6.8	115	56	0
leg, whole:							
roasted, lean w/fat	279	28.1	0	17.6	115	49	0
roasted, lean only	205	31.4	0	7.9	113	51	0
loin chop:							
broiled, lean w/fat	357	26.6	0	27.1	127	56	0
broiled, lean only	226	33.2	0	9.3	129	62	0
rib:							
roasted, lean w/fat	386	21.5	0	32.6	113	49	0
roasted, lean only	222	27.7	0	11.5	107	54	0

Food and Measure	cal.	prot. (gms)	carbo. (gms)	fat (gms)	chol. (mgs)	sod. (mgs)	fiber (gms)
Lamb, New Zealand *(cont.)*							
shoulder:							
braised, lean w/fat	405	32.0	0	29.8	139	58	0
braised, lean only	323	38.6	0	17.6	144	64	0
Lambsquarters,							
boiled, drained,							
chopped, 1/2 cup	29	2.9	4.5	.6	0	m.q.	1.9 d
Lard, pork, 1 tbsp.	115	0	0	12.8	12	tr.	0
Lasagna entree,							
canned or pack-							
aged:							
(Hormel Micro Cup),							
7.5 oz.	250	8.0	25.0	13.0	23	949	m.q.
Italian *(Hormel Top*							
Shelf), 10 oz. . . .	350	23.0	30.0	16.0	60	840	m.q.
w/meat sauce:							
(Dinty Moore Ameri-							
can Classics),							
10 oz.	320	16.0	33.0	14.0	35	870	m.q.
(Healthy Choice),							
7.5 oz.	220	15.0	29.0	5.0	25	530	m.q.
(Libby's Diner),							
7.75 oz.	200	9.0	29.0	5.0	15	790	m.q.
Lasagna entree,							
freeze-dried *(Moun-*							
tain House), 1 cup*	240	14.0	23.0	10.0	m.q.	630	m.q.
Lasagna entree, fro-							
zen:							
(Celentano), 10 oz. . .	400	18.0	51.0	14.0	80	650	7.0 d
(Celentano Great							
Choice), 10 oz. . .	260	18.0	42.0	2.5	20	650	2.0 d
(Dining Lite), 9 oz. . .	240	13.0	36.0	5.0	25	800	m.q.
(Freezer Queen),							
10 oz.	320	12.0	41.0	11.0	20	1060	m.q.
(On-Cor), 8 oz.	232	12.0	34.0	5.0	m.q.	1135	m.q.
(Stouffer's), 10 oz. . .	340	18.0	40.0	12.0	m.q.	840	m.q.
(Tyson Gourmet Selec-							
tion), 11.5 oz. . . .	380	20.0	47.0	14.0	m.q.	840	m.q.

Food and Measure	cal.	prot. (gms)	carbo. (gms)	fat (gms)	chol. (mgs)	sod. (mgs)	fiber (gms)
(Weight Watchers), 10.25 oz.	270	24.0	29.0	6.0	5	510	m.q.
cheese:							
(Dining Lite), 9 oz.	260	14.0	36.0	6.0	30	800	m.q.
Italian *(Weight Watchers),* 11 oz.	290	28.0	29.0	7.0	20	510	m.q.
three *(The Budget Gourmet),* 10 oz.	390	23.0	36.0	17.0	70	640	m.q.
Florentine *(Weight Watchers Smart Ones),* 11 oz. . . .	220	18.0	34.0	1.0	10	460	m.q.
garden *(Weight Watchers),* 11 oz.	260	19.0	30.0	7.0	15	430	m.q.
w/meat sauce:							
(Banquet Family), 7 oz.	270	15.0	30.0	10.0	m.q.	m.q.	m.q.
(The Budget Gourmet Light and Healthy), 9.4 oz.	290	18.0	30.0	11.0	30	720	m.q.
(Dining Lite), 9 oz.	240	13.0	36.0	5.0	25	800	m.q.
(Freezer Queen Family), 7 oz. . .	200	8.0	28.0	6.0	m.q.	730	m.q.
(Healthy Choice), 10 oz.	260	18.0	37.0	5.0	20	420	m.q.
(Lean Cuisine), 10.25 oz.	280	20.0	36.0	6.0	25	560	m.q.
(Swanson), 10 oz.	410	25.0	44.0	15.0	m.q.	1080	m.q.
primavera *(Celentano Great Choice),* 10 oz.	240	17.0	33.0	7.0	20	600	7.0 d
sausage, Italian *(The Budget Gourmet),* 10 oz.	430	20.0	34.0	23.0	45	830	m.q.
tuna, w/spinach noodles and vegetables *(Lean Cuisine),* 9.75 oz.	240	16.0	29.0	7.0	20	520	m.q.

Food and Measure	cal.	prot. (gms)	carbo. (gms)	fat (gms)	chol. (mgs)	sod. (mgs)	fiber (gms)
Lasagna entree, frozen *(cont.)*							
vegetable:							
(The Budget Gour-							
met Light and							
Healthy), 10.5 oz.	290	16.0	36.0	10.0	15	770	m.q.
(On-Cor), 8 oz. . . .	229	11.0	34.0	5.0	n.a.	815	m.q.
(Stouffer's), 10.5 oz.	430	20.0	35.0	23.0	n.a.	820	m.q.
zucchini:							
(Healthy Choice							
Quick Meal),							
11.5 oz.	250	14.0	41.0	3.0	15	400	m.q.
(Lean Cuisine),							
11 oz.	260	17.0	34.0	6.0	20	520	m.q.
Lasagna sheets, fro-							
zen, precooked							
(Aunt Vi's), 4 oz. . .	190	9.0	36.0	0	0	15	2.0 d
Leek:							
fresh:							
raw, 9.9-oz. leek	76	1.9	17.6	.4	0	25	2.2 d
raw, trimmed,							
chopped, 1/2 cup	32	.8	7.4	.2	0	10	.9 d
boiled, drained,							
chopped, 1/2 cup	16	.4	4.0	.1	0	6	.4 c
freeze-dried, 1 tbsp.	1	<.1	.2	tr.	0	tr.	<.1 c
Lemon:							
21/8"-diam. lemon,							
3.9 oz. w/peel . . .	22	1.3	11.6	.3	0	3	m.q.
1 wedge, 1/4 medium	5	.3	2.9	.1	0	1	m.q.
peeled, 21/8"-diam.							
lemon	17	.6	5.4	.2	0	1	1.6 d
peel, 1 tbsp.	—[1]	.1	1.0	<.1	0	0	.6 d
Lemon dill seasoning							
(McCormick/Schill-							
ing Bag'n Season),							
1 pkg.	161	3.0	15.0	11.0	0	2035	m.q.

[1] *Cannot be calculated; no digestibility value for peel.*

Food and Measure	cal.	prot. (gms)	carbo. (gms)	fat (gms)	chol. (mgs)	sod. (mgs)	fiber (gms)
Lemon herb season-							
ing *(McCormick/*							
Schilling Spice							
Blends), 1 tsp. . . .	6	.2	.7	.2	0	615	n.a.
Lemon juice:							
fresh, 1 tbsp.	4	.1	1.3	0	0	tr.	.1 d
bottled or chilled							
(ReaLemon)	6	0	2.0	0	0	10	(0)
frozen*, 1 fl. oz.:							
(Minute Maid) . . .	8	0	2.0	0	0	0	(0)
(Sunkist)	7	.1	2.0	.1	0	<1	(0)
Lemon pepper,							
1 tsp.:							
(Lawry's Spice Blends)	6	.2	1.2	.1	0	340	.1 c
(McCormick/Schilling							
Parsley Patch) . . .	10	.4	2.0	.2	0	8	m.q.
(McCormick/Schilling							
Spice Blends) . . .	7	m.q.	.8	.2	0	618	m.q.
Lemon pepper mari-							
nade *(Lawry's),*							
1 oz.	20	.4	2.1	1.2	n.a.	800	n.a.
Lemon soufflé mix,							
flavor *(Knorr),*							
1 serving dry . . .	40	3.6	5.2	.3	<1	175	n.a.
Lemon-lime drink							
mix* *(Kool-Aid),*							
8 fl. oz.	100	0	25.0	0	0	0	0
Lemonade:							
canned or bottled:							
(Crush), 11.5 fl. oz.	140	0	35.0	0	0	4	(0)
(R.W. Knudsen Nat-							
ural), 8 fl. oz. . .	100	<1.0	26.0	<1.0	0	(0)	n.a.
(Kool-Aid Koolers),							
8.45 fl. oz.	120	0	32.0	0	0	10	(0)
(Santa Cruz Natural),							
8 fl. oz.	60	<1.0	21.0	<1.0	0	(0)	n.a.
(Shasta), 12 fl. oz.	168	0	42.0	0	0	165	0

Food and Measure	cal.	prot. (gms)	carbo. (gms)	fat (gms)	chol. (mgs)	sod. (mgs)	fiber (gms)
Lemonade, canned or bottled *(cont.)*							
(Shasta Plus),							
12 fl. oz.	172	0	43.0	0	0	58	0
(Sunkist), 8 fl. oz.	141	0	36.0	0	0	0	(0)
(Welch's), 6 fl. oz.	100	0	24.0	0	0	20	(0)
(Wylers), 6 fl. oz.	60	(0)	16.0	(0)	0	35	(0)
chilled *(Tropicana),*							
6 fl. oz.	100	<1.0	22.0	<1.0	0	35	(0)
chilled, regular, country style, or pink *(Minute Maid),*							
6 fl. oz.	80	0	21.0	0	0	20	(0)
frozen* *(Sunkist),*							
8 fl. oz.	92	.1	24.2	0	0	1	(0)
mix*, 8 fl. oz.:							
(Kool-Aid)	100	0	25.0	0	0	10	0
(Kool-Aid Presweetened)* . . .	70	0	17.0	0	0	0	0
regular or pink *(Wylers* Crystals)	80	(0)	20.0	(0)	0	50	(0)
Lemonade fruit blends, 8 fl. oz., except as noted:							
cherry:							
(Boku)	120	0	29.0	0	0	30	0
(R.W. Knudsen) . .	105	<1.0	31.0	<1.0	0	(0)	m.q.
dark sweet *(Santa Cruz Natural)* . .	60	<1.0	20.0	<1.0	0	(0)	m.q.
cranberry:							
(R.W. Knudsen) . .	115	<1.0	29.0	<1.0	0	(0)	m.q.
(Minute Maid),							
6 fl. oz.	90	0	23.0	0	0	20	(0)
(Santa Cruz Natural)	100	<1.0	24.0	<1.0	0	(0)	m.q.
Concord grape–wild blackberry *(Santa Cruz Natural)* . . .	60	<1.0	22.0	<1.0	0	(0)	m.q.
raspberry:							
(R.W. Knudsen) . .	110	<1.0	28.0	<1.0	0	(0)	m.q.

Food and Measure	cal.	prot. (gms)	carbo. (gms)	fat (gms)	chol. (mgs)	sod. (mgs)	fiber (gms)
(Minute Maid), 6 fl. oz.	90	0	23.0	0	0	20	(0)
or strawberry *(Santa Cruz Natural)* . .	60	<1.0	20.0	<1.0	0	(0)	m.q.
strawberry *(R.W. Knudsen)*	90	<1.0	21.0	<1.0	0	(0)	m.q.
Lentil, dry:							
green *(Arrowhead Mills),* 2 oz.	190	13.0	35.0	1.0	0	9	8.8 d
red *(Arrowhead Mills),* 2 oz.	195	14.0	34.0	1.0	0	10	8.8 d
boiled, 1/2 cup	115	8.9	19.9	.4	0	2	7.8 d
Lentil, sprouted, raw, 1/2 cup	40	3.4	8.4	.2	0	4	1.2 c
Lentil dishes:							
canned, hearty, w/vegetables *(Health Valley Fast Menu Fat Free),* 5 oz. . .	80	9.0	12.0	<1.0	0	140	10.3 d
mix*, 10 oz.:							
and couscous *(Fantastic Only a Pinch)*	220	13.0	47.0	1.0	0	120	10.0 d
curried, w/rice *(Fantastic)*	220	12.0	44.0	2.0	0	490	8.0 d
pilaf, w/couscous *(Fantastic Leapin' Lentils)*	225	12.0	42.0	1.0	0	490	9.0 d
Lentil rice loaf, frozen *(Natural Touch),* 2.5"-slice	200	8.0	18.0	11.0	0	420	m.q.
Lettuce:							
bibb or Boston:							
1 head, 5" diam.	21	2.1	3.8	.4	0	8	1.6 d
2 inner leaves . . .	2	.2	.4	<.1	0	1	.2 d
cos or romaine:							
1 inner leaf	2	.2	.2	<.1	0	1	.2 d
shredded, 1/2 cup	4	.5	.7	.1	0	2	.7 d

Food and Measure	cal.	prot. (gms)	carbo. (gms)	fat (gms)	chol. (mgs)	sod. (mgs)	fiber (gms)
Lettuce (cont.)							
iceberg:							
1 head, 6″ diam.	70	5.4	11.3	1.0	0	48	7.5 d
1 leaf, .7 oz.	3	.2	.4	<.1	0	2	.3 d
limestone (Frieda's),							
1 oz.	4	.3	.7	.1	0	3	m.q.
looseleaf, shredded,							
1/2 cup	5	.4	1.0	.1	0	3	.5 d
Lima beans:							
fresh, 1/2 cup:							
raw, trimmed . . .	88	5.3	15.7	.7	0	6	3.8 d
boiled, drained . .	104	5.8	20.1	.3	0	14	4.5 d
canned, 1/2 cup:							
(Green Giant/Joan of Arc Butter Beans)	70	6.0	12.0	0	0	450	4.0 d
(Stokely)	80	5.0	16.0	0	0	390	m.q.
green (Allens/Butterfield/Sunshine)	90	5.0	15.0	<1.0	0	370	m.q.
green and white (Allens)	90	5.0	15.0	<1.0	0	370	m.q.
large (Allens Butterbeans)	110	5.0	18.0	<1.0	0	370	4.0 d
frozen, 3.3 oz., except as noted:							
baby (Green Giant Harvest Fresh), 1/2 cup	80	6.0	18.0	0	0	170	4.0 d
baby (Seabrook) . .	130	7.0	24.0	0	0	125	2.0 c
baby, butter (Seabrook)	140	7.0	26.0	1.0	0	213	2.0 c
Fordhook (Seabrook)	100	6.0	19.0	0	0	71	2.0 c
speckled (Seabrook)	120	7.0	23.0	0	0	19	2.0 c
tiny (Seabrook) . .	110	6.0	21.0	1.0	0	144	2.0 c
in butter sauce (Green Giant), 1/2 cup	100	6.0	17.0	3.0	5	390	4.5 d

Food and Measure	cal.	prot. (gms)	carbo. (gms)	fat (gms)	chol. (mgs)	sod. (mgs)	fiber (gms)
Lima beans, mature, 1/2 cup:							
baby, boiled	115	7.3	21.2	.3	0	2	7.0 d
large, boiled	108	7.3	19.6	.4	0	2	6.6 d
canned, w/liquid . . .	95	5.9	17.9	.2	0	403	5.8 d
Lime:							
2"-diam. lime	20	.5	7.1	.1	0	1	1.9 d
peeled, seeded, 1 oz.	9	.2	3.0	.1	0	1	.8 d
Lime cooler, tropical (R.W. Knudsen), 8 fl. oz.	130	<1.0	32.0	<1.0	0	(0)	n.a.
Lime juice, 1 tbsp.:							
fresh	4	.1	1.4	<.1	0	tr.	.1 d
bottled (ReaLime) . .	3	0	1.0	0	0	5	(0)
sweetened (Rose's)	24	<1.0	6.0	<1.0	0	3	(0)
Limeade:							
(Minute Maid), 6 fl. oz.	70	0	19.0	0	0	0	(0)
Key lime (Boku), 8 fl. oz.	110	0	28.0	0	0	30	0
Ling, meat only:							
raw, 4 oz.	99	21.5	0	.7	m.q.	153	0
baked, broiled, or microwaved, 4 oz. . .	126	27.6	0	.9	m.q.	196	0
Ling cod, meat only:							
raw, 4 oz.	96	20.0	0	1.2	59	67	0
baked, broiled, or microwaved, 4 oz. . .	124	25.7	0	1.5	76	86	0
Linguine, see "Pasta"							
Linguine entrée, frozen:							
w/clam sauce (Lean Cuisine), 95/8 oz.	280	17.0	36.0	8.0	30	560	m.q.
w/scallops and clams (The Budget Gourmet Light and Healthy), 9.5 oz. . .	280	14.0	34.0	10.0	45	710	m.q.
w/shrimp (Healthy Choice), 9.5 oz. . .	230	13.0	40.0	2.0	60	420	m.q.

Food and Measure	cal.	prot. (gms)	carbo. (gms)	fat (gms)	chol. (mgs)	sod. (mgs)	fiber (gms)
Linguine entree *(cont.)*							
w/shrimp and clams							
(The Budget Gour-							
met), 10 oz.	270	12.0	35.0	9.0	50	1160	m.q.
Liquor[1], 1 fl. oz.:							
80 proof	65	0	tr.	0	0	tr.	0
86 proof	70	0	tr.	0	0	tr.	0
90 proof	74	0	tr.	0	0	tr.	0
100 proof	83	0	tr.	0	0	tr.	0
Little Caesars,							
1 serving:							
Baby Pan!Pan!	525	28.0	53.0	22.0	60	1180	m.q.
Crazy Bread, 1 piece	98	4.0	18.0	1.0	2	119	1.0 d
Crazy Sauce	63	3.0	11.0	1.0	0	360	4.0 d
Pizza!Pizza!, 1 slice:							
cheese:							
round, small . . .	138	9.0	14.0	5.0	15	200	2.0 d
round, medium	154	10.0	16.0	5.0	15	220	3.0 d
round, large . . .	169	11.0	18.0	6.0	15	240	3.0 d
square, small . .	188	10.0	22.0	6.0	20	380	3.0 d
square, medium	185	10.0	22.0	6.0	20	370	3.0 d
square, large . .	188	10.0	22.0	6.0	20	380	3.0 d
cheese and pepper-							
oni:							
round, small . . .	151	10.0	14.0	6.0	15	240	2.0 d
round, medium	168	11.0	16.0	7.0	20	270	3.0 d
round, large . . .	185	12.0	18.0	7.0	20	300	3.0 d
square, small . .	204	11.0	22.0	8.0	20	435	3.0 d
square, medium	201	11.0	22.0	8.0	23	430	3.0 d
square, large . .	204	11.0	22.0	8.0	20	430	3.0 d
Slice!Slice!	756	48.0	71.0	31.0	90	1260	m.q.
salads:							
antipasto, small . .	96	6.0	8.0	5.0	10	320	2.0 d
Greek, small	85	4.0	6.0	5.0	10	400	1.0 d
tossed, small . . .	37	2.0	7.0	1.0	0	85	2.0 d

[1] *Includes all pure distilled liquors (bourbon, brandy, gin, rum, Scotch, tequila, vodka, whiskey, etc.).*

Food and Measure	cal.	prot. (gms)	carbo. (gms)	fat (gms)	chol. (mgs)	sod. (mgs)	fiber (gms)
sandwiches:							
ham and cheese	553	32.0	47.0	27.0	50	1580	4.0 d
Italian	615	29.0	47.0	35.0	55	1580	4.0 d
tuna	610	33.0	51.0	31.0	75	1080	6.0 d
turkey	450	24.0	49.0	17.0	45	1590	3.0 d
veggie	784	38.0	48.0	47.0	95	920	4.0 d
Liver:							
beef, pan-fried, 4 oz.	246	30.3	8.9	9.1	547	120	0
chicken, simmered:							
4 oz.	178	27.6	1.0	6.2	716	58	0
chopped, 1 cup . .	219	34.1	1.2	7.6	883	71	0
duck, raw, 1 oz. . . .	39	5.3	1.0	1.3	146	m.q.	0
goose, raw, 1 oz. . .	38	4.6	1.8	1.2	m.q.	40	0
lamb, pan-fried, 4 oz.	270	29.0	4.3	14.3	559	141	0
pork, braised, 4 oz.	187	29.5	4.3	5.0	403	56	0
turkey, simmered:							
4 oz.	192	27.2	3.9	6.7	710	73	0
chopped, 1 cup . .	237	33.6	4.8	8.3	876	89	0
veal (calves), braised,							
4 oz.	187	24.5	3.1	7.8	636	60	0
Liver cheese *(Oscar*							
Mayer), 1 slice . . .	120	6.0	<1.0	10.0	80	420	0
Liver loaf *(Kahn's),*							
1 slice	170	6.0	3.0	15.0	m.q.	370	0
Liver pâté, see							
"Pâté"							
Liver sausage (see							
also "Braunschwei-							
ger"):							
(Jones Dairy Farm),							
.8-oz. slice	80	3.0	tr.	7.0	43	200	0
(Jones Dairy Farm							
Chub),* 1 oz.	80	4.5	tr.	6.5	67	270	0
lowfat *(Jones Dairy*							
Farm Chub), 1 oz.	50	5.0	tr.	3.0	76	270	0

Food and Measure	cal.	prot. (gms)	carbo. (gms)	fat (gms)	chol. (mgs)	sod. (mgs)	fiber (gms)
Lobster, northern, meat only:							
raw, 4 oz.	102	21.3	.6	1.0	108	m.q.	0
boiled or steamed:							
4 oz.	111	23.2	1.5	.7	82	431	0
1 cup, 5.1 oz. . . .	142	29.7	1.9	.9	104	551	0
"Lobster," imitation *(Louis Kemp Lobster Delights),* 2 oz. . .	50	6.0	5.0	<1.0	m.q.	320	0
Lobster, spiny, see "Spiny lobster"							
Lobster Newburg, frozen *(Stouffer's),* 6.5 oz.	380	14.0	9.0	32.0	m.q.	870	m.q.
Lobster sauce, rock, canned *(Progresso),* 1/2 cup	120	4.0	11.0	8.0	10	430	2.0 d
Loganberry:							
fresh, 1 cup	89	1.4	21.5	.9	0	1	4.3 c
frozen, 1/2 cup	40	1.1	9.6	.2	0	1	3.6 d
Long John Silver's:							
à la carte:							
chicken, light herb, 3.5 oz.	120	22.0	<1.0	4.0	60	570	0
Chicken Planks, 1 piece	120	8.0	11.0	6.0	15	400	m.q.
fish, batter dipped, 1 piece	180	12.0	12.0	11.0	30	490	m.q.
fish, lemon crumb, baked, 5 oz. . . .	150	29.0	4.0	1.0	110	370	n.a.
shrimp, batter dipped, 1 piece	30	1.0	2.0	2.0	10	80	n.a.
Chicken Planks, w/fries, 2 pieces	490	19.0	50.0	26.0	30	1290	m.q.
sandwiches, 1 serving:							
chicken, batter dipped, no sauce	280	14.0	39.0	8.0	15	790	m.q.

Food and Measure	cal.	prot. (gms)	carbo. (gms)	fat (gms)	chol. (mgs)	sod. (mgs)	fiber (gms)
fish, batter dipped, no sauce	340	18.0	40.0	13.0	30	890	m.q.
soup and side dishes:							
coleslaw, fork drained, 3.4 oz.	140	1.0	20.0	6.0	15	260	m.q.
Corn Cobette, w/prep, 1 piece	140	3.0	18.0	8.0	0	0	m.q.
fries, 3 oz.	250	3.0	28.0	15.0	0	500	m.q.
green beans, 3.5 oz.	20	1.0	3.0	<1.0	0	320	m.q.
hushpuppy, 1 piece	70	2.0	10.0	2.0	<5	25	m.q.
rice, 4 oz.	160	3.0	30.0	3.0	0	340	m.q.
roll, 1 piece	110	4.0	23.0	<1.0	0	170	m.q.
seafood chowder, w/cod, 7 oz. . .	140	11.0	10.0	6.0	20	590	m.q.
seafood gumbo, w/cod, 7 oz. . .	120	9.0	4.0	8.0	25	740	m.q.
finger food:							
Chicken Planks, 2 pieces	240	16.0	22.0	12.0	30	790	m.q.
fish, batter dipped, 1 piece	180	12.0	12.0	11.0	30	490	m.q.
salads, no dressing or crackers:							
ocean chef	110	12.0	13.0	1.0	40	730	m.q.
seafood	380	15.0	12.0	31.0	55	980	m.q.
small	14	<1.0	3.0	<1.0	0	10	m.q.
condiments:							
catsup, .32 oz. . .	12	<1.0	2.0	0	0	135	m.q.
honey mustard sauce, .42 oz. . .	20	<1.0	5.0	<1.0	0	60	n.a.
Italian dressing, creamy, 1 oz. . .	30	<1.0	<1.0	3.0	n.a.	280	n.a.
malt vinegar, .28 oz.	1	0	0	<1.0	0	15	0
ranch dressing, 1 oz.	180	<1.0	<1.0	19.0	<5	230	n.a.
sea salad dressing, 1 oz.	140	<1.0	2.0	15.0	<5	160	n.a.

Food and Measure	cal.	prot. (gms)	carbo. (gms)	fat (gms)	chol. (mgs)	sod. (mgs)	fiber (gms)
***Long John Silver's,* condiments** *(cont.)*							
seafood sauce,							
.42 oz.	14	<1.0	3.0	<1.0	0	180	n.a.
sweet 'n sour							
sauce, .42 oz. . . .	20	<1.0	5.0	<1.0	0	45	n.a.
tartar sauce, .42 oz.	50	<1.0	2.0	5.0	0	35	n.a.
desserts, 1 serving:							
apple pie	320	3.0	45.0	13.0	<5	420	m.q.
brownie, walnut . .	440	5.0	54.0	22.0	20	150	m.q.
cherry pie	360	4.0	55.0	13.0	5	200	m.q.
cookie:							
chocolate chip	230	3.0	35.0	9.0	10	170	m.q.
oatmeal raisin . .	160	3.0	15.0	10.0	15	150	m.q.
lemon pie	340	7.0	60.0	9.0	45	130	m.q.
Longan, shelled:							
fresh, seeded, 1 oz.	17	.4	4.3	<.1	0	tr.	.3 d
dried, 1 oz.	81	1.4	21.0	.1	0	14	.6 c
Loquat:							
1 medium, .6 oz. . .	5	<.1	1.2	<.1	0	tr.	.2 d
peeled, seeded, 1 oz.	13	.1	3.4	.1	0	<1	.5 d
Lotus root:							
raw, trimmed, 1 oz.	16	.7	4.9	<.1	0	11	1.4 d
boiled, drained, 4 oz.	75	1.8	18.2	.1	0	51	3.5 d
Lotus seed:							
raw, 1 oz.	25	1.2	4.9	.2	0	tr.	.2 c
dried, 1 oz.	94	4.4	18.3	.6	0	1	.7 c
fried, 1 cup	106	4.9	20.6	.6	0	1	.8 c
Lox, see "Salmon, Chinook"							
Lunch combinations							
(Lunchables), 1 pkg:							
bologna and American	490	18.0	18.0	38.0	75	1520	<1.0 d
chicken and:							
Monterey Jack . .	360	21.0	17.0	23.0	60	1590	1.0 d
Monterey Jack,							
fudge	390	19.0	31.0	21.0	55	1220	<1.0 d
roast beef, deluxe	380	24.0	21.0	22.0	70	1600	1.0 d

Food and Measure	cal.	prot. (gms)	carbo. (gms)	fat (gms)	chol. (mgs)	sod. (mgs)	fiber (gms)
turkey, deluxe . . .	380	23.0	21.0	23.0	70	1560	<1.0 d
ham and:							
cheddar	380	20.0	18.0	25.0	80	1680	<1.0 d
honey, American,							
pudding	410	19.0	34.0	23.0	55	1400	<1.0 d
honey, chicken,							
deluxe	370	24.0	24.0	20.0	65	1680	1.0 d
roast beef, deluxe	400	24.0	21.0	24.0	70	1750	<1.0 d
Swiss	350	22.0	17.0	22.0	65	1660	<1.0 d
Swiss, cookies . .	380	18.0	27.0	22.0	45	1070	1.0 d
salami and mozzarella	420	22.0	17.0	29.0	60	1220	1.0 d
turkey and:							
cheddar	370	22.0	17.0	24.0	65	1600	1.0 d
ham, deluxe	360	23.0	21.0	21.0	65	1850	<1.0 d
smoked, Monterey							
Jack	360	20.0	19.0	22.0	60	1630	1.0 d
spreadable:							
ham, garden vegeta-							
ble	370	14.0	33.0	20.0	55	1110	<1.0 d
honey ham, herb							
and chive	380	15.0	33.0	20.0	50	1130	<1.0 d
turkey, green onion	370	14.0	34.0	20.0	45	1010	2.0 d
smoked turkey,							
ranch and herb	360	15.0	31.0	19.0	45	930	2.0 d
Luncheon meat (see							
also specific list-							
ings):							
spiced loaf, 1 slice:							
(Oscar Mayer) . . .	70	4.0	2.0	5.0	20	340	0
(Kahn's)	80	3.0	1.0	7.0	m.q.	240	0
canned:							
(Deviled Spam),							
1 oz.	78	4.0	<2.0	7.0	20	260	0
(Spam), 1 oz. . . .	86	4.0	<2.0	8.0	20	376	0
(Spam Less Salt),							
2 oz.	176	8.0	1.0	15.0	38	550	0
(Spam Lite), 2 oz.	140	8.0	1.0	12.0	43	560	0

Food and Measure	cal.	prot. (gms)	carbo. (gms)	fat (gms)	chol. (mgs)	sod. (mgs)	fiber (gms)
Luncheon "meat," vegetarian, canned, 1/2″ slice:							
(LaLoma Nuteena) . .	160	8.0	6.0	12.0	0	110	m.q.
(Worthington Numete)	150	7.0	7.0	11.0	0	410	m.q.
(Worthington Protose)	180	17.0	9.0	8.0	0	470	m.q.
Lupin, boiled, 1/2 cup	98	12.9	8.2	2.4	0	3	2.3 d
Lychees, shelled, 1 oz.:							
raw, seeded	19	.2	4.7	.1	0	<1	.4 d
raw, peeled *(Frieda's)*	18	.3	4.6	.1	0	1	m.q.
dried	79	1.1	20.0	.3	0	1	1.3 d

M

Food and Measure	cal.	prot. (gms)	carbo. (gms)	fat (gms)	chol. (mgs)	sod. (mgs)	fiber (gms)
Macadamia nut:							
raw *(Frieda's)*, 1 oz.	196	2.2	4.5	20.3	0	m.q.	m.q.
dried, shelled:							
1 oz.	199	2.4	3.9	20.9	0	1	2.6 d
1 cup	940	11.1	18.4	98.8	0	6	12.5 d
oil-roasted, 1 oz. . . .	204	2.1	3.7	21.7	0	2	.5 c
roasted, salted *(Master Choice)*, 1 oz. . . .	200	2.0	4.0	22.0	0	100	m.q.
Macaroni (see also "Pasta"):							
uncooked:							
2 oz.	211	7.3	42.6	.9	0	4	1.4 d
elbow, 1 cup . . .	389	13.4	78.4	1.7	0	8	2.5 d
cooked:							
4 oz.	160	5.4	32.1	.8	0	1	1.8 d
elbow, 1 cup . . .	197	6.7	39.7	.9	0	1	2.2 d
small shells, 1 cup	162	5.5	32.6	.8	0	1	1.8 d
spirals, 1 cup . . .	189	6.4	38.0	.9	0	1	2.1 d
vegetable (tricolor), 4 oz.	145	5.1	30.2	.1	0	7	4.9 d
whole-wheat, 4 oz.	141	6.0	30.1	.6	0	3	5.0 d
Macaroni and cheese, see "Macaroni dinner" and "Macaroni entree"							
Macaroni dinner, and cheese, frozen *(Swanson)*, 12.25 oz.	340	10.0	49.0	12.0	m.q.	960	m.q.

Food and Measure	cal.	prot. (gms)	carbo. (gms)	fat (gms)	chol. (mgs)	sod. (mgs)	fiber (gms)
Macaroni entree, canned or packaged, 7.5 oz., except as noted:							
and beef, in sauce (Libby's Diner), 7.75 oz.	230	10.0	34.0	6.0	20	670	m.q.
and cheese:							
(Franco-American), 7.35 oz.	160	6.0	24.0	6.0	m.q.	880	m.q.
(Hormel Micro Cup)	260	12.0	28.0	11.0	45	650	m.q.
(Libby's Diner) . . .	360	14.0	27.0	22.0	35	1020	m.q.
small, w/tomato sauce (Mothers Choice)	150	5.0	29.0	1.0	0	923	1.0 d
Macaroni entree, frozen:							
and beef:							
(Healthy Choice Quick Meal), 8.5 oz.	200	12.0	32.0	3.0	15	420	m.q.
(Weight Watchers), 9 oz.	220	14.0	31.0	4.0	10	510	m.q.
w/cheese (Swanson), 9 oz.	260	19.0	26.0	9.0	m.q.	1040	m.q.
w/tomatoes (Stouffer's), 11.5 oz.	340	21.0	38.0	12.0	m.q.	1440	m.q.
in tomato sauce (Lean Cuisine), 10 oz.	250	14.0	35.0	6.0	25	540	m.q.
and cheese:							
(Banquet Casserole), 6.5 oz.	290	8.0	30.0	14.0	m.q.	760	m.q.
(Banquet Family), 7 oz.	260	10.0	28.0	11.0	m.q.	m.q.	m.q.
(The Budget Gourmet Side Dish), 5.75 oz.	230	9.0	22.0	12.0	35	570	m.q.

Food and Measure	cal.	prot. (gms)	carbo. (gms)	fat (gms)	chol. (mgs)	sod. (mgs)	fiber (gms)
(Freezer Queen),							
11.5 oz.	320	13.0	59.0	4.0	10	1090	m.q.
(Freezer Queen							
Family), 4.5 oz.	110	3.0	19.0	2.0	m.q.	420	m.q.
(Green Giant One							
Serving), 5.7 oz.	220	10.0	27.0	8.0	25	480	1.5 d
(Healthy Choice							
Quick Meal), 9 oz.	280	12.0	45.0	6.0	20	520	m.q.
(Lean Cuisine), 9 oz.	290	15.0	37.0	9.0	30	550	m.q.
(Morton Casserole),							
6.5 oz.	290	8.0	30.0	14.0	m.q.	760	m.q.
(On-Cor), 8 oz. . .	161	8.0	27.0	3.0	m.q.	1065	m.q.
(Stouffer's), 6 oz.	250	11.0	23.0	13.0	m.q.	640	m.q.
(Swanson), 7 oz. . .	200	7.0	24.0	8.0	m.q.	740	m.q.
(Swanson Entrees),							
9 oz.	220	10.0	25.0	9.0	m.q.	820	m.q.
(Weight Watchers),							
9 oz.	280	15.0	43.0	6.0	20	550	m.q.
cheddar/Parmesan							
(The Budget							
Gourmet),							
10.5 oz.	330	19.0	49.0	8.0	30	760	m.q.
nacho *(Healthy*							
Choice Quick							
Meal), 9 oz. . . .	280	13.0	44.0	5.0	20	560	m.q.
Macaroni entree							
mix*, 1/2 cup, ex-							
cept as noted:							
and cheese:							
(Fantastic Foods)[1]	167	6.0	20.0	7.0	m.q.	305	2.6 d
(Fantastic Foods)[2]	122	6.0	20.0	2.0	4	260	2.6 d
(Kraft Deluxe Din-							
ner), 3/4 cup . . .	260	11.0	36.0	8.0	20	590	m.q.
(Kraft Dinner),							
3/4 cup	290	9.0	34.0	13.0	5	530	m.q.

[1] *Prepared with whole milk and salted butter.*
[2] *Prepared with skim milk, without butter.*

Food and Measure	cal.	prot. (gms)	carbo. (gms)	fat (gms)	chol. (mgs)	sod. (mgs)	fiber (gms)
Macaroni entree mix, and cheese *(cont.)*							
(Kraft Family Size Dinner), 3/4 cup	290	9.0	34.0	13.0	5	490	m.q.
Parmesan *(Fantastic Foods)*[1]	162	6.0	21.0	6.0	m.q.	340	2.6 d
Parmesan *(Fantastic Foods)*[2]	113	6.0	20.0	1.0	2	295	2.6 d
rotini, w/broccoli *(Velveeta)*	210	10.0	24.0	8.0	25	730	m.q.
shells *(Velveeta* Dinner), 3/4 cup . . .	210	10.0	25.0	8.0	20	570	m.q.
shells, w/bacon *(Velveeta* Bits of Bacon)	240	11.0	27.0	10.0	25	690	m.q.
shells, Mexican *(Velveeta* Touch of Mexico)	210	10.0	27.0	8.0	20	630	m.q.
spiral *(Kraft* Dinner), 3/4 cup	340	9.0	36.0	18.0	10	600	m.q.
salad, creamy *(Suddenly Salad)*	180	4.0	21.0	9.0	n.a.	280	m.q.
Mace, ground, 1 tsp.	8	.1	.9	.6	0	1	.3 d
Mackerel, meat only:							
Atlantic:							
raw, 4 oz.	232	21.1	0	15.8	80	102	0
baked, broiled, or microwaved, 4 oz.	297	27.0	0	20.2	85	94	0
king:							
raw, 4 oz.	119	23.0	0	2.3	61	179	0
baked, broiled, or microwaved, 4 oz.	152	29.5	0	2.9	77	230	0
Pacific and jack:							
raw, 4 oz.	179	22.8	0	9.0	53	98	0
baked, broiled, or microwaved, 4 oz.	228	29.2	0	11.5	68	125	0

[1] *Prepared with whole milk and salted butter.*

[2] *Prepared with skim milk, without butter.*

Food and Measure	cal.	prot. (gms)	carbo. (gms)	fat (gms)	chol. (mgs)	sod. (mgs)	fiber (gms)
Spanish:							
raw, 4 oz.	158	21.9	0	7.2	86	67	0
baked, broiled, or							
microwaved, 4 oz.	179	26.8	0	7.2	83	75	0
Mackerel, canned,							
jack, drained, 4 oz.	177	26.3	0	7.1	90	430	0
Mahi mahi, see "Dolphin fish"							
Mai tai mixer (Holland House):							
bottled, 4.5 fl. oz. . . .	144	<1.0	36.0	<1.0	0	270	(0)
instant, .56 oz.	64	<1.0	16.0	<1.0	0	4	(0)
Malt cooler (Bartles & Jaymes), 6 fl. oz.:							
berry	103	<.1	16.2	.1	0	2	0
berry, light	74	<.1	15.6	.1	0	1	0
cherry, black	97	.1	15.0	.1	0	2	0
cherry, black, light . .	71	<.1	14.4	.1	0	1	0
peach	103	<.1	16.2	.1	0	2	0
strawberry	100	<.1	15.6	.1	0	2	0
tropical	110	<.1	18.0	.1	0	2	0
tropical light	75	<.1	15.6	.1	0	1	0
Malted milk powder, 3 heaping tsp.:							
(Carnation Original)	90	2.0	16.0	2.0	4	105	m.q.
natural	87	2.3	15.9	1.7	4	103	.1 d
chocolate	79	1.1	18.4	.8	1	53	.2 d
chocolate (Carnation)	80	1.0	18.0	1.0	1	55	m.q.
Mammy apple, peeled, seeded, 1 oz.	14	.1	3.5	.1	0	4	.9 d
Manicotti entree, frozen:							
cheese (Healthy Choice), 9.25 oz.	220	15.0	34.0	3.0	30	310	m.q.
vegetable, marinara (On-Cor), 8 oz. . .	200	12.0	26.0	6.0	n.a.	1070	m.q.

Food and Measure	cal.	prot. (gms)	carbo. (gms)	fat (gms)	chol. (mgs)	sod. (mgs)	fiber (gms)
Mango:							
10.6-oz. fruit	135	1.1	35.2	.6	0	4	3.7 d
peeled *(Frieda's)*, 1 oz.	19	.2	4.8	.1	0	2	m.q.
peeled, sliced, 1/2 cup	54	.4	14.0	.2	0	2	1.5 d
Mango flavored drink							
mix* *(Tang)*, 6 fl. oz.	80	0	20.0	0	0	0	0
Mango nectar:							
(Kern's), 6 fl. oz. . . .	110	0	28.0	0	0	0	m.q.
(Libby's), 6 fl. oz. . .	110	0	26.0	0	0	0	m.q.
Mango-peach juice							
(R.W. Knudsen),							
8 fl. oz.	110	<1.0	29.0	<1.0	0	(0)	m.q.
Manhattan mixer,							
bottled *(Holland*							
House), 1 fl. oz. . .	28	<1.0	7.0	<1.0	0	5	0
Manicotti, frozen							
(Celentano), 7 oz.	410	19.0	31.0	19.0	100	630	7.0 d
Manicotti entree, fro-							
zen, 10 oz., except							
as noted:							
(Celentano Great							
Choice)	250	16.0	41.0	2.5	20	650	3.0 d
cheese:							
(Weight Watchers),							
9.25 oz.	260	17.0	31.0	8.0	25	510	m.q.
(The Budget Gour-							
met)	440	20.0	36.0	24.0	75	740	m.q.
Florentine *(Celentano*							
Great Choice) . . .	210	15.0	29.0	6.0	35	600	5.0 d
w/sauce *(Celentano)*	450	24.0	41.0	21.0	85	910	9.0 d
Maple sugar, see							
"Sugar, maple"							
Maple syrup, 1 tbsp.:							
(Cary's/Maple							
Orchards/MacDon-							
ald's)	50	0	13.0	<1.0	0	<5	0
imitation *(Cary's* Sugar							
Free)	10	0	2.0	0	0	20	0

Food and Measure	cal.	prot. (gms)	carbo. (gms)	fat (gms)	chol. (mgs)	sod. (mgs)	fiber (gms)
Margarine, 1 tbsp., except as noted:							
(Diet *Mazola*)	50	0	0	6.0	0	130	0
(*Land O'Lakes*)	100	0	0	11.0	0	100	0
(*Mazola*)	100	0	0	11.0	0	100	0
(*Parkay*)	100	0	0	11.0	0	105	0
blend, see "spreads," below:							
safflower (*Hain*) . . .	100	0	0	11.0	0	170	0
safflower (*Hain* Unsalted)	100	0	0	11.0	0	<5	0
soft:							
(*Chiffon* Cup) . . .	90	0	0	10.0	0	95	0
(*Chiffon* Stick) . . .	100	0	0	11.0	0	105	0
(*Chiffon* Unsalted)	90	0	0	10.0	0	0	0
(Diet *Parkay*)	50	0	0	6.0	0	110	0
(*Nucoa*)	90	0	0	10.0	0	150	0
(*Parkay*)	100	0	0	11.0	0	105	0
spread:							
(*Country Cottage Farms* Extra Light)	45	0	2.0	4.0	0	75	0
(*Country Cottage Farms* Extra Light Unsalted)	50	0	0	6.0	0	0	0
(*Country Cottage Farms* Light) . . .	60	0	0	7.0	0	130	0
(*Country Morning* Light)	70	0	0	7.0	10	85	0
(*Country Morning* Stick)	100	0	0	11.0	10	100	0
(*Country Morning* Soft)	90	0	0	10.0	10	80	0
(*Kraft* Touch of Butter Bowl)	50	0	0	6.0	0	110	0
(*Kraft* Touch of Butter Stick)	90	0	0	10.0	0	110	0
(*Land O'Lakes* Soft)	80	0	0	8.0	0	80	0
(*Land O'Lakes* Stick)	100	0	0	11.0	0	95	0

Food and Measure	cal.	prot. (gms)	carbo. (gms)	fat (gms)	chol. (mgs)	sod. (mgs)	fiber (gms)
Margarine, spread *(cont.)*							
(Land O'Lakes Un-							
salted Stick) . . .	100	0	0	11.0	0	0	0
(Nucanola 52% Soft)	70	0	0	7.0	0	90	0
(Nucanola 64%							
Stick)	80	0	0	9.0	0	90	0
(Parkay 50% Vege-							
table Oil)	60	0	0	7.0	0	110	0
squeeze *(Parkay)* . . .	90	0	0	10.0	0	110	0
whipped:							
(Chiffon)	70	0	0	8.0	0	80	0
(Miracle Brand Cup)	60	0	0	7.0	0	70	0
(Miracle Brand Stick)	70	0	0	7.0	0	65	0
(Parkay Cup)	70	0	0	7.0	0	70	0
(Parkay Stick) . . .	70	0	0	7.0	0	65	0
Margarita mixer:							
bottled *(Holland*							
House), 3 fl. oz. . . .	72	<1.0	18.0	<1.0	0	276	(0)
bottled, strawberry							
(Holland House),							
3.5 fl. oz.	98	<1.0	24.0	<1.0	0	10	(0)
frozen, w/liquor* *(Ba-*							
cardi), 7 fl. oz. . . .	160	0	24.0	0	0	5	(0)
instant *(Holland*							
House), .56 oz. dry	56	<1.0	14.0	<1.0	0	4	(0)
instant, strawberry							
(Holland House),							
.56 oz. dry	64	<1.0	16.0	<1.0	0	<1	(0)
Marinade, see spe-							
cific listings							
Marjoram, dried,							
1 tsp.	2	.1	.4	<.1	0	tr.	.1 d
Marmalade, see "Jam							
and preserves"							
Marrow squash, raw,							
trimmed, 1 oz. . . .	4	.2	1.0	<.1	0	n.a.	.1 c

Food and Measure	cal.	prot. (gms)	carbo. (gms)	fat (gms)	chol. (mgs)	sod. (mgs)	fiber (gms)
Marshmallow topping:							
(Smucker's), 2 tbsp.	120	0	29.0	0	0	0	0
creme (Kraft), 1 oz.	90	0	23.0	0	0	20	0
plain or raspberry (Marshmallow Fluff), 1 heaping tsp. . . .	60	0	15.0	0	0	20	0
Matzo, see "Crackers"							
Matzo meal, see "Cracker crumbs and meal"							
Mayonnaise, 1 tbsp.:							
(Bennett's Real) . . .	110	0	1.0	12.0	m.q.	65	0
(Blue Plate)	100	0	0	11.0	10	80	0
(Cains All Natural) . .	100	0	0	11.0	5	75	0
(Hain)	110	0	0	12.0	5	70	0
(Hain Light Low Sodium)	60	0	2.0	6.0	10	95	0
(Hain Real No Salt)	110	0	0	12.0	5	5	0
(Hellman's/Best Foods)	100	0	0	11.0	5	80	0
(Hellman's/Best Foods Light)	50	0	1.0	5.0	5	115	0
(Kraft)	100	0	0	12.0	5	70	0
(Kraft Light)	50	0	1.0	5.0	0	110	0
(Master Choice) . . .	100	0	0	12.0	5	80	0
(Rokeach)	100	0	0	11.0	10	70	0
(Smartbeat Fat Free)	10	0	3.0	0	0	115	0
canola (Hain)	100	0	<1.0	11.0	5	100	0
canola (Hain Reduced Calorie)	60	0	2.0	5.0	0	160	0
canola, corn, or soy (Smartbeat Light)	40	0	1.0	4.0	0	110	0
cholesterol free (Hellmann's)	50	0	1.0	5.0	0	80	0
eggless (Hain No Salt)	110	0	0	12.0	0	<5	0
safflower (Hain) . . .	110	0	0	12.0	5	70	0

Food and Measure	cal.	prot. (gms)	carbo. (gms)	fat (gms)	chol. (mgs)	sod. (mgs)	fiber (gms)
Mayonnaise *(cont.)*							
soy *(Featherweight Soyamaise)*	100	0	0	11.0	5	3	0
tofu *(Nasoya Nayonaise)*	35	0	1.0	3.0	0	100	(0)
McDonald's, 1 serving:							
breakfast biscuit:							
w/bacon, egg, and cheese	440	15.0	33.0	26.0	240	1215	m.q.
w/biscuit spread . .	260	5.0	32.0	13.0	1	730	m.q.
w/sausage	420	12.0	32.0	28.0	44	1040	m.q.
w/sausage and egg	505	19.0	33.0	33.0	260	1210	m.q.
breakfast dishes:							
burrito	280	12.0	21.0	17.0	135	580	m.q.
eggs, scrambled . .	140	12.0	1.0	10.0	425	290	0
hash browns	130	1.0	15.0	7.0	0	330	m.q.
hotcakes, w/syrup and margarine . .	440	8.0	74.0	12.0	8	685	m.q.
sausage	160	7.0	0	15.0	43	310	0
breakfast muffin:							
Egg McMuffin . . .	280	18.0	28.0	11.0	235	710	m.q.
English, w/spread .	170	5.0	26.0	4.0	0	285	m.q.
Sausage McMuffin	345	15.0	27.0	20.0	57	770	m.q.
Sausage McMuffin, w/egg	430	21.0	27.0	25.0	270	920	m.q.
danish:							
apple	390	6.0	51.0	17.0	25	370	m.q.
cinnamon raisin . .	440	6.0	58.0	21.0	34	430	m.q.
iced cheese	390	7.0	42.0	21.0	47	420	m.q.
raspberry	410	6.0	62.0	16.0	26	310	m.q.
muffin, fat-free apple bran	180	5.0	40.0	0	0	200	m.q.
sandwiches:							
Big Mac	500	25.0	42.0	26.0	100	890	m.q.
cheeseburger . . .	305	15.0	30.0	13.0	50	725	m.q.
chicken fajita . . .	190	11.0	20.0	8.0	35	310	m.q.
Filet-O-Fish	370	14.0	38.0	18.0	50	730	m.q.

Food and Measure	cal.	prot. (gms)	carbo. (gms)	fat (gms)	chol. (mgs)	sod. (mgs)	fiber (gms)
hamburger	255	12.0	30.0	9.0	37	490	m.q.
McChicken	415	19.0	39.0	20.0	50	830	m.q.
McLean Deluxe . .	320	22.0	35.0	10.0	60	670	m.q.
McLean Deluxe,							
w/cheese	370	24.0	35.0	14.0	75	890	m.q.
McRib	460	26.0	44.0	20.0	55	1020	m.q.
Quarter Pounder	410	23.0	34.0	20.0	85	645	m.q.
Quarter Pounder,							
w/cheese	510	28.0	34.0	28.0	115	1110	m.q.
Chicken McNuggets:							
4 piece	180	13.0	11.0	10.0	35	390	m.q.
6 piece	270	20.0	17.0	15.0	55	580	m.q.
9 piece	405	30.0	25.0	22.0	85	870	m.q.
McNuggets sauces:							
barbeque, 1.12 oz.	50	0	12.0	.5	0	340	n.a.
honey, .5 oz. . . .	45	0	12.0	0	0	0	0
hot mustard,							
1.05 oz.	70	0	8.0	3.6	5	250	n.a.
sweet and sour,							
1.12 oz.	60	0	14.0	.2	0	190	n.a.
french fries:							
small	220	3.0	26.0	12.0	0	110	m.q.
medium	320	4.0	36.0	17.0	0	150	m.q.
large	400	6.0	46.0	22.0	0	200	m.q.
salads:							
chef	170	17.0	8.0	9.0	111	400	m.q.
chicken, chunky . .	150	25.0	7.0	4.0	78	230	m.q.
garden	50	4.0	6.0	2.0	65	70	m.q.
side	30	2.0	4.0	1.0	33	35	m.q.
salad dressing:							
blue cheese, 1/5 pkt.	50	0	1.0	4.0	7	150	n.a.
ranch, 1/4 pkt. . . .	55	0	1.0	5.0	5	130	n.a.
red French, reduced							
calorie, 1/4 pkt.	40	0	5.0	2.0	0	115	n.a.
Thousand Island,							
1/5 pkt.	45	0	4.0	3.0	8	100	n.a.
vinaigrette, lite,							
1/4 pkt.	12	0	2.0	.5	0	60	n.a.

Food and Measure	cal.	prot. (gms)	carbo. (gms)	fat (gms)	chol. (mgs)	sod. (mgs)	fiber (gms)
McDonald's *(cont.)*							
pies and cookies:							
baked apple pie . .	280	3.0	35.0	15.0	0	90	m.q.
cookies, Chocolaty							
Chip	330	4.0	42.0	15.0	4	280	m.q.
cookies, *McDonald-*							
land	290	4.0	47.0	9.0	0	300	m.q.
shakes, lowfat:							
chocolate	320	11.0	66.0	1.7	10	240	(0)
strawberry	320	11.0	67.0	1.3	10	170	(0)
vanilla	290	11.0	60.0	1.3	10	170	0
yogurt, frozen, lowfat:							
cone, vanilla	105	4.0	22.0	1.0	3	80	m.q.
sundae, hot caramel	270	7.0	59.0	3.0	13	180	n.a.
sundae, hot fudge	240	7.0	50.0	3.0	6	170	(0)
sundae, strawberry	210	6.0	49.0	1.0	5	95	(0)
Meat, see specific list-ings							
Meat, potted, canned:							
(Hormel), 1 oz.	53	4.0	<2.0	4.0	23	280	0
(Libby's), 1.83 oz. . .	110	7.0	0	9.0	m.q.	320	0
"Meat" loaf, vegetar-ian, mix:							
(LaLoma Savory Din-ner Loaf), 1/4 cup	50	9.0	4.0	0	0	380	m.q.
(Natural Touch), 4 oz.	180	21.0	7.0	7.0	0	25	m.q.
Meat loaf dinner, fro-zen:							
(Armour Classics), 11.25 oz.	360	20.0	32.0	17.0	65	1170	m.q.
(Banquet Extra Help-ing), 16.25 oz. . . .	640	30.0	60.0	34.0	85	3320	m.q.
(Freezer Queen), 9.5 oz.	260	13.0	23.0	13.0	20	810	m.q.
(Swanson 4 Compart-ment), 10 oz. . . .	370	15.0	38.0	18.0	m.q.	930	m.q.
(Swanson Hungry Man), 16.5 oz.	660	30.0	60.0	33.0	m.q.	1850	m.q.

Food and Measure	cal.	prot. (gms)	carbo. (gms)	fat (gms)	chol. (mgs)	sod. (mgs)	fiber (gms)
Meat loaf entree, frozen:							
(Banquet Healthy Balance), 11 oz. . . .	270	15.0	36.0	7.0	30	800	m.q.
(Banquet Meals), 9.5 oz.	340	11.0	32.0	19.0	35	1220	m.q.
(On-Cor), 8 oz.	518	25.0	15.0	40.0	m.q.	1860	m.q.
gravy, whipped potato (Stouffer's Homestyle), 9⅞ oz. . . .	360	20.0	20.0	35.0	m.q.	970	m.q.
w/macaroni and cheese (Lean Cuisine), 9⅜ oz. . . .	280	26.0	26.0	8.0	55	540	m.q.
w/tomato sauce (Banquet Entree Express), 7 oz.	330	16.0	16.0	22.0	m.q.	1330	m.q.
Meat loaf seasoning mix:							
(French's), 1/7 pkg. . .	14	1.0	3.0	0	0	690	n.a.
(French's Roasting Bag), 1/6 pkg. . . .	20	2.0	3.0	0	0	490	n.a.
(Lawry's Seasoning Blends), 1 pkg. . .	355	15.5	64.5	1.2	0	6547	1.8 c
(McCormick/Schilling Bag'n Season), 1 pkg.	111	.6	26.0	.7	n.a.	3090	m.q.
Meat marinade mix (French's), 1/16 pkg.	4	0	1.0	0	0	270	n.a.
Meat tenderizer, unseasoned (Tone's), 1 tsp.	7	0	1.2	.2	0	1760	tr.d
"Meatball," vegetarian:							
canned (LaLoma Tender Rounds), 6 pieces	120	15.0	7.0	4.0	0	310	m.q.

Food and Measure	cal.	prot. (gms)	carbo. (gms)	fat (gms)	chol. (mgs)	sod. (mgs)	fiber (gms)
"Meatball," vegetarian *(cont.)*							
canned *(Worthington Non-Meat Balls)*, 3 pieces	100	6.0	5.0	6.0	0	210	m.q.
frozen *(LaLoma Savory Meatballs)*, 7 pieces	190	22.0	7.0	8.0	0	420	m.q.
Meatball dinner, Swedish, frozen *(Armour Classics)*, 11.25 oz.	330	19.0	23.0	18.0	80	1140	m.q.
Meatball entree, Swedish, frozen:							
(On-Cor), 8 oz.	295	21.0	7.0	21.0	m.q.	1500	n.a.
in cream sauce *(Swanson)*, 8.5 oz.	350	18.0	26.0	19.0	m.q.	740	m.q.
in gravy w/pasta *(Lean Cuisine)*, 9 1/8 oz. . .	290	23.0	31.0	8.0	55	550	m.q.
in gravy w/parsley noodles *(Stouffer's)*, 9.25 oz.	490	22.0	42.0	26.0	m.q.	790	m.q.
w/noodles *(The Budget Gourmet)*, 10 oz.	590	24.0	37.0	38.0	145	920	m.q.
sauce and *(Dining Lite)*, 9 oz.	280	14.0	34.0	10.0	55	660	m.q.
Meatball seasoning mix, Swedish *(McCormick/Schilling)*, 1/4 pkg.	57	2.0	11.0	1.0	n.a.	1054	n.a.
Meatball stew, canned, *(Dinty Moore)*, 8 oz. . . .	240	11.0	14.0	16.0	30	980	m.q.
Melon balls, cantaloupe and honeydew, frozen, 1/2 cup	28	.7	6.9	.2	0	27	.6 d
Menudo seasoning mix *(Gebhardt)*, 1 tsp.	5	<1.0	1.0	<1.0	0	310	<1.0 d

Food and Measure	cal.	prot. (gms)	carbo. (gms)	fat (gms)	chol. (mgs)	sod. (mgs)	fiber (gms)
Mesquite marinade							
(Lawry's), 2 tbsp.	24	3.0	3.0	.4	0	4142	.1 c
Mesquite seasoning							
(Tone's), 1 tsp. . . .	13	.1	3.2	<.1	0	467	n.a.
Mexican bean,							
canned, 1/2 cup:							
(Allens/Brown Beauty)	140	8.0	24.0	<1.0	0	330	5.0 d
(Old El Paso Mexe-							
Beans)	163	10.0	31.0	1.0	0	627	13.0 d
Mexican bean dip							
(Hain), 4 tbsp. . . .	60	4.0	9.0	1.0	5	260	n.a.
Mexican dinner, fro-							
zen (see also spe-							
cific listings):							
(Patio Fiesta), 12 oz.	460	16.0	54.0	20.0	30	1990	m.q.
(Swanson Hungry							
Man), 20 oz.	820	25.0	88.0	41.0	m.q.	2080	m.q.
style:							
(Banquet Extra							
Helping), 19 oz.	680	25.0	102.0	25.0	5	3930	m.q.
(Patio), 13.25 oz.	540	15.0	64.0	25.0	45	1940	m.q.
combination (Swan-							
son 4 Compart-							
ment), 13.25 oz.	490	19.0	61.0	18.0	m.q.	1680	m.q.
Mexican entree, fro-							
zen:							
combination (Banquet							
Meals), 11 oz. . . .	380	14.0	54.0	12.0	15	1340	m.q.
style (Banquet Meals),							
11 oz.	410	12.0	53.0	17.0	20	1330	m.q.
Mexican seasoning:							
(Tone's), 1 tsp.	6	.3	1.3	.1	tr.	4185	.4 d
rice (Lawry's Season-							
ing Blends), 1 pkg.	94	3.9	17.0	2.0	0	3246	2.1 c
Milk, 8 fl. oz., except							
as noted:							
buttermilk, cultured	99	8.1	11.7	2.2	9	257	0
whole, 3.3% fat . . .	150	8.0	11.4	8.2	33	120	0

Food and Measure	cal.	prot. (gms)	carbo. (gms)	fat (gms)	chol. (mgs)	sod. (mgs)	fiber (gms)
Milk *(cont.)*							
lowfat:							
2% fat	121	8.1	11.7	4.7	18	122	0
2%, protein fortified	137	9.7	13.5	4.9	19	145	0
1% fat	102	8.0	11.7	2.6	10	123	0
1%, protein fortified	119	9.7	13.6	2.9	10	143	0
skim	86	8.4	11.9	.4	4	126	0
Milk, canned:							
condensed, sweet:							
1 tbsp.	61	1.5	10.4	1.7	6	24	0
(Borden), 1/3 cup	320	7.0	54.0	8.0	m.q.	115	0
(Carnation), 1/3 cup	320	7.0	56.0	8.0	24	110	0
(Eagle/Meadow							
Gold), 3 tbsp. . . .	190	4.0	32.0	5.0	25	65	0
filled dairy blend							
(Magnolia), 3 tbsp.	190	4.0	33.0	5.0	<5	60	0
evaporated, 1/2 cup:							
(Carnation)	170	8.0	12.0	10.0	37	135	0
(Pet/Dairymate) . .	170	8.0	12.0	10.0	36	140	0
filled *(Pet/Dairymate)*	150	8.0	12.0	8.0	5	140	0
imitation, filled							
(Diehl)	150	8.0	12.0	8.0	5	135	0
lowfat *(Carnation)*	110	8.0	12.0	3.0	10	140	0
skim *(Carnation* Lite)	100	9.0	14.0	<1.0	5	150	0
skim *(Pet/Dairymate*							
Light)	100	9.0	14.0	<1.0	5	150	0
Milk, chocolate, see							
"Chocolate milk"							
Milk, dry:							
buttermilk:							
sweet cream, 1 cup	464	41.2	58.8	6.9	83	621	0
sweet cream,							
1 tbsp.	25	2.2	3.2	.4	5	34	0
whole, 1 oz.	141	7.5	10.9	7.6	27	105	0
whole, 1 cup	635	33.7	49.2	34.2	124	475	0
nonfat:							
regular, 1 cup . . .	435	43.4	62.4	.9	24	642	0
instant, 3.2-oz. pkt.	244	23.9	35.5	.5	12	373	0

Food and Measure	cal.	prot. (gms)	carbo. (gms)	fat (gms)	chol. (mgs)	sod. (mgs)	fiber (gms)
instant *(Carnation)*, 5 level tbsp. . . .	80	8.0	12.0	0	5	125	0
Milk, goat's, 1 cup	168	8.7	10.9	10.1	28	122	0
"Milk," imitation:							
fluid[1], 1 cup	150	4.3	15.0	8.3	tr.	191	0
soy, see "Soy milk"							
Milk, sheep's, 1 cup	264	14.7	13.1	17.2	m.q.	108	0
Milk beverage, see "Milk shake" and specific flavors							
Milkfish, meat only:							
raw, 4 oz.	168	23.3	0	7.6	59	m.q.	0
baked, broiled or microwaved, 4 oz. . .	215	29.8	0	9.8	76	m.q.	0
Milk shake, frozen, chocolate *(MicroMagic)*, 1 shake . .	290	7.0	46.0	8.0	40	90	(0)
Milk shake mix *(Weight Watchers)*:							
chocolate fudge, 1 pkt.	70	6.0	11.0	<1.0	n.a.	150	n.a.
orange sherbet, 1 pkt.	70	6.0	12.0	<1.0	n.a.	210	n.a.
Millet:							
raw, 1 oz.	107	3.1	20.7	1.2	0	1	2.4 d
cooked, 4 oz.	135	4.0	26.8	1.1	0	2	1.5 d
hulled, raw *(Arrowhead Mills)*, 1 oz.	90	3.0	21.0	1.0	0	tr.	1.8 d
Millet flour *(Arrowhead Mills)*, 2 oz.	185	6.0	41.0	2.0	0	1	3.7 d
Mincemeat, see "Pie filling"							
Miso:							
1 oz.	58	3.3	7.9	1.7	0	1034	1.5 d
1/2 cup	284	16.3	38.6	8.4	0	5032	7.6 d

---

[1] *Containing a blend of hydrogenated vegetable oils.*

Food and Measure	cal.	prot. (gms)	carbo. (gms)	fat (gms)	chol. (mgs)	sod. (mgs)	fiber (gms)
Molasses, 1 tbsp., except as noted:							
bead *(La Choy)*, 1/2 tsp.	7	<1.0	2.0	<1.0	0	1	0
dark *(Brer Rabbit)* . .	60	0	14.0	0	0	15	0
gold *(Grandma's)* . :	68	<1.0	17.0	<1.0	0	28	0
green *(Grandma's)* . .	68	<1.0	17.0	<1.0	0	57	0
light *(Brer Rabbit)* . .	60	0	14.0	0	0	10	0
Monkfish, meat only:							
raw, 4 oz.	86	16.4	0	1.7	29	21	0
baked, broiled, or microwaved, 4 oz. . . .	110	21.0	0	2.2	36	26	0
Monosodium glutamate *(Tone's)*, 1 tsp.	0	0	0	0	0	638	0
Mortadella, beef and pork, 1 oz.	88	4.6	.9	7.2	16	353	0
Mostaccioli entree, frozen:							
w/meat sauce *(Banquet Family)*, 7 oz.	170	7.0	28.0	3.0	m.q.	m.q.	m.q.
w/meatballs *(On-Cor)*, 8 oz.	220	8.0	30.0	8.0	m.q.	1090	m.q.
Mothbean, boiled, 4 oz.	133	8.9	23.8	.6	0	11	1.5 c
Mother's loaf, pork, 1 oz.	80	3.4	2.1	6.3	13	320	(0)
Mousse, frozen *(Weight Watchers Sweet Celebrations)*, 1 serving:							
chocolate	150	6.0	26.0	3.0	5	160	n.a.
chocolate caramel, triple	170	4.0	31.0	4.0	5	120	n.a.
praline pecan	160	5.0	25.0	4.0	5	140	n.a.

Food and Measure	cal.	prot. (gms)	carbo. (gms)	fat (gms)	chol. (mgs)	sod. (mgs)	fiber (gms)
Mousse mix *(Knorr),* 1 serving dry:							
dark chocolate	75	1.1	8.2	4.1	0	37	n.a.
milk chocolate	80	1.1	9.9	4.2	0	40	n.a.
white chocolate . . .	70	.9	8.2	3.5	0	40	n.a.
Muffin, 1 piece, except as noted:							
(Arnold Bran'nola) . .	160	6.0	30.0	1.0	0	220	2.0 d
(Arnold Extra Crisp)	130	4.0	26.0	1.0	0	230	1.0 d
apple:							
(Awrey's), 1.5 oz.	130	2.0	17.0	6.0	20	210	0
spice *(Health Valley)*	130	4.0	30.0	<1.0	0	110	5.1 d
streusel *(Awrey's)*	340	6.0	50.0	13.0	35	540	1.0 d
streusel *(Hostess 97% Fat Free)* . .	100	1.0	23.0	1.0	0	160	1.0 d
banana:							
(Health Valley) . . .	130	4.0	29.0	<1.0	0	110	4.5 d
nut *(Awrey's Grande)*	370	4.0	55.0	15.0	30	400	1.0 d
walnut, mini *(Hostess),* 5 pieces . .	260	3.0	27.0	16.0	40	160	.6 d
blueberry:							
(Awrey's), 1.5 oz.	130	2.0	18.0	5.0	10	180	1.0 d
(Awrey's Grande)	360	5.0	52.0	14.0	35	480	2.0 d
(Hostess 97% Fat Free)	100	2.0	21.0	1.0	0	160	1.0 d
apple *(Health Valley Twin Pack)* . . .	140	4.0	32.0	<1.0	0	100	5.0 d
mini *(Hostess),* 5 pieces	240	3.0	29.0	13.0	40	180	.7 d
carrot *(Health Valley Twin Pack)*	130	4.0	30.0	<1.0	0	110	5.0 d
cinnamon apple, mini *(Hostess),* 5 pieces	160	2.0	17.0	9.0	0	100	m.q.
cranberry *(Awrey's)*	120	2.0	20.0	4.0	10	210	0
corn *(Awrey's),* 1.5 oz.	130	2.0	20.0	5.0	15	270	0
English:							
(Pepperidge Farm)	140	5.0	27.0	1.0	0	220	m.q.

Food and Measure	cal.	prot. (gms)	carbo. (gms)	fat (gms)	chol. (mgs)	sod. (mgs)	fiber (gms)
Muffin, English *(cont.)*							
(Roman Meal) . . .	134	5.7	24.6	1.2	0	329	2.5 d
(Tastykake)	130	5.0	26.0	1.0	0	240	m.q.
(Thomas')	130	4.0	25.0	1.0	0	210	1.0 d
(Wonder Rounds)	120	5.0	24.0	1.0	0	290	1.5 d
bran nut *(Thomas')*	140	5.0	23.0	3.0	0	200	4.0 d
cinnamon raisin							
(Oatmeal Goodness)	140	6.0	26.0	2.0	0	190	2.1 d
cinnamon raisin *(Pepperidge Farm)* . . .	150	4.0	29.0	2.0	0	200	m.q.
cinnamon raisin *(Tastykake)*	150	4.0	31.0	1.0	0	150	m.q.
cinnamon–raisin bran *(Pepperidge Farm Wholesome Choice)*	120	5.0	28.0	1.0	0	120	4.0 d
honey & oatmeal *(Oatmeal Goodness)*	140	6.0	24.0	2.0	0	210	1.6 d
honey wheat *(Thomas')*	120	5.0	21.0	1.0	0	200	3.0 d
oat bran *(Thomas',* 12 pk.)	120	4.0	26.0	1.0	0	210	3.0 d
onion *(Thomas')* . . .	130	4.0	27.0	1.0	0	190	2.0 d
raisin *(Thomas')* . . .	150	4.0	30.0	1.0	0	200	2.0 d
raisin *(Wonder* Rounds)	140	4.0	26.0	2.0	0	220	1.6 d
rye *(Thomas')*	120	5.0	24.0	1.0	0	210	3.0 d
sandwich size *(Thomas')*	210	7.0	42.0	2.0	0	330	2.0 d
sourdough *(Tastykake)*	130	5.0	25.0	1.0	0	210	m.q.
sourdough *(Thomas')*	130	4.0	26.0	1.0	0	220	2.0 d
sourdough *(Wonder* Rounds)	120	5.0	24.0	1.0	0	240	1.6 d
white, country *(Pepperidge Farm Wholesome Choice)*	130	5.0	26.0	1.0	0	150	2.0 d
oat bran:							
(Hostess)	160	2.0	21.0	7.0	0	150	1.5 d

Food and Measure	cal.	prot. (gms)	carbo. (gms)	fat (gms)	chol. (mgs)	sod. (mgs)	fiber (gms)
almond date (Health Valley Fancy Fruit)	140	4.0	31.0	<1.0	0	80	8.2 d
banana´nut (Hostess)	140	2.0	20.0	5.0	0	160	1.0 d
blueberry (Health Valley Fancy Fruit)	140	4.0	32.0	<1.0	0	100	7.5 d
raisin (Health Valley Fancy Fruit) . . .	140	4.0	31.0	<1.0	0	90	7.7 d
raisin:							
(Arnold)	160	6.0	33.0	1.0	0	220	2.0 d
bran (Awrey's), 1.5 oz.	110	2.0	18.0	4.0	15	170	1.0 d
bran (Awrey's Grande)	320	5.0	50.0	12.0	35	470	3.0 d
raspberry (Health Valley Twin Pack) . . .	130	4.0	30.0	<1.0	0	110	5.0 d
sourdough (Arnold)	130	4.0	25.0	1.0	0	250	1.0 d
Muffin, frozen or refrigerated, 1 piece:							
apple oatmeal (Pepperidge Farm Wholesome Choice)	120	4.0	28.0	4.0	0	190	3.0 d
apple spice (Healthy Choice)	190	3.0	40.0	4.0	0	90	m.q.
banana nut:							
(Healthy Choice) . .	180	3.0	32.0	6.0	0	80	m.q.
(Weight Watchers)	170	3.0	32.0	5.0	10	250	m.q.
blueberry:							
(Healthy Choice) . .	190	3.0	39.0	4.0	0	110	m.q.
(Pepperidge Farm Wholesome Choice)	130	3.0	27.0	2.0	0	190	2.0 d
(Weight Watchers)	170	3.0	32.0	5.0	10	220	m.q.
bran, harvest honey (Weight Watchers)	160	3.0	32.0	4.0	5	150	m.q.
corn (Pepperidge Farm Wholesome Choice)	150	4.0	28.0	3.0	0	180	1.0 d

Food and Measure	cal.	prot. (gms)	carbo. (gms)	fat (gms)	chol. (mgs)	sod. (mgs)	fiber (gms)
Muffin, frozen or refrigerated *(cont.)*							
English:							
(Roman Meal) . . .	132	4.6	28.7	1.0	0	190	2.6 d
honey nut oat bran							
(Roman Meal) . .	161	4.9	31.5	2.7	0	228	2.2 d
raisin bran *(Pepper-*							
idge Farm Whole-							
some Choice) . . .	140	4.0	30.0	2.0	0	260	4.0 d
Muffin mix*, 1 piece:							
apple cinnamon:							
(Betty Crocker) . .	120	2.0	18.0	4.0	25	140	m.q.
(Robin Hood/Gold							
Medal Pouch) . .	170	3.0	24.0	7.0	35	220	m.q.
banana *(Robin Hood/*							
Gold Medal Pouch)	170	3.0	22.0	8.0	35	200	m.q.
banana nut *(Betty*							
Crocker)	120	2.0	18.0	4.0	20	150	m.q.
blueberry:							
(Betty Crocker Twice							
the Blueberries)	120	2.0	18.0	4.0	20	140	m.q.
(Duncan Hines) . .	120	2.0	21.0	3.0	n.a.	185	m.q.
(Duncan Hines							
Bakery Style) . .	190	2.0	32.0	6.0	n.a.	250	m.q.
(Pillsbury Lovin'							
Lites)	100	3.0	21.0	1.0	0	160	m.q.
(Robin Hood/Gold							
Medal Pouch) . .	170	3.0	25.0	6.0	m.q.	240	m.q.
wild *(Betty Crocker)*	120	2.0	19.0	4.0	20	150	m.q.
wild *(Betty Crocker*							
Light)	90	2.0	20.0	1.0	20	140	m.q.
caramel *(Robin Hood/*							
Gold Medal Pouch)	170	3.0	24.0	7.0	35	240	m.q.
cinnamon streusel							
(Betty Crocker) . .	200	3.0	27.0	9.0	25	240	m.q.
cinnamon swirl							
(Duncan Hines							
Bakery Style) . . .	200	2.0	32.0	7.0	n.a.	245	m.q.

Food and Measure	cal.	prot. (gms)	carbo. (gms)	fat (gms)	chol. (mgs)	sod. (mgs)	fiber (gms)
corn:							
(Dromedary)	120	3.0	20.0	4.0	n.a.	270	m.q.
(Robin Hood/Gold Medal Pouch) . .	180	3.0	27.0	7.0	m.q.	310	m.q.
blue (Arrowhead Mills)	110	4.0	15.0	4.0	tr.	m.q.	2.6 d
honey bran (Robin Hood/Gold Medal Pouch)	170	5.0	25.0	5.0	m.q.	240	m.q.
oat bran:							
(Arrowhead Mills Wheat Free) . . .	100	5.0	11.0	5.0	tr.	m.q.	4.5 d
(Betty Crocker) . .	180	4.0	26.0	7.0	35	250	m.q.
apple spice (Arrowhead Mills) . . .	120	6.0	15.0	4.0	tr.	m.q.	5.4 d
wheat bran (Arrowhead Mills)	270	10.0	43.0	7.0	tr.	m.q.	10.5 d
Mulberry:							
10 berries, .5 oz. . .	7	.2	1.5	.1	0	2	.3 d
1/2 cup	31	1.0	6.9	.3	0	7	1.2 d
Mullet, striped, meat only:							
raw, 4 oz.	133	22.0	0	4.3	56	74	0
baked, broiled, or microwaved, 4 oz. . .	170	28.1	0	5.5	71	81	0
Mung beans:							
dry (Arrowhead Mills), 2 oz.	50	4.0	7.0	1.0	0	2	10.9 d
boiled, 1/2 cup	107	7.1	19.3	.4	0	2	7.7 d
Mung beans, sprouted, fresh:							
raw, 1 oz.	9	.9	1.7	.1	0	2	.5 d
boiled, drained, 1/2 cup	13	1.3	2.6	.1	0	6	.5 d
Mungo beans, boiled, 1/2 cup	95	6.8	16.5	.5	0	7	5.8 d

Food and Measure	cal.	prot. (gms)	carbo. (gms)	fat (gms)	chol. (mgs)	sod. (mgs)	fiber (gms)
Mushroom:							
fresh:							
raw, pieces, 1/2 cup	9	.7	1.6	.2	0	1	.4 d
boiled, drained,							
pieces, 1/2 cup	21	1.7	4.0	.4	0	2	1.7 d
canned, 1/4 cup, ex-							
cept as noted:							
all cuts (B in B) . .	12	1.0	2.0	0	0	240	1.0 d
all cuts (Green Gi-							
ant)	12	1.0	2.0	0	0	220	1.0 d
w/garlic, sliced							
(B in B)	12	1.0	2.0	0	0	200	1.0 d
in butter sauce							
(Green Giant),							
1/2 cup	30	2.0	4.0	1.0	n.a.	330	.6 d
straw (Green Giant)	12	1.0	2.0	0	0	290	1.0 d
frozen:							
whole (Birds Eye							
Deluxe), 2.6 oz.	20	2.0	4.0	0	0	0	2.0 d
battered (Qwik-							
Krisp), 7 pieces	140	3.0	13.0	8.0	20	350	1.0 d
breaded (Ore-Ida),							
2.67 oz.	120	3.0	12.0	7.0	<5	440	m.q.
breaded (Stilwell),							
5 pieces	90	3.0	13.0	2.5	0	190	2.0 d
Mushroom, enoki:							
trimmed, 1 oz.	10	.4	2.2	.1	0	1	m.q.
1 large, 4 1/8" long . .	2	.1	.4	<.1	0	tr.	m.q.
Mushroom, Japanese							
honey, trimmed							
(Frieda's), 1 oz. . .	9	.6	1.2	<.1	0	m.q.	m.q.
Mushroom, oyster,							
fresh or dried							
(Frieda's), 1 oz. . .	7	.6	1.3	.1	0	1	.2 d
Mushroom, shiitake:							
fresh:							
raw (Frieda's), 1 oz.	48	2.1	3.2	.3	0	m.q.	.7 d

Food and Measure	cal.	prot. (gms)	carbo. (gms)	fat (gms)	chol. (mgs)	sod. (mgs)	fiber (gms)
cooked, 4 medium or 1/2 cup pieces	40	1.1	10.4	.2	0	3	1.5 d
dried, 4 medium, .5 oz.	44	1.4	11.3	.2	0	2	1.7 d
Mushroom, Yama-biko honshimeji *(Frieda's)*, 1 oz. . .	3	.6	1.2	.1	0	m.q.	m.q.
Mushroom gravy: canned, 2 oz. or 1/4 cup:							
(Franco-American)	25	(0)	3.0	1.0	n.a.	290	n.a.
(Heinz HomeStyle)	25	1.0	3.0	1.0	<1	340	n.a.
and wine *(Pepper-idge Farm)* . . .	30	1.0	4.0	1.0	n.a.	270	n.a.
mix: *(French's)*, 1/4 pkg.	18	0	3.0	1.0	0	230	n.a.
(LaLoma Gravy Quik), 2 tbsp.* . .	10	<1.0	2.0	<1.0	0	160	n.a.
(McCormick/Schill-ing), 1/4 cup* . .	19	.5	3.0	.5	n.a.	270	n.a.
Mushroom and herb dip *(Breakstone's Gourmet)*, 2 tbsp.	50	1.0	2.0	4.0	10	150	n.a.
Mussel, blue, meat only:							
raw, 4 oz.	98	13.5	4.2	2.5	32	324	0
raw, 1 cup	129	17.9	5.5	3.4	42	429	0
boiled or steamed, 4 oz.	195	27.0	8.4	5.1	64	418	0
Mustard, prepared, 1 tbsp., except as noted:							
(Kraft Pure)	11	1.0	1.0	1.0	0	160	0
blend *(Hellmann's Dijonnaise)*, 1 tsp.	12	0	1.0	1.0	0	70	0
brown: *(Heinz Spicy)* . . .	14	<1.0	1.0	1.0	0	115	0

Food and Measure	cal.	prot. (gms)	carbo. (gms)	fat (gms)	chol. (mgs)	sod. (mgs)	fiber (gms)
Mustard, brown *(cont.)*							
(Gulden's Spicy),							
1/4 oz.	8	0	0	0	0	45	0
creamy mild *(Gul-*							
den's), 1/4 oz. . . .	6	0	0	0	0	60	0
Dijon:							
(French's), 1 tsp.	8	0	0	1.0	0	140	0
(Grey Poupon) . . .	18	0	0	1.0	0	450	0
w/horseradish:							
(French's)	16	1.0	1.0	1.0	0	265	n.a.
(Kraft)	14	1.0	1.0	1.0	0	135	0
hot *(Gulden's* Diablo),							
1/4 oz.	8	0	0	0	0	55	0
Medford *(French's)*	16	1.0	1.0	1.0	0	240	n.a.
mild, yellow *(Heinz)*	8	1.0	1.0	<1.0	0	175	0
w/onion *(French's),*							
1 tsp.	8	0	2.0	0	0	70	n.a.
spicy *(French's* Bold'n							
Spicy), 1 tsp. . . .	6	0	0	0	0	50	n.a.
stone ground:							
(Hain)	14	1.0	1.0	1.0	0	185	n.a.
(Hain No Salt) . . .	14	1.0	1.0	1.0	0	10	n.a.
yellow *(French's)* . . .	10	1.0	1.0	1.0	0	180	n.a.
Mustard greens:							
fresh, chopped:							
raw, 1 oz. or 1/2 cup	7	.8	1.4	.1	0	7	.6 d
boiled, drained,							
1/2 cup	11	1.6	1.5	.2	0	11	1.4 d
canned *(Allens/Sun-*							
shine), 1/2 cup . . .	20	1.0	2.0	<1.0	0	40	1.0 d
frozen, chopped:							
(Frosty Acres),							
3.3 oz.	20	2.0	3.0	0	0	20	1.0 c
(Seabrook), 3.3 oz.	20	2.0	3.0	0	0	20	1.0 c
Mustard powder							
(Spice Islands),							
1 tsp.	9	.5	.3	.6	0	<1	<.1 c

Food and Measure	cal.	prot. (gms)	carbo. (gms)	fat (gms)	chol. (mgs)	sod. (mgs)	fiber (gms)
Mustard seed, yellow, 1 tsp.	15	.8	1.2	1.0	0	tr.	.2 d
Mustard spinach:							
raw, chopped, 1/2 cup	17	1.7	2.9	.2	0	m.q.	.8 c
boiled, drained, chopped, 1/2 cup	14	1.5	2.5	.2	0	m.q.	.7 c
Mustard tallow, 1 tbsp.	115	0	0	12.8	13	0	0

N

Food and Measure	cal.	prot. (gms)	carbo. (gms)	fat (gms)	chol. (mgs)	sod. (mgs)	fiber (gms)
Nacho, mix, regular or jalapeño *(Tio Sancho* Microwave Snacks):							
chips, 4 oz.	567	8.5	74.4	26.1	n.a.	590	4.0 c
cheese sauce, 3.5 oz.	247	14.5	2.3	20.0	m.q.	995	.4 c
Nacho dip, see "Cheese dip"							
Natto, 1/2 cup	187	15.6	12.6	9.7	0	6	4.8 d
Navy beans, 1/2 cup:							
boiled	129	7.9	24.0	.5	0	1	3.3 d
canned, w/liquid . . .	148	9.9	26.8	.6	0	587	6.7 d
canned *(Allens)* . . .	160	8.0	24.0	<1.0	0	380	5.0 d
Navy beans, sprouted:							
raw, 1/2 cup	35	3.2	6.8	.4	0	m.q.	1.3 c
boiled, drained, 4 oz.	88	8.0	17.0	.9	0	m.q.	3.3 c
Nectarine:							
1 medium, 21/2" diam.	67	1.3	16.0	.6	0	tr.	2.2 d
sliced, 1/2 cup	34	.7	8.1	.3	0	tr.	1.1 d
New England Brand sausage *(Oscar Mayer)*, 2 slices . .	60	8.0	<1.0	2.5	25	570	0
New Zealand spinach, chopped:							
raw, 1 oz. or 1/2 cup	4	.4	.7	.1	0	37	.2 c
boiled, drained, 1/2 cup	11	1.2	2.0	.2	0	97	.6 c
Newburg sauce, w/sherry, canned *(Snow's)*, 1/3 cup	120	3.0	10.0	8.0	n.a.	520	0

Food and Measure	cal.	prot. (gms)	carbo. (gms)	fat (gms)	chol. (mgs)	sod. (mgs)	fiber (gms)
Newberg sauce mix							
(Knorr), 1 serving							
dry	20	.7	2.9	.6	0	170	n.a.
Noodle, Chinese:							
(Azumaya), 1 oz. . . .	81	3.0	16.6	.3	0	111	m.q.
cellophane or long							
rice, dry, 2 oz. . . .	199	.1	48.8	<.1	0	6	<.1 c
chow mein, 1/2 cup	119	1.9	13.0	6.9	0	99	.9 d
chow mein, narrow *(La*							
Choy), 1/2 cup . . .	150	3.0	16.0	8.0	0	230	<1.0 d
chow mein, wide *(La*							
Choy), 1/2 cup . . .	150	3.0	16.0	8.0	0	300	<1.0 d
fried *(Frieda's* Crispy,							
1 oz.	130	4.0	18.0	5.0	0	180	m.q.
rice *(La Choy)*, 1/2 cup	130	2.0	21.0	5.0	0	420	<1.0 d
Noodle, egg:							
uncooked, 2 oz.:							
(Creamette)	220	8.0	40.0	3.0	55	15	m.q.
(Herb's Organic) . .	230	10.0	40.0	2.0	60	5	m.q.
(Prince)	210	8.0	40.0	2.0	65	35	m.q.
cooked:							
1 cup	212	7.6	39.7	2.4	53	11	1.8 d
spinach, 1 cup . .	211	8.1	38.8	2.5	52	20	3.7 d
precooked, frozen:							
(Aunt Vi's), 4 oz. . . .	75	4.0	13.0	1.0	10	30	1.0 d
Noodle, Japanese:							
(Azumaya), 1 oz. . . .	80	2.9	16.6	.2	0	117	m.q.
soba, dry, 2 oz. . . .	192	8.2	42.5	.4	0	451	m.q.
soba, cooked, 1 cup	113	5.8	24.4	.1	0	40	m.q.
somen, dry, 2 oz. . .	203	6.5	42.2	.5	0	1049	2.4 d
somen, cooked, 1 cup	230	7.0	48.5	.3	0	284	.4 c
udon, dry, 2 oz. . . .	159	3.9	32.3	.7	0	340	m.q.
udon, cooked, 4 oz. .	115	2.8	23.0	.6	0	51	m.q.
Noodle and chicken							
dinner, frozen							
(Swanson), 10.5 oz.	250	6.0	31.0	11.0	m.q.	660	m.q.

Food and Measure	cal.	prot. (gms)	carbo. (gms)	fat (gms)	chol. (mgs)	sod. (mgs)	fiber (gms)
Noodle and chicken dishes:							
canned or packaged:							
(Dinty Moore American Classics),							
10 oz.	230	17.0	24.0	7.0	65	1020	m.q.
(Hormel Micro Cup),							
7.5 oz.	174	7.0	19.0	7.0	29	1009	m.q.
freeze-dried (Mountain House), 1 cup* . .	200	13.0	28.0	4.0	m.q.	970	m.q.
Noodle dishes, mix*, 1/2 cup, except as noted:							
Alfredo:							
(Lipton Noodles and Sauce)	200	6.0	22.0	10.0	m.q.	600	m.q.
broccoli (Lipton Noodles and Sauce)	180	7.0	22.0	7.0	m.q.	570	m.q.
beef (Lipton Noodles and Sauce)	180	5.0	22.0	7.0	m.q.	570	m.q.
broccoli au gratin (Noodle Roni) . . .	170	6.0	23.0	6.0	n.a.	530	m.q.
butter:							
(Lipton Noodles and Sauce)	190	5.0	22.0	10.0	m.q.	520	m.q.
and herb (Lipton Noodles and Sauce)	190	5.0	22.0	9.0	m.q.	520	m.q.
carbonara Alfredo (Lipton Noodles and Sauce)	200	6.0	22.0	10.0	m.q.	530	m.q.
cheddar, white, shells (Noodle Roni) . . .	180	5.0	23.0	8.0	m.q.	450	m.q.
cheddar bacon (Lipton Noodles and Sauce)	160	6.0	22.0	6.0	m.q.	580	m.q.

Food and Measure	cal.	prot. (gms)	carbo. (gms)	fat (gms)	chol. (mgs)	sod. (mgs)	fiber (gms)
cheese:							
(*Lipton* Noodles and Sauce)	190	5.0	24.0	8.0	m.q.	530	m.q.
w/egg noodles (*Kraft Dinner*), 3/4 cup	340	10.0	37.0	17.0	50	670	m.q.
fettuccine (*Noodle Roni*)	230	6.0	22.0	12.0	m.q.	600	m.q.
chicken:							
(*Lipton* Noodles and Sauce)	180	5.0	22.0	8.0	m.q.	450	m.q.
broccoli (*Lipton* Noodles and Sauce)	190	6.0	24.0	9.0	m.q.	500	m.q.
creamy (*Lipton* Noodles and Sauce)	190	6.0	23.0	9.0	m.q.	470	m.q.
w/egg noodles (*Kraft Dinner*), 3/4 cup	240	8.0	32.0	9.0	45	1050	m.q.
garlic, creamy (*Noodle Roni*)	250	6.0	24.0	15.0	n.a.	600	m.q.
w/herbs, angel hair (*Noodle Roni*) . . .	200	5.0	26.0	8.0	n.a.	510	m.q.
Parmesan:							
(*Lipton* Noodles and Sauce)	210	6.0	22.0	11.0	m.q.	480	m.q.
(*Noodle Roni* Parmesano) . . .	190	6.0	24.0	8.0	m.q.	460	m.q.
angel hair (*Noodle Roni*)	210	6.0	26.0	9.0	m.q.	580	m.q.
Romanoff (*Lipton* Noodles and Sauce) . .	200	6.0	22.0	11.0	m.q.	590	m.q.
sour cream and chive (*Lipton* Noodles and Sauce)	190	5.0	23.0	9.0	m.q.	500	m.q.
Stroganoff (*Lipton* Noodles and Sauce)	180	5.0	20.0	8.0	m.q.	490	m.q.

Food and Measure	cal.	prot. (gms)	carbo. (gms)	fat (gms)	chol. (mgs)	sod. (mgs)	fiber (gms)
Noodle entree, frozen:							
and beef, w/gravy *(Banquet* Family), 7 oz.	180	11.0	20.0	6.0	m.q.	m.q.	m.q.
Romanoff *(Stouffer's)*, 6 oz.	240	9	22.0	13.0	m.q.	670	m.q.
Nut topping (see also specific listings), 1 oz.:							
(Fisher Fancy)	170	5.0	7.0	15.0	0	60	m.q.
oil-roasted, w/peanuts *(Fisher)*	160	6.0	7.0	14.0	0	115	m.q.
Nutmeg, ground, 1 tsp.	12	.1	1.1	.8	0	tr.	.5 d
Nuts, see specific listings							
Nuts, mixed, 1 oz.:							
(Flavor House Deluxe)	170	5.0	5.0	15.0	0	125	2.0 d
dry-roasted:							
w/peanuts	169	4.9	7.2	14.6	0	3	2.6 d
w/peanuts, salted	169	4.9	7.2	14.6	0	190	2.6 d
(Fisher)	170	6.0	7.0	15.0	0	125	m.q.
(Flavor House)	160	6.0	8.0	12.0	0	200	2.0 d
oil-roasted:							
w/peanuts	175	4.8	6.1	16.0	0	3	2.8 d
w/peanuts, salted	175	4.8	6.1	16.0	0	185	2.8 d
(Fisher)	170	6.0	6.0	16.0	0	110	m.q.
(Fisher Lightly Salted)	170	6.0	6.0	16.0	0	50	m.q.
(Flavor House)	170	6.0	4.0	14.0	0	125	2.0 d
cashews and almonds, oil-roasted *(Fisher)*	170	5.0	6.0	15.0	0	95	m.q.
peanuts and cashews, honey-roasted *(Fisher)*	150	5.0	6.0	13.0	0	105	m.q.

O

Food and Measure	cal.	prot. (gms)	carbo. (gms)	fat (gms)	chol. (mgs)	sod. (mgs)	fiber (gms)
Oat (see also "Cereal"):							
whole-grain, 1 oz. . . .	110	4.8	18.8	2.0	0	1	m.q.
flakes (*Arrowhead Mills*), 2 oz.	220	10.0	39.0	4.0	0	1	8.1 d
rolled or oatmeal:							
dry, 1 oz.	109	4.5	19.0	1.8	0	1	2.9 d
cooked, 1 cup . . .	145	6.0	25.2	2.4	0	1	.4 c
steel cut (*Arrowhead Mills*), 2 oz.	220	10.0	37.0	4.0	0	1	2.8 d
Oat bran:							
raw, 1 oz.	70	4.9	18.8	2.0	0	1	4.5 d
cooked, 1 cup	87	7.0	25.1	1.9	0	2	.8 c
Oat flour (*Arrowhead Mills*), 2 oz.	200	7.0	43.0	1.0	0	1	8.3 d
Oat groats (*Arrowhead Mills*), 2 oz.	220	8.0	38.0	4.0	0	tr.	5.6 d
Ocean perch, Atlantic, meat only:							
raw, 4 oz.	107	21.1	0	1.9	48	85	0
baked, broiled, or microwaved, 4 oz. . .	137	27.1	0	2.4	61	109	0
Ocean perch, frozen:							
(*Van de Kamp's* Natural), 4 oz.	130	20.0	0	5.0	40	65	0
battered (*Gorton's* Crispy), 2 pieces	300	11.0	19.0	20.0	25	580	m.q.
breaded (*Van de Kamp's* Light), 1 piece	280	17.0	21.0	14.0	35	450	m.q.

Food and Measure	cal.	prot. (gms)	carbo. (gms)	fat (gms)	chol. (mgs)	sod. (mgs)	fiber (gms)
Octopus, meat only:							
raw, 4 oz.	93	16.9	2.5	1.2	55	m.q.	0
boiled or steamed,							
4 oz.	186	33.8	5.0	2.4	109	m.q.	0
Oheloberry, 1/2 cup	20	.3	4.8	.2	0	1	.9 c
Oil, 1 tbsp., except as noted:							
almond, cocoa butter, corn, cottonseed, hazelnut, nutmeg butter, oat, palm, palm kernel, or poppyseed	120	0	0	13.6	0	0	0
avocado or mustard	124	0	0	14.0	0	0	0
butter	112	<.1	0	12.7	33	n.a.	0
coconut	117	0	0	13.6	0	0	0
cod liver:							
1 tbsp.	123	0	0	13.6	78	n.a.	0
regular/mint (Hain)	120	0	0	14.0	85	0	0
cherry (Hain)	120	0	0	14.0	75	0	0
w/garlic (Hain)	120	0	0	14.0	0	0	0
herring	123	0	0	13.6	104	n.a.	0
olive, peanut, safflower, sesame, soybean, sunflower, vegetable, or walnut	120	0	0	14.0	0	0	0
plain, butter flavor or olive, spray (PAM), 1/3 of 10″ skillet . .	2	0	0	1.0	0	0	0
popcorn (Orville Redenbacher Gourmet)	120	0	0	14.0	0	0	0
pumpkinseed capsules (Hain), 1 capsule	12	0	0	1.0	0	0	0
salmon	123	0	0	13.6	66	n.a.	0
sardine	123	0	0	13.6	97	n.a.	0
sesame, hot pepper (Eden)	120	0	0	14.0	0	0	0

Food and Measure	cal.	prot. (gms)	carbo. (gms)	fat (gms)	chol. (mgs)	sod. (mgs)	fiber (gms)
Okara, see "Tofu"							
Okra:							
fresh:							
raw, sliced, 1/2 cup	19	1.0	3.8	.1	0	4	1.3 d
boiled, drained,							
8 pods, 3" × 5/8"	27	1.6	6.1	.1	0	5	2.1 d
boiled, drained,							
sliced, 1/2 cup . .	25	1.5	5.8	.1	0	4	2.0 d
canned, cut *(Allens),*							
1/2 cup	15	1.0	2.0	<1.0	0	430	2.0 d
canned, w/tomatoes							
(Allens), 1/2 cup . .	15	1.0	3.0	<1.0	0	520	2.0 d
frozen:							
boiled, drained,							
sliced, 1/2 cup . .	34	1.9	7.5	.3	0	3	2.6 d
whole *(Seabrook),*							
3.3 oz.	30	2.0	7.0	0	0	2	1.0 c
whole *(Stilwell),*							
9 pieces	35	1.0	6.0	.5	0	15	4.0 d
whole, baby *(Frosty*							
Acres), 3.3 oz.	30	2.0	7.0	0	0	2	1.0 c
cut *(Seabrook),*							
3.3 oz.	25	1.0	6.0	0	0	3	1.0 c
cut *(Stilwell),* 3/4 cup							
or 3 oz.	25	2.0	4.0	0	0	15	3.0 d
breaded *(Ore-Ida),*							
3 oz.	170	3.0	17.0	10.0	<5	600	m.q.
breaded *(Stilwell*							
Light), 21 pieces							
or 3 oz.	70	2.0	14.0	1.0	0	250	1.0 d
Old-fashioned mixer,							
bottled *(Holland*							
House), 1 fl. oz. . .	32	<1.0	8.0	<1.0	0	6	(0)
Old-fashioned loaf							
(Oscar Mayer),							
1 slice	60	4.0	2.0	5.0	15	340	0

Food and Measure	cal.	prot. (gms)	carbo. (gms)	fat (gms)	chol. (mgs)	sod. (mgs)	fiber (gms)
Olive, pickled, 1/2 oz., except as noted:							
Alfonso *(Krinos)* . . .	30	0	1.0	3.0	0	360	0
Calamata *(Krinos)* . .	40	0	2.0	4.0	0	260	0
green, w/pits:							
10 small	33	.4	.4	3.6	0	686	.7 d
10 large	45	.5	.5	4.9	0	926	1.0 d
10 giant	76	.9	.9	8.3	0	1572	1.7 d
green, pitted, 1 oz.	33	.4	.4	3.6	0	680	.7 d
green, Greek, cracked *(Krinos)*	15	0	1.0	1.0	0	410	0
Nafplion *(Krinos)* . . .	20	0	2.0	1.0	0	300	0
ripe, all varieties, except Spanish *(Vlasic)*	18	0	1.0	2.0	0	110	m.q.
ripe, oil-cured:							
(Progresso), 5 medium	60	<1.0	3.0	5.0	0	280	m.q.
imported *(Krinos)*	70	0	3.0	6.0	0	390	0
ripe, salt-cured, Greek style:							
10 medium	65	.4	1.7	6.9	0	631	m.q.
10 extra large . . .	89	.6	2.3	9.5	0	868	m.q.
pitted, 1 oz.	96	.6	2.5	10.2	0	932	m.q.
imported *(Krinos)*	30	0	1.0	2.5	0	310	0
ripe, Spanish, all varieties *(Vlasic)*	14	0	1.0	0	n.a.	300	m.q.
royal *(Krinos)*	30	0	1.0	2.5	0	290	0
Olive loaf *(Oscar Mayer)*, 1 slice . . .	60	3.0	3.0	4.0	10	380	0
Olive oil, see "Oil"							
Olive salad *(Progresso)*, 1/2 cup . .	130	<1.0	5.0	14.0	0	870	2.0 d
Omelet, see "Egg breakfast"							
Onion, mature:							
fresh or stored:							
raw, 1 oz.	11	.3	2.4	<.1	0	1	.5 d

Food and Measure	cal.	prot. (gms)	carbo. (gms)	fat (gms)	chol. (mgs)	sod. (mgs)	fiber (gms)
raw, chopped, ½ cup	30	.9	6.9	0.1	0	2	1.4 d
raw, chopped, 1 tbsp.	4	.1	.9	<.1	0	tr.	.2 d
boiled, drained, chopped, ½ cup	47	1.4	10.7	.2	0	3	1.5 d
in jars, 1 oz.:							
cocktail (Vlasic) . .	4	0	1.0	0	0	420	m.q.
cocktail, spiced (Vlasic)	4	0	1.0	0	0	410	m.q.
sweet (Heinz) . . .	40	0	9.0	0	0	165	m.q.
wild, marinated, (Krinos Volvi)	15	0	2.0	.5	0	230	1.0 d
frozen:							
whole, small (Seabrook), 3.3 oz.	35	1.0	8.0	0	0	9	1.0 c
chopped, boiled, drained, 1 tbsp.	4	.1	1.0	<.1	0	2	.2 d
chopped (Ore-Ida), 2 oz.	20	<1.0	4.0	<1.0	0	5	m.q.
chopped (Seabrook), 1 oz.	8	0	2.0	0	0	2	0
w/cream sauce (Birds Eye), 5 oz.	70	2.0	12.0	3.0	m.q.	340	1.0 d
rings, see "Onion rings"							
Onion, dried:							
flakes, 1 tbsp.	16	.5	4.2	<.1	0	1	.5 d
minced (Lawry's Spice Blends), 1 tsp. . . .	7	.4	1.6	.2	0	1	.6 c
Onion, green (scallion), raw, trimmed, w/top:							
chopped, ½ cup . .	16	.9	3.7	.1	0	8	1.3 d
chopped, 1 tbsp. . .	2	.1	.4	<.1	0	1	.2 d
Onion, Welsh, trimmed, 1 oz.	10	.5	1.8	.1	0	n.a.	.3 c

Food and Measure	cal.	prot. (gms)	carbo. (gms)	fat (gms)	chol. (mgs)	sod. (mgs)	fiber (gms)
Onion dip, 2 tbsp., except as noted:							
creamy *(Kraft Premium)*	45	1.0	2.0	4.0	10	160	n.a.
French:							
(Breakstone's/Sealtest)	50	1.0	2.0	5.0	15	140	n.a.
(Frito-Lay's)	50	1.0	3.0	4.0	10	180	n.a.
(Kraft)	60	1.0	3.0	4.0	0	240	n.a.
(Kraft Premium) . .	45	1.0	2.0	4.0	10	150	n.a.
green *(Kraft)*	60	1.0	3.0	4.0	0	170	n.a.
toasted *(Breakstone's* Gourmet)	50	1.0	2.0	5.0	10	170	n.a.
mix, chive *(Knorr),* 1 serving dry . . .	5	.1	.7	.1	0	110	n.a.
Onion flavor snack, rings *(Tom's),* 3/4 oz.	120	1.0	12.0	8.0	0	270	n.a.
Onion gravy:							
canned *(Heinz),* 2 oz.	25	0	4.0	1.0	n.a.	150	n.a.
mix:							
(French's), 1/4 pkg.	20	0	4.0	1.0	0	240	n.a.
(LaLoma Gravy Quik), 2 tbsp.* . .	10	<1.0	2.0	<1.0	0	120	n.a.
(McCormick/Schilling), 1/4 cup* . .	22	.6	3.6	.6	n.a.	337	n.a.
Onion powder *(Spice Islands),* 1 tsp. . . .	8	.2	1.7	<.1	0	1	.1 d
Onion ring batter mix, *(Golden Dipt),* 1 oz.	100	2.0	22.0	0	0	570	m.q.
Onion rings, frozen:							
(Ore-Ida Onion Ringers), 2 oz.	150	2.0	17.0	9.0	0	90	m.q.
(Qwik-Krisp Natural Cut), 4 pieces . . .	155	3.0	22.0	7.0	0	405	2.0 d
(Stilwell Crispy Crunchy), 6 pieces	220	2.0	30.0	10.0	0	650	5.0 d

Food and Measure	cal.	prot. (gms)	carbo. (gms)	fat (gms)	chol. (mgs)	sod. (mgs)	fiber (gms)
battered:							
(Farm Rich), 4 oz.	260	3.0	32.0	13.0	n.a.	580	m.q.
(Mrs. Paul's Crispy), 2 oz.	150	2.0	15.0	10.0	n.a.	180	m.q.
beer *(Stilwell)*, 4 pieces	200	4.0	21.0	11.0	0	360	2.0 d
Onion salt *(Tone's)*, 1 tsp.	1	.1	.4	tr.	0	1599	<.1 d
Onion seeds, salad, sprouted *(Shaw's* Premium), 2 oz. . .	11	1.0	0	<1.0	0	85	3.0 d
Opossum, meat only, roasted, 4 oz. . . .	251	34.2	0	11.6	m.q.	m.q.	0
Orange:							
California navel:							
2⁷/₈″-diam. orange	65	1.4	16.3	.1	0	1	3.4 d
sections w/out membrane, 1/2 cup	38	.9	9.6	.1	0	1	2.0 d
California Valencia:							
2⁵/₈″-diam. orange	59	1.3	14.4	.4	0	0	2.9 d
sections w/out membrane, 1/2 cup	44	.9	10.7	.3	0	0	2.2 d
Florida:							
2¹¹/₁₆″-diam. orange	69	1.1	17.4	.3	0	1	3.6 d
sections w/out membrane, 1/2 cup	42	.7	10.7	.2	0	1	2.2 d
peel, 1 tbsp.	—[1]	.1	1.5	<.1	0	0	.2 d
Orange, mandarin, see "Tangerine"							
Orange drink:							
canned:							
(Hi-C), 6 fl. oz. . . .	90	0	23.0	0	0	20	(0)

[1] *Cannot be calculated; no digestibility value for peel.*

Food and Measure	cal.	prot. (gms)	carbo. (gms)	fat (gms)	chol. (mgs)	sod. (mgs)	fiber (gms)
Orange drink, canned *(cont.)*							
(Kool-Aid Kool Bursts), 6.75 oz.	130	0	34.0	0	0	10	0
mix*:							
(Kool-Aid), 8 fl. oz.	100	0	25.0	0	0	0	0
(Kool-Aid Presweetened)*, 8 fl. oz. . .	70	0	18.0	0	0	5	0
(Tang), 6 fl. oz. . .	70	0	19.0	0	0	0	0
(Tang Sugar Free)*, 6 fl. oz.	6	0	1.0	0	0	0	0
Orange float *(R.W. Knudsen)*, 8 fl. oz.	120	2.0	27.0	<1.0	0	(0)	n.a.
Orange fruit juice blend *(Mott's)*, 11.5 fl. oz.	200	2.0	46.0	<1.0	0	10	n.a.
Orange juice, 6 fl. oz., except as noted:							
fresh	83	1.3	19.3	.4	0	2	.4 d
canned or bottled:							
(Libby's)	80	1.0	20.0	0	0	0	m.q.
(Minute Maid) . . .	80	1.0	20.0	0	0	20	m.q.
(Ocean Spray 100%)	80	0	19.0	0	0	15	m.q.
(R.W. Knudsen), 8 fl. oz.	90	1.0	22.0	<1.0	0	(0)	m.q.
(Tree Top)	90	1.0	22.0	0	0	5	m.q.
blend *(Minute Maid)*	90	1.0	22.0	0	0	20	(0)
blend *(Welch's)* . .	90	0	22.0	0	0	20	m.q.
chilled:							
6 fl. oz.	82	1.5	18.8	.5	0	2	.4 d
(Tropicana)	80	1.0	16.0	<1.0	0	20	m.q.
(Tropicana Pure Premium)*	80	1.0	19.0	<1.0	0	0	m.q.
all varieties, except Premium Choice *(Minute Maid)* . .	80	1.0	20.0	0	0	20	m.q.

Food and Measure	· cal.	prot. (gms)	carbo. (gms)	fat (gms)	chol. (mgs)	sod. (mgs)	fiber (gms)
regular or country style (Minute Maid Premium Choice)	90	1.0	21.0	0	0	0	m.q.
frozen*:							
6 fl. oz.	84	1.3	20.1	.1	0	2	.4 d
(TreeSweet)	84	1.0	20.0	0	0	15	m.q.
all varieties (Minute Maid)	80	1.0	20.0	0	0	0	m.q.
cocktail (Ocean Spray)	100	0	25.0	0	0	15	m.q.
Orange juice drink:							
canned, 8.45 fl. oz., except as noted:							
(Kool-Aid Koolers)	110	0	30.0	0	0	10	(0)
(Shasta Plus), 12 fl. oz.	184	0	46.0	0	0	58	0
(Tang Fruit Box) . .	130	0	32.0	0	0	10	(0)
tropical (Tang Fruit Box)	150	0	37.0	0	0	10	(0)
chilled, 6 fl. oz.:							
(Bright & Early) . .	90	0	21.0	0	0	20	(0)
(Tropicana)	90	<1.0	22.0	<1.0	0	35	(0)
frozen* (Bright & Early), 6 fl. oz. . . .	90	0	21.0	0	0	5	(0)
Orange sauce, Mandarin (La Choy), 1 tbsp.	24	<.1	6.1	tr.	0	38	.1 d
Orange-banana juice:							
(Chiquita), 6 fl. oz. . .	90	0	22.0	0	0	20	m.q.
(Smucker's Naturally 100%), 8 fl. oz. . .	120	0	30.0	0	0	10	m.q.
Orange-banana juice drink (Boku), 6 fl. oz.	90	0	22.0	0	0	0	0
Orange-banana nectar (Kern's), 6 fl. oz.	110	1.0	25.0	0	0	0	m.q.

Food and Measure	cal.	prot. (gms)	carbo. (gms)	fat (gms)	chol. (mgs)	sod. (mgs)	fiber (gms)
Orange-cranberry juice (Master Choice Tropical Shakers), 6 fl. oz.	100	0	25.0	0	0	15	m.q.
Orange-cranberry juice drink, 6 fl. oz.:							
(Ocean Spray Refreshers)	100	0	26.0	0	0	15	(0)
(Tropicana)	100	<1.0	23.0	<1.0	0	25	(0)
(Tropicana Twister Light)	25	<1.0	4.0	<1.0	0	30	(0)
Orange-grapefruit juice, canned, 6 fl. oz.	80	1.1	19.1	.2	0	6	.2 d
Orange-kiwi-passion fruit juice (Tropicana), 6 fl. oz. . . .	80	1.0	17.0	<1.0	0	35	m.q.
Orange-mango juice:							
(R.W. Knudsen), 8 fl. oz.	110	<1.0	24.0	<1.0	0	(0)	m.q.
drink (Tropicana Twister), 6 fl. oz. . .	90	<1.0	21.0	<1.0	0	45	(0)
Orange-passion fruit juice drink (Tropicana Twister), 6 fl. oz.	80	<1.0	19.0	<1.0	0	35	(0)
Orange-peach juice (Master Choice Tropical Shakers), 6 fl. oz.	100	0	25.0	0	0	15	m.q.
Orange-peach juice drink, 6 fl. oz.:							
(Boku)	90	0	22.0	0	0	0	0
(Tropicana Twister) . .	90	<1.0	21.0	<1.0	0	35	(0)
Orange-peach-mango juice (Tropicana), 6 fl. oz. . . .	80	1.0	19.0	<1.0	0	20	m.q.

Food and Measure	cal.	prot. (gms)	carbo. (gms)	fat (gms)	chol. (mgs)	sod. (mgs)	fiber (gms)
Orange-pineapple juice *(Tropicana)*, 6 fl. oz.	80	1.0	19.0	<1.0	0	15	m.q.
Orange-raspberry juice *(Master Choice Tropical Shakers)*, 6 fl. oz.	100	0	25.0	0	0	15	m.q.
Orange-raspberry juice drink, 6 fl. oz.:							
(Tropicana Twister) . .	80	<1.0	20.0	<1.0	0	30	(0)
(Tropicana Twister Light)	30	<1.0	6.0	<1.0	0	30	(0)
Orange-strawberry-banana juice, 6 fl. oz.:							
(Master Choice Tropical Shakers)	100	0	25.0	0	0	15	m.q.
(Tropicana)	80	1.0	18.0	<1.0	0	25	m.q.
Orange-strawberry-banana juice drink, 6 fl. oz.:							
(Tropicana Twister) . .	80	<1.0	20.0	<1.0	0	45	(0)
(Tropicana Twister Light)	25	<1.0	6.0	<1.0	0	20	(0)
Orange-strawberry-guava juice drink *(Tropicana Twister)*, 6 fl. oz.	80	<1.0	20.0	<1.0	0	40	(0)
Oregano, dried *(Spice Islands)*, 1 tsp. . . .	6	.2	1.0	.1	0	<1	.2 d
Oriental 5-spice *(Tone's)*, 1 tsp. . .	9	.3	1.9	.3	0	2	.5 d
Oriental seasoning and coating mix *(McCormick/Schilling Bag'n Season)*, 1 pkg.	152	5.0	31.0	8.0	n.a.	1912	m.q.

Food and Measure	cal.	prot. (gms)	carbo. (gms)	fat (gms)	chol. (mgs)	sod. (mgs)	fiber (gms)
Oyster, meat only:							
Eastern, wild:							
raw, 1 lb.	310	32.0	17.7	11.1	238	957	0
raw, 6 medium,							
3 oz.	57	5.9	3.3	2.1	44	177	0
baked, broiled, or							
microwaved, 4 oz.	82	9.4	5.4	2.2	56	277	0
steamed or							
poached, 4 oz.	155	16.0	8.9	5.6	119	478	0
Eastern, farmed:							
raw, 4 oz.	67	5.9	6.3	1.8	29	202	0
baked, broiled, or							
microwaved, 4 oz.	90	7.9	8.3	2.4	43	185	0
Pacific:							
raw, 4 oz.	93	10.7	5.6	2.6	m.q.	120	0
raw, boiled, or							
steamed, 1 me-							
dium	41	4.7	2.5	1.2	m.q.	53	0
boiled or steamed,							
4 oz.	185	21.4	11.2	5.2	m.q.	240	0
Oyster, canned, Eastern:							
(Bumble Bee), 1 cup	218	25.4	15.4	5.3	m.q.	185	0
wild, w/liquid, 4 oz.	78	8.0	4.4	2.8	62	127	0
wild, w/liquid, 1 cup	170	17.5	9.7	6.1	136	277	0
Oyster plant, see "Salsify"							
Oyster stew, see "Soup"							

P

Food and Measure	cal.	prot. (gms)	carbo. (gms)	fat (gms)	chol. (mgs)	sod. (mgs)	fiber (gms)
P&B loaf *(Kahn's)*, 1 slice	40	5.0	1.0	2.0	m.q.	270	0
Pancake, frozen, 3 pieces:							
(Aunt Jemima Original)	210	6.0	38.0	4.0	n.a.	700	1.5 d
(Hungry Jack Microwave Original) . . .	240	5.0	49.0	4.0	10	570	2.0 d
blueberry *(Hungry Jack Microwave)*	230	5.0	47.0	4.0	10	550	1.0 d
buttermilk *(Hungry Jack Microwave)*	260	5.0	51.0	4.0	10	590	1.0 d
buttermilk or plain *(Downyflake)*	280	5.0	45.0	9.0	n.a.	920	m.q.
oat bran *(Hungry Jack Microwave)*	230	6.0	45.0	4.0	10	580	3.0 d
wheat, harvest *(Hungry Jack Microwave)*	230	6.0	46.0	4.0	10	560	3.0 d
Pancake batter, frozen*, 3 pancakes, 4″ each:							
(Aunt Jemima Original)	180	6.0	36.0	2.0	n.a.	640	m.q.
buttermilk *(Aunt Jemima)*	180	6.0	36.0	2.0	n.a.	650	m.q.
Pancake breakfast, frozen:							
w/bacon *(Swanson Great Starts)*, 4.5 oz.	400	13.0	43.0	20.0	m.q.	1030	m.q.

Food and Measure	cal.	prot. (gms)	carbo. (gms)	fat (gms)	chol. (mgs)	sod. (mgs)	fiber (gms)
Pancake breakfast (cont.)							
blueberry, w/sausage, on a stick (Jimmy Dean Flapsticks), 1 piece	170	4.0	15.0	10.0	15	280	m.q.
mini (Swanson Breakfast Blast), 4.25 oz.	300	6.0	51.0	8.0	n.a.	580	m.q.
w/sausages (Swanson Great Starts), 6 oz.	470	14.0	53.0	23.0	m.q.	940	m.q.
w/sausage, on a stick (Jimmy Dean Flapsticks), 1 piece . .	170	4.0	13.0	12.0	15	290	m.q.
silver dollar, w/sausages (Swanson Budget), 3.75 oz.	320	10.0	36.0	16.0	m.q.	680	m.q.
and vegetarian links (Morningstar Farms), 4 oz.	240	11.0	31.0	8.0	0	700	m.q.
Pancake and waffle mix*, 3 pancakes, 4″ each, except as noted:							
(Bisquick Shake'N Pour Original) . . .	250	6.0	49.0	3.0	0	880	m.q.
(Hungry Jack Extra Lights)	190	5.0	28.0	6.0	55	490	.5 d
(Hungry Jack Extra Lights Complete)	180	4.0	38.0	3.0	0	730	1.0 d
apple cinnamon (Bisquick Shake'N Pour)	240	6.0	47.0	3.0	0	880	m.q.
blueberry:							
(Bisquick Shake'N Pour)	280	6.0	52.0	5.0	0	910	m.q.
wild (Hungry Jack)	320	6.0	41.0	14.0	45	820	m.q.
buttermilk:							
(Betty Crocker) . .	280	8.0	39.0	10.0	m.q.	810	m.q.
(Bisquick Shake'N Pour)	250	6.0	49.0	3.0	0	880	m.q.

Food and Measure	cal.	prot. (gms)	carbo. (gms)	fat (gms)	chol. (mgs)	sod. (mgs)	fiber (gms)
(Hungry Jack) . . .	210	6.0	28.0	9.0	55	560	.5 d
(Hungry Jack Complete)	180	5.0	38.0	1.0	5	720	1.0 d
(Robin Hood/Gold Medal Pouch), 1/8 mix	110	5.0	16.0	3.0	m.q.	270	m.q.
kamut (Arrowhead Mills), 1/4 cup . . .	130	7.0	26.0	1.0	0	330	4.0 d
whole grain (Arrowhead Mills), 1/2 cup	290	11.0	58.0	2.0	0	620	10.0 d
wild rice (Arrowhead Mills), 2.5 oz. dry	250	6.0	53.0	2.0	0	110	4.3 d
Pancake syrup (see also "Maple syrup"), 2 tbsp., except as noted:							
table blends:							
1 tbsp.	57	0	15.1	0	0	17	0
w/butter, 1 tbsp.	59	0	14.8	.3	1	20	0
w/2% maple, 1 tbsp.	53	0	13.9	0	0	12	0
(Country Kitchen) . .	100	0	27.0	0	0	40	(0)
(Country Kitchen Lite)	50	0	13.0	0	0	85	(0)
(Hungry Jack)	100	0	26.0	0	0	25	0
(Hungry Jack Lite) . .	50	0	14.0	0	0	105	0
(Log Cabin)	100	0	26.0	0	0	35	(0)
(Log Cabin Lite) . . .	50	0	13.0	0	0	90	(0)
(Vermont Maid), 1 tbsp.	50	0	13.0	0	0	5	(0)
butter flavor (Country Kitchen)	100	0	27.0	0	0	100	(0)
Pancreas, braised:							
beef, 4 oz.	307	30.7	0	19.5	m.q.	68	0
lamb, 4 oz.	265	25.9	0	17.1	454	59	0
pork, 4 oz.	248	32.3	0	12.2	357	48	0
veal (calf), 4 oz. . . .	290	33.0	0	16.6	m.q.	m.q.	0

Food and Measure	cal.	prot. (gms)	carbo. (gms)	fat (gms)	chol. (mgs)	sod. (mgs)	fiber (gms)
Papaya:							
1 lb. papaya,							
3¹/₂″ × 5¹/₈″	117	1.9	29.8	.4	0	8	5.5 d
peeled:							
cubed, ¹/₂ cup . . .	27	.4	6.9	.1	0	2	1.3 d
(Frieda's), 1 oz. . .	11	.2	2.8	<.1	0	1	m.q.
Papaya concentrate							
(R.W. Knudsen),							
1.5 fl. oz.	90	<1.0	22.0	<1.0	0	37	m.q.
Papaya cream *(R.W.*							
Knudsen), 2 fl. oz.	25	<1.0	6.0	<1.0	0	16	m.q.
Papaya nectar:							
canned, 6 fl. oz. . . .	107	.3	27.2	.3	0	9	1.1 d
(Kern's), 6 fl. oz. . . .	110	0	27.0	0	0	5	m.q.
(R.W. Knudsen),							
8 fl. oz.	100	<1.0	26.0	<1.0	0	(0)	m.q.
(Libby's), 6 fl. oz. . .	110	0	28.0	0	0	10	m.q.
Papaya-lime juice							
(R.W. Knudsen),							
8 fl. oz.	115	1.0	29.0	1.0	0	(0)	m.q.
Paprika, 1 tsp. . . .	6	.3	1.2	.3	0	1	.4 d
Parsley:							
fresh:							
10 sprigs	4	.3	.6	.1	0	6	.3 d
chopped, ¹/₂ cup . .	11	.9	1.9	.2	0	17	1.0 d
dried, 1 tsp.	1	.1	.2	.1	0	1	<.1 d
freeze-dried, 1 tbsp. .	1	.1	.2	<.1	0	2	<.1 d
Parsley root, 1 oz. .	3	.8	.7	.2	0	28	.4 d
Parsley seasoning, all							
purpose *(McCor-*							
mick/Schilling Pars-							
ley Patch), ¹/₂ tsp.	3	.2	.5	0	0	2	m.q.
Parsnip:							
raw, sliced, ¹/₂ cup	50	.8	12.1	.2	0	7	3.3 d
boiled, drained:							
1 medium, 9″ × 2¹/₄″							
diam.	130	2.1	31.3	.5	0	17	6.4 d
sliced, ¹/₂ cup . . .	63	1.0	15.2	.2	0	8	3.1 d

Food and Measure	cal.	prot. (gms)	carbo. (gms)	fat (gms)	chol. (mgs)	sod. (mgs)	fiber (gms)
Passion fruit, purple:							
1 medium	18	.4	4.2	.1	0	n.a.	1.9 d
trimmed, 1 oz.	27	.6	6.6	.2	0	n.a.	2.9 d
trimmed *(Frieda's)*, 1 oz.	26	.6	6.0	.2	0	8	m.q.
Passion fruit juice, 6 fl. oz.:							
fresh, purple	95	.7	25.2	.1	0	n.a.	.4 d
fresh, yellow	111	1.2	26.8	.3	0	11	.4 d
cocktail, frozen* *(Welch's Orchard Tropicals)*	100	0	25.0	0	0	20	0
Passion fruit-orange nectar *(Libby's Ripe)*, 8 fl. oz. . . .	150	0	36.0	0	0	10	m.q.
Passion fruit-raspberry juice *(R.W. Knudsen)*, 8 fl. oz.	130	<1.0	32.0	<1.0	0	(0)	m.q.
Pasta, dry (see also "Macaroni" and specific listings):							
uncooked, 2 oz.:							
plain	211	7.3	42.6	.9	0	4	1.4 d
all varieties *(Master Choice)*	210	7.0	42.0	1.0	0	0	m.q.
(Ronzoni)	210	7.0	41.0	1.0	0	<5	m.q.
kamut ribbons *(Eden)*	190	10.0	31.0	1.0	0	0	m.q.
pepper, bell, and basil fettuccine *(Herb's* Organic)	220	10.0	40.0	2.0	60	5	m.q.
sesame rice spirals *(Eden)*	212	10.0	40.0	1.0	0	0	m.q.
spinach ribbons *(Eden)*	210	10.0	40.0	1.0	0	5	m.q.
vegetable spirals *(Eden)*	228	8.0	44.0	<1.0	0	0	m.q.

Food and Measure	cal.	prot. (gms)	carbo. (gms)	fat (gms)	chol. (mgs)	sod. (mgs)	fiber (gms)
Pasta *(cont.)*							
cooked, 1 cup:							
plain	197	6.7	39.7	.9	0	1	2.4 d
corn	176	3.7	39.1	1.0	0	1	3.4 d
spinach	183	6.4	36.6	.9	0	20	m.q.
whole wheat	174	7.5	37.2	.6	0	4	6.3 d
Pasta, refrigerated:							
uncooked:							
w/egg, 2 oz.	163	6.4	31.0	1.3	41	15	m.q.
fettuccine or lin- guine *(Contadina)*, 3 oz.	260	12.0	45.0	4.0	75	35	m.q.
spaghetti style *(Con- tadina)*, 3 oz. . .	260	9.0	48.0	3.0	0	25	m.q.
spinach, w/egg, 2 oz.	164	6.4	31.6	1.2	41	15	m.q.
cooked:							
w/egg, 4 oz.	149	5.8	28.3	1.2	37	7	m.q.
spinach, w/egg, 4 oz.	147	5.7	28.4	1.1	37	7	m.q.
Pasta, frozen (see also specific listings) yolkless, precooked *(Aunt Vi's)*, 4 oz. . .	150	7.0	29.0	0	0	5	2.0 d
Pasta dinner (see also specific list- ings), frozen, w/tur- key and vegetables *(Swanson)*, 11.25 oz.	310	22.0	36.0	9.0	35	670	m.q.
Pasta dishes, canned or packaged (see also specific list- ings):							
broccoli marinara *(Del Monte Pasta Clas- sics)*, 3/4 cup . . .	70	2.0	13.0	1.0	n.a.	470	m.q.

Food and Measure	cal.	prot. (gms)	carbo. (gms)	fat (gms)	chol. (mgs)	sod. (mgs)	fiber (gms)
Italian style (Del Monte Pasta Classics), 3/4 cup	70	2.0	11.0	1.0	n.a.	450	m.q.
w/meatballs, in tomato sauce (Franco-American CircusO's), 7³/₈ oz. . .	210	9.0	26.0	8.0	m.q.	950	m.q.
spirals, and chicken (Libby's Diner), 7.75 oz.	120	8.0	16.0	3.0	15	910	m.q.
in tomato and cheese sauce (Franco-American CircusO's), 7.5 oz. . .	160	5.0	31.0	2.0	n.a.	860	m.q.
Pasta dishes, frozen (see also "Pasta entree" and specific listings), 1/2 cup, except as noted:							
Alfredo, w/broccoli (The Budget Gourmet Side Dish), 5.5 oz.	210	8.0	22.0	10.0	30	630	m.q.
creamy cheddar (Green Giant Pasta Accents)	90	4.0	14.0	3.0	5	280	2.0 d
Dijon (Green Giant Garden Gourmet Right for Lunch), 9.5 oz.	260	7.0	21.0	17.0	55	630	4.0 d
garden herb seasoning (Green Giant Pasta Accents)	80	3.0	12.0	3.0	5	290	3.0 d
garlic seasoning (Green Giant Pasta Accents)	100	3.0	14.0	4.0	5	260	2.0 d

Food and Measure	cal.	prot. (gms)	carbo. (gms)	fat (gms)	chol. (mgs)	sod. (mgs)	fiber (gms)
Pasta dishes, frozen *(cont.)*							
Florentine *(Green Giant Garden Gourmet Right for Lunch)*, 9.5 oz.	230	14.0	27.0	9.0	25	840	4.0 d
Parmesan, w/sweet peas *(Green Giant One Serving)*, 5.5 oz.	160	9.0	21.0	5.0	10	420	2.5 d
primavera *(Green Giant Pasta Accents)*	110	5.0	15.0	4.0	5	190	2.5 d
Pasta dishes, mix* (see also "Salad mix" and specific listings), 1/2 cup, except as noted:							
Alfredo *(McCormick/ Schilling Pasta Prima)*	253	7.0	27.0	13.0	n.a.	1178	m.q.
cheese:							
cheddar, tangy *(Hain Pasta & Sauce)*	190	7.0	19.0	11.0	15	340	3.5 d
cheddar broccoli *(Kraft Pasta & Cheese)*	180	6.0	19.0	8.0	30	620	m.q.
cheddar broccoli *(Lipton Pasta and Sauce)*	200	6.0	25.0	9.0	m.q.	530	m.q.
Parmesan *(Kraft Pasta & Cheese)*	180	6.0	19.0	8.0	30	630	m.q.
Parmesan, creamy *(Hain Pasta & Sauce)*	160	7.0	20.0	7.0	10	400	3.0 d
three cheese w/vegetables *(Kraft Pasta & Cheese)*	180	6.0	19.0	8.0	25	630	m.q.
chicken w/herbs *(Kraft Pasta & Cheese)*	170	5.0	21.0	7.0	25	550	m.q.

Food and Measure	cal.	prot. (gms)	carbo. (gms)	fat (gms)	chol. (mgs)	sod. (mgs)	fiber (gms)
dill, creamy, multibran (*Hain* Pasta & Sauce)	150	6.0	22.0	6.0	<5	370	5.0 d
garlic, creamy:							
(*Lipton* Pasta & Sauce)	220	6.0	28.0	9.0	m.q.	520	m.q.
(*McCormick/Schilling Pasta Prima*)	277	9.0	44.0	7.0	n.a.	791	m.q.
herb and garlic (*Mc-Cormick/Schilling Pasta Prima*)	326	9.0	45.0	12.0	m.q.	869	m.q.
herb tomato (*Lipton* Pasta & Sauce)	180	5.0	26.0	7.0	m.q.	420	m.q.
Italian:							
herb (*Hain* Pasta & Sauce)	170	7.0	18.0	10.0	10	350	4.0 d
multibran (*Hain* Pasta & Sauce)	120	5.0	17.0	7.0	5	390	5.0 d
marinara (*McCormick/ Schilling Pasta Prima*)	329	9.0	55.0	8.0	n.a.	432	m.q.
pesto (*McCormick/ Schilling Pasta Prima*)	193	6.0	29.0	6.0	n.a.	356	m.q.
primavera:							
(*Hain* Pasta & Sauce)	180	6.0	19.0	10.0	15	360	2.5 d
(*McCormick/Schilling Pasta Prima*), ¾ cup	244	10.0	32.0	9.0	n.a.	625	m.q.
salsa, multibran (*Hain* Pasta & Sauce) . .	130	4.0	18.0	7.0	0	390	5.0 d
seafood, creamy (*Mc-Cormick/Schilling Pasta Prima*)	209	21.0	9.0	10.0	n.a.	850	m.q.
sour cream w/chives (*Kraft* Pasta & Cheese)	180	5.0	22.0	8.0	25	360	m.q.

Food and Measure	cal.	prot. (gms)	carbo. (gms)	fat (gms)	chol. (mgs)	sod. (mgs)	fiber (gms)
Pasta dishes, mix *(cont.)*							
Swiss, creamy *(Hain Pasta & Sauce)*	180	7.0	20.0	9.0	10	390	3.5 d
tomato basil *(McCormick/Schilling Pasta Prima)*, 3/4 cup	175	5.0	21.0	8.0	n.a.	737	m.q.
Pasta entree, frozen, (see also "Pasta dishes, frozen" and specific listings):							
baked, and cheese *(Celentano)*, 10 oz.	480	22.0	63.0	19.0	30	810	8.0 d
w/chicken:							
cacciatore *(Healthy Choice Extra Portion)*, 12.5 oz.	310	26.0	47.0	3.0	35	430	m.q.
teriyaki *(Healthy Choice Extra Portion)*, 12.6 oz.	350	24.0	58.0	3.0	45	370	m.q.
Italiano							
(Healthy Choice Extra Portion), 12 oz.	350	16.0	59.0	5.0	30	530	m.q.
(Weight Watchers Ultimate 200), 8 oz.	190	17.0	19.0	4.0	5	450	m.q.
Portafino *(Weight Watchers Smart Ones)*, 9.5 oz.	160	8.0	30.0	1.0	0	220	m.q.
Romanoff supreme *(Weight Watchers)*, 9 oz.	230	12.0	29.0	7.0	20	540	m.q.
w/shrimp and vegetables *(Healthy Choice Extra Portion)*, 12.5 oz.	270	16.0	44.0	4.0	50	490	m.q.
trio *(Tyson Gourmet Selection)*, 11 oz.	450	21.0	53.0	17.0	n.a.	890	m.q.

Food and Measure	cal.	prot. (gms)	carbo. (gms)	fat (gms)	chol. (mgs)	sod. (mgs)	fiber (gms)
vegetable, Italiano *(Healthy Choice Quick Meal)*, 10 oz.	220	7.0	46.0	1.0	0	330	m.q.
Pasta salad, see "Salad mix"							
Pasta sauce (see also "Tomato sauce" and specific listings), 4 oz.:							
(Eden)	80	3.0	14.0	2.0	0	350	m.q.
(Hunt's Chunky) . . .	50	1.0	12.0	<1.0	0	470	2.0 d
(Hunt's Homestyle)	60	2.0	10.0	2.0	0	530	2.0 d
(Hunt's Traditional) . .	70	2.0	12.0	2.0	0	530	2.0 d
(Pastorelli Italian Chef)	100	4.0	13.0	4.0	0	660	4.0 d
(Prego)	120	2.0	20.0	4.0	n.a.	540	m.q.
(Prego Low Sodium)	100	2.0	11.0	5.0	n.a.	25	m.q.
(Progresso)	110	3.0	13.0	5.0	<5	660	m.q.
(Ragú Old World) . .	80	2.0	9.0	4.0	0	740	m.q.
(Ragú Thick & Hearty)	100	2.0	15.0	3.0	0	460	m.q.
w/beef and pork *(Classico D'Abruzzi)* . .	80	3.0	7.0	4.0	10	540	m.q.
cheese:							
four *(Classico Di Parma)*	70	2.0	7.0	4.0	<5	440	m.q.
four *(Master Choice Quattro Formaggi)*	60	3.0	8.0	1.0	1	560	m.q.
three *(Prego)* . . .	100	3.0	17.0	2.0	n.a.	410	m.q.
garden combination *(Prego Extra Chunky)*	80	2.0	14.0	2.0	n.a.	420	m.q.
garden harvest or chunky mushroom *(Ragú Today's Recipe)*	50	2.0	8.0	1.0	0	370	m.q.
garden medley or garlic and basil *(Ragú Fino Italian)*	80	2.0	12.0	3.0	0	490	m.q.

Pasta sauce (cont.)

Food and Measure	cal.	prot. (gms)	carbo. (gms)	fat (gms)	chol. (mgs)	sod. (mgs)	fiber (gms)
marinara:							
(Hain)	40	2.0	9.0	1.0	0	400	3.0 d
(Master Choice) . .	80	2.0	10.0	4.0	0	649	m.q.
(Prego)	100	2.0	10.0	6.0	0	620	m.q.
(Progresso)	90	4.0	9.0	5.0	1	520	<5.0 d
(Ragú Old World)	80	2.0	7.0	5.0	0	740	m.q.
meat or meat flavor:							
(Hunt's)	70	2.0	12.0	2.0	2	570	2.0 d
(Hunt's Homestyle)	60	3.0	9.0	2.0	2	570	2.0 d
(Master Choice Bolognese)	90	3.0	14.0	2.0	m.q.	721	m.q.
(Prego)	120	2.0	20.0	4.0	m.q.	580	m.q.
(Progresso)	110	4.0	13.0	5.0	5	660	m.q.
(Ragú Old World)	80	2.0	7.0	5.0	2	740	m.q.
meatless (Master Choice Pomodoro)	70	2.0	12.0	1.0	0	725	m.q.
mushroom:							
(Hain)	40	2.0	8.0	1.0	0	360	3.0 d
(Hunt's)	70	2.0	12.0	2.0	0	560	2.0 d
(Hunt's Homestyle)	50	2.0	10.0	1.0	0	530	2.0 d
(Prego)	120	2.0	20.0	4.0	n.a.	550	m.q.
(Progresso)	110	3.0	13.0	5.0	5	630	m.q.
(Ragú Thick & Hearty)	100	2.0	15.0	3.0	0	460	m.q.
super (Ragú Chunky Garden Style) . .	110	2.0	15.0	5.0	0	500	m.q.
mushroom and green pepper (Prego Extra Chunky)	90	2.0	14.0	3.0	n.a.	410	m.q.
mushroom and onion (Prego Extra Chunky)	100	2.0	13.0	4.0	n.a.	490	m.q.
mushroom and pepper (Master Choice Giardino)	80	2.0	12.0	3.0	0	777	m.q.

Food and Measure	cal.	prot. (gms)	carbo. (gms)	fat (gms)	chol. (mgs)	sod. (mgs)	fiber (gms)
mushroom w/extra spice (Prego Extra Chunky)	100	2.0	17.0	3.0	n.a.	450	m.q.
mushroom and tomato (Prego Extra Chunky)	100	2.0	16.0	3.0	n.a.	480	m.q.
w/olives and mushrooms (Classico Di Sicilia)	50	2.0	7.0	2.0	0	470	m.q.
onion and garlic (Prego)	100	2.0	15.0	4.0	n.a.	510	m.q.
Parmesan (Ragú Fino Italian)	90	3.0	12.0	3.0	2	540	m.q.
w/peppers, sweet, and onions (Classico Di Salerno)	70	1.0	7.0	4.0	0	360	m.q.
w/red pepper, spicy (Classico Di Roma Arrabbiata)	50	2.0	6.0	2.0	0	250	m.q.
sausage and green pepper (Prego Extra Chunky)	160	3.0	19.0	8.0	m.q.	500	m.q.
tomato:							
and basil (Classico Di Napoli)	60	2.0	6.0	3.0	0	340	m.q.
and basil (Prego)	100	2.0	18.0	2.0	n.a.	370	m.q.
garlic and onions (Ragú Chunky Garden Style) . .	110	2.0	15.0	5.0	0	500	m.q.
and herbs (Ragú Fino Italian) . . .	90	2.0	13.0	3.0	0	490	m.q.
and herbs (Ragú Today's Recipe) . .	50	2.0	8.0	1.0	0	370	m.q.
onion, garlic (Prego Extra Chunky) . .	100	2.0	14.0	5.0	n.a.	480	m.q.
w/zinfandel (Sutter Home)	100	2.0	11.0	5.0	0	520	m.q.

Food and Measure	cal.	prot. (gms)	carbo. (gms)	fat (gms)	chol. (mgs)	sod. (mgs)	fiber (gms)
Pasta sauce, frozen or refrigerated:							
meatless (Bodin's), 3.4 oz.	60	5.0	10.0	0	0	340	1.0 d
tomato, chunky (Contadina Light), 5 oz.	50	2.0	9.0	0	0	570	m.q.
Pasta sauce mix, 1 pkg., except as noted:							
(Lawry's Rich & Thick)	147	3.5	28.1	2.2	<1	2172	.5 c
(McCormick/Schilling), ¼ pkg.	32	1.0	6.0	.3	n.a.	615	m.q.
(Spatini), 1 cup* . . .	64	1.5	10.0	5.1	<1	960	<.1 c
w/mushrooms (Lawry's)	143	5.2	26.0	1.5	<1	2015	2.1 c
Pastrami:							
(Healthy Deli), 1 oz.	36	5.6	.8	1.1	15	290	0
(Hillshire Farm Deli Select), 1 oz.	31	6.0	<1.0	.4	m.q.	290	0
turkey, see "Turkey pastrami"							
Pastry dough (see also "Pie crust"):							
sheet, puff pastry (Pepperidge Farm), ¼ piece	260	4.0	22.0	17.0	n.a.	290	m.q.
shell, 1 piece:							
patty (Pepperidge Farm)	210	3.0	16.0	15.0	n.a.	180	m.q.
puff pastry, mini (Pepperidge Farm)	50	1.0	4.0	4.0	n.a.	40	m.q.
tart (Stilwell)	100	2.0	9.0	7.0	0	65	2.0 d
Pâté, canned:							
1 oz.	90	4.0	.4	7.9	m.q.	198	0
1 tbsp.	41	1.9	.2	3.6	m.q.	91	0
chicken liver, 1 oz. . .	57	3.8	1.9	3.7	m.q.	m.q.	0
chicken liver, 1 tbsp.	26	1.8	.9	1.7	m.q.	m.q.	0

Food and Measure	cal.	prot. (gms)	carbo. (gms)	fat (gms)	chol. (mgs)	sod. (mgs)	fiber (gms)
goose liver, smoked, 1 oz.	131	3.2	1.3	12.4	43	m.q.	0
goose liver, smoked, 1 tbsp.	60	1.5	.6	5.7	20	m.q.	0
liver (Sells), 2¼ oz.	190	8.0	3.0	16.0	m.q.	460	n.a.
Pea pod, Chinese, see "Peas, edible-podded"							
Peach, ½ cup, except as noted:							
fresh:							
2½"-diam. peach, 4 per lb.	37	.6	9.7	.1	0	tr.	1.7 d
pulp, sliced	37	.6	9.4	.1	0	1	1.7 d
canned:							
(Hunt's), 4 oz. . . .	90	<1.0	23.0	<1.0	0	7	<1.0 d
(Stokely)	70	0	18.0	0	0	10	m.q.
spiced, heavy syrup, whole	90	.5	24.3	.1	0	5	1.2 d
canned, freestone, halves or slices:							
in extra heavy syrup	126	.6	34.1	<.1	0	11	.4 c
or yellow cling, in heavy syrup . . .	95	.6	25.5	.1	0	8	.4 c
canned, yellow cling, halves or slices, except as noted:							
in water	29	.5	7.5	.1	0	4	1.2 d
in water (Libby's)	30	0	8.0	0	0	5	m.q.
in juice	55	.8	14.3	<.1	0	6	1.2 d
in juice, diced (Del Monte Fruit Naturals)	60	0	16.0	0	0	10	1.0 d
in extra light syrup, diced (Del Monte Lite)	60	0	16.0	0	0	10	1.0 d
in light syrup . . .	68	.6	18.3	<.1	0	7	1.3 d

Food and Measure	cal.	prot. (gms)	carbo. (gms)	fat (gms)	chol. (mgs)	sod. (mgs)	fiber (gms)
Peach, canned, yellow cling *(cont.)*							
in heavy syrup							
(Libby's)	100	0	25.0	0	0	10	m.q.
in heavy syrup,							
diced *(Del Monte)*	100	0	24.0	0	0	10	1.0 d
dried:							
(Del Monte), 2 oz.	140	2.0	35.0	0	0	<10	m.q.
sulfured, halves . .	192	2.9	49.1	.6	0	6	6.6 d
sulfured, 10 halves,							
4.6 oz.	311	4.7	79.7	1.0	0	9	10.7 d
freeze-dried *(Mountain House Fruit Crisps)*,							
1/4 cup	60	0	15.0	0	0	5	m.q.
frozen, sliced, sweetened	118	.8	30.0	.2	0	8	1.8 d
Peach butter							
(Smucker's), 1 tsp.	15	0	4.0	0	0	0	m.q.
Peach daiquiri mixer, frozen*, w/rum *(Bacardi)*, 7 fl. oz. . . .	200	0	33.0	0	0	5	n.a.
Peach drink, canned *(Hi-C)*, 6 fl. oz. . . .	100	0	24.0	0	0	20	(0)
Peach juice:							
(Smucker's Naturally 100%), 8 fl. oz. . .	120	0	30.0	0	0	10	m.q.
orchard blend *(Dole Pure & Light)*,							
6 fl. oz.	90	0	24.0	0	0	10	m.q.
Peach nectar:							
canned, 6 fl. oz. . . .	101	.5	26.0	<.1	0	13	1.1 d
(Kern's), 6 fl. oz. . . .	110	1.0	26.0	0	0	0	m.q.
(R.W. Knudsen),							
8 fl. oz.	107	<1.0	32.0	<1.0	0	(0)	m.q.
(Libby's), 6 fl. oz. . .	100	0	24.0	0	0	5	m.q.
(Libby's Ripe), 8 fl. oz.	130	0	32.0	0	0	5	m.q.
Peanut, shelled, 1 oz., except as noted:							
(Beer Nuts)	170	7.0	7.0	14.0	0	80	2.0 d

Food and Measure	cal.	prot. (gms)	carbo. (gms)	fat (gms)	chol. (mgs)	sod. (mgs)	fiber (gms)
unroasted	159	7.2	4.5	13.8	0	5	2.4 d
boiled, salted	90	3.8	6.0	6.2	0	213	2.5 d
dry-roasted:							
1 oz.	164	6.6	6.0	13.9	0	2	2.3 d
1/2 cup	428	17.3	15.7	36.3	0	4	5.8 d
salted	164	6.6	6.0	13.9	0	228	2.3 d
(Fisher)	160	7.0	6.0	14.0	0	210	m.q.
(Fisher Lightly Salted)	160	7.0	6.0	14.0	0	100	m.q.
(Flavor House)	160	8.0	4.0	14.0	0	200	2.0 d
honey-roasted:							
(Eagle Honey Roast)	170	7.0	7.0	13.0	0	140	m.q.
(Fisher)	150	6.0	5.0	13.0	0	115	m.q.
dry-roasted (Fisher)	150	7.0	4.0	13.0	0	110	m.q.
dry- or oil-roasted (Flavor House)	160	7.0	8.0	12.0	0	60	1.0 d
oil-roasted:							
1 oz.	163	7.4	5.3	13.8	0	2	2.6 d
1/2 cup	419	19.0	13.6	35.5	0	4	6.6 d
salted	163	7.4	5.3	13.8	0	121	2.5 d
(Fisher)	160	7.0	6.0	14.0	0	130	m.q.
(Fisher Lightly Salted)	160	7.0	6.0	14.0	0	65	m.q.
butter toffee (Flavor House)	150	3.0	20.0	7.0	0	80	<1.0 d
flavored, hot (Tom's)	170	7.0	5.0	13.0	0	240	m.q.
party, oil-roasted (Flavor House)	170	8.0	4.0	14.0	0	125	2.0 d
red skin (Tom's), 1 1/8-oz. pkg.	190	9.0	5.0	16.0	0	170	m.q.
Spanish:							
(Flavor House)	160	8.0	3.0	14.0	0	125	2.0 d
raw (Fisher)	160	7.0	5.0	14.0	0	m.q.	m.q.
dry-roasted (Planters)	160	7.0	6.0	14.0	0	200	m.q.
roasted (Fisher)	170	8.0	5.0	14.0	0	130	m.q.
toasted (Tom's), 1 1/8-oz. pkg.	190	8.0	6.0	16.0	0	140	m.q.

Food and Measure	cal.	prot. (gms)	carbo. (gms)	fat (gms)	chol. (mgs)	sod. (mgs)	fiber (gms)
Peanut butter,							
2 tbsp.:							
chunky:							
2 tbsp.	188	7.7	6.9	16.0	0	156	2.1 d
(*Jif* Extra Crunchy)	180	9.0	6.0	16.0	0	130	m.q.
(*Peter Pan* Crunchy)	190	9.0	5.0	16.0	0	120	2.0 d
(*Simply Jif* Extra							
Crunchy)	180	9.0	5.0	16.0	0	50	m.q.
(*Skippy* Super							
Chunk)	190	9.0	4.0	17.0	0	130	.6 c
(*Smucker's* Chunky							
Natural)	200	8.0	6.0	16.0	0	125	m.q.
chunky or creamy:							
(*Arrowhead Mills*)	190	9.0	6.0	16.0	0	tr.	4.5 d
(*Peter Pan* Salt Free)	190	9.0	5.0	17.0	0	0	2.0 d
(*Roaster Fresh*) . .	166	8.0	5.0	14.0	0	2	m.q.
creamy:							
2 tbsp.	188	7.9	6.6	16.0	0	153	1.9 d
(*Jif*)	180	9.0	6.0	16.0	0	155	m.q.
(*Peter Pan* Creamy)	190	9.0	6.0	16.0	0	150	2.0 d
(*Simply Jif*)	180	9.0	5.0	16.0	0	65	m.q.
(*Skippy* Creamy) . .	190	9.0	4.0	17.0	0	150	.6 c
(*Smucker's* Natural)	200	8.0	6.0	16.0	0	125	m.q.
(*Smucker's* No Salt							
Added Natural)	200	8.0	6.0	16.0	0	<10	m.q.
honey sweetened							
(*Smucker's*) . . .	200	7.0	7.0	16.0	0	150	m.q.
jelly and, see "Jelly							
and peanut butter"							
Peanut butter flavor							
baking chips							
(*Reese's*), 1/4 cup	230	9.0	19.0	13.0	5	90	m.q.
Peanut butter–cara-							
mel topping							
(*Smucker's*), 2 tbsp.	150	3.0	29.0	2.0	0	120	m.q.
Peanut flour, 1 cup:							
defatted	196	31.3	20.8	.3	0	9	2.4 c
defatted, salted . . .	196	31.3	20.8	.3	0	108	2.4 c

Food and Measure	cal.	prot. (gms)	carbo. (gms)	fat (gms)	chol. (mgs)	sod. (mgs)	fiber (gms)
lowfat	257	20.3	18.8	13.1	0	0	m.q.
Pear, 1/2 cup, except as noted:							
fresh, w/peel:							
Bartlett, 1 medium, 21/2 per lb. . . .	98	.7	25.1	.7	0	1	4.0 d
sliced	49	.3	12.5	.3	0	1	2.0 d
canned, halves or slices, except as noted:							
(Hunt's), 4 oz. . . .	90	<1.0	22.0	<1.0	0	6	<1.0 d
(Stokely)	90	0	23.0	0	0	10	m.q.
in water	36	.2	9.5	<.1	0	3	2.4 d
in water (Libby's)	35	0	10.0	0	0	10	m.q.
in juice	62	.4	16.0	.1	0	5	2.5 d
in extra light syrup, diced (Del Monte Lite)	60	0	15.0	0	0	10	1.0 d
in light syrup . . .	72	.2	19.0	<.1	0	7	2.5 d
in heavy syrup . . .	94	.3	24.4	.2	0	7	2.6 d
in heavy syrup, diced (Del Monte)	100	0	24.0	0	0	10	1.0 d
in heavy syrup (Libby's)	90	0	23.0	0	0	10	m.q.
dried, sulfured:							
2 oz.	149	1.1	39.5	.4	0	4	4.3 d
halves	236	1.7	62.7	.6	0	5	6.8 d
freeze-dried (Mountain House Fruit Crisps), 1/4 cup	60	0	14.0	0	0	0	m.q.
Pear, Asian, whole, 1 medium, 21/4″ × 21/2″ diam.	51	.6	13.0	.3	0	(0)	4.4 d
Pear juice, (R.W. Knudsen), 8 fl. oz.	110	<1.0	28.0	<1.0	0	(0)	m.q.
Pear nectar:							
canned, 6 fl. oz. . . .	112	.2	29.6	<.1	0	7	1.1 d
(Kern's), 6 fl. oz. . . .	120	0	28.0	0	0	0	m.q.

Food and Measure	cal.	prot. (gms)	carbo. (gms)	fat (gms)	chol. (mgs)	sod. (mgs)	fiber (gms)
Pear nectar *(cont.)*							
(Libby's), 6 fl. oz. . .	110	0	28.0	0	0	0	m.q.
Peas, see specific list-							
ings							
Peas, cream, canned,							
(Allens/East Texas							
Fair), 1/2 cup	90	7.0	14.0	<1.0	0	440	3.0 d
Peas, crowder:							
canned *(Allens/East*							
Texas Fair), 1/2 cup	80	5.0	15.0	<1.0	0	370	4.0 d
frozen *(Seabrook)*,							
3 oz.	130	8.0	23.0	1.0	0	m.q.	1.0 c
Peas, edible-podded:							
fresh:							
raw, 1/2 cup	30	2.0	5.4	.1	0	3	1.9 d
boiled, drained,							
1/2 cup	34	2.6	5.6	.2	0	3	2.2 d
sugar snap							
(Frieda's), 1 oz.	15	1.0	3.4	.1	0	m.q.	m.q.
frozen:							
boiled, drained,							
1/2 cup	42	2.8	7.2	.3	0	4	2.4 d
(Green Giant Sugar							
Snap), 1/2 cup . .	30	2.0	8.0	0	0	0	2.0 d
Chinese *(Chun*							
King), 1.5 oz. . . .	20	1.0	3.0	0	0	<10	m.q.
Chinese *(Seabrook)*,							
2 oz.	20	2.0	4.0	0	0	n.a.	m.q.
snow *(La Choy)*,							
3 oz.	35	2.0	6.0	<1.0	0	10	m.q.
mix*, Oriental snow,							
w/rice *(Fantastic)*,							
10 oz.	160	5.0	30.0	2.0	0	490	3.0 d
Peas, field, canned,							
1/2 cup:							
(Allens)	100	7.0	18.0	<1.0	0	370	m.q.
w/snaps *(Allens)* . . .	70	6.0	13.0	<1.0	0	340	4.0 d

Food and Measure	cal.	prot. (gms)	carbo. (gms)	fat (gms)	chol. (mgs)	sod. (mgs)	fiber (gms)
Peas, green or sweet, 1/2 cup, except as noted:							
fresh:							
raw, in pod, 1 lb.	140	9.3	24.9	.7	0	8	8.8 d
raw, shelled	58	3.9	10.4	.3	0	3	3.7 d
boiled, drained . .	67	4.3	12.5	.2	0	2	4.4 d
canned:							
dry early June *(Crest Top)*	80	5.0	15.0	<1.0	0	320	5.0 d
sweet *(Green Giant 50% Less Salt)*	50	4.0	11.0	0	0	195	3.0 d
sweet *(Stokely)* . .	60	4.0	10.0	0	0	320	m.q.
sweet, w/pearl onions *(Green Giant)*	50	4.0	11.0	0	0	510	4.0 d
very young, small, early *(Green Giant)*	50	3.0	12.0	0	0	390	3.0 d
very young, small, sweet *(Green Giant)*	50	4.0	12.0	0	0	390	4.0 d
very young, tender, sweet *(Green Giant)*	50	4.0	11.0	0	0	390	4.0 d
freeze-dried* *(Mountain House)*	70	4.0	12.0	1.0	0	90	m.q.
frozen:							
(Frosty Acres), 3.3 oz.	80	5.0	13.0	0	0	91	2.0 c
(Seabrook), 3.3 oz.	80	5.0	13.0	0	0	91	2.0 c
Le Sueur baby, early *(Green Giant Harvest Fresh)* . . .	60	4.0	12.0	1.0	0	140	3.0 d
Le Sueur baby, early *(Green Giant Select)*	60	4.0	13.0	0	0	115	4.0 d
sweet *(Green Giant)*	50	4.0	11.0	0	0	95	4.0 d

Food and Measure	cal.	prot. (gms)	carbo. (gms)	fat (gms)	chol. (mgs)	sod. (mgs)	fiber (gms)
Peas, green or sweet, frozen (cont.)							
sweet (Green Giant Harvest Fresh)	50	4.0	12.0	0	0	135	3.0 d
tiny (Frosty Acres), 3.3 oz.	60	4.0	11.0	0	0	127	2.0 c
frozen in butter sauce:							
Le Sueur baby, early (Green Giant) . .	80	5.0	14.0	2.0	5	440	3.0 d
Le Sueur baby, early (Green Giant One Serving), 4.5 oz.	90	5.0	17.0	2.0	5	400	5.0 d
sweet (Green Giant)	80	5.0	14.0	2.0	5	410	4.0 d
tender, sweet (Bird's Eye)	80	4.0	12.0	2.0	5	170	3.0 d
Peas, green, combinations, frozen or packaged, 1/2 cup:							
and carrots, see "Peas and carrots"							
Le Sueur style (Green Giant Valley Combinations)	70	4.0	12.0	2.0	0	400	2.0 d
and mushrooms:							
(Del Monte Vegetable Classics) . . .	70	3.0	9.0	2.0	n.a.	430	m.q.
Le Sueur early peas (Green Giant Select)	60	4.0	11.0	0	0	95	4.0 d
and water chestnuts Oriental (The Budget Gourmet Side Dish), 1 serving	110	5.0	14.0	4.0	5	400	m.q.
Peas lady, canned, w/or w/out snaps (Allens/Sunshine) 1/2 cup	90	7.0	14.0	<1.0	0	440	m.q.

Food and Measure	cal.	prot. (gms)	carbo. (gms)	fat (gms)	chol. (mgs)	sod. (mgs)	fiber (gms)
Peas, pepper,							
canned, *(Allens/East*							
Texas Fair), 1/2 cup	90	6.0	15.0	<1.0	0	530	4.0 d
Peas, purple hull:							
canned *(Allens/East*							
Texas Fair), 1/2 cup	100	7.0	18.0	<1.0	0	350	4.0 d
frozen *(Frosty Acres)*,							
3.3 oz.	130	9.0	23.0	0	0	6	m.q.
Peas, sprouted, ma-							
ture seeds:							
raw, 1/2 cup	77	5.3	17.0	.4	0	12	1.7 c
boiled, drained, 4 oz.	134	8.0	24.8	.6	0	3	3.7 d
Peas, white acre,							
canned *(Allens/East*							
Texas Fair), 1/2 cup	90	7.0	14.0	<1.0	0	440	m.q.
Peas and carrots:							
canned *(Stokely)*,							
1/2 cup	50	3.0	9.0	0	0	320	m.q.
frozen, 3.3 oz.:							
(Frosty Acres)	60	3.0	11.0	0	0	75	1.0 c
(Seabrook)	60	3.0	11.0	0	0	75	1.0 c
Pecan, shelled:							
raw, ground or							
chopped *(Fisher)*,							
1 oz.	190	2.0	5.0	19.0	0	0	m.q.
dried:							
1 oz.	190	2.2	5.2	19.2	0	tr.	2.2 d
halves, 1 cup . . .	721	8.4	19.7	73.1	0	1	8.2 d
chopped, 1 cup . .	794	9.2	21.7	80.5	0	1	9.0 d
dry-roasted:							
1 oz.	187	2.3	6.3	18.4	0	tr.	.5 c
salted, 1 oz.	187	2.3	6.3	18.4	0	221	.5 c
oil-roasted:							
1 oz.	195	2.0	4.6	20.2	0	tr.	.5 c
salted, 1 oz.	195	2.0	4.6	20.2	0	214	.5 c
Pecan flour, 1 oz. . . .	93	9.1	14.4	.4	0	tr.	.4 c

Food and Measure	cal.	prot. (gms)	carbo. (gms)	fat (gms)	chol. (mgs)	sod. (mgs)	fiber (gms)
Pecan topping, in syrup *(Smucker's),* 2 tbsp.	130	2.0	28.0	1.0	0	0	m.q.
Pectin, unsweetened, dry, 1.75-oz. pkg.	163	.1	45.2	.1	0	100	n.a.
Penne entree, frozen, w/sauce, Italian sausage *(The Budget Gourmet),* 10 oz.	320	13.0	54.0	9.0	5	590	m.q.
Pepper, ground, 1 tsp.:							
black	5	.2	1.4	.1	0	1	.6 d
chili *(Spice Islands)*	9	.3	1.2	.3	0	<1	.3 c
red or cayenne . . .	6	.2	1.0	.3	0	1	.5 d
white	7	.3	1.7	.1	0	tr.	.1 c
seasoned (see also specific listings):							
(Lawry's Spice Blends)	9	.3	1.8	.1	0	5	.2 c
(McCormick/Schilling All Pepper)	6	.1	1.0	0	0	426	m.q.
pizza *(Lawry's* Spice Blends)	2	1.5	3.2	.2	n.a.	11	m.q.
Pepper, banana, 1 oz.:							
hot or mild, chunks or rings *(Vlasic)*	4	0	1.0	0	0	480	m.q.
sweet, rings *(Vlasic)*	8	0	2.0	0	0	170	m.q.
Pepper, bell, see "Pepper, sweet"							
Pepper, cherry:							
(Progresso), 1/2 cup	190	0	3.0	20.0	0	130	1.0 d
(Vlasic), 1 oz.	8	0	2.0	0	0	480	m.q.
pickled *(Progresso),* 1/2 cup	130	0	3.0	12.0	0	110	1.0 d

Food and Measure	cal.	prot. (gms)	carbo. (gms)	fat (gms)	chol. (mgs)	sod. (mgs)	fiber (gms)
Pepper, chili:							
raw, green and red, w/out seeds:							
1 medium, 1.6 oz.	18	.9	4.3	.1	0	3	.7 d
chopped, 1/2 cup	30	1.5	7.1	.2	0	5	1.1 d
canned:							
w/liquid, chopped, 1/2 cup	17	.6	4.2	.1	0	m.q.	1.3 d
green, whole *(Old El Paso)*, 1 chili . .	8	<1.0	1.0	<1.0	0	105	m.q.
green, chopped *(Old El Paso)*, 2 tbsp.	8	<1.0	2.0	<1.0	0	70	m.q.
hot, Mexican *(Vlasic)*, 1 oz. . .	8	0	2.0	0	0	470	m.q.
mild *(Vlasic)*, 1 oz.	8	0	2.0	0	0	480	m.q.
Pepper, jalapeño:							
all styles *(Ortega)*, 1 oz.	10	0	3.0	0	0	20	m.q.
marinated *(La Victoria)*, 1 1/2 pieces	10	0	2.0	0	0	300	m.q.
nacho *(La Victoria)*, 14 pieces	5	0	1.0	0	0	330	m.q.
Pepper, pepper-oncini:							
(Progresso Tuscan), 1/2 cup	20	0	7.0	0	0	5	1.0 d
salad *(Vlasic)*, 1 oz.	4	0	1.0	0	0	440	m.q.
Pepper, piccalilli *(Progresso)*, 1/2 cup	190	<1.0	4.0	20.0	0	220	1.0 d
Pepper, stuffed, entree, frozen:							
(On-Cor), 8 oz.	168	9.0	15.0	8.0	n.a.	1135	m.q.
(Stouffer's Single Serving), 10 oz. . . .	220	10.0	28.0	8.0	n.a.	1010	m.q.
green, w/beef, tomato sauce *(Stouffer's)*, 7.75 oz.	200	9.0	22.0	8.0	m.q.	650	m.q.

Food and Measure	cal.	prot. (gms)	carbo. (gms)	fat (gms)	chol. (mgs)	sod. (mgs)	fiber (gms)
Pepper, stuffed *(cont.)*							
sweet red *(Celentano)*,							
13 oz.	350	28.0	28.0	20.0	n.a.	710	m.q.
Pepper, sweet:							
fresh, green and red:							
raw, 1 medium,							
3¾″ × 3″ diam.	20	.7	4.8	.1	0	1	1.3 d
raw, chopped,							
½ cup	13	.4	3.2	.1	0	1	.9 d
boiled, drained,							
1 medium	20	.7	4.9	.1	0	1	.9 d
boiled, drained,							
chopped, ½ cup	19	.6	4.6	.1	0	1	.8 d
fresh, yellow, raw:							
1 large, 5″ × 3″							
diam.	50	1.9	11.8	.4	0	3	m.q.
10 strips, 1.8 oz.	14	.5	3.3	.1	0	1	m.q.
canned or jars, (see							
also "Pimiento"):							
roasted *(Progresso)*,							
½ cup	20	<1.0	5.0	<1.0	0	2	1.7 d
fried *(Progresso)*,							
½ jar	37	<1.0	4.0	3.0	0	17	1.0 d
salad *(B&G)*, 1 oz.	10	0	3.0	0	0	240	m.q.
freeze-dried, 1 tbsp.	1	.1	.3	<.1	0	1	.1 d
frozen, 1 oz.:							
chopped	6	.3	1.3	.1	0	1	.5 d
green *(Seabrook)*	6	0	1.0	0	0	1	m.q.
red *(Seabrook)* . . .	8	0	1.0	0	0	n.a.	m.q.
Pepper rings, hot							
(Vlasic), 1 oz. . . .	4	0	1.0	0	0	480	m.q.
Pepper sauce, hot:							
(Gebhardt), ½ tsp.	<1	<1.0	<1.0	<1.0	0	55	<1.0 d
(Pickapeppa), 1 tbsp.	4	0	4.0	0	0	95	n.a.
(Tabasco), 2 fl. oz. . .	7	.4	.7	.2	0	404	(0)
cayenne *(Maull's)*,							
1 tsp.	4	0	1.0	0	0	200	0

Food and Measure	cal.	prot. (gms)	carbo. (gms)	fat (gms)	chol. (mgs)	sod. (mgs)	fiber (gms)
Pepper sauce mix *(Knorr)*, 1 serving							
dry	25	.7	3.4	.8	0	350	m.q.
Peppercorn sauce mix*, green *(McCormick/Schilling McCormick Collection)*,							
1/4 cup	86	1.0	4.0	4.0	n.a.	546	n.a.
Peppered loaf:							
(Kahn's), 1 slice . . .	40	5.0	1.0	2.0	m.q.	340	(0)
(Oscar Mayer), 1 oz.	43	4.8	1.3	2.1	13	361	(0)
Pepperoni, 1 oz., except as noted:							
(Hormel/Rosa Grande)	138	6.0	<2.0	13.0	29	460	0
(Oscar Mayer),							
15 slices	140	6.0	0	13.0	25	550	0
sliced *(Hormel Deli)*	135	6.0	<2.0	12.0	32	480	0
sliced *(Pillow Pack)*	140	5.0	1.0	13.0	30	450	0
Perch, meat only:							
raw, 4 oz.	103	22.0	0	1.1	102	70	0
baked, broiled, or microwaved, 4 oz. . . .	133	28.2	0	1.3	130	90	0
ocean, see "Ocean perch"							
Perch entree, frozen, battered *(Van de Kamp's)*, 2 pieces	310	12.0	18.0	21.0	30	500	m.q.
Persimmon, 1 oz., except as noted:							
Japanese:							
fresh, 1 medium, 2 1/2" × 3 1/2" . . .	118	1.0	31.2	.3	0	3	6.0 d
dried	78	.4	20.8	.2	0	1	4.1 d
California, dried *(Frieda's)*	67	1.8	.1	m.q.	0	m.q.	m.q.
fuyu, fresh *(Frieda's)*	22	.2	5.6	.1	0	2	m.q.
hachiya, fresh, trimmed *(Frieda's)*	36	.2	10.1	.1	0	<1	m.q.

Food and Measure	cal.	prot. (gms)	carbo. (gms)	fat (gms)	chol. (mgs)	sod. (mgs)	fiber (gms)
Persimmon *(cont.)*							
native, fresh, 1 medium, 1.1 oz. . . .	32	.2	8.4	.1	0	tr.	.4 c
Pesto dip mix*							
(Knorr), 1 tbsp. . .	30	<1.0	1.0	3.0	5	75	n.a.
Pheasant, raw:							
meat w/skin, 4 oz. . .	205	25.7	0	10.5	m.q.	45	0
meat only:							
4 oz.	151	26.7	0	4.1	m.q.	42	0
1/2 breast, 6.4 oz.	243	44.4	0	5.9	m.q.	60	0
1 leg, 3.8 oz. . . .	143	23.8	0	4.6	m.q.	48	0
Phyllo, see "Fillo pastry"							
Picante beans, canned, *(Allens/East Texas Fair)*, 1/2 cup	80	6.0	15.0	<1.0	0	600	5.0 d
Picante sauce (see also "Salsa"):							
(Frito-Lay's), 1 oz. . .	10	0	3.0	0	0	160	m.q.
(Gebhardt), 1 tbsp. .	4	0	1.0	0	0	120	m.q.
(Old El Paso Thick'n Chunky), 2 tbsp. . . .	6	<1.0	1.0	0	m.q.	310	<1.0 d
(Tabasco), 1 oz. . . .	12	.4	2.9	<.1	0	206	.4 d
hot:							
(Chi-Chi's), 1 oz.	10	<2.0	2.0	<2.0	<2	268	m.q.
(Rosarita Chunky), 3 tbsp.	18	<1.0	4.0	<1.0	0	515	<1.0 d
medium:							
(Chi-Chi's), 1 oz.	8	<2.0	2.0	<2.0	<2	192	m.q.
(Rosarita Chunky), 3 tbsp.	16	<1.0	4.0	<1.0	0	650	<1.0 d
mild:							
(Chi-Chi's), 1 oz.	9	<2.0	2.0	<2.0	<2	198	m.q.
(Rosarita Chunky), 3 tbsp.	25	1.0	5.0	<1.0	0	630	<1.0 d

Food and Measure	cal.	prot. (gms)	carbo. (gms)	fat (gms)	chol. (mgs)	sod. (mgs)	fiber (gms)
Pickle, 1 oz., except as noted:							
bread and butter:							
(Mrs. Fanning's), 2 slices, 2/3 oz.	15	0	3.0	0	0	140	m.q.
(Vlasic)	25	0	6.0	0	0	170	m.q.
slices *(Claussen)* . .	20	0	4.0	0	0	170	m.q.
chips *(Vlasic)* . . .	25	0	6.0	0	0	170	m.q.
chunks *(Vlasic* Old Fashioned) . . .	24	0	6.0	0	0	135	m.q.
stix *(Vlasic)*	20	0	5.0	0	0	130	m.q.
sweet *(Vlasic* Sweet Butter Chips Half Salt)	30	0	7.0	0	0	85	m.q.
zesty chips *(Vlasic)*	45	0	11.0	0	0	220	m.q.
dill:							
(New Morning Kosher), 1.1 oz. . .	6	0	1.0	0	0	410	m.q.
(New Morning Kosher No Salt), 1.1 oz.	6	0	1.0	0	0	0	m.q.
(Vlasic Original) . .	4	0	1.0	0	0	390	m.q.
all varieties, except halves *(Vlasic* Deli)	4	0	1.0	0	0	310	m.q.
whole, 33/4″ long, 2.3 oz.	12	.4	2.7	.1	0	833	.8 d
baby or crunchy, zesty *(Vlasic)* . .	4	0	1.0	0	0	280	m.q.
baby, gherkins, spears, or snack chunks *(Vlasic* Kosher)	4	0	1.0	0	0	220	m.q.
crunchy *(Vlasic* Kosher)	4	0	1.0	0	0	390	m.q.
halves *(Vlasic* Deli)	4	0	1.0	0	0	300	m.q.
spears *(New Morning* Kosher), 1.1 oz.	4	0	1.0	0	0	350	m.q.

Food and Measure	cal.	prot. (gms)	carbo. (gms)	fat (gms)	chol. (mgs)	sod. (mgs)	fiber (gms)
Pickle, dill *(cont.)*							
spears or crunchy *(Vlasic* Kosher Half Salt)	4	0	1.0	0	0	110	m.q.
spears or snack chunks, Polish or zesty *(Vlasic)* . .	4	0	1.0	0	0	280	m.q.
hamburger chips *(Vlasic* Kosher) . . .	4	0	1.0	0	0	180	m.q.
hamburger chips, half salt *(Vlasic)*	4	0	1.0	0	0	180	m.q.
no garlic, spears or crunchy *(Vlasic)* . .	4	0	1.0	0	0	220	m.q.
sour	3	.1	.6	.1	0	342	.3 d
sweet:							
midget *(Vlasic)* . . .	45	0	10.0	0	0	220	m.q.
whole, gherkins, or chips *(Vlasic)* . .	45	0	10.0	0	0	170	m.q.
Pickle loaf, 1 slice:							
(Kahn's)	80	3.0	2.0	7.0	m.q.	280	(0)
(Kahn's Family Pack)	70	3.0	2.0	6.0	m.q.	220	(0)
beef *(Kahn's* Family Pack)	60	2.0	1.0	5.0	m.q.	210	(0)
Pickle and pimiento loaf *(Oscar Mayer),* 1 slice	60	3.0	4.0	4.0	10	360	0
Pickle relish, see "Relish"							
Pickling spice *(Tone's),* 1 tsp. . .	10	.3	1.2	.6	n.a.	1	.3 d
Pie, frozen, 1/6 pie, except as noted:							
apple:							
(Banquet Family Size)	250	2.0	37.0	11.0	n.a.	290	m.q.
(Mrs. Smith's 8")	270	2.0	40.0	11.0	0	300	1.0 d
(Mrs. Smith's 9"), 1/8 pie	370	2.0	50.0	18.0	0	430	2.0 d

Food and Measure	cal.	prot. (gms)	carbo. (gms)	fat (gms)	chol. (mgs)	sod. (mgs)	fiber (gms)
(Mrs. Smith's 10"),							
¹/₁₀ pie	280	2.0	43.0	12.0	0	310	1.0 d
(Sara Lee Home-style), 3.7 oz. . .	260	2.0	37.0	12.0	0	250	m.q.
apple, Dutch:							
(Mrs. Smith's 8")	310	3.0	48.0	13.0	0	270	1.0 d
(Mrs. Smith's 10"),							
¹/₁₀ pie	320	3.0	50.0	12.0	0	270	1.0 d
(Sara Lee Home-style), 3.7 oz. . .	290	2.0	41.0	13.0	0	280	m.q.
crumb *(Mrs. Smith's 9"),* ¹/₉ pie	300	2.0	48.0	12.0	0	240	2.0 d
apple-cranberry *(Mrs. Smith's 8")*	280	2.0	43.0	11.0	0	290	1.0 d
banana cream:							
(Banquet)	180	2.0	21.0	10.0	n.a.	150	m.q.
(Pet-Ritz)	170	2.0	22.0	9.0	n.a.	155	m.q.
berry *(Mrs. Smith's 8")*	280	2.0	44.0	11.0	0	340	0
blackberry *(Mrs. Smith's 8")*	280	2.0	43.0	11.0	0	310	0
blackberry or blue-berry *(Banquet* Fam-ily Size)	270	3.0	40.0	11.0	n.a.	350	m.q.
blueberry: *(Mrs. Smith's 8")*	260	2.0	39.0	11.0	0	320	1.0 d
blueberry cheese yo-gurt *(Mrs. Smith's 7"),* ¹/₄ pie	270	3.0	48.0	8.0	10	260	1.0 d
Boston cream, see "Cake, frozen"							
cherry:							
(Banquet Family Size)	250	3.0	36.0	11.0	n.a.	260	m.q.
(Mrs. Smith's 8")	270	2.0	41.0	11.0	0	320	1.0 d
(Mrs. Smith's 9"), ¹/₈ pie	320	3.0	48.0	13.0	0	350	1.0 d
(Mrs. Smith's 10"), ¹/₁₀ pie	290	2.0	44.0	11.0	0	330	1.0 d

Food and Measure	cal.	prot. (gms)	carbo. (gms)	fat (gms)	chol. (mgs)	sod. (mgs)	fiber (gms)
Pie, frozen (cont.)							
chocolate cream:							
(Banquet)	190	2.0	24.0	10.0	n.a.	110	m.q.
(Pet-Ritz)	190	1.0	27.0	8.0	n.a.	145	m.q.
coconut cream:							
(Banquet)	190	2.0	22.0	11.0	n.a.	120	m.q.
(Pet-Ritz)	190	2.0	27.0	8.0	n.a.	145	m.q.
coconut custard:							
(Mrs. Smith's 8")	230	6.0	30.0	10.0	65	290	0
(Mrs. Smith's 10"),							
1/10 pie	230	7.0	30.0	10.0	70	280	0
French silk cream (Mrs. Smith's 8"),							
1/5 pie	410	3.0	55.0	21.0	5	250	1.0 d
lemon cream:							
(Banquet)	170	2.0	23.0	9.0	n.a.	120	m.q.
(Pet-Ritz)	190	2.0	26.0	9.0	n.a.	150	m.q.
lemon meringue (Mrs. Smith's 8"), 1/5 pie	300	3.0	54.0	8.0	65	220	0
mince:							
(Mrs. Smith's 8")	300	2.0	48.0	11.0	0	400	2.0 d
(Mrs. Smith's 10"),							
1/10 pie	320	2.0	51.0	12.0	0	410	2.0 d
mincemeat (Banquet Family Size)	260	3.0	38.0	11.0	n.a.	370	m.q.
Neapolitan cream (Pet-Ritz)	180	1.0	17.0	10.0	n.a.	185	m.q.
peach:							
(Banquet Family Size)	245	3.0	35.0	11.0	n.a.	280	m.q.
(Mrs. Smith's 8")	260	2.0	37.0	11.0	0	310	1.0 d
(Mrs. Smith's 9"),							
1/8 pie	310	3.0	46.0	13.0	0	350	1.0 d
peach cheese yogurt (Mrs. Smith's 7"),							
1/4 pie	270	3.0	46.0	8.0	10	240	1.0 d

Food and Measure	cal.	prot. (gms)	carbo. (gms)	fat (gms)	chol. (mgs)	sod. (mgs)	fiber (gms)
pecan:							
(Mrs. Smith's 8"),							
1/5 pie	520	5.0	73.0	23.0	70	450	1.0 d
(Mrs. Smith's 10"),							
1/8 pie	500	5.0	68.0	23.0	60	460	1.0 d
pumpkin:							
(Banquet Family							
Size)	200	3.0	29.0	8.0	n.a.	350	m.q.
(Mrs. Smith's 8")	220	5.0	36.0	7.0	40	290	1.0 d
(Mrs. Smith's),							
1/10 pie	230	5.0	38.0	7.0	45	300	1.0 d
hearty (Mrs. Smith's							
8")	230	4.0	37.0	8.0	50	290	2.0 d
raspberry, red (Mrs.							
Smith's 8")	280	2.0	43.0	11.0	0	310	0
strawberry (Mrs.							
Smith's 8"), 1/5 pie	220	2.0	44.0	4.0	0	150	2.0 d
strawberry banana yo-							
gurt (Mrs. Smith's							
7"), 1/4 pie	240	3.0	48.0	5.0	0	190	1.0 d
strawberry cream:							
(Banquet)	170	2.0	22.0	9.0	n.a.	120	m.q.
(Pet-Ritz)	170	2.0	20.0	9.0	n.a.	145	m.q.
strawberry-rhubarb							
(Mrs. Smith's 8")	280	2.0	44.0	11.0	0	380	0
Pie, snack, 1 piece:							
apple:							
(Drake's)	210	2.0	29.0	10.0	0	135	m.q.
(Hostess)	430	3.0	60.0	20.0	15	390	2.0 d
(Tastykake)	300	3.0	46.0	12.0	0	340	2.0 d
French (Hostess)	430	3.0	60.0	20.0	15	390	2.0 d
French (Tastykake)	350	3.0	63.0	11.0	0	220	2.0 d
banana creme (Tas-							
tykake)	380	5.0	54.0	16.0	25	430	2.0 d
blackberry or blue-							
berry (Hostess) . .	420	4.0	59.0	18.0	15	360	2.4 d
blueberry:							
(Drake's)	210	2.0	30.0	10.0	0	135	m.q.

Food and Measure	cal.	prot. (gms)	carbo. (gms)	fat (gms)	chol. (mgs)	sod. (mgs)	fiber (gms)
Pie, snack, blueberry *(cont.)*							
(Tastykake)	310	3.0	55.0	9.0	0	410	2.0 d
cherry:							
(Drake's)	220	2.0	30.0	10.0	0	135	m.q.
(Hostess)	460	4.0	65.0	20.0	15	380	2.4 d
(Tastykake)	300	3.0	49.0	10.0	0	310	2.0 d
coconut creme *(Tas-tykake)*	380	5.0	46.0	20.0	65	420	2.0 d
lemon:							
(Drake's)	210	2.0	27.0	11.0	0	115	m.q.
(Hostess)	440	4.0	60.0	20.0	30	370	1.4 d
(Tastykake)	320	4.0	48.0	13.2	40	380	2.0 d
lemon lime *(Tastykake)*	320	4.0	49.0	13.0	45	310	1.0 d
marshmallow, banana *(Little Debbie)* . . .	170	1.0	28.0	6.0	0	85	m.q.
marshmallow, choco-late *(Little Debbie)*	170	2.0	27.0	6.0	0	75	m.q.
oatmeal creme *(Little Debbie)*	160	2.0	24.0	8.0	0	170	m.q.
peach:							
(Hostess)	420	4.0	60.0	19.0	15	360	2.0 d
(Tastykake)	300	3.0	47.0	12.0	0	360	3.0 d
pineapple cheese *(Tas-tykake)*	340	5.0	54.0	13.0	20	410	2.0 d
pumpkin *(Tastykake)*	320	5.0	46.0	14.0	30	520	2.0 d
raisin creme *(Little Debbie)*	140	0	23.0	5.0	0	115	m.q.
strawberry:							
(Hostess)	410	4.0	56.0	19.0	15	360	2.2 d
(Tastykake)	340	3.0	57.0	11.0	0	300	1.0 d
(Tastykake Tasty Klair)	400	6.0	51.0	20.0	55	320	2.0 d
Pie, snack, frozen *(Weight Watchers Sweet Celebrations),* 1 piece:							
chocolate mocha . .	160	6.0	29.0	4.0	5	150	m.q.
Mississippi mud . . .	160	3.0	28.0	4.0	5	130	m.q.

Food and Measure	cal.	prot. (gms)	carbo. (gms)	fat (gms)	chol. (mgs)	sod. (mgs)	fiber (gms)
Pie crust shell (see also "Pastry dough"), 1/6 shell, except as noted:							
frozen or refrigerated:							
(Oronoque)	120	2.0	9.0	8.0	0	115	m.q.
(Pet-Ritz)	110	2.0	9.0	8.0	0	115	m.q.
(Pet-Ritz, 95/8") . .	170	2.0	15.0	11.0	7	180	m.q.
(Pillsbury All Ready), 1/8 of 2-crust pie	240	2.0	24.0	15.0	15	270	m.q.
(Stilwell), 1/8 shell	90	1.0	9.0	5.0	0	60	1.0 d
cookie crumb:							
(Nilla), 3/4 oz. . .	110	1.0	14.0	6.0	5	50	m.q.
(Oreo), 3/4 oz. . .	110	1.0	14.0	6.0	0	140	m.q.
deep dish *(Pet-Ritz/ Oronoque)*	130	2.0	11.0	9.0	0	130	m.q.
deep dish *(Stilwell),* 1/8 shell	100	1.0	10.0	6.0	0	70	1.0 d
graham cracker:							
(Honeymaid), 3/4 oz.	110	1.0	15.0	6.0	0	100	m.q.
(Pet-Ritz), ...	110	1.0	8.0	6.0	7	80	m.q.
(Stilwell)	150	1.0	17.0	9.0	0	65	1.0 d
vegetable shortening:							
(Pet-Ritz)	120	2.0	11.0	8.0	0	80	m.q.
deep dish *(Pet-Ritz)*	140	2.0	12.0	9.0	0	75	m.q.
mix:							
(Betty Crocker), 1/16 pkg.	120	1.0	10.0	8.0	0	150	m.q.
(Pillsbury), 1/8 mix*	200	3.0	20.0	13.0	0	300	m.q.
Pie filling, canned (see also "Pudding, mix"), 1/3 cup, except as noted:							
apple *(Comstock)* . .	90	0	22.0	0	0	75	2.0 d
blueberry *(Comstock)*	100	0	25.0	0	0	15	1.0 d

Food and Measure	cal.	prot. (gms)	carbo. (gms)	fat (gms)	chol. (mgs)	sod. (mgs)	fiber (gms)
Pie filling, canned *(cont.)*							
cherry *(Comstock)* . . .	90	0	23.0	0	0	25	1.0 d
mincemeat:							
(Borden None Such)	.200	1.0	48.0	1.0	0	280	m.q.
w/brandy and rum *(Borden None Such)*	210	1.0	49.0	1.0	0	260	m.q.
condensed *(Borden None Such),* 1/4 pkg.	220	1.0	50.0	2.0	0	310	m.q.
pumpkin, mix *(Libby's),* 1 cup . .	260	2.0	64.0	.3	0	440	m.q.
Pierogi, frozen *(Golden),* 3 pieces:							
potato cheese	250	8.0	38.0	8.0	35	260	2.0 d
potato onion	210	6.0	36.0	6.0	n.a.	220	1.0 d
Pigeon, see "Squab"							
Pigeon peas, 1/2 cup, except as noted:							
fresh:							
raw	105	5.5	18.4	1.3	0	4	3.2 d
boiled, drained . .	86	4.6	15.0	1.1	0	3	2.2 c
mature, boiled	102	5.7	19.5	.3	0	5	3.9 d
Pig's feet:							
simmered, 4 oz. . . .	220	21.8	0	14.1	113	m.q.	0
pickled:							
cured, 1 oz.	58	3.8	<.1	4.6	26	m.q.	0
(Penrose), 6 oz. . .	220	19.0	2.0	15.0	m.q.	2890	0
Pig's knuckles, pickled *(Penrose),* 6 oz.	290	23.0	1.0	21.0	m.q.	2380	0
Pike:							
northern, meat only:							
raw, 4 oz.	100	21.8	0	.8	44	44	0
baked, broiled, or microwaved, 4 oz.	128	28.0	0	1.0	57	56	0
walleye, meat only, raw, 4 oz.	105	21.7	0	1.4	98	58	0

Food and Measure	cal.	prot. (gms)	carbo. (gms)	fat (gms)	chol. (mgs)	sod. (mgs)	fiber (gms)
baked, broiled, or microwaved, 4 oz.	135	27.8	0	1.8	125	74	0
Pili nut, dried:							
shelled, 1 oz.	204	3.1	1.1	22.6	0	4	.8 c
shelled, 1 cup	863	13.0	4.8	95.5	0	4	3.4 c
Pimiento, all varieties, drained (Dromedary), 1 oz.	10	0	2.0	0	0	5	m.q.
Pimiento spread:							
(Price's), 1 oz.	80	3.0	2.0	6.0	n.a.	m.q.	n.a.
(Price's Light), 1 oz.	50	4.0	2.0	3.0	10	230	0
Piña colada mixer:							
bottled (Holland House), 4.5 fl. oz.	144	<1.0	36.0	<1.0	0	18	(0)
frozen*, w/rum (Bacardi), 7 fl. oz. . . .	260	1.0	37.0	6.0	0	25	(0)
instant (Holland House), .56 oz. dry	75	<1.0	12.0	3.0	0	<1	(0)
Pine nuts, dried:							
pignolia:							
1 oz.	146	6.8	4.0	14.4	0	1	1.3 d
1 tbsp.	51	2.4	1.4	5.1	0	tr.	.5 d
(Krinos), .5 oz. . . .	90	5.0	0	7.5	0	5	1.0 d
(Progresso), 1 tbsp.	60	3.0	1.0	5.0	0	0	m.q.
pinyon:							
1 oz.	161	3.3	5.5	17.3	0	20	3.0 d
10 kernels	6	.1	.2	.6	0	1	.1 d
Pineapple, 1/2 cup, except as noted:							
fresh:							
diced	39	.3	9.6	.3	0	<1	.9 d
baby, trimmed (Frieda's Sugarloaf), 1 oz.	14	.1	3.9	.1	0	<1	m.q.
canned, in juice:							
4 oz.	68	.5	17.8	.1	0	1	.8 d
(Dole)	70	0	18.0	<1.0	0	10	m.q.

Food and Measure	cal.	prot. (gms)	carbo. (gms)	fat (gms)	chol. (mgs)	sod. (mgs)	fiber (gms)
Pineapple *(cont.)*							
canned, in heavy syrup:							
4 oz.	88	.4	22.9	.1	0	1	.8 d
(Dole)	90	0	23.0	0	0	10	m.q.
chunks, tidbits or crushed	100	.5	25.8	.1	0	2	.9 d
canned, w/mandarin orange *(Dole)* . . .	80	0	19.0	<1.0	0	5	m.q.
frozen, sweetened, chunks	104	.5	27.1	.1	0	2	1.3 d
Pineapple float *(R.W. Knudsen)*, 8 fl. oz.	130	2.0	31.0	<1.0	0	(0)	m.q.
Pineapple juice, 6 fl. oz., except as noted:							
canned or bottled:							
6 fl. oz.	105	.6	25.9	.2	0	2	.2 d
(R.W. Knudsen), 8 fl. oz.	110	<1.0	25.0	<1.0	0	(0)	m.q.
(Mott's), 11.5 fl. oz.	204	<1.0	51.0	<1.0	0	<1	m.q.
(Tree Top)	100	0	24.0	0	0	0	m.q.
chilled *(Dole)*	90	0	22.0	0	0	5	m.q.
chilled or frozen* *(Minute Maid)*	90	1.0	23.0	0	0	0	m.q.
frozen*	97	.7	23.9	.1	0	2	.2 d
frozen* *(Dole)*	90	0	22.0	0	0	10	m.q.
Pineapple juice drink, frozen* *(Bright & Early)*, 6 fl. oz. . . .	90	0	23.0	0	0	0	(0)
Pineapple nectar *(Libby's)*, 6 fl. oz.	110	0	27.0	0	0	30	m.q.
Pineapple topping:							
(Kraft), 1 tbsp.	50	0	13.0	0	0	0	m.q.
(Smucker's), 2 tbsp.	130	0	32.0	0	0	0	m.q.

Food and Measure	cal.	prot. (gms)	carbo. (gms)	fat (gms)	chol. (mgs)	sod. (mgs)	fiber (gms)
Pineapple-banana juice cocktail, frozen* *(Welch's Orchard Tropicals),* 6 fl. oz.	100	0	24.0	0	0	20	(0)
Pineapple-coconut juice *(R.W. Knudsen),* 8 fl. oz. . . .	110	<1.0	24.0	<1.0	0	(0)	m.q.
Pineapple-grapefruit juice *(Dole),* 6 fl. oz.	90	1.0	22.0	0	0	10	m.q.
Pineapple-grapefruit juice drink:							
(Tropicana), 6 fl. oz.	100	<1.0	24.0	<1.0	0	10	(0)
regular or pink *(Del Monte),* 6 fl. oz. . .	90	0	24.0	0	0	50	(0)
Pineapple-orange drink:							
(Crush), 11.5 fl. oz.	160	<1.0	39.0	<1.0	0	0	0
(Mott's), 10 fl. oz. . .	160	<1.0	39.0	<1.0	0	0	0
Pineapple-orange juice:							
(Dole), 6 fl. oz.	90	1.0	22.0	0	0	10	m.q.
chilled or frozen* *(Minute Maid)*	90	1.0	23.0	0	0	0	m.q.
Pineapple-orange-banana juice, 6 fl. oz.:							
chilled *(Dole)*	100	0	23.0	0	0	10	m.q.
frozen* *(Dole)*	90	1.0	21.0	0	0	5	m.q.
Pineapple-orange-guava juice, 6 fl. oz.:							
chilled *(Dole)*	100	<1.0	21.0	0	0	10	m.q.
frozen* *(Dole)*	100	<1.0	22.0	0	0	10	m.q.
Pineapple-passion-fruit-banana juice, chilled or frozen* *(Dole),* 6 fl. oz.	100	<1.0	21.0	0	0	10	m.q.

Food and Measure	cal.	prot. (gms)	carbo. (gms)	fat (gms)	chol. (mgs)	sod. (mgs)	fiber (gms)
Pink bean, boiled,							
1/2 cup	125	7.6	23.5	.4	0	2	4.5 d
Pinto bean, 1/2 cup,							
except as noted:							
dry (Arrowhead Mills),							
2 oz.	200	13.0	36.0	1.0	0	3	11.2 d
boiled	117	7.0	21.8	.4	0	1	7.3 d
canned:							
w/liquid	93	5.5	17.5	.4	0	499	4.2 d
(Eden)	110	6.0	20.0	<1.0	0	20	6.4 d
(Eden No Salt							
Added)	70	6.0	17.0	<1.0	0	15	6.0 d
(Gebhardt), 4 oz.	100	6.0	19.0	<1.0	0	600	5.0 d
(Green Giant/Joan							
of Arc)	90	6.0	20.0	1.0	0	280	5.0 d
(Hain), 4 oz.	70	7.0	15.0	1.0	0	220	6.0 d
(Old El Paso) . . .	100	6.0	19.0	0	0	320	8.0 d
(Progresso)	110	8.0	21.0	<1.0	0	410	6.5 d
dry	93	5.5	17.5	.4	0	499	1.5 c
dry (Allens/East Texas							
Fair)	110	5.0	18.0	<1.0	0	350	5.0 d
frozen (Seabrook),							
3.2 oz.	160	9.0	29.0	0	0	m.q.	m.q.
Pinto bean, sprouted,							
boiled, drained,							
4 oz.	25	2.1	4.6	.4	0	58	1.1 c
Pinto bean mix*, and							
rice (Fantastic),							
10 oz.	190	9.0	44.0	2.0	0	490	8.0 d
Pistachio nut[1]:							
dried:							
in shell, 1 lb.	1309	46.7	56.3	109.7	0	13	24.5 d
1 oz.	164	5.8	7.1	13.7	0	2	3.1 d
dry-roasted:							
in shell, salted, 1 lb.	1429	35.2	64.9	124.5	0	1840	25.5 d
1 oz.	172	4.2	7.8	15.0	0	2	3.1 d

[1] Shelled, except as noted.

Food and Measure	cal.	prot. (gms)	carbo. (gms)	fat (gms)	chol. (mgs)	sod. (mgs)	fiber (gms)
1 cup	776	19.1	35.2	67.6	0	8	13.8 d
salted, 1 oz.	172	4.2	7.8	15.0	0	221	3.1 d
natural or red tint							
(Fisher), 1 oz. . . .	170	5.0	7.0	14.0	0	85	m.q.
Pitanga:							
1 medium, .3 oz. . .	2	.1	.5	<.1	0	tr.	<.1 c
1/2 cup	29	.7	6.5	.3	0	3	.5 c
Pizza, frozen:							
Canadian bacon:							
(Totino's Party),							
1/2 pie	330	15.0	42.0	13.0	10	860	3.0 d
(Jeno's Crisp'N							
Tasty), 1/2 pie . .	240	10.0	28.0	10.0	5	680	1.0 d
cheese:							
(Ellio's Healthy							
Slices), 1 slice . .	160	9.0	25.0	2.0	5	390	m.q.
(Ellio's 9 Slice),							
1/9 pie	180	8.0	24.0	6.0	m.q.	420	m.q.
(Ellio's Round 16"),							
1/6 pie	180	8.0	24.0	6.0	m.q.	420	m.q.
(Ellio's 3 Slice),							
1/3 pie	180	8.0	24.0	6.0	m.q.	420	m.q.
(Jeno's Crisp'N							
Tasty), 1/2 pie . .	240	11.0	28.0	10.0	10	500	1.0 d
(Pillsbury Oven							
Lovin'), 1/2 pie . .	250	11.0	24.0	12.0	10	430	m.q.
(Totino's Micro-							
wave), 1 pie . . .	250	11.0	30.0	10.0	15	550	m.q.
(Totino's Pan Pizza),							
1/6 pie	290	15.0	35.0	10.0	20	440	m.q.
(Totino's Party),							
1/2 pizza	290	13.0	40.0	10.0	15	530	2.0 d
(Totino's Party) Fam-							
ily Size), 1/3 pie .	320	14.0	43.0	11.0	15	580	2.0 d
(Weight Watchers),							
6.03-oz. pkg. . .	300	24.0	36.0	7.0	10	310	m.q.
double (Ellio's 6							
Slice), 1/6 pie . .	230	12.0	22.0	12.0	m.q.	530	m.q.

Food and Measure	cal.	prot. (gms)	carbo. (gms)	fat (gms)	chol. (mgs)	sod. (mgs)	fiber (gms)
Pizza, frozen, cheese *(cont.)*							
extra *(Ellio's 3 Slice)*,							
1/3 pie	200	9.0	26.0	9.0	m.q.	440	m.q.
cheese, four *(Master*							
Choice), 1/4 pie . .	310	16.0	30.0	14.0	m.q.	320	m.q.
cheese, three:							
(Pappalo's 9"),							
1/2 pie	350	21.0	47.0	11.0	30	640	4.0 d
(Pappalo's 12"),							
1/4 pie	310	20.0	41.0	7.0	30	440	4.0 d
(Pappalo's Pan),							
1/5 pie	310	20.0	39.0	8.0	30	490	3.0 d
Chicken Suprema							
(Ellio's Healthy							
Slices), 1 slice . .	160	10.0	24.0	3.0	5	360	m.q.
combination:							
(Jeno's Crisp'N							
Tasty), 1/2 pie . .	280	10.0	27.0	15.0	15	680	1.0 d
(MicroMagic Deep							
Dish), 1 pie . . .	605	14.0	60.0	34.0	28	1280	m.q.
(Pillsbury Oven							
Lovin'), 1/2 pie . .	310	13.0	26.0	18.0	20	580	m.q.
(Totino's Micro-							
wave), 1 pie . . .	290	9.0	34.0	13.0	15	780	m.q.
(Totino's Party),							
1/2 pie	370	15.0	43.0	17.0	20	920	3.0 d
(Totino's Party Fam-							
ily Size), 1/3 pie	400	17.0	47.0	18.0	20	990	3.0 d
(Weight Watchers							
Deluxe), 7.32 oz.	320	25.0	36.0	9.0	10	370	m.q.
garden style *(Ellio's*							
Healthy Slices),							
1 slice	150	8.0	25.0	2.0	5	370	m.q.
hamburger:							
(Jeno's Crisp'N							
Tasty), 1/2 pie . .	280	11.0	28.0	14.0	15	640	1.0 d
(Totino's Party),							
1/2 pie	350	16.0	37.0	17.0	15	780	3.0 d

Food and Measure	cal.	prot. (gms)	carbo. (gms)	fat (gms)	chol. (mgs)	sod. (mgs)	fiber (gms)
Mexican style (Master Choice), 1/4 pie . .	330	16.0	28.0	17.0	m.q.	470	m.q.
pepperoni:							
(Banquet), 1 pie . .	470	11.0	45.0	27.0	35	970	m.q.
(Ellio's 3 Slice), 1/3 pie	230	10.0	24.0	11.0	20	580	m.q.
(Jeno's Crisp'N Tasty), 1/2 pie . .	280	10.0	28.0	15.0	15	710	1.0 d
(MicroMagic Deep Dish), 1 pie . . .	610	15.0	65.0	32.0	42	1300	m.q.
(Pappalo's 9"), 1/2 pie	390	23.0	47.0	14.0	45	870	4.0 d
(Pappalo's 12"), 1/4 pie	350	22.0	40.0	11.0	45	700	4.0 d
(Pappalo's Pan), 1/5 pie	350	22.0	40.0	11.0	50	720	3.0 d
(Pillsbury Oven Lovin'), 1/2 pie . .	300	13.0	25.0	17.0	25	620	m.q.
(Tombstone Light), 1/2 pie	190	13.0	22.0	6.0	15	500	2.0 d
(Totino's Micro-wave), 1 pie . . .	270	10.0	29.0	13.0	15	680	m.q.
(Totino's Pan Pizza), 1/6 pie	330	16.0	35.0	15.0	30	620	m.q.
(Totino's Party), 1/2 pie	380	14.0	41.0	19.0	15	980	3.0 d
(Totino's Party Family Size), 1/3 pie	410	16.0	44.0	20.0	20	1060	3.0 d
(Weight Watchers), 6.08 oz.	320	25.0	36.0	8.0	15	550	m.q.
sausage:							
(Banquet), 1 pie . .	500	11.0	48.0	29.0	35	860	m.q.
(Jeno's Crisp'N Tasty), 1/2 pie . .	280	10.0	27.0	15.0	10	640	1.0 d
(MicroMagic Deep Dish), 1 pie . . .	590	15.0	62.0	31.0	18	1250	m.q.
(Pappalo's 9"), 1/2 pie	380	22.0	47.0	13.0	40	680	4.0 d

Food and Measure	cal.	prot. (gms)	carbo. (gms)	fat (gms)	chol. (mgs)	sod. (mgs)	fiber (gms)
Pizza, frozen, sausage *(cont.)*							
(Pappalo's 12"),							
1/4 pie	350	22.0	39.0	12.0	40	600	4.0 d
(Pappalo's Pan),							
1/5 pie	350	22.0	39.0	11.0	40	530	3.0 d
(Pillsbury Oven Lovin'), 1/2 pie . .	290	12.0	26.0	16.0	15	510	m.q.
(Totino's Micro- wave), 1 pie . . .	280	10.0	31.0	13.0	10	680	m.q.
(Totino's Pan Pizza),							
1/6 pie	320	16.0	35.0	13.0	20	500	m.q.
(Totino's Party),							
1/2 pie	370	15.0	44.0	17.0	10	800	3.0 d
(Totino's Party Fam- ily Size), 1/3 pie	410	16.0	48.0	18.0	15	870	4.0 d
sausage and pepper- oni:							
(Banquet), 1 pie . .	470	12.0	43.0	27.0	40	930	m.q.
(Master Choice),							
1/4 pie	340	16.0	28.0	19.0	m.q.	490	m.q.
(Pappalo's 9"),							
1/2 pie	390	23.0	45.0	15.0	45	650	4.0 d
(Pappalo's 12"),							
1/4 pie	360	23.0	40.0	12.0	45	730	4.0 d
(Pappalo's Pan),							
1/5 pie	360	22.0	40.0	12.0	45	630	3.0 d
(Totino's Pan Pizza),							
1/6 pie	330	16.0	35.0	15.0	25	560	m.q.
supreme:							
(Pappalo's 9"),							
1/2 pie	400	25.0	46.0	16.0	45	700	4.0 d
(Pappalo's 12"),							
1/4 pie	350	22.0	38.0	12.0	45	640	4.0 d
(Pappalo's Pan),							
1/5 pie	340	22.0	37.0	12.0	45	610	3.0 d
(Pillsbury Oven Lovin'), 1/2 pie . .	310	13.0	27.0	18.0	20	570	m.q.

Food and Measure	cal.	prot. (gms)	carbo. (gms)	fat (gms)	chol. (mgs)	sod. (mgs)	fiber (gms)
(Tombstone Light), 1/2 pie	190	13.0	23.0	6.0	15	530	2.0 d
(Tombstone Light 12"), 1/5 pie . . .	250	16.0	30.0	9.0	20	670	4.0 d
spinach *(Master Choice Gourmet)*, 1/4 pie	300	16.0	29.0	14.0	m.q.	320	m.q.
vegetable:							
(Tombstone Light), 1/2 pie	170	11.0	22.0	5.0	5	340	2.0 d
(Tombstone Light 12"), 1/5 pie . . .	220	13.0	31.0	6.0	10	500	3.0 d
mixed *(Ellio's Healthy Slices)*, 1 slice	150	7.0	24.0	2.0	5	370	m.q.
Pizza, croissant crust, frozen *(Pepperidge Farm)*, 1 pie:							
cheese	430	15.0	41.0	23.0	m.q.	640	m.q.
deluxe	440	16.0	43.0	23.0	m.q.	790	m.q.
pepperoni	420	14.0	43.0	22.0	m.q.	690	m.q.
Pizza, French bread, frozen, 1 piece, except as noted:							
Canadian bacon *(Stouffer's)*, 1/2 pkg.	370	18.0	40.0	15.0	m.q.	1070	m.q.
cheese:							
(Healthy Choice), 5.6 oz.	290	19.0	46.0	4.0	15	390	m.q.
(Lean Cuisine), 51/8 oz.	300	17.0	38.0	9.0	15	310	m.q.
(Pillsbury Oven Lovin')	350	17.0	40.0	14.0	15	700	m.q.
(Stouffer's), 1/2 pkg.	350	16.0	40.0	14.0	m.q.	630	m.q.
double *(Stouffer's)*, 1/2 pkg.	420	22.0	43.0	18.0	m.q.	850	m.q.

Food and Measure	cal.	prot. (gms)	carbo. (gms)	fat (gms)	chol. (mgs)	sod. (mgs)	fiber (gms)
Pizza, French bread, cheese *(cont.)*							
double *(Stouffer's Lunch Express)*	420	18.0	48.0	17.0	m.q.	790	m.q.
three *(Lean Cuisine)*, 5.5 oz.	330	23.0	38.0	10.0	20	350	m.q.
combination *(Pillsbury Oven Lovin')*	420	18.0	41.0	21.0	30	910	m.q.
deluxe:							
(Healthy Choice), 6.35 oz.	330	23.0	41.0	7.0	35	500	m.q.
(Lean Cuisine), 6 1/8 oz.	350	22.0	40.0	11.0	30	580	m.q.
(Stouffer's), 1/2 pkg.	420	21.0	40.0	19.0	m.q.	950	m.q.
(Stouffer's Lunch Express)	450	19.0	41.0	23.0	m.q.	940	m.q.
hamburger *(Stouffer's)*, 1/2 pkg.	410	23.0	39.0	18.0	m.q.	650	m.q.
pepperoni:							
(Healthy Choice), 6 oz.	310	20.0	38.0	7.0	30	470	m.q.
(Lean Cuisine), 5.25 oz.	340	19.0	41.0	11.0	25	580	m.q.
(Pillsbury Oven Lovin')	410	18.0	40.0	21.0	35	980	m.q.
(Stouffer's), 1/2 pkg.	400	19.0	39.0	19.0	m.q.	880	m.q.
pepperoni and mushroom *(Stouffer's)*, 1/2 pkg.	410	19.0	40.0	19.0	m.q.	920	m.q.
sausage:							
(Lean Cuisine), 6 oz.	350	22.0	42.0	10.0	35	600	m.q.
(Pillsbury Oven Lovin')	400	18.0	41.0	20.0	25	830	m.q.
(Stouffer's), 1/2 pkg.	430	20.0	40.0	21.0	m.q.	840	m.q.
Italian turkey *(Healthy Choice)*, 6.35 oz.	330	23.0	48.0	5.0	25	390	m.q.

Food and Measure	cal.	prot. (gms)	carbo. (gms)	fat (gms)	chol. (mgs)	sod. (mgs)	fiber (gms)
sausage and pepperoni *(Stouffer's)*, 1/2 pkg.	460	23.0	41.0	23.0	m.q.	920	m.q.
vegetable deluxe *(Stouffer's)*, 1/2 pkg.	420	18.0	41.0	20.0	m.q.	830	m.q.
Pizza chips, cheese *(Keebler Pizzarias)*, 1 oz.	140	3.0	18.0	6.0	<5	200	m.q.
Pizza crust (see also "Bread shell"):							
(Pillsbury All Ready), 1/8 crust	90	3.0	16.0	1.0	0	170	m.q.
mix *(Robin Hood Pouch)*, 1/6 mix . .	110	3.0	22.0	1.0	0	220	m.q.
Pizza Hut, 1 slice, 1/8 pie:							
hand-tossed:							
beef	261	15.4	27.8	9.8	25	795	2.7 d
cheese	253	15.4	27.5	9.0	25	593	2.5 d
Meat Lover's . . .	321	15.9	28.0	14.6	42	1106	2.7 d
pepperoni	253	19.8	27.7	9.7	25	738	2.2 d
Pepperoni Lover's	335	19.3	27.9	16.2	43	981	2.7 d
pork	270	15.3	27.9	10.8	25	803	2.7 d
sausage, Italian . .	313	15.6	27.5	15.5	38	871	2.5 d
supreme	289	16.6	28.3	12.1	29	894	3.2 d
super supreme . .	276	17.3	28.3	10.4	32	980	2.8 d
Veggie Lover's . . .	222	12.7	28.2	6.6	17	641	2.9 d
pan pizza:							
beef	288	9.9	26.6	18.2	25	675	2.7 d
cheese	279	14.4	26.2	13.0	25	473	2.5 d
Meat Lover's . . .	347	14.9	26.7	23.0	42	986	2.7 d
pepperoni	280	8.3	26.4	18.1	25	618	2.2 d
Pepperoni Lover's	362	13.8	26.6	24.7	43	861	2.7 d
pork	296	9.8	26.7	19.2	25	683	2.7 d
sausage, Italian . .	399	14.6	26.2	23.9	38	751	2.5 d
supreme	315	15.6	27.0	16.1	29	774	3.2 d
super supreme . .	302	11.9	27.0	18.8	32	860	2.8 d
Veggie Lover's . . .	249	7.2	26.9	15.0	17	521	2.9 d

Food and Measure	cal.	prot. (gms)	carbo. (gms)	fat (gms)	chol. (mgs)	sod. (mgs)	fiber (gms)
Pizza Hut *(cont.)*							
Thin 'n Crispy:							
beef	231	13.3	19.8	10.9	25	705	2.3 d
cheese	223	13.3	19.4	10.2	25	503	2.1 d
Meat Lover's . . .	298	13.9	19.7	16.2	44	1069	2.3 d
pepperoni	230	12.1	19.6	11.5	26	678	1.8 d
Pepperoni Lover's	320	18.0	19.9	18.7	46	949	2.3 d
pork	240	13.2	19.8	11.9	25	713	2.3 d
sausage, Italian . .	282	13.5	19.4	16.6	38	781	2.1 d
supreme	262	14.7	20.2	13.6	30	819	2.8 d
super supreme . .	253	16.0	20.3	12.0	35	700	2.5 d
Veggie Lover's . . .	192	10.6	20.1	7.7	17	551	2.5 d
Pizza mix, Mexican *(Tio Sancho):*							
sauce, 2 oz.	14	1.4	.2	.4	n.a.	3350	n.a.
tortilla, 1 piece	125	3.3	24.0	1.9	n.a.	569	m.q.
Pizza pocket, frozen, 4.5 oz., except as noted:							
combo *(Hot Pockets)*	340	12.0	38.0	15.0	30	700	m.q.
deluxe:							
(Lean Pockets) . . .	290	13.0	34.0	11.0	30	660	m.q.
(Weight Watchers Ultimate 200), 4 oz.	200	15.0	25.0	5.0	5	400	m.q.
pepperoni:							
(Hot Pockets) . . .	350	14.0	39.0	16.0	35	790	m.q.
(Jeno's)	370	12.0	35.0	20.0	25	790	m.q.
sausage:							
(Hot Pockets) . . .	350	13.0	36.0	17.0	35	490	m.q.
(Jeno's)	360	11.0	35.0	19.0	15	660	m.q.
sausage and pepperoni *(Jeno's)*	360	12.0	35.0	20.0	20	710	m.q.
supreme *(Jeno's)* . .	370	12.0	36.0	19.0	20	720	m.q.
Pizza roll, frozen *(Jeno's Pizza Rolls),* 3 oz.:							
cheese	200	9.0	30.0	5.0	20	370	1.4 d

Food and Measure	cal.	prot. (gms)	carbo. (gms)	fat (gms)	chol. (mgs)	sod. (mgs)	fiber (gms)
combination	220	10.0	26.0	9.0	15	230	1.9 d
hamburger	220	10.0	28.0	8.0	20	310	2.0 d
pepperoni	220	9.0	26.0	9.0	20	350	1.8 d
sausage	210	9.0	26.0	7.0	15	340	1.6 d
Pizza sauce:							
(Contadina Pizza Squeeze), 1/4 cup	30	1.0	5.0	1.0	n.a.	330	m.q.
(Contadina Quick & Easy), 1/4 cup . . .	30	1.0	5.0	1.0	n.a.	330	m.q.
(Master Choice), 3 tbsp.	20	1.0	4.0	1.0	0	312	m.q.
(Pastorelli Continental Chef), 1/4 cup . . .	45	2.0	5.0	2.0	0	390	3.0 d
(Pastorelli Italian Chef), 2 oz.	50	1.0	5.0	3.0	0	380	2.0 d
(Ragú), 3 tbsp.	25	1.0	3.0	1.0	0	200	m.q.
w/cheese, garlic and basil, or traditional *(Ragú Pizza Quick)*, 3 tbsp.	35	1.0	3.0	2.0	0	330	m.q.
w/Italian cheese *(Contadina)*, 1/4 cup . .	30	1.0	5.0	1.0	m.q.	380	m.q.
w/pepperoni *(Contadina)*, 1/4 cup . .	40	1.0	5.0	2.0	m.q.	360	m.q.
pepperoni *(Master Choice)*, 3 tbsp. . . .	25	1.0	4.0	1.0	m.q.	310	m.q.
tomato, chunky *(Ragú Pizza Quick)*, 3 tbsp.	35	1.0	5.0	1.0	0	220	m.q.
Plantain:							
raw:							
1 medium, 9.7 oz.	218	2.3	57.1	.7	0	7	4.1 d
sliced, 1/2 cup . . .	91	1.0	23.6	.3	0	3	1.7 d
(Frieda's), 1 oz. . .	34	.3	8.8	.1	0	1	m.q.
cooked, sliced, 1/2 cup	89	.6	24.0	.1	0	4	1.8 d
Plum:							
fresh:							
pitted, sliced, 1/2 cup	46	.7	10.7	.5	0	1	1.2 d

Food and Measure	cal.	prot. (gms)	carbo. (gms)	fat (gms)	chol. (mgs)	sod. (mgs)	fiber (gms)
Plum, fresh *(cont.)*							
Japanese or hybrid,							
1 medium, 2¹/₈″	36	.5	8.6	.4	0	tr.	1.0 d
canned in juice:							
¹/₂ cup	73	.7	19.1	<.1	0	2	1.3 d
3 plums and 2 tbsp.							
liquid	55	.5	14.4	<.1	0	1	1.0 d
canned in light syrup:							
¹/₂ cup	79	.5	20.5	.1	0	25	1.3 d
3 plums and 2³/₄							
tbsp. liquid . . .	83	.5	21.7	.1	0	26	1.3 d
canned in heavy							
syrup:							
¹/₂ cup	115	.5	30.0	.1	0	25	1.3 d
3 plums and 2³/₄							
tbsp. liquid . . .	119	.5	30.9	.1	0	26	1.3 d
(Stokely), ¹/₂ cup	130	0	30.0	0	0	25	m.q.
Plum sauce, tangy *(La*							
Choy), 1 oz.	45	.1	10.8	.1	0	17	m.q.
Poi, ¹/₂ cup	134	.5	32.7	.2	0	14	.5 d
Poke greens, canned							
(Allens), ¹/₂ cup . .	15	2.0	2.0	<1.0	0	0	1.0 d
Pokeberry shoots:							
raw, ¹/₂ cup	18	2.1	3.0	.3	0	n.a.	1.4 d
boiled, drained,							
¹/₂ cup	16	1.9	2.5	.3	0	n.a.	1.2 d
Polenta mix *(Fantas-*							
tic), 4 oz.	110	3.0	19.0	2.5	2	234	.3 d
Polish sausage (see							
also "Kielbasa")							
(Hillshire Farm),							
2 oz.	190	7.0	2.0	17.0	m.q.	520	0
Pollock, meat only:							
Atlantic:							
raw, 4 oz.	104	22.1	0	1.1	80	98	0
baked, broiled, or							
microwaved, 4 oz.	134	28.3	0	1.4	103	125	0

Food and Measure	cal.	prot. (gms)	carbo. (gms)	fat (gms)	chol. (mgs)	sod. (mgs)	fiber (gms)
walleye:							
raw, 4 oz.	91	19.5	0	.9	81	112	0
baked, broiled, or							
microwaved, 4 oz.	128	26.7	0	1.3	109	132	0
Pomegranate:							
1 medium, 9.7 oz. . .	104	1.5	26.4	.5	0	5	.9 d
trimmed (Frieda's),							
1 oz.	18	.1	4.6	.1	0	1	m.q.
Pomegranate juice							
(R.W. Knudsen),							
8 fl. oz.	85	<1.0	21.0	<1.0	0	(0)	m.q.
Pompano, Florida,							
meat only:							
raw, 4 oz.	186	21.0	0	10.7	57	74	0
baked, broiled, or mi-							
crowaved, 4 oz. . .	239	26.4	0	13.8	73	86	0
Popcorn, popped:							
(Chesters), 1/2 oz. . .	70	1.0	9.0	3.0	0	200	m.q.
(Jiffy Pop Pan Pop-							
corn), 4 cups . . .	130	3.0	16.0	6.0	0	270	2.0 d
(Kettle Poppins),							
1/2 oz.	70	2.0	9.0	2.5	0	40	1.0 d
(Orville Redenbacher's							
Gourmet Hot Air),							
3 cups	40	1.0	10.0	<1.0	0	0	3.0 d
(Orville Redenbacher's							
Gourmet Original/							
White), 3 cups . . .	80	1.0	10.0	4.0	0	0	3.0 d
(Tom's Natural), 3/4 oz.	110	2.0	13.0	6.0	n.a.	280	m.q.
brewer's yeast (Kettle							
Poppins), 1/2 oz. . .	70	2.0	8.0	2.5	0	40	1.0 d
butter (Cape Cod),							
1/2 oz.	80	1.0	7.0	5.0	0	110	1.0 d
butter flavor:							
(Jiffy Pop Pan Pop-							
corn), 4 cups . .	130	3.0	16.0	6.0	0	270	2.0 d
(Smartfood Light),							
1/2 oz.	70	1.0	9.0	3.0	5	105	m.q.

Food and Measure	cal.	prot. (gms)	carbo. (gms)	fat (gms)	chol. (mgs)	sod. (mgs)	fiber (gms)
Popcorn *(cont.)*							
butter toffee, w/pea-							
nuts *(Cracker Jack)*,							
1 oz.	130	2.0	20.0	5.0	n.a.	125	m.q.
caramel:							
(Tom's), 1.6 oz. . .	190	1.0	40.0	3.0	n.a.	130	n.a.
w/peanuts *(Cracker*							
Jack), 1 oz. . . .	120	2.0	22.0	3.0	0	85	m.q.
caramel crunch *(Flavor*							
House), 1.1 oz. . .	120	1.0	26.0	1.0	0	70	1.0 d
cheddar, white,							
1/2 oz., except as							
noted:							
(Flavor House),							
1.1 oz.	170	3.0	13.0	12.0	5	360	2.0 d
(Kettle Poppins) . .	70	2.0	9.0	2.5	1	120	m.q.
(Smartfood)	80	1.0	7.0	5.0	5	130	m.q.
(Tom's), 11/4 oz. . .	110	2.0	12.0	6.0	n.a.	450	m.q.
cheese flavor:							
(Tom's), 1.5-oz. pkg.	130	2.0	14.0	7.0	n.a.	410	m.q.
cheddar *(Chee·tos)*,							
1/2 oz.	80	1.0	6.0	6.0	0	160	m.q.
cheddar *(Chesters)*,							
1/2 oz.	80	1.0	7.0	5.0	0	180	m.q.
honey caramel *(Kee-*							
bler Pop Deluxe),							
1 oz.	120	<1.0	22.0	3.0	0	180	m.q.
air popped, 3 cups:							
white *(Jolly Time)*	60	2.0	15.0	<1.0	0	0	4.0 d
yellow *(Jolly Time)*	60	2.0	14.0	<1.0	0	0	4.0 d
Popcorn, microwave,							
popped, 3 cups, ex-							
cept as noted:							
(Chesters Natural) . .	110	1.0	13.0	7.0	0	170	m.q.
plain or butter flavor							
(Jiffy Pop Pan),							
4 cups	130	3.0	16.0	6.0	0	270	2.0 d
(Jolly Time Natural)	120	2.0	15.0	7.0	0	125	3.0 d

Food and Measure	cal.	prot. (gms)	carbo. (gms)	fat (gms)	chol. (mgs)	sod. (mgs)	fiber (gms)
(Jolly Time Natural Light)	70	2.0	13.0	2.0	0	110	3.0 d
(Orville Redenbacher's Gourmet Natural)	100	2.0	11.0	6.0	0	200	3.0 d
(Orville Redenbacher's Gourmet Salt Free)	100	2.0	11.0	6.0	0	0	3.0 d
(Orville Redenbacher's Light Natural) . . .	70	2.0	8.0	3.0	0	115	3.0 d
(Pop • Secret)	100	2.0	11.0	6.0	0	170	2.0 d
(Pop • Secret Light)	70	2.0	12.0	3.0	0	160	2.0 d
(Pop Weaver's Natural/ Butter), 4 cups . .	140	3.0	20.0	8.0	0	230	4.0 d
plain or butter flavor *(Jiffy Pop)*, 4 cups	140	3.0	17.0	7.0	0	270	m.q.
butter flavor:							
(Chesters)	120	2.0	13.0	7.0	0	180	m.q.
(Jolly Time)	90	2.0	13.0	5.0	0	95	3.0 d
(Jolly Time Light)	60	2.0	12.0	2.0	0	105	3.0 d
(Orville Redenbacher's Gourmet)	100	2.0	11.0	6.0	0	240	3.0 d
(Orville Redenbacher's Gourmet Salt Free)	100	2.0	11.0	6.0	0	0	3.0 d
(Orville Redenbacher's Lite) . .	70	2.0	8.0	3.0	0	110	3.0 d
(Pop • Secret) . . .	100	2.0	11.0	6.0	0	170	2.0 d
(Pop • Secret Light)	70	2.0	12.0	3.0	0	115	2.0 d
salt free *(Pop • Secret)* . .	100	2.0	11.0	6.0	0	<5	2.0 d
butter toffee *(Orville Redenbacher's* Gourmet), 2¹/2 cups	210	2.0	26.0	12.0	<1	85	2.0 d
caramel *(Orville Redenbacher's* Gourmet), 2¹/2 cups	240	2.0	29.0	14.0	<1	90	2.0 d
cheddar: *(Jolly Time)*	180	3.0	17.0	11.0	0	200	m.q.

Food and Measure	cal.	prot. (gms)	carbo. (gms)	fat (gms)	chol. (mgs)	sod. (mgs)	fiber (gms)
Popcorn, microwave, cheddar *(cont.)*							
(Orville Reden-							
bacher's Gourmet)	130	2.0	14.0	8.0	2	280	3.0 d
cheese *(Chesters)* . .	110	2.0	11.0	8.0	0	230	m.q.
sour cream 'n onion							
(Orville Reden-							
bacher's Gourmet)	160	2.0	12.0	12.0	0	270	3.0 d
Popcorn cake, plain							
or butter flavor							
(Quaker), 1 piece	35	1.0	7.0	0	0	55	m.q.
Popcorn seasoning:							
(Tone's), 1 tsp.	0	0	0	0	0	2455	0
(McCormick/Schilling							
Parsley Patch),							
1 tsp.	10	.6	3.0	0	0	4	n.a.
Poppyseed, 1 tsp.	15	.5	.7	1.3	0	1	.8 d
Porgy, see "Scup"							
Pork, meat only,							
4 oz., except as							
noted:							
leg, see "Ham"							
loin, whole:							
braised, lean w/fat	417	30.8	0	31.6	116	74	0
braised, lean only	310	37.4	0	16.6	119	85	0
broiled, lean w/fat	392	26.7	0	30.9	107	75	0
broiled, lean only	291	31.6	0	17.3	108	85	0
roasted, lean w/fat	362	26.6	0	27.5	102	71	0
roasted, lean only	272	30.5	0	15.8	102	78	0
loin, blade:							
braised, lean w/fat	465	27.2	0	38.7	122	78	0
braised, lean only	355	33.7	0	23.3	128	92	0
broiled, lean w/fat	446	23.4	0	38.4	111	76	0
broiled, lean only	340	28.2	0	24.3	113	87	0
roasted, lean w/fat	413	23.9	0	34.5	102	69	0
roasted, lean only	316	28.0	0	21.9	101	77	0
loin, center:							
braised, lean w/fat	401	33.3	0	28.7	121	58	0
braised, lean only	308	39.4	0	15.5	126	62	0

Food and Measure	cal.	prot. (gms)	carbo. (gms)	fat (gms)	chol. (mgs)	sod. (mgs)	fiber (gms)
broiled, lean w/fat	358	31.1	0	25.1	110	79	0
broiled, lean w/fat, 3.1 oz. (3.7 oz. raw chop w/bone)	275	23.9	0	19.2	84	61	0
broiled, lean only	262	36.3	0	11.9	111	88	0
broiled, lean only, 2.5 oz. (3.7 oz. raw chop w/bone and fat)	166	23.0	0	7.5	71	56	0
roasted, lean w/fat	346	28.8	0	24.7	103	73	0
roasted, lean only	272	32.3	0	14.8	103	78	0
loin, center rib:							
braised, lean w/fat	416	32.4	0	30.8	108	54	0
braised, lean only	314	39.1	0	16.4	110	59	0
broiled, lean w/fat	389	27.9	0	29.9	106	69	0
broiled, lean only	293	32.7	0	16.9	107	76	0
roasted, lean w/fat	361	28.1	0	26.8	92	50	0
roasted, lean only	278	32.0	0	15.6	86	52	0
loin, top:							
braised, lean w/fat	432	31.4	0	33.1	108	53	0
braised, lean only	314	39.1	0	16.4	110	59	0
broiled, lean w/fat	408	26.9	0	32.5	105	67	0
broiled, lean only	293	32.7	0	16.9	107	76	0
roasted, lean only	278	32.0	0	15.6	90	52	0
shoulder, whole:							
roasted, lean w/fat	370	25.0	0	29.1	109	77	0
roasted, lean only	277	28.8	0	17.0	110	86	0
shoulder, arm (picnic):							
roasted, lean w/fat	375	25.3	0	29.6	107	79	0
roasted, lean w/fat, diced, 1 cup . .	463	31.3	0	36.5	132	97	0
roasted, lean only	259	30.3	0	14.3	108	91	0
roasted, lean only, diced, 1 cup . .	319	37.4	0	17.7	133	112	0
shoulder, Boston blade:							
braised, lean w/fat	421	29.9	0	32.5	126	76	0
braised, lean only	333	35.3	0	19.9	132	85	0

Food and Measure	cal.	prot. (gms)	carbo. (gms)	fat (gms)	chol. (mgs)	sod. (mgs)	fiber (gms)
Pork, shoulder, Boston blade *(cont.)*							
broiled, lean w/fat	397	24.8	0	32.3	117	85	0
broiled, lean only	311	28.5	0	20.9	119	95	0
roasted, lean only	290	27.6	0	19.1	111	83	0
shoulder, butt, boneless, smoked *(Oscar Mayer Sweet Morsel)*, 3 oz.	210	12.0	2.0	18.0	55	800	0
sirloin:							
braised, lean w/fat	399	31.7	0	29.2	120	61	0
braised, lean only	296	38.0	0	14.8	125	67	0
broiled, lean w/fat	375	27.4	0	28.6	110	62	0
broiled, lean w/fat, 3 oz. (3.7 oz. raw chop w/bone) . .	278	20.3	0	21.2	81	46	0
broiled, lean only	276	32.1	0	15.4	111	68	0
broiled, lean only, 2.4 oz. (3.7 oz. raw chop w/bone and fat)	165	19.2	0	9.2	67	41	0
roasted, lean w/fat	330	28.4	0	23.1	103	67	0
roasted, lean only	268	31.2	0	14.9	102	70	0
spareribs, lean w/fat, braised, 6.3 oz. (1 lb. raw w/bone) . .	703	51.4	0	53.6	214	165	0
tenderloin, lean only, roasted	188	32.6	0	5.5	105	76	0
Pork, cured (see also "Ham"), 4 oz.:							
arm (picnic), roasted:							
lean w/fat	318	23.2	0	24.2	66	1216	0
lean only	193	28.3	0	8.0	54	1396	0
blade roll, lean w/fat, roasted	325	19.6	.4	26.6	76	1103	0
Pork belly, raw, 1 oz.	147	2.7	0	15.1	20	9	0
Pork dinner, loin of, frozen *(Swanson)*, 10.75 oz.	270	19.0	26.0	10.0	m.q.	810	m.q.

Food and Measure	cal.	prot. (gms)	carbo. (gms)	fat (gms)	chol. (mgs)	sod. (mgs)	fiber (gms)
Pork entree, canned:							
chow mein *(La Choy Bi-Pack)*, 3/4 cup	80	5.0	7.0	4.0	14	950	2.0 d
sweet and sour *(La Choy)*, 3/4 cup . . .	250	6.0	48.0	4.0	18	1540	1.0 d
Pork entree, freeze-dried*, sweet and sour, w/rice *(Mountain House)*, 1 cup	270	12.0	44.0	6.0	m.q.	730	m.q.
Pork entree, frozen, sweet and sour *(Chun King)*, 13 oz.	400	11.0	78.0	5.0	25	1460	m.q.
Pork entree sauce, see "Entree sauce"							
Pork fat, roasted, 1 oz.	167	2.2	0	17.5	24	177	0
Pork gravy:							
canned, 1/4 cup, 2 oz.:							
(Franco- American)	40	(0)	3.0	3.0	n.a.	330	n.a.
(Heinz Home Style)	25	1.0	3.0	1.0	<1	310	.1 d
mix:							
(French's), 1/4 pkg.	20	0	3.0	0	0	150	n.a.
(McCormick/Schilling), 1/4 cup* . .	20	.6	4.0	.6	n.a.	297	n.a.
Pork sandwich, barbecue, frozen *(Hormel Quick Meal)*, 4.3 oz.	350	16.0	40.0	14.0	65	550	m.q.
Pork seasoning and coating mix:							
(French's Roasting Bag), 1/5 pkg. . . .	25	1.0	6.0	0	0	250	n.a.
(Shake'n Bake), 1/8 pkt.	40	1.0	8.0	1.0	0	310	m.q.
barbecue *(Shake'n Bake)*, 1/8 pkt. . . .	35	0	8.0	0	0	260	m.q.
extra crispy *(Oven Fry)*, 1/8 pkt.	60	2.0	10.0	1.0	0	350	m.q.

Food and Measure	cal.	prot. (gms)	carbo. (gms)	fat (gms)	chol. (mgs)	sod. (mgs)	fiber (gms)
Pork seasoning and coating mix *(cont.)*							
chop *(McCormick/ Schilling Bag'n Season)*, 1 pkg.	102	1.1	24.0	.6	0	3518	m.q.
hot and spicy *(Shake'n Bake)*, 1/8 pkt. . . .	45	1.0	8.0	1.0	0	220	m.q.
spareribs *(McCormick/ Schilling Bag'n Season)*, 1 pkg.	185	.3	42.0	1.5	n.a.	3690	m.q.
Pork skins, fried:							
(Baken-ets), 1 oz. . .	160	12.0	2.0	10.0	25	850	n.a.
hot'n spicy *(Baken-ets)*, 1 oz.	150	17.0	1.0	9.0	25	750	n.a.
Pork and beans, see "Baked beans" and specific listings							
Pot roast, see "Beef dinner" and "Beef entree"							
Pot roast seasoning mix:							
(French's Roasting Bag), 1/7 pkg. . . .	18	1.0	4.0	0	0	230	n.a.
(Lawry's Seasoning Blends), 1 pkg. . .	122	3.7	25.0	.7	0	4008	.5 c
(McCormick/Schilling Bag'n Season), 1 pkg.	55	4.0	9.0	.6	0	3071	m.q.
onion *(French's Roasting Bag)*, 1/7 pkg.	18	1.0	4.0	0	0	10	n.a.
Potato:							
raw:							
unpeeled, 1 lb. . .	269	7.1	61.2	.3	0	21	5.4 d
peeled, 2 1/2"-diam.	88	2.3	20.1	.1	0	7	1.8 d
peeled, diced, 1/2 cup	59	1.6	13.5	.1	0	5	1.2 d

Food and Measure	cal.	prot. (gms)	carbo. (gms)	fat (gms)	chol. (mgs)	sod. (mgs)	fiber (gms)
baked in skin, 1 medium, 4³/4″ × 2¹/3″ diam.	220	4.7	51.0	.2	0	16	4.8 d
baked w/out skin:							
4 oz.	105	2.2	24.4	.1	0	6	1.7 d
¹/2 cup	57	1.2	13.2	.1	0	3	.9 d
boiled in skin, baby (Frieda's), 4 oz. . .	86	2.4	19.4	.1	0	3	m.q.
boiled in skin, peeled:							
2¹/2″-diam.	119	2.5	27.4	.1	0	6	2.4 d
4 oz.	99	2.1	22.8	.1	0	5	2.0 d
¹/2 cup	68	1.5	15.7	.1	0	3	1.4 d
boiled w/out skin:							
2¹/2″-diam.	116	2.3	27.0	.1	0	7	2.4 c
4 oz.	98	1.9	22.7	.1	0	6	2.0 c
¹/2 cup	67	1.3	15.6	.1	0	4	1.4 d
microwaved in skin: 1 medium,							
4³/4″ × 2¹/3″ diam.	212	4.9	48.7	.2	0	16	1.6 c
4 oz.	119	2.8	27.4	.1	0	9	.9 c
peeled, ¹/2 cup . .	78	1.6	18.2	.1	0	5	.3 c
skin only, 2 oz. . .	75	2.5	16.8	.1	0	9	1.8 c
mashed, w/whole milk:							
¹/2 cup	81	2.0	18.4	.6	2	318	2.1 d
w/butter, ¹/2 cup	111	2.0	17.5	4.4	13	309	2.1 d
w/margarine, ¹/2 cup	111	2.0	17.5	4.4	2	309	2.1 d
Potato, canned:							
w/liquid, 4 oz.	45	1.5	9.8	.2	0	341	1.8 d
drained, 1.2-oz. potato	21	.5	4.8	.1	0	m.q.	.1 c
(Stokely), ¹/2 cup . . .	50	2.0	11.0	0	0	360	m.q.
whole:							
(Allens/Butterfield), ¹/2 cup	50	1.0	10.0	<1.0	0	230	m.q.
new (Hunt's), 4 oz.	70	2.0	15.0	<1.0	0	230	<1.0 d
sliced (Allens/Butterfield), ¹/2 cup . . .	50	2.0	9.0	<1.0	0	350	m.q.
diced (Allens/Butterfield), ¹/2 cup . . .	50	2.0	9.0	<1.0	0	290	m.q.

Food and Measure	cal.	prot. (gms)	carbo. (gms)	fat (gms)	chol. (mgs)	sod. (mgs)	fiber (gms)
Potato, freeze-dried,							
hash brown *(Mountain House)*, 1 cup*	150	2.0	36.0	0	n.a.	80	m.q.
Potato, frozen (see also "Potato dishes, frozen"), 3 oz., except as noted:							
whole, white, boiled *(Seabrook)*, 3.2 oz.	60	2.0	13.0	0	0	5	0
diced and hash shred *(Seabrook)*, 4 oz.	80	2.0	19.0	0	0	41	0
fried or french-fried:							
(Ore-Ida)	170	2.0	23.0	7.0	0	10	m.q.
(Ore-Ida Country Style Dinner Fries)	110	2.0	20.0	2.0	0	10	m.q.
(Ore-Ida Crispers!)	220	2.0	24.0	13.0	0	490	m.q.
(Ore-Ida Crispy Crowns)	190	2.0	21.0	11.0	0	390	m.q.
(Ore-Ida Golden Fries)	120	2.0	20.0	3.0	0	10	m.q.
(Ore-Ida Golden Twirls)	160	2.0	22.0	7.0	0	15	m.q.
battered *(Ore-Ida Zesties!)*	160	2.0	21.0	8.0	0	300	m.q.
cottage cut *(Ore-Ida)*	130	2.0	21.0	4.0	0	15	m.q.
crinkle cut *(Micro-Magic)*	220	3.0	27.0	10.5	0	45	1.0 d
crinkle cut *(Ore-Ida Deep Fries)* . . .	160	2.0	23.0	7.0	0	10	m.q.
crinkle cut *(Ore-Ida Golden Crinkles)*	120	2.0	21.0	3.0	0	10	m.q.
crinkle cut *(Ore-Ida Lites)*	90	2.0	17.0	2.0	0	10	m.q.
crinkle cut *(Ore-Ida Microwave)*, 3.5 oz.	190	3.0	27.0	8.0	0	10	m.q.
crinkle cut *(Ore-Ida Pixie Crinkles)* . .	140	2.0	21.0	5.0	0	15	m.q.

Food and Measure	cal.	prot. (gms)	carbo. (gms)	fat (gms)	chol. (mgs)	sod. (mgs)	fiber (gms)
seasoned (Ore-Ida Crispy Crunchers)	180	2.0	23.0	9.0	0	410	m.q.
shoestring (Ore-Ida)	150	2.0	23.0	6.0	0	15	m.q.
sticks (MicroMagic Tater Sticks), 4 oz.	260	2.0	29.0	15.5	0	460	1.0 d
wedges (Ore-Ida Home Style Potato Wedges) . .	110	2.0	19.0	2.0	0	10	m.q.
hash brown:							
(MicroMagic Okray)	60	1.0	14.0	0	0	25	1.0 d
(Ore-Ida Golden Patties), 2.5 oz.	130	1.0	16.0	7.0	0	210	m.q.
(Ore-Ida Microwave), 2 oz.	110	1.0	13.0	6.0	0	120	m.q.
(Ore-Ida Southern Style)	70	1.0	16.0	<1.0	0	15	m.q.
(Ore-Ida Toaster), 1.75 oz.	100	1.0	12.0	5.0	0	230	m.q.
w/cheddar (Ore-Ida Cheddar Browns)	90	3.0	14.0	2.0	<5	330	m.q.
shredded (Ore-Ida)	70	2.0	15.0	<1.0	0	15	m.q.
mashed (Simplot Singles), 4 oz.	90	2.0	21.0	0	0	210	1.0 d
O'Brien (Ore-Ida) . . .	60	1.0	13.0	<1.0	0	10	m.q.
puffs:							
(Ore-Ida Tater Tots)	160	2.0	21.0	8.0	0	280	m.q.
w/bacon flavor (Ore-Ida Tater Tots) . .	150	2.0	21.0	7.0	0	390	m.q.
(Ore-Ida Tater Tots Microwave), 4 oz.	210	3.0	28.0	9.0	0	370	m.q.
w/onion (Ore-Ida Tater Tots)	150	2.0	21.0	7.0	0	370	m.q.
Potato, mix*, 1/2 cup, except as noted:							
American cheese (Betty Crocker Homestyle)	150	3.0	21.0	6.0	m.q.	620	m.q.

Food and Measure	cal.	prot. (gms)	carbo. (gms)	fat (gms)	chol. (mgs)	sod. (mgs)	fiber (gms)
Potato, mix *(cont.)*							
au gratin:							
(Betty Crocker) . .	150	3.0	21.0	6.0	m.q.	580	m.q.
(Fantastic Foods)[1]	201	6.0	24.0	9.0	m.q.	561	1.7 d
(Fantastic Foods)[2]	138	6.0	24.0	2.0	6	495	1.7 d
(Idahoan)	130	3.0	18.0	5.0	m.q.	475	m.q.
(Kraft Potatoes & Cheese)	130	4.0	19.0	5.0	40	570	m.q.
broccoli *(Betty Crocker* Homestyle)	140	3.0	19.0	6.0	m.q.	550	m.q.
broccoli *(Kraft* Potatoes & Cheese)	150	5.0	20.0	5.0	40	530	m.q.
tangy *(Pillsbury)* . .	140	3.0	20.0	6.0	15	520	1.0 d
bacon and cheddar *(Betty Crocker* Twice Baked)	200	6.0	21.0	10.0	m.q.	580	m.q.
cheddar:							
(Betty Crocker Homestyle) . . .	150	3.0	21.0	6.0	m.q.	530	m.q.
'N bacon *(Betty Crocker)*	150	3.0	21.0	6.0	m.q.	540	m.q.
and bacon *(Pillsbury)*	140	3.0	19.0	6.0	15	480	1.0 d
classic *(Idahoan)*	140	3.0	21.0	5.0	m.q.	500	m.q.
mild, w/onion *(Betty Crocker* Twice Baked)	200	5.0	20.0	11.0	m.q.	650	m.q.
smoky *(Betty Crocker)*	140	3.0	21.0	5.0	m.q.	580	m.q.
cheese, two *(Kraft* Potatoes & Cheese)	130	4.0	19.0	4.0	10	540	m.q.
country style:							
(Fantastic Foods)	91	3.0	19.0	.3	n.a.	221	1.7 d

[1] *Prepared with whole milk and salted butter.*

[2] *Prepared with skim milk, no butter.*

Food and Measure	cal.	prot. (gms)	carbo. (gms)	fat (gms)	chol. (mgs)	sod. (mgs)	fiber (gms)
w/butter (Fantastic Foods)	124	3.0	19.0	4.0	m.q.	260	1.7 d
hash brown:							
(Betty Crocker) . .	160	2.0	24.0	6.0	n.a.	450	m.q.
(Idahoan Quick One-Pan)	140	2.0	18.0	7.0	m.q.	400	m.q.
julienne (Betty Crocker)	130	3.0	19.0	5.0	m.q.	580	m.q.
mashed:							
(Country Store), 1/3 cup flakes . .	70	1.0	16.0	0	0	10	m.q.
(Hungry Jack Flakes)	130	2.0	17.0	6.0	0	260	1.0 d
(Idahoan Complete)	80	1.0	17.0	1.0	0	175	m.q.
(Idahoan)	140	3.0	16.0	7.0	m.q.	320	m.q.
(Pillsbury Idaho Granules)	120	2.0	16.0	5.0	0	190	1.0 d
(Pillsbury Idaho Spuds)	130	3.0	16.0	6.0	0	370	1.0 d
(Potato Buds) . . .	130	3.0	17.0	6.0	m.q.	360	m.q.
pancake, see "Potato pancake"							
ranch, creamy (Idahoan)	130	2.0	18.0	5.0	n.a.	400	m.q.
scalloped:							
(Betty Crocker) . .	140	3.0	20.0	5.0	n.a.	570	m.q.
(Idahoan)	140	3.0	20.0	5.0	m.q.	425	m.q.
(Kraft Potatoes & Cheese)	140	4.0	20.0	5.0	25	500	m.q.
cheesy (Betty Crocker Homestyle)	150	3.0	20.0	6.0	m.q.	560	m.q.
cheesy (Pillsbury)	150	3.0	20.0	6.0	15	540	1.0 d
w/ham (Betty Crocker Scalloped'N Ham) . .	170	4.0	22.0	7.0	m.q.	620	m.q.
w/ham (Kraft Potatoes & Cheese)	150	5.0	20.0	5.0	15	510	m.q.

Food and Measure	cal.	prot. (gms)	carbo. (gms)	fat (gms)	chol. (mgs)	sod. (mgs)	fiber (gms)
Potato, mix, scalloped *(cont.)*							
white sauce, creamy							
(Pillsbury)	150	3.0	20.0	6.0	15	470	1.0 d
sour cream, chives:							
(Betty Crocker) . .	150	3.0	20.0	6.0	m.q.	520	m.q.
(Betty Crocker Twice							
Baked)	200	5.0	19.0	11.0	m.q.	570	m.q.
(Kraft Potatoes &							
Cheese)	150	5.0	20.0	5.0	10	610	m.q.
(Pillsbury)	150	3.0	20.0	6.0	15	500	1.0 d
Western *(Idahoan)* . .	120	2.0	18.0	4.0	m.q.	400	m.q.
Potato, stuffed, see							
"Potato dishes, fro-							
zen"							
Potato, sweet, see							
"Sweet potato"							
Potato chips and							
crisps, 1 oz., ex-							
cept as noted:							
(Kettle Chips No Salt)	150	2.0	15.0	9.0	0	10	m.q.
(Krunchers!)	150	2.0	16.0	9.0	0	170	m.q.
(Lay's)	150	1.0	15.0	10.0	0	170	1.1 d
(Lay's Crunch Tators)	150	2.0	17.0	8.0	0	120	1.1 d
(Lay's Unsalted) . . .	150	2.0	15.0	10.0	0	10	1.1 d
(Mr. Phipps Original)	120	2.0	20.0	4.0	0	260	m.q.
(Munchos)	160	1.0	15.0	10.0	0	230	m.q.
(No Fries)	120	2.0	24.0	2.0	0	240	m.q.
(O'Boisies)	150	1.0	16.0	9.0	0	180	m.q.
(Pringles)	160	2.0	14.0	11.0	0	170	m.q.
(Pringles Light)	130	1.0	17.0	6.0	0	100	m.q.
(Pringles Rippled) . .	160	2.0	14.0	11.0	0	150	m.q.
(Ripplin's Original) . .	150	1.0	16.0	9.0	0	180	m.q.
(Ruffles)	150	2.0	15.0	10.0	0	135	1.1 d
(Ruffles Light)	130	2.0	19.0	6.0	0	140	1.1 d
(Tom's), 1⅛-oz. pkg.	180	2.0	16.0	12.0	0	260	m.q.
Alfredo *(Krunchers!)*	150	2.0	16.0	9.0	0	200	m.q.
au gratin *(King Kold)*	150	2.0	15.0	8.0	n.a.	220	m.q.

Food and Measure	cal.	prot. (gms)	carbo. (gms)	fat (gms)	chol. (mgs)	sod. (mgs)	fiber (gms)
barbecue flavor:							
(Mr. Phipps)	120	2.0	20.0	4.0	0	320	m.q.
(Pringles)	160	2.0	14.0	11.0	0	200	m.q.
(Pringles Light) . .	130	1.0	17.0	6.0	0	100	m.q.
(Ripplin's)	150	1.0	16.0	9.0	0	200	m.q.
(Tom's), 1 1/8-oz. pkg.	180	2.0	16.0	12.0	0	300	m.q.
plain or Kansas City (Lay's Bar-B-Q)	150	1.0	15.0	9.0	0	270	1.1 d
Cajun (Lay's Crunch Tators Amazin' Cajun)	150	2.0	17.0	8.0	0	150	1.1 d
cheddar:							
(Lay's)	150	2.0	14.0	10.0	0	300	1.1 d
(O'Boisies)	150	2.0	15.0	10.0	0	130	m.q.
New York (Kettle Chips)	150	2.0	15.0	9.0	0	100	m.q.
and sour cream (Ruffles)	160	2.0	15.0	10.0	0	250	1.1 d
cheese (Pringles Cheezums)	160	2.0	14.0	11.0	0	190	m.q.
dill (King Kold)	150	2.0	16.0	8.0	n.a.	340	m.q.
hot (Lay's Flamin' Hot)	150	2.0	15.0	9.0	0	190	1.1 d
jalapeño:							
(Krunchers!)	150	2.0	16.0	9.0	0	250	m.q.
(Lay's Crunch Tators Hoppin' Jalapeño)	140	1.0	18.0	7.0	0	200	1.1 d
jack (Kettle Chips)	150	2.0	15.0	9.0	0	110	m.q.
lightly salted or sea salt (Kettle Chips)	150	2.0	15.0	9.0	0	80	m.q.
mesquite:							
(Krunchers!)	150	2.0	16.0	9.0	0	200	m.q.
(Lay's Crunch Tators Mighty Mesquite)	150	2.0	17.0	8.0	0	135	1.1 d
grill (Ruffles B-B-Q)	160	2.0	15.0	10.0	0	270	1.1 d
Monterey Jack flavor (Ruffles Cheese Attack)	160	2.0	15.0	10.0	0	200	1.1 d

Food and Measure	cal.	prot. (gms)	carbo. (gms)	fat (gms)	chol. (mgs)	sod. (mgs)	fiber (gms)
Potato chips and crisps (cont.)							
ranch:							
(Lay's Tangy Ranch)	160	2.0	15.0	10.0	0	210	1.1 d
(Pringles Light) . .	130	1.0	17.0	6.0	0	110	m.q.
(Ripplin's)	150	2.0	13.0	10.0	0	200	m.q.
(Ruffles)	160	2.0	15.0	10.0	0	220	1.1 d
salsa w/mesquite, sea salt and vinegar, or yogurt and green onion (Kettle Chips)	150	2.0	15.0	9.0	0	120	m.q.
salt and vinegar:							
(Krunchers!)	150	2.0	16.0	9.0	0	290	m.q.
(Lay's)	150	1.0	14.0	10.0	0	390	1.1 d
sea salt and vinegar (Eagle Ripples) . .	150	2.0	16.0	9.0	0	140	m.q.
sour cream and onion:							
(Krunchers!)	150	2.0	16.0	9.0	<5	220	m.q.
(Lay's)	160	2.0	15.0	10.0	0	220	1.1 d
(Lay's Crunch Tators Supreme Sour Cream)	150	2.0	16.0	8.0	0	180	1.1 d
(Mr. Phipps)	120	2.0	20.0	4.0	0	300	m.q.
(O'Boisies)	150	2.0	15.0	9.0	0	190	m.q.
(Pringles)	160	2.0	14.0	11.0	0	135	m.q.
(Pringles Light) . .	130	1.0	17.0	6.0	0	110	m.q.
(Ruffles)	160	2.0	15.0	10.0	0	220	1.1 d
(Ruffles Light) . . .	130	3.0	18.0	6.0	0	190	1.1 d
(Tom's), 1 1/8-oz. pkg.	180	2.0	16.0	12.0	2	200	m.q.
vinegar and salt (Tom's), 1 1/8-oz. pkg.	180	2.0	18.0	12.0	0	370	m.q.
Potato dishes, frozen:							
au gratin (Stouffer's), 5.75 oz.	170	5.0	17.0	9.0	n.a.	670	m.q.
baked, w/broccoli: and cheddar (Lean Cuisine), 10 3/8 oz.	290	14.0	37.0	9.0	20	590	m.q.

Food and Measure	cal.	prot. (gms)	carbo. (gms)	fat (gms)	chol. (mgs)	sod. (mgs)	fiber (gms)
and cheese *(The Budget Gourmet Light and Healthy),* 10.5 oz.	300	13.0	40.0	10.0	30	740	m.q.
and cheese *(Ore-Ida Topped Baked),* 5.63 oz.	160	5.0	25.0	4.0	<5	400	m.q.
and cheese *(Weight Watchers),* 10.5 oz.	270	10.0	43.0	6.0	5	570	m.q.
and ham *(Weight Watchers),* 11.5 oz.	240	19.0	30.0	5.0	15	520	m.q.
baked, butter *(Ore-Ida Twice Baked),* 5 oz.	200	4.0	28.0	8.0	0	460	m.q.
baked, cheddar *(Ore-Ida Twice Baked),* 5 oz.	210	5.0	28.0	9.0	<5	570	m.q.
baked, chicken divan *(Weight Watchers),* 11.25 oz.	280	17.0	38.0	7.0	30	480	m.q.
baked, w/sour cream: *(Lean Cuisine),* 10 3/8 oz.	220	9.0	33.0	6.0	15	580	m.q.
and chives *(Ore-Ida Twice Baked),* 5 oz.	190	4.0	27.0	8.0	0	430	m.q.
baked, turkey, home-style *(Weight Watchers),* 11.25 oz. . . .	230	17.0	27.0	7.0	45	510	m.q.
baked, vegetable primavera: *(Ore-Ida Topped Baked),* 6.13 oz.	160	6.0	23.0	5.0	<5	390	m.q.
(Weight Watchers), 11.15 oz.	320	11.0	49.0	9.0	5	500	m.q.

Food and Measure	cal.	prot. (gms)	carbo. (gms)	fat (gms)	chol. (mgs)	sod. (mgs)	fiber (gms)
Potato dishes, frozen *(cont.)*							
baked, wedges, w/broccoli and cheese *(Healthy Choice)*, 9.5 oz. . . .	240	8.0	41.0	5.0	15	510	m.q.
and broccoli, w/cheese sauce *(Green Giant* One Serving), 5.5 oz. . . .	130	4.0	19.0	4.0	5	580	2.0 d
casserole, garden *(Healthy Choice Quick Meal)*, 9.25 oz.	180	12.0	23.0	4.0	20	360	m.q.
cheddared:							
(The Budget Gourmet Side Dish), 5.5 oz.	260	7.0	22.0	16.0	35	600	m.q.
w/broccoli *(The Budget Gourmet* Side Dish), 5 oz.	150	6.0	14.0	7.0	20	410	m.q.
pancake, see "Potato pancake"							
scalloped *(Stouffer's)*, 5.75 oz.	130	4.0	16.0	6.0	m.q.	610	m.q.
stuffed, three cheese *(The Budget Gourmet* Side Dish), 5.75 oz.	220	7.0	23.0	11.0	30	470	m.q.
Potato dishes, packaged, au gratin *(Green Giant Pantry Express)*, 1/2 cup	120	3.0	17.0	5.0	5	430	1.5 d
Potato flakes *(Arrowhead Mills)*, 2 oz.	140	5.0	44.0	0	0	24	m.q.
Potato flour, 1 cup	628	14.3	143.0	1.4	0	61	10.9 d
Potato pancake:							
frozen *(Golden)*, 1 piece	80	2.0	11.0	3.0	5	210	1.0 d

Food and Measure	cal.	prot. (gms)	carbo. (gms)	fat (gms)	chol. (mgs)	sod. (mgs)	fiber (gms)
frozen, Mexican (Golden), 1 piece	70	2.0	11.0	2.0	5	170	m.q.
mix* (Pillsbury), 3 cakes, 3″ each	90	3.0	16.0	2.0	55	420	1.0 d
Potato planks, catsup flavor (Durkee), 1 oz.	160	2.0	14.0	11.0	0	630	m.q.
Potato salad seasoning (Tone's), 1 tsp.	5	.2	.3	.2	0	1498	.1 d
Potato sticks, 1 oz., except as noted:							
1 oz.	148	1.9	15.1	9.8	0	71	.3 c
(Allens/Butterfield), 1/2 cup	140	1.0	16.0	8.0	0	190	m.q.
(Durkee)	160	2.0	16.0	9.0	0	210	m.q.
plain or cheddar (Andy Capp's Pub Fries)	140	2.0	18.0	6.0	0	290	m.q.
bacon and cheddar (Tom's), 7/8 oz. . .	130	2.0	15.0	7.0	n.a.	270	m.q.
hot:							
(Andy Capp's Fries)	130	2.0	20.0	5.0	0	200	m.q.
(Tom's Fries)	150	2.0	17.0	6.0	n.a.	290	m.q.
salt'n vinegar (Andy Capp's)	140	2.0	17.0	7.0	0	260	m.q.
Poultry, see specific listings							
Poultry seasoning, 1 tsp.	5	.1	1.0	.1	0	tr.	.2 d
Pout, ocean, meat only:							
raw, 4 oz.	90	18.9	0	1.0	59	69	0
baked, broiled, or microwaved, 4 oz. . .	116	24.2	0	1.3	76	88	0
Preserves, see "Jam and preserves"							
Pretzel (see also "Crackers"), 1 oz., except as noted:							
hard, plain	108	2.6	22.5	1.0	0	486	.9 d

Food and Measure	cal.	prot. (gms)	carbo. (gms)	fat (gms)	chol. (mgs)	sod. (mgs)	fiber (gms)
Pretzel *(cont.)*							
(Andy Capp's Pub							
Pretzels)	110	3.0	23.0	1.0	0	500	m.q.
(Mr. Salty Mini)	110	3.0	21.0	1.0	0	450	m.q.
cheddar *(Combos),*							
1.8 oz.	240	5.0	34.0	9.0	n.a.	580	m.q.
chips:							
(Mr. Phipps)	120	2.0	20.0	2.0	0	620	m.q.
fat free *(Mr. Phipps)*	100	2.0	22.0	0	0	620	m.q.
lightly salted *(Mr.*							
Phipps)	120	2.0	22.0	2.0	0	400	m.q.
sesame *(Mr. Phipps)*	120	2.0	20.0	4.0	0	500	m.q.
Dutch *(Mr. Salty)* . . .	110	3.0	22.0	1.0	0	440	m.q.
nacho *(Combos),*							
1.8 oz.	240	5.0	34.0	9.0	n.a.	620	m.q.
pizza *(Combos),*							
1.8 oz.	240	5.0	35.0	9.0	n.a.	550	m.q.
sticks:							
(Eagle)	110	3.0	22.0	2.0	0	570	m.q.
(Mr. Salty)	110	3.0	22.0	1.0	0	600	m.q.
sticks or twists *(Mr.*							
Salty Fat Free) . . .	110	3.0	23.0	0	0	380	m.q.
twists *(Mr. Salty)* . . .	110	3.0	21.0	2.0	0	580	m.q.
whole wheat, hard . .	103	3.1	23.0	.7	0	58	.5 c
Pretzel, frozen							
(Super-Pretzel),							
1 piece	170	7.0	37.0	0	0	140	3.0 d
Prickly pear:							
1 medium, 4.8 oz. . . .	42	.8	9.9	.5	0	6	3.7 d
(Frieda's), 1 oz.	12	.1	3.1	<.1	0	1	m.q.
Prosciutto, boneless,							
(Hormel Deli), 1 oz. .	65	8.0	<2.0	4.0	23	524	0
Protein shake mix:							
(Naturade Mega Pro-							
tein), 1 oz.	100	25.0	0	0	0	150	n.a.
(Naturade N-R-G Pro-							
tein+), 1.1 oz.	115	26.0	2.0	0	0	185	n.a.

Food and Measure	cal.	prot. (gms)	carbo. (gms)	fat (gms)	chol. (mgs)	sod. (mgs)	fiber (gms)
carob or vanilla *(Naturade* N-R-G), 1 oz.	100	24.0	1.0	0	n.a.	195	n.a.
Prune:							
canned, in heavy syrup:							
pitted, 4 oz.	119	1.0	31.5	.2	0	3	4.3 d
1/2 cup	123	1.0	32.5	.2	0	3	4.4 d
5 medium and 2 tbsp. liquid . .	90	.8	23.9	.2	0	2	3.3 d
dehydrated:							
uncooked, 1/2 cup	224	2.4	58.8	.5	0	4	1.9 c
cooked, 1/2 cup . .	158	1.7	41.6	.3	0	3	1.4 c
dried, 2 oz., except as noted:							
(Dole)	140	1.0	36.0	1.0	0	<10	m.q.
(Sunsweet)	120	1.0	32.0	0	0	<10	m.q.
w/pits, 1/2 cup . . .	193	2.1	50.5	.4	0	3	5.7 d
pitted, 10 prunes	201	2.2	52.7	.4	0	3	6.0 d
pitted *(Sunsweet)*	140	1.0	36.0	0	0	<10	m.q.
dried, stewed, w/pits, unsweetened, 1/2 cup	113	1.2	29.8	.2	0	2	7.0 d
Prune juice:							
6 fl. oz.	136	1.2	33.5	.1	0	8	1.9 d
(R.W. Knudsen Organic), 8 fl. oz. . .	170	1.0	42.0	1.0	0	(0)	m.q.
(Mott's All Natural), 6 fl. oz.	136	1.0	34.0	<1.0	0	8	m.q.
(Mott's Country Style), 6 fl. oz.	149	1.0	37.0	<1.0	0	7	m.q.
(Sunsweet), 6 fl. oz.	130	1.0	33.0	0	0	<20	m.q.
Pudding, ready-to-serve, 4 oz., except as noted:							
banana *(Hunt's Snack Pack),* 4.25 oz. . .	145	2.0	22.0	6.0	1	180	0

Food and Measure	cal.	prot. (gms)	carbo. (gms)	fat (gms)	chol. (mgs)	sod. (mgs)	fiber (gms)
Pudding, ready-to-serve *(cont.)*							
butterscotch:							
(Hunt's Snack Pack),							
4.25 oz.	170	2.0	27.0	6.0	1	210	0
(Swiss Miss)	180	2.0	29.0	6.0	5	135	0
butterscotch-choco-							
late-vanilla swirl							
(Jell-O Pudding							
Snacks)	180	3.0	28.0	6.0	0	190	n.a.
chocolate:							
(Hershey's)	180	3.0	29.0	5.0	0	260	n.a.
(Hershey's Special							
Dark)	180	4.0	30.0	5.0	0	135	n.a.
(Hunt's Snack Pack),							
4.25 oz.	170	2.0	26.0	6.0	1	120	0
(Hunt's Snack Pack							
Light)	100	3.0	20.0	2.0	1	120	0
(Jell-O Free Pudding							
Snacks)	100	3.0	24.0	0	0	200	n.a.
(Swiss Miss)	180	2.0	29.0	6.0	5	160	0
fudge *(Hunt's Snack*							
Pack), 4.25 oz.	165	2.0	27.0	6.0	1	125	0
fudge *(Swiss Miss)*	220	3.0	38.0	6.0	5	180	0
parfait *(Swiss Miss)*	170	3.0	27.0	6.0	1	200	0
regular or fudge							
(Jell-O Pudding							
Snacks)	160	3.0	28.0	5.0	0	200	n.a.
regular or fudge							
(Swiss Miss Light)	100	3.0	20.0	1.0	0	120	0
sundae *(Swiss Miss)*	220	2.0	36.0	7.0	5	140	0
chocolate and almond							
(Hershey's)	180	3.0	29.0	6.0	0	210	m.q.
chocolate caramel:							
(Hershey's Cara-							
mello)	180	3.0	28.0	6.0	0	170	n.a.
swirl *(Jell-O* Pudding							
Snacks)	170	3.0	28.0	6.0	0	190	n.a.

Food and Measure	cal.	prot. (gms)	carbo. (gms)	fat (gms)	chol. (mgs)	sod. (mgs)	fiber (gms)
chocolate marshmal-low *(Hunt's Snack Pack)*, 4.25 oz.	165	2.0	26.0	6.0	1	125	0
chocolate mint *(Hershey's York Peppermint Pattie)*	180	3.0	29.0	6.0	0	210	n.a.
chocolate/mint or chocolate/vanilla swirl *(Jell-O Free Pudding Snacks)*	100	3.0	24.0	0	0	220	n.a.
chocolate and vanilla *(Hershey's Kisses)*	180	3.0	29.0	6.0	0	210	n.a.
chocolate-vanilla swirl *(Jell-O Pudding Snacks)*	170	3.0	28.0	6.0	0	190	n.a.
lemon *(Hunt's Snack Pack)*, 4.25 oz.	150	<1.0	30.0	4.0	0	75	<1.0
tapioca:							
(Hunt's Snack Pack), 4.25 oz.	150	2.0	23.0	5.0	1	125	0
(Hunt's Snack Pack Light)	100	2.0	18.0	2.0	1	105	0
(Jell-O Pudding Snacks)	170	3.0	29.0	4.0	0	180	n.a.
(Swiss Miss)	160	2.0	27.0	5.0	5	170	0
vanilla:							
(Hunt's Snack Pack), 4.25 oz.	170	2.0	27.0	6.0	1	150	0
(Jell-O Free Pudding Snacks)	100	3.0	23.0	0	0	250	n.a.
(Jell-O Pudding Snacks)	160	3.0	25.0	5.0	0	180	n.a.
(Swiss Miss)	190	2.0	30.0	7.0	5	140	0
(Swiss Miss Light)	100	2.0	20.0	1.0	0	105	0
parfait *(Swiss Miss)*	180	2.0	29.0	6.0	1	150	0
sundae *(Swiss Miss)*	220	2.0	36.0	7.0	5	180	0

Food and Measure	cal.	prot. (gms)	carbo. (gms)	fat (gms)	chol. (mgs)	sod. (mgs)	fiber (gms)
Pudding, ready-to-serve *(cont.)*							
vanilla-chocolate parfait *(Swiss Miss Light)*	100	2.0	20.0	1.0	0	110	0
vanilla-chocolate swirl *(Jell-O* Pudding Snacks)	180	3.0	28.0	6.0	0	190	n.a.
Pudding, frozen:							
almond *(Imagine Foods* Dream), 4 oz.	150	1.0	31.0	2.0	0	30	m.q.
banana, butterscotch, or lemon *(Imagine Foods* Dream), 4 oz.	120	1.0	30.0	0	0	5	n.a.
butterscotch *(Rich's),* 3 oz.	130	2.0	18.0	6.0	0	130	0
carob *(Imagine Foods* Dream), 4 oz. . . .	130	1.0	31.0	0	0	30	n.a.
chocolate:							
(Imagine Foods Dream), 4 oz. . . .	170	1.0	39.0	0	0	30	n.a.
(Rich's), 3 oz. . . .	140	2.0	19.0	7.0	1	120	.2 d
coconut *(Imagine Foods* Dream), 4 oz.	150	1.0	32.0	2.0	0	10	n.a.
vanilla *(Rich's),* 3 oz.	130	2.0	18.0	6.0	0	160	0
Pudding bar, frozen *(Jell-O* Pudding Pops), 1 bar:							
chocolate	80	2.0	13.0	2.0	0	85	n.a.
chocolate, double swirl or fudge . . .	80	2.0	13.0	2.0	0	90	n.a.
chocolate, milk . . .	80	2.0	13.0	2.0	0	55	n.a.
chocolate-vanilla swirl	80	2.0	13.0	2.0	0	70	n.a.
vanilla	80	2.0	13.0	2.0	0	55	n.a.
Pudding mix*, 1/2 cup, except as noted:							
banana cream:							
(Jell-O), 1/6 recipe	100	3.0	17.0	3.0	10	160	n.a.

Food and Measure	cal.	prot. (gms)	carbo. (gms)	fat (gms)	chol. (mgs)	sod. (mgs)	fiber (gms)
(Jell-O Instant) . . .	160	4.0	28.0	4.0	15	410	n.a.
butter pecan (Jell-O Instant)	170	4.0	28.0	5.0	15	410	n.a.
butterscotch:							
(Jell-O)	170	4.0	30.0	4.0	15	190	n.a.
(Jell-O Instant) . . .	160	4.0	28.0	4.0	15	450	n.a.
caramel, creme (Knorr Dessert Mix), 1 serving mix and sauce dry	115	.1	274	.4	4	15	n.a.
chocolate:							
(Jell-O)	160	5.0	28.0	4.0	15	170	n.a.
(Jell-O Instant) . . .	180	4.0	31.0	4.0	15	480	n.a.
milk (Jell-O)	160	4.0	28.0	4.0	15	170	n.a.
milk (Jell-O Instant)	180	5.0	31.0	5.0	15	470	n.a.
chocolate fudge:							
(Jell-O)	160	5.0	28.0	4.0	15	170	n.a.
(Jell-O Instant) . . .	180	5.0	31.0	5.0	15	440	n.a.
coconut:							
cream (Jell-O), 1/6 recipe	110	3.0	16.0	4.0	10	140	n.a.
cream (Jell-O Instant)	180	4.0	27.0	6.0	15	320	n.a.
custard, golden egg (Jell-O Americana)	150	5.0	24.0	4.0	15	190	n.a.
flan (Jell-O)	150	4.0	26.0	4.0	15	65	n.a.
lemon:							
(Jell-O), 1/6 recipe	170	2.0	38.0	2.0	90	95	n.a.
(Jell-O Instant) . . .	170	4.0	29.0	4.0	15	360	n.a.
pistachio (Jell-O Instant)	170	4.0	28.0	5.0	15	410	n.a.
raspberry or strawberry (Salada Danish Dessert)	130	0	32.0	0	0	5	n.a.
rennet custard:							
chocolate (Junket)	120	5.0	15.0	4.0	m.q.	65	n.a.
raspberry or strawberry (Junket) . .	120	4.0	16.0	4.0	m.q.	60	n.a.

Food and Measure	cal.	prot. (gms)	carbo. (gms)	fat (gms)	chol. (mgs)	sod. (mgs)	fiber (gms)
Pudding mix, rennet custard *(cont.)*							
vanilla *(Junket)* . . .	120	4.0	16.0	4.0	m.q.	65	n.a.
rice *(Jell-O Americana)*	170	5.0	30.0	4.0	15	160	n.a.
tapioca:							
vanilla *(Jell-O Americana)*	150	4.0	26.0	4.0	15	170	n.a.
vanilla *(Royal)* . . .	160	4.0	27.0	4.0	m.q.	150	n.a.
vanilla:							
(Jell-O)	160	4.0	27.0	4.0	15	200	n.a.
(Jell-O Instant) . . .	170	4.0	29.0	4.0	15	410	n.a.
French *(Jell-O)* . . .	170	4.0	30.0	4.0	15	190	n.a.
French *(Jell-O Instant)*	160	4.0	28.0	4.0	15	400	n.a.
Puff pastry, see "Pastry dough"							
Pummelo:							
1 medium, 5½" diam.	228	4.6	58.6	.2	0	7	6.1 d
sections, ½ cup . . .	36	.7	9.1	<.1	0	1	1.0 d
trimmed *(Frieda's)*, 1 oz.	11	.2	2.7	<.1	0	<1	m.q.
Pumpkin:							
fresh, pulp, ½ cup:							
raw, 1" cubes . . .	15	.6	3.8	.1	0	1	1.0 d
boiled, drained, mashed	24	.9	6.0	.1	0	2	1.0 c
canned, ½ cup:							
(Libby's)	42	1.4	10.1	.4	0	6	3.8 d
w/ or w/out winter squash	41	1.3	9.9	.3	0	6	3.4 d
Pumpkin butter *(Smucker's* Autumn Harvest)*, 1 tsp. . .	12	0	3.0	0	0	14	m.q.
Pumpkin flower:							
raw, ½ cup	3	.2	.5	<.1	0	1	.1 c
boiled, drained, ½ cup	10	.7	2.2	.1	0	4	.6 d
Pumpkin leaf:							
raw, ½ cup	4	.6	.5	.1	0	2	.2 c

Food and Measure	cal.	prot. (gms)	carbo. (gms)	fat (gms)	chol. (mgs)	sod. (mgs)	fiber (gms)
boiled, drained,							
½ cup	7	1.0	1.2	.1	0	3	.9 d
Pumpkin pie spice,							
1 tsp.	6	.1	1.2	.2	0	1	.3 d
Pumpkin seeds:							
roasted, in shell:							
1 oz. or 85 seeds	127	5.3	15.3	5.5	0	5	10.2 c
1 cup	285	11.9	34.4	12.4	0	12	23.0 c
salted, 1 oz.	127	5.3	15.3	5.5	0	163	10.2 c
roasted, shelled:							
1 oz.	148	9.4	3.8	12.0	0	5	1.8 d
salted, 1 oz.	148	9.4	3.8	12.0	0	163	1.8 d
dried, shelled, 1 oz. or							
142 kernels	154	7.0	5.1	13.0	0	5	.6 c
Punch, see "Fruit punch" and specific fruit listings							
Purslane:							
raw, ½ cup	4	.3	.7	<.1	0	10	.2 c
boiled, drained,							
½ cup	10	.9	2.1	.1	0	26	.5 c

Q

Food and Measure	cal.	prot. (gms)	carbo. (gms)	fat (gms)	chol. (mgs)	sod. (mgs)	fiber (gms)
Quail, raw:							
meat w/skin:							
1 quail, 3.8 oz.							
(4.3 oz. w/bone)	210	21.4	0	13.1	m.q.	58	0
1 oz.	54	5.6	0	3.4	m.q.	15	0
meat only:							
1 quail, 3.2 oz.							
(4.3 oz. w/bone							
and skin)	123	20.0	0	4.2	m.q.	47	0
1 oz.	38	6.2	0	1.3	m.q.	14	0
breast meat only:							
1 breast, 2 oz. . . .	69	12.7	0	1.8	m.q.	31	0
1 oz.	35	6.4	0	.8	m.q.	16	0
Quince:							
1 medium, 5.3 oz. . . .	53	.4	14.1	.1	0	4	1.7 d
peeled, seeded, 1 oz.	16	.1	4.3	<.1	0	1	.5 d
pineapple, peeled,							
seeded *(Frieda's)*,							
1 oz.	16	.1	4.3	<.1	0	1	m.q.
Quincy's, 1 serving:							
chicken breast, grilled	124	25.7	2.4	1.4	m.q.	140	n.a.
steak:							
filet	331	40.0	0	12.0	m.q.	159	0
ribeye	665	31.0	0	60.0	m.q.	205	0
ribeye, thick	865	60.0	0	78.0	m.q.	298	0
sirloin club	283	44.0	0	10.0	m.q.	160	0
sirloin, petite	446	26.0	0	37.0	m.q.	118	0
sirloin, regular . . .	649	38.0	0	54.0	m.q.	206	0
sirloin, large	852	50.0	0	70.0	m.q.	241	0
T-bone	1612	71.0	0	159.0	m.q.	389	0

Food and Measure	cal.	prot. (gms)	carbo. (gms)	fat (gms)	chol. (mgs)	sod. (mgs)	fiber (gms)
trout, rainbow, grilled	237	34.3	0	10.2	m.q.	50	0
side dishes:							
broccoli spears . .	108	9.0	13.5	1.0	0	30	m.q.
peppers and onions	87	1.0	10.0	5.0	n.a.	111	m.q.
potato, baked . . .	372	8.0	86.0	.5	0	45	m.q.
yeast roll	158	2.0	29.4	3.9	n.a.	283	m.q.
Quinoa:							
1 oz.	106	3.7	19.5	1.6	0	n.a.	1.7 d
(Eden), 2 oz.	200	8.0	38.0	4.0	0	<30	4.3 d

R

Food and Measure	cal.	prot. (gms)	carbo. (gms)	fat (gms)	chol. (mgs)	sod. (mgs)	fiber (gms)
Rabbit, meat only:							
domesticated:							
roasted, 4 oz. . . .	223	33.0	0	9.1	93	53	0
stewed, 4 oz. . . .	234	34.5	0	9.5	98	42	0
stewed, diced,							
1 cup	288	42.5	0	11.8	120	52	0
wild, stewed:							
4 oz.	196	37.4	0	4.0	139	51	0
diced, 1 cup	242	46.2	0	4.9	172	63	0
Radicchio, fresh:							
trimmed, 1 oz.	7	.4	1.3	.1	0	6	m.q.
1 medium leaf, .3 oz.	2	.1	.4	<.1	0	2	m.q.
shredded, 1/2 cup . .	5	.3	.9	.1	0	4	m.q.
Radish:							
10 medium, 3/4"–1"							
diam.	7	.3	1.6	.2	0	11	.7 d
sliced, 1/2 cup	10	.4	2.1	.3	0	14	.9 d
Radish, black, 1 oz.	5	.3	1.0	<.1	0	5	m.q.
Radish, Oriental:							
raw, 1 medium,							
7" × 21/4" diam. . .	62	2.0	13.9	.3	0	71	5.4 d
raw, sliced, 1/2 cup	8	.3	1.8	<.1	0	9	.7 d
boiled, drained, sliced,							
1/2 cup	13	.5	2.5	.2	0	10	1.2 d
dried, 1 oz.	77	2.2	18.0	.2	0	79	2.4 c
Radish, white-icicle:							
1 medium, .6 oz. . .	2	.2	.5	<.1	0	3	.1 c
sliced, 1/2 cup	7	.6	1.3	.1	0	8	.4 c

Food and Measure	cal.	prot. (gms)	carbo. (gms)	fat (gms)	chol. (mgs)	sod. (mgs)	fiber (gms)
Raisin, 1/2 cup, except as noted:							
golden seedless:							
not packed	219	2.5	57.7	.3	0	9	2.9 d
(Dole)	250	3.0	66.0	0	0	25	m.q.
seeded, not packed	214	1.8	56.9	.4	0	21	4.9 d
seedless:							
not packed	217	2.3	57.4	.3	0	9	2.9 d
(Cinderella Thompson)	250	3.0	66.0	0	0	15	m.q.
(Dole)	250	3.0	66.0	0	0	15	m.q.
(Sun • Maid)	290	3.0	69.0	0	0	<15	m.q.
Ranch dip mix*, dry, cracked pepper *(Knorr),* 1 serving	6	.2	.8	.2	<1	100	n.a.
Raspberry, red:							
1 pint	154	2.8	36.1	1.7	0	tr.	21.2 d
1/2 cup	31	.6	7.1	.3	0	tr.	4.2 d
frozen:							
sweetened, 1/2 cup	129	.9	32.7	.2	0	1	5.5 d
in syrup *(Birds Eye),* 5 oz.	100	1.0	25.0	1.0	0	0	4.0 d
Raspberry drink mix*, 8 fl. oz.:							
(Kool-Aid)	100	0	25.0	0	0	25	0
(Kool-Aid Presweetened)	70	0	18.0	0	0	0	0
Raspberry float *(R.W. Knudsen),* 8 fl. oz.	130	2.0	31.0	<1.0	0	(0)	n.a.
Raspberry juice:							
blend, 6 fl. oz.:							
(Chiquita Raspberry Passion)	110	0	26.0	0	0	30	(0)
(Dole Pure & Light Country Raspberry)	87	.3	24.0	.2	0	15	(0)
red *(Smucker's* Naturally 100%), 8 fl. oz.	120	0	30.0	0	0	10	(0)

Food and Measure	cal.	prot. (gms)	carbo. (gms)	fat (gms)	chol. (mgs)	sod. (mgs)	fiber (gms)
Raspberry nectar, red *(R.W. Knudsen)*, 8 fl. oz.	120	<1.0	30.0	<1.0	0	(0)	m.q.
Raspberry-cranberry juice *(Master Choice)*, 6 fl. oz. . . .	90	0	21.0	0	0	<20	m.q.
Raspberry-peach juice *(R.W. Knudsen)*, 8 fl. oz. . . .	115	<1.0	28.0	<1.0	0	(0)	m.q.
Raspberry-tamarind dipping sauce *(Helen's Tropical Exotics)*, 2 tbsp. . . .	50	0	11.0	1.0	0	0	1.0 d
Ravioli, canned or packaged, 7.5 oz., except as noted:							
beef:							
(Hormel Micro Cup)	270	9.0	34.0	11.0	20	920	m.q.
in meat sauce *(Franco-American RavioliO's)*	250	10.0	35.0	8.0	m.q.	930	m.q.
in sauce *(Libby's Diner)*	240	13.0	35.0	5.0	15	890	m.q.
mini *(Hormel Kid's Kitchen)*	230	10.0	34.0	6.0	15	870	m.q.
Ravioli, frozen or re-frigerated:							
(Celentano), 6.5 oz.	400	21.0	61.0	9.0	100	390	m.q.
cheese *(Contadina)*, 3 oz.	270	13.0	30.0	11.0	75	360	m.q.
mini *(Celentano)*, 4 oz.	270	13.0	42.0	6.0	30	150	2.0 d
Ravioli entree, cheese, frozen:							
(The Budget Gourmet Light and Healthy), 9.5 oz.	290	12.0	34.0	13.0	30	750	m.q.

Food and Measure	cal.	prot. (gms)	carbo. (gms)	fat (gms)	chol. (mgs)	sod. (mgs)	fiber (gms)
baked, 9 oz., except as noted:							
(Healthy Choice) . .	250	14.0	44.0	2.0	20	420	m.q.
(Weight Watchers)	240	18.0	27.0	6.0	30	370	m.q.
w/tomato sauce (Lean Cuisine), 8.5 oz.	240	13.0	30.0	7.0	55	430	m.q.
Rax, 1 serving:							
sandwiches:							
beef, bacon'n cheddar	523	24.0	37.0	32.0	42	1042	m.q.
chicken breast, country fried . .	618	23.0	49.0	29.0	45	1078	m.q.
chicken breast, grilled	402	25.0	26.0	23.0	69	872	m.q.
Philly melt	396	25.0	40.0	16.0	27	1055	m.q.
Rax, regular	262	18.0	25.0	10.0	15	707	m.q.
roast beef, deluxe	498	21.0	39.0	30.0	36	864	m.q.
side dishes:							
french fries, 3.25 oz.	282	3.0	36.0	14.0	3	75	m.q.
potato, baked, plain	264	6.0	61.0	0	0	15	m.q.
potato, baked, plain, w/margarine . . .	364	6.0	61.0	11.0	0	115	m.q.
salads, no dressing:							
grilled chicken garden	202	19.0	14.0	9.0	32	747	m.q.
gourmet garden . .	134	7.0	13.0	6.0	2	350	m.q.
salad dressings:							
French, 2 oz. . . .	275	0	20.0	22.0	0	442	n.a.
Italian, light, 2 oz.	63	0	8.0	3.0	0	294	n.a.
sauces:							
barbecue, 1 pkt. . . .	11	0	3.0	0	0	158	n.a.
cheddar cheese, 1 oz.	29	<1.0	4.0	<1.0	0	225	n.a.
mushroom, 1 oz.	16	1.0	1.0	<1.0	0	113	n.a.
chocolate chip cookie, 2 pieces	262	4.0	36.0	12.0	5	192	m.q.

Food and Measure	cal.	prot. (gms)	carbo. (gms)	fat (gms)	chol. (mgs)	sod. (mgs)	fiber (gms)
Rax (cont.)							
chocolate shake,							
16 oz.	445	9.0	77.0	12.0	35	248	(0)
Colombo yogurt							
shakes:							
candy cane	320	9.0	62.0	4.0	0	160	n.a.
blackberry	270	9.0	58.0	1.0	0	160	n.a.
buckeye/peanut but-							
ter kiss	660	15.0	63.0	41.0	1	300	n.a.
cherry, chocolate							
covered	540	10.0	72.0	23.0	0	200	(0)
chocolate, fat free	310	10.0	66.0	<1.0	0	180	(0)
chocolate chip . .	480	10.0	57.0	23.0	0	160	(0)
mint chocolate chip	570	10.0	80.0	23.0	0	170	(0)
mocha	350	9.0	64.0	7.0	0	200	n.a.
orange, cool	360	9.0	35.0	4.0	0	160	n.a.
peach	320	9.0	60.0	4.0	0	160	n.a.
vanilla, fat free . . .	220	9.0	44.0	<1.0	0	140	0
strawberry, fat free	300	9.0	64.0	<1.0	0	150	(0)
Red beans, canned:							
(Allens), 1/2 cup . . .	80	5.0	17.0	<1.0	0	360	5.0 d
(Green Giant/Joan of							
Arc), 1/2 cup	90	6.0	19.0	1.0	0	340	5.0 d
small *(Hunt's),* 4 oz.	90	6.0	18.0	<1.0	0	560	6.0 d
Red bean mix*:							
and rice *(Fantastic* Ca-							
jun), 10 oz.	190	10.0	44.0	2.0	0	490	9.0 d
(Mahatma), 3/4 cup . .	200	4.0	44.0	0	0	920	m.q.
Red snapper, see							
"Snapper"							
Redfish, see "Ocean							
perch"							
Refried beans,							
canned, 4 oz., ex-							
cept as noted:							
4 oz.	121	7.1	21.0	1.2	n.a.	481	6.0 d
1/2 cup	134	7.9	23.3	1.4	n.a.	534	6.7 d

Food and Measure	cal.	prot. (gms)	carbo. (gms)	fat (gms)	chol. (mgs)	sod. (mgs)	fiber (gms)
(Chi-Chi's), 7.5 oz. . . .	250	9.0	29.0	11.0	5	930	m.q.
(Gebhardt)	100	7.0	20.0	2.0	2	490	6.8 d
(Old El Paso)	80	6.0	15.0	2.0	<5	430	5.0 d
w/bacon (Rosarita) . .	110	7.0	20.0	2.0	14	560	6.0 d
w/nacho cheese							
(Rosarita)	110	7.0	20.0	2.0	2	490	6.0 d
w/green chilies:							
(Old El Paso),							
1/4 cup	49	3.0	8.0	<1.0	n.a.	252	2.5 d
(Rosarita)	90	6.0	18.0	2.0	0	460	6.0 d
jalapeño (Gebhardt)	115	6.0	19.0	2.0	2	270	6.8 d
w/onions (Rosarita)	110	7.0	21.0	2.0	0	490	6.0 d
plain or vegetarian							
(Rosarita)	100	7.0	18.0	6.0	0	480	6.0 d
w/sausage (Old El							
Paso), 1/4 cup . . .	180	6.0	8.0	8.0	m.q.	300	m.q.
spicy (Rosarita) . . .	100	7.0	19.0	6.0	0	500	6.0 d
vegetarian:							
(Hain)	70	6.0	15.0	1.0	0	280	5.0 d
(Old El Paso) . . .	70	6.0	15.0	1.0	0	590	5.0 d
Refried beans, mix*,							
w/butter (Fantastic							
Instant), 1/2 cup . .	176	8.0	23.0	6.0	m.q.	373	12.0 d
Relish, 1 oz., except							
as noted:							
corn (New Morning)	36	0	8.0	0	0	0	m.q.
dill (Vlasic)	2	0	m.q.	0	0	450	m.q.
hamburger:							
1 cup	316	1.5	84.1	1.3	0	2676	8.0 d
1 tbsp.	19	.1	5.2	.1	0	164	.5 d
(Heinz)	30	0	7.0	0	0	325	m.q.
(Vlasic)	35	0	9.0	0	0	260	m.q.
hot dog:							
1 cup	222	3.7	57.0	1.1	0	2664	2.2 c
1 tbsp.	14	.2	3.5	.1	0	164	.1 c
(Heinz)	35	0	8.0	0	0	200	m.q.
(Vlasic)	40	0	8.0	0	0	260	m.q.

Food and Measure	cal.	prot. (gms)	carbo. (gms)	fat (gms)	chol. (mgs)	sod. (mgs)	fiber (gms)
Relish *(cont.)*							
India *(Heinz)*	35	0	9.0	0	0	215	m.q.
India *(Vlasic)*	30	0	8.0	0	0	260	m.q.
jalapeño *(Old El Paso)*,							
2 tbsp.	16	1.0	4.0	0	0	100	1.0 d
piccalilli:							
(Heinz)	30	0	7.0	0	0	145	m.q.
(New Morning) . . .	20	0	6.0	0	0	180	m.q.
green tomato or hot							
(Vlasic)	35	0	8.0	0	0	180	m.q.
pickle *(Claussen)*,							
1 tbsp.	15	0	3.0	0	0	85	m.q.
sweet:							
1 cup	318	.9	85.5	1.2	0	1980	2.1 c
1 tbsp.	19	.1	5.3	.1	0	122	.1 c
(Heinz)	35	0	9.0	0	0	205	m.q.
(New Morning) . . .	28	0	8.0	0	0	130	m.q.
(Vlasic)	35	0	8.0	0	0	260	m.q.
pickle, uncooked							
(Claussen), 1 oz.	25	<1.0	5.0	<1.0	0	160	m.q.
Rennet *(Junket)*,							
1 tablet	1	0	0	0	0	165	n.a.
Rennet custard, see							
"Pudding mix"							
Rhubarb:							
fresh:							
diced, 1/2 cup . . .	13	.6	2.8	.1	0	2	1.1 d
regular or hot house							
(Frieda's), 1 oz.	5	.2	1.0	<.1	0	1	m.q.
frozen, cooked, sweet-							
ened, 1/2 cup . . .	139	.5	37.4	.1	0	2	2.4 d
Rib sauce *(Dip n'Joy*							
Saucey Rib), 1 oz.	60	0	14.0	0	0	250	n.a.

Food and Measure	cal.	prot. (gms)	carbo. (gms)	fat (gms)	chol. (mgs)	sod. (mgs)	fiber (gms)
Rice, cooked*[1] (see also "Rice dishes, mix"), 1/2 cup, except as noted:							
basmati:							
brown (*Arrowhead Mills*), 2 oz. dry	200	4.0	44.0	1.0	0	3	3.1 d
brown (*Arrowhead Mills* Indian), 2 oz. dry	200	6.0	43.0	1.0	0	35	m.q.
brown (*Fantastic Foods*)......	110	3.0	23.0	.5	0	18	.4 d
brown (*Master Choice Texmati*)	110	3.0	23.0	0	0	0	1.0 d
white (*Arrowhead Mills* Indian), 2 oz. dry	190	6.0	44.0	1.0	0	25	m.q.
white (*Fantastic Foods*)......	105	3.0	22.0	.5	0	12	.3 d
white (*Master Choice Texmati*)	100	2.0	22.0	0	0	0	.2 d
white (*Texmati*) ..	82	3.0	31.0	0	0	0	m.q.
white and wild (*Master Choice Texmati*)	80	2.0	20.0	0	0	0	1.0 d
brown, long grain:							
(*Arrowhead Mills*), 2 oz. dry	200	4.0	44.0	1.0	0	3	3.1 d
(*Carolina/Mahatma/ River*)	100	2.0	23.0	0	0	0	m.q.
(*Uncle Ben's* Whole Grain), 1.3 oz. dry	130	3.2	27.6	.9	0	1	1.0 d
(*Uncle Ben's* Fast Cooking Whole Grain), .9 oz. dry	89	1.9	19.6	.6	0	10	.8 d

[1] Prepared without butter or salt.

Food and Measure	cal.	prot. (gms)	carbo. (gms)	fat (gms)	chol. (mgs)	sod. (mgs)	fiber (gms)
Rice *(cont.)*							
brown, medium or short grain *(Arrowhead Mills)*, 2 oz. dry	200	4.0	44.0	1.0	0	3	3.4 d
brown, instant *(Minute)*	120	3.0	26.0	1.0	0	5	m.q.
glutinous or sweet . .	117	2.5	25.4	.3	0	7	1.2 d
jasmine *(Fantastic Foods)*	100	2.5	22.0	.3	0	8	.3 d
jasmine, brown *(Fantastic Foods)*	105	2.5	23.0	.4	0	10	.4 d
white, long grain:							
1/2 cup	103	2.2	22.3	.3	0	tr.	.1 c
(Carolina/Mahatma/ River/Water Maid)	100	2.0	22.0	0	0	0	m.q.
parboiled *(Success)*	90	2.0	20.0	0	0	0	m.q.
parboiled *(Uncle Ben's Converted)*, 1.2 oz. dry . . .	123	3.0	27.2	.3	0	1	.3 d
white, long grain, instant:							
(Carolina/Mahatma)	110	2.0	23.0	0	0	0	m.q.
(Minute/Minute Premium), 2/3 cup	120	3.0	27.0	0	0	0	m.q.
(Minute Boil-in-Bag)	90	2.0	21.0	0	0	0	m.q.
(Uncle Ben's Boil-in-Bag), 1 oz. dry	94	2.0	21.6	.2	0	9	.5 d
(Uncle Ben's Fast Cook), 1.1 oz. dry	111	2.4	25.1	.2	0	10	.4 d
white, medium grain	120	2.2	26.6	.2	0	tr.	.1 c
Rice, wild, see "Wild rice"							
Rice beverage *(Rice Dream)*, 8 fl. oz.:							
carob lite	150	1.0	32.0	3.0	0	80	n.a.
chocolate	190	1.0	44.0	3.0	0	80	n.a.
organic original lite	130	1.0	28.0	2.0	0	80	n.a.
vanilla lite	130	1.0	30.0	2.0	0	80	n.a.

Food and Measure	cal.	prot. (gms)	carbo. (gms)	fat (gms)	chol. (mgs)	sod. (mgs)	fiber (gms)
Rice bran, crude,							
1 cup	262	11.1	41.2	17.3	0	4	17.4 d
Rice cake, 1 piece, except as noted:							
plain:							
(Hain Mini), 1/2 oz.	50	1.0	12.0	<1.0	0	20	0
(Hain Mini No Salt), 1/2 oz.	50	1.0	12.0	<1.0	0	5	m.q.
(Hain No Salt) . . .	40	<1.0	8.0	<1.0	0	<5	m.q.
brown, .3-oz. piece	35	.7	7.3	.3	0	26	.2 c
or 5-grain *(Hain)* . .	40	<1.0	8.0	<1.0	0	10	m.q.
w/popcorn *(Hain)*	35	1.0	8.0	0	0	55	m.q.
apple cinnamon:							
(Crispy Cakes) . . .	35	1.0	7.0	<1.0	0	50	m.q.
(Hain Mini), 1/2 oz.	60	1.0	12.0	<1.0	0	15	0
(Hollywood Mini), 1/2 oz.	50	1.0	12.0	<1.0	0	5	m.q.
apple spice *(Mini Crispys)*, 1.1 oz. . . .	120	2.0	25.0	1.0	0	50	m.q.
barbecue:							
(Hain Mini), 1/2 oz.	70	1.0	10.0	3.0	0	50	0
(Mini Crispys), 1.1 oz.	120	2.0	24.0	2.0	0	100	m.q.
butter flavor, w/pop- corn *(Hain)*	45	1.0	8.0	1.0	0	60	m.q.
cheese:							
(Hain Mini), 1/2 oz.	60	1.0	10.0	2.0	<5	100	m.q.
(Hollywood Mini), 1/2 oz.	60	1.0	10.0	2.0	0	80	m.q.
cheddar, white, w/popcorn *(Hain)*	45	1.0	8.0	1.0	<5	150	m.q.
nacho *(Hain* Mini), 1/2 oz.	70	1.0	10.0	2.0	<5	90	m.q.
nacho, w/popcorn *(Hain)*	45	1.0	8.0	1.0	<5	60	m.q.
honey almond *(Mini Crispys)*, 1.1 oz. . . .	120	2.0	26.0	<1.0	0	50	m.q.

Food and Measure	cal.	prot. (gms)	carbo. (gms)	fat (gms)	chol. (mgs)	sod. (mgs)	fiber (gms)
Rice cake (cont.)							
honey nut, 1/2 oz.:							
(Hain Mini)	60	1.0	11.0	1.0	0	55	m.q.
(Hollywood Mini) . .	60	1.0	11.0	1.0	0	55	m.q.
pizza (Crispy Cakes)	35	1.0	7.0	<1.0	n.a.	50	m.q.
popcorn, 1/2 oz.:							
(Hain Mini)	60	1.0	11.0	1.0	0	40	m.q.
butter flavor (Hain							
Mini)	60	1.0	10.0	2.0	0	50	m.q.
cheddar, mild (Hain							
Mini)	60	1.0	10.0	2.0	0	70	m.q.
ranch:							
(Crispy Cakes) . . .	35	1.0	7.0	<1.0	n.a.	60	m.q.
(Hain Mini), 1/2 oz.	70	1.0	9.0	3.0	0	90	m.q.
sesame:							
(Hain)	40	<1.0	8.0	<1.0	0	10	m.q.
(Hain No Salt) . . .	40	<1.0	8.0	<1.0	0	<5	m.q.
teriyaki (Hain Mini),							
1/2 oz.	50	1.0	11.0	<1.0	0	110	m.q.
toasted (Crispy Cakes)	30	1.0	7.0	<1.0	0	15	m.q.
vegetable, garden							
(Crispy Cakes) . . .	35	1.0	7.0	<1.0	0	45	m.q.
Rice chips, brown							
(Eden), 1 oz.	130	2.0	19.0	5.0	0	197	m.q.
Rice dishes, canned,							
fried (La Choy),							
3/4 cup	190	4.0	41.0	1.0	0	820	<1.0 d
Rice dishes, freeze-							
dried, and chicken							
(Mountain House),							
1 cup*	400	13.0	41.0	13.0	m.q.	1170	m.q.
Rice dishes, frozen							
(see also specific							
listings):							
(Green Giant Rice							
Originals Rice Med-							
ley), 1/2 cup	100	3.0	19.0	1.0	5	310	m.q.

Food and Measure	cal.	prot. (gms)	carbo. (gms)	fat (gms)	chol. (mgs)	sod. (mgs)	fiber (gms)
and broccoli, au gratin *(Freezer Queen Family)*, 4.5 oz. . .	120	3.0	21.0	2.0	n.a.	1090	m.q.
and broccoli, in cheese sauce:							
(Green Giant One Serving), 5.5 oz.	160	5.0	26.0	5.0	5	490	2.0 d
(Green Giant Rice Originals), 1/2 cup	120	3.0	18.0	4.0	5	510	m.q.
Florentine *(Green Giant Rice Originals)*, 1/2 cup	140	4.0	22.0	4.0	10	400	m.q.
fried, 8 oz.:							
w/chicken *(Chun King)*	260	14.0	41.0	4.0	75	1460	m.q.
w/pork *(Chun King)*	270	10.0	44.0	6.0	55	1210	m.q.
Oriental, w/vegetables *(The Budget Gourmet Side Dish)*, 5.75 oz.	230	4.0	28.0	12.0	20	420	m.q.
pilaf:							
(Green Giant Rice Originals), 1/2 cup	110	2.0	21.0	1.0	2	530	m.q.
w/green beans *(The Budget Gourmet Side Dish)*, 5.5 oz.	230	4.0	30.0	11.0	10	510	m.q.
white and wild *(Green Giant Rice Originals)*, 1/2 cup . . .	130	3.0	24.0	2.0	0	540	m.q.
Rice dishes, mix:							
1/2 cup[1], except as noted:							
almondine *(Hain 3-Grain Side Dish)*	130	3.0	17.0	5.0	0	260	m.q.

[1] Prepared without butter or margarine, except as noted.

Food and Measure	cal.	prot. (gms)	carbo. (gms)	fat (gms)	chol. (mgs)	sod. (mgs)	fiber (gms)
Rice dishes, mix *(cont.)*							
au gratin, herbed *(Country Inn)*, 1.2 oz. dry	119	3.4	23.6	1.5	3	361	.7 d
beef flavor:							
(Lipton Rice and Sauce)	150	3.0	25.0	3.0	m.q.	630	m.q.
(Rice-A-Roni) . . .	150	4.0	24.0	4.0	n.a.	530	m.q.
almond *(Mahatma)*	100	2.0	20.0	0	n.a.	340	m.q.
broccoli *(Lipton Rice and Sauce)* . . .	140	3.0	24.0	3.0	m.q.	550	m.q.
Oriental *(Success)*	100	2.0	19.0	0	n.a.	370	m.q.
beef and mushroom *(Rice-A-Roni)*	150	4.0	26.0	3.0	n.a.	740	m.q.
broccoli:							
almondine *(Country Inn)*, 1.2 oz. dry	124	3.8	24.5	1.5	<1	337	.8 d
au gratin *(Country Inn)*, 1.1 oz. dry	116	3.6	22.2	1.8	3	342	.9 d
au gratin *(Rice-A-Roni 1/3 Less Salt)*	160	4.0	24.0	6.0	5	280	m.q.
and cheddar, white *(Country Inn)*, 1.2 oz. dry . . .	131	4.0	23.8	2.6	3	288	.8 d
and cheese *(Success)*	120	6.0	23.0	<1.0	n.a.	310	m.q.
brown, 2 oz. dry:							
(Arrowhead Mills Quick Brown Rice)	200	4.0	43.0	1.0	0	0	2.8 d
Spanish *(Arrowhead Mills Quick Brown Rice)*	150	4.0	30.0	1.0	0	145	2.8 d
vegetable herb *(Arrowhead Mills Quick Brown Rice)*	150	4.0	30.0	1.0	0	85	4.0 d
brown and wild:							
(Success)	120	3.0	23.0	0	n.a.	500	m.q.

Food and Measure	cal.	prot. (gms)	carbo. (gms)	fat (gms)	chol. (mgs)	sod. (mgs)	fiber (gms)
herb (Arrowhead Mills Quick Brown Rice), 2 oz. dry	140	4.0	28.0	1.0	0	64	4.0 d
Cajun (Lipton Rice and Sauce)	150	4.0	26.0	3.0	n.a.	630	m.q.
cheddar broccoli (Lipton Rice and Sauce)	180	3.0	25.0	7.0	m.q.	550	m.q.
chicken flavor:							
(Lipton Rice and Sauce)	150	3.0	25.0	4.0	m.q.	500	m.q.
(Rice-A-Roni) . . .	150	3.0	24.0	4.0	n.a.	520	m.q.
(Rice-A-Roni 1/3 Less Salt)	130	3.0	24.0	2.0	0	340	m.q.
(Success Classic)	100	2.0	19.0	0	n.a.	410	m.q.
broccoli (Golden Sauté)	130	4.0	25.0	2.0	0	570	m.q.
broccoli (Lipton Rice and Sauce) . . .	150	4.0	25.0	4.0	m.q.	500	m.q.
broccoli (Rice-A-Roni)	150	4.0	25.0	3.0	n.a.	650	m.q.
creamy (Lipton Rice and Sauce) . . .	190	3.0	27.0	8.0	m.q.	490	m.q.
creamy, and mushroom (Country Inn), 1.3 oz. dry	138	3.9	24.5	3.2	2	380	1.0 d
creamy, and wild rice (Country Inn), 1.3 oz. dry . . .	135	4.2	26.8	1.5*	4	340	.6 d
drumstick, w/margarine (Minute) . . .	150	3.0	25.0	4.0	0	690	m.q.
sesame (Mahatma)	100	2.0	20.0	0	n.a.	620	m.q.
stock (Country Inn), 1.2 oz. dry . . .	123	4.2	23.9	1.4	3	269	.5 d
and vegetables (Rice-A-Roni) . .	140	3.0	24.0	3.0	n.a.	750	m.q.
and vegetables, homestyle (Country Inn), 1.3 oz. dry	139	4.1	24.1	3.3	7	298	.9 d

Food and Measure	cal.	prot. (gms)	carbo. (gms)	fat (gms)	chol. (mgs)	sod. (mgs)	fiber (gms)
Rice dishes, mix (cont.)							
Florentine (Country Inn), 1.2 oz. dry . .	121	3.7	23.9	1.6	3	354	.9 d
fried:							
(Minute)	160	3.0	25.0	5.0	0	550	m.q.
w/almonds (Rice-A-Roni) . .	170	4.0	26.0	6.0	n.a.	760	m.q.
beef flavor (Golden Sauté)	120	4.0	22.0	2.0	0	490	m.q.
chicken flavor (Golden Sauté)	130	4.0	23.0	2.0	0	490	m.q.
Oriental (Golden Sauté)	130	4.0	23.0	2.0	n.a.	600	m.q.
green bean almondine (Country Inn), 1.2 oz. dry	128	3.9	24.8	1.8	2	280	.8 d
herb and butter:							
(Golden Sauté) . .	120	3.0	23.0	2.0	0	450	m.q.
(Lipton Rice and Sauce)	140	3.0	24.0	5.0	m.q.	480	m.q.
(Rice-A-Roni) . . .	130	3.0	22.0	4.0	n.a.	670	m.q.
long grain and wild:							
(Lipton Rice and Sauce Original)	150	4.0	26.0	3.0	n.a.	560	m.q.
(Near East)	130	3.0	21.0	4.0	n.a.	430	m.q.
(Uncle Ben's Original), 1 oz. dry . .	96	3.2	20.6	.4	<1	363	.6 d
(Uncle Ben's Original Fast Cook), 1 oz. dry	101	3.2	22.0	.4	1	450	.8 d
w/butter (Minute)	150	3.0	25.0	4.0	10	570	m.q.
chicken stock sauce (Uncle Ben's), 1.3 oz. dry . . .	133	4.4	25.4	2.0	5	601	1.1 d
mushroom and herbs (Lipton Rice and Sauce) . . .	150	4.0	26.0	3.0	n.a.	360	m.q.
Mexican (Old El Paso)	140	2.0	28.0	2.0	0	370	m.q.

Food and Measure	cal.	prot. (gms)	carbo. (gms)	fat (gms)	chol. (mgs)	sod. (mgs)	fiber (gms)
mushroom, Oriental (*Hain* 3-Grain Goodness)	120	4.0	15.0	5.0	n.a.	300	m.q.
pilaf:							
(*Lipton* Rice and Sauce)	170	4.0	26.0	6.0	m.q.	470	m.q.
(*Mahatma* Classic)	100	3.0	20.0	0	n.a.	470	m.q.
(*Near East*)	140	3.0	21.0	5.0	n.a.	450	m.q.
(*Rice-A-Roni*) . . .	160	4.0	26.0	4.0	n.a.	670	m.q.
(*Success*)	120	2.0	24.0	0	n.a.	410	m.q.
basmati, tomato and herb (*Knorr*), 1 serving dry . .	150	3.4	32.6	.5	0	390	1.0 d
beef flavor (*Near East*)	140	3.0	21.0	5.0	n.a.	470	m.q.
brown, w/miso (*Quick Pilaf*) . . .	109	3.0	22.0	1.0	0	265	.5 d
brown, w/miso, w/butter (*Quick Pilaf*)	150	3.0	22.0	5.5	m.q.	312	.5 d
chicken flavor (*Near East*)	140	3.0	21.0	5.0	n.a.	420	m.q.
jasmine, w/lemon and herbs (*Knorr*), 1 serving dry . .	130	3.1	27.9	.8	0	370	.4 d
lentil (*Near East*) . .	170	6.0	21.0	7.0	n.a.	430	m.q.
medley, and carrots (*Knorr*), 1 serving dry	95	2.3	20.0	.3	0	360	.5 d
Spanish, brown (*Quick Pilaf*) . . .	109	3.0	22.0	1.0	0	251	.5 d
Spanish, brown, w/ butter (*Quick Pilaf*)	150	3.0	22.0	5.5	m.q.	298	.5 d
vegetable (*Country Inn*), 1.2 oz. dry	115	3.1	24.8	.7	1	357	.7 d
wheat (*Near East*)	150	3.0	21.0	6.0	n.a.	380	m.q.

Food and Measure	cal.	prot. (gms)	carbo. (gms)	fat (gms)	chol. (mgs)	sod. (mgs)	fiber (gms)
Rice dishes, mix (cont.)							
Spanish:							
(Lipton Rice and							
Sauce)	140	3.0	25.0	3.0	m.q.	560	m.q.
(Mahatma Authentic)	100	2.0	20.0	0	n.a.	190	m.q.
(Rice-A-Roni),							
1/7 pkg. dry . . .	110	3.0	22.0	1.0	n.a.	480	m.q.
(Success)	110	3.0	23.0	0	n.a.	460	m.q.
and beans (Fantastic							
Only a Pinch),							
10 oz.	214	9.0	48.0	2.0	0	120	8.0 d
vegetable blend, gar-							
den (Uncle Ben's),							
1.3 oz. dry	128	3.6	26.5	1.2	1	601	.9 d
yellow:							
(Rice-A-Roni) . . .	150	3.0	25.0	4.0	n.a.	580	m.q.
saffron (Mahatma)	100	2.0	21.0	0	n.a.	480	m.q.
wild (Mahatma) . . .	100	2.0	20.0	0	n.a.	480	m.q.
Rice flour:							
brown, 1 cup	574	11.4	120.8	4.4	0	12	7.3 d
brown (Arrowhead							
Mills), 2 oz.	200	4.0	44.0	1.0	0	3	3.1 d
white, 1 cup	578	9.4	126.6	2.2	0	1	3.9 d
Rigatoni entree, fro-							
zen:							
baked, w/meat sauce							
and cheese (Lean							
Cuisine), 9 oz. . . .	210	14.0	29.0	4.0	25	560	m.q.
w/chicken and vegeta-							
bles (Healthy Choice							
Extra Portion), 12.5							
oz.	360	31.0	50.0	4.0	60	430	m.q.
in cream sauce,							
w/broccoli and							
chicken (The Budget							
Gourmet Light and							
Healthy), 10.8 oz.	290	19.0	44.0	7.0	30	710	m.q.

Food and Measure	cal.	prot. (gms)	carbo. (gms)	fat (gms)	chol. (mgs)	sod. (mgs)	fiber (gms)
in meat sauce *(Healthy Choice)*, 9.5 oz. . . .	240	16.0	34.0	6.0	30	540	m.q.
w/meat sauce *(Stouffer's* Home-style), 12 oz.	400	21.0	49.0	13.0	m.q.	860	m.q.
Roast, vegetarian, frozen *(Worthington* Dinner Roast), 2 oz.	120	7.0	5.0	8.0	0	440	m.q.
Robert sauce *(Escoffier)*, 1 tbsp.	20	0	5.0	0	0	70	m.q.
Rockfish, meat only:							
raw, 4 oz.	107	21.3	0	1.8	39	68	0
baked, broiled, or microwaved, 4 oz. . . .	137	27.3	0	2.3	50	87	0
Roe (see also "Caviar"):							
raw, 1 oz.	40	6.3	.4	1.8	106	m.q.	0
raw, 1 tbsp.	22	3.6	.2	1.0	60	m.q.	0
baked, broiled or microwaved, 4 oz. . . .	231	32.5	2.2	9.3	543	m.q.	0
carp *(Krinos* Tarama), 1 tbsp.	20	3.0	0	.5	50	700	0
Roll (see also "Roll, sweet"), 1 piece, except as noted:							
(Arnold Bakery Light)	80	4.0	21.0	<2.0	0	190	4.0 d
(Arnold Bran'nola Buns)	100	5.0	20.0	1.0	0	160	3.0 d
(Francisco 8")	210	7.0	39.0	3.0	0	260	m.q.
(Wonder Bakery Style)	140	5.0	24.0	2.0	0	280	m.q.
(Wonder Enriched Buns)	70	3.0	13.0	1.0	0	160	.7 d
assorted *(Brownberry* Hearth)	110	4.0	20.0	2.0	m.q.	m.q.	m.q.
brown and serve: *(Pepperidge Farm* Hearth)	50	2.0	10.0	1.0	0	100	0
(Roman Meal) . . .	70	2.6	11.8	1.3	0	136	1.2 d

Food and Measure	cal.	prot. (gms)	carbo. (gms)	fat (gms)	chol. (mgs)	sod. (mgs)	fiber (gms)
Roll, brown and serve *(cont.)*							
Bavarian wheat							
(Bread du Jour)	80	3.0	15.0	1.0	0	180	1.6 d
plain or buttermilk							
(Wonder)	70	1.0	14.0	1.0	0	135	.6 d
club *(Pepperidge*							
Farm)	100	3.0	19.0	1.0	0	190	0
Italian, crusty *(Bread*							
du Jour)	80	4.0	16.0	1.0	0	190	.8 d
sourdough *(Fran-*							
cisco)	100	3.0	19.0	1.0	0	120	m.q.
crescent, butter *(Pep-*							
peridge Farm Heat							
& Serve)	110	2.0	13.0	6.0	15	150	0
croissant, see "Crois-							
sant"							
dinner:							
(August Bros.) . . .	90	6.0	18.0	1.0	0	170	m.q.
(Pepperidge Farm							
Country Style) . .	50	2.0	9.0	1.0	0	90	0
(Pepperidge Farm							
Party)	30	1.0	5.0	1.0	0	50	0
(Roman Meal) . . .	69	2.8	11.8	1.1	0	139	1.2 d
(Wonder)	80	2.0	14.0	1.0	0	140	.6 d
parker house *(Pep-*							
peridge Farm) . .	60	2.0	9.0	1.0	5	80	0
plain or sesame *(Ar-*							
nold)	50	2.0	9.0	1.0	<5	80	1.0 d
poppy seed finger							
(Pepperidge Farm)	50	2.0	8.0	2.0	0	80	0
potato *(Pepperidge*							
Farm Hearty) . .	90	2.0	14.0	3.0	0	125	1.0 d
sesame seed finger							
(Pepperidge Farm)	60	2.0	9.0	2.0	0	85	0
wheat or white							
(Home Pride) . .	70	2.0	10.0	2.0	<5	120	.7 d
egg, Dutch *(Arnold)*	130	4.0	21.0	3.0	0	180	2.0 d
French style:							
(Francisco 6") . . .	210	7.0	39.0	3.0	0	260	m.q.

Food and Measure	cal.	prot. (gms)	carbo. (gms)	fat (gms)	chol. (mgs)	sod. (mgs)	fiber (gms)
(Pepperidge Farm)	100	4.0	20.0	1.0	0	230	0
mini (Francisco) . .	130	4.0	24.0	2.0	n.a.	140	m.q.
7 grain (Pepperidge Farm)	100	5.0	18.0	2.0	0	270	1.0 d
sourdough (Pepper- idge Farm) . . .	100	4.0	19.0	1.0	0	240	0
hamburger:							
(Arnold)	120	4.0	20.0	2.0	0	190	2.0 d
(Pepperidge Farm)	130	5.0	22.0	2.0	0	240	0
(Roman Meal) . . .	112	4.5	19.2	1.8	0	226	1.9 d
(Wonder Light) . . .	80	4.0	14.0	1.0	0	210	4.6 d
hoagie, soft (Pepper- idge Farm)	210	8.0	34.0	5.0	0	320	1.0 d
honey wheat (Wonder Buns)	130	5.0	22.0	2.0	0	230	2.1 d
hot dog:							
(Arnold), 12 oz. . . .	110	4.0	21.0	2.0	0	160	1.0 d
(Arnold Bran'nola)	110	4.0	18.0	2.0	0	170	1.0 d
(Arnold New En- gland)	110	4.0	20.0	2.0	0	160	1.0 d
(Pepperidge Farm)	140	5.0	24.0	3.0	0	270	0
(Roman Meal) . . .	105	4.2	18.0	1.6	0	211	1.8 d
(Wonder Light) . . .	80	4.0	14.0	1.0	0	210	4.6 d
Dijon (Pepperidge Farm)	160	5.0	23.0	5.0	0	230	2.0 d
sliced (Brownberry)	110	4.0	21.0	2.0	0	210	1.0 d
Italian (Savoni 8") . .	210	8.0	38.0	3.0	0	m.q.	3.0 d
kaiser:							
(Arnold Deli)	170	5.0	34.0	2.0	0	m.q.	m.q.
(August Bros.) . . .	170	6.0	35.0	1.0	0	310	2.0 d
(Brownberry Hearth)	150	5.0	26.0	3.0	10	320	2.0 d
(Francisco 6") . . .	180	6.0	34.0	m.q.	m.q.	230	m.q.
onion:							
(Arnold Deli)	170	5.0	34.0	2.0	0	m.q.	m.q.
(Arnold Premium)	180	7.0	38.0	1.0	0	340	2.0 d
(August Bros.) . . .	160	6.0	33.0	1.0	0	310	2.0 d
soft (Arnold)	140	5.0	28.0	3.0	0	200	2.0 d
pan (Wonder)	80	2.0	14.0	1.0	0	140	.6 d

Food and Measure	cal.	prot. (gms)	carbo. (gms)	fat (gms)	chol. (mgs)	sod. (mgs)	fiber (gms)
Roll (cont.)							
pan Cubano (Arnold Agusto)	230	7.0	43.0	3.0	0	500	2.0 d
party, petite (Arnold), 2 pieces	70	2.0	10.0	2.0	m.q.	70	1.0 d
potato (Arnold)	140	5.0	25.0	2.0	0	210	2.0 d
sandwich:							
(Arnold)	110	4.0	18.0	3.0	0	170	2.0 d
(Roman Meal) . . .	184	7.2	31.4	3.0	0	389	3.4 d
onion w/poppy seeds (Pepperidge Farm) . . .	150	5.0	26.0	3.0	0	260	0
potato (Pepperidge Farm)	160	4.0	28.0	4.0	0	260	1.0 d
sesame (Arnold) . .	130	4.0	23.0	3.0	0	220	2.0 d
w/sesame seeds (Pepperidge Farm)	140	5.0	23.0	3.0	0	230	0
wheat (Brownberry)	130	5.0	23.0	3.0	0	230	2.0 d
white (Brownberry)	130	4.0	23.0	3.0	0	220	2.0 d
sesame (August Bros.)	170	6.0	35.0	1.0	0	310	2.0 d
sourdough:							
(Francisco)	100	3.0	19.0	1.0	0	120	m.q.
(Wonder Bakery Style)	150	6.0	25.0	2.0	0	300	m.q.
sub (Levy Old Country)	180	6.0	34.0	2.0	0	230	m.q.
twist, golden (Pepperidge Farm Heat & Serve)	110	2.0	14.0	5.0	5	150	0
wheat:							
(Arnold Old Fashioned), 2 pieces	80	2.0	11.0	3.0	m.q.	98	m.q.
(Wonder Bakery Style)	150	6.0	25.0	2.0	0	300	m.q.
white (Arnold Old Fashioned), 2 pieces	80	2.0	11.0	3.0	m.q.	85	m.q.
Roll, frozen or refrigerated (see also "Roll, sweet"), 1 piece:							
butterflake (Pillsbury)	140	3.0	20.0	5.0	5	530	m.q.

Food and Measure	cal.	prot. (gms)	carbo. (gms)	fat (gms)	chol. (mgs)	sod. (mgs)	fiber (gms)
crescent (Pillsbury) . .	100	2.0	11.0	6.0	0	230	m.q.
homestyle (Rich's) . .	70	2.0	13.0	1.0	0	140	m.q.
Parkerhouse (Bridg-ford), 1 oz.	90	3.0	16.0	1.0	0	170	m.q.
ranch, white (Bridg-ford), 1.5 oz.	135	4.5	24.0	1.5	0	255	m.q.
Roll, mix, 1 piece:							
hot (Dromedary) . . .	239	6.0	41.0	5.0	n.a.	410	m.q.
hot (Pillsbury)	120	4.0	21.0	2.0	15	210	m.q.
Roll, sweet, (see also "Bun, sweet"), 1 piece:							
(Tastykake Tasty Twist)	18	0	3.0	1.0	n.a.	n.a.	m.q.
apple cinnamon (Aunt Fanny's Old Fash-ioned)	180	4.0	34.0	4.0	5	125	1.5 d
caramel nut (Aunt Fanny's)	190	4.0	33.0	6.0	5	125	1.0 d
cinnamon:							
(Aunt Fanny's), 2 oz.	190	4.0	34.0	5.0	5	160	1.0 d
(Aunt Fanny's Duos)	180	4.0	32.0	5.0	5	150	1.0 d
(Awrey's Homestyle)	240	4.0	40.0	7.0	5	200	1.0 d
(Sara Lee Deluxe)	230	3.0	31.0	11.0	n.a.	220	m.q.
swirl (Awrey's Grande)	340	4.0	46.0	16.0	10	370	1.0 d
twirl (Aunt Fanny's)	110	2.0	16.0	4.0	0	85	m.q.
fruit roll (Aunt Fanny's Dixie)	180	3.0	34.0	4.0	5	120	1.0 d
pecan twirl:							
(Aunt Fanny's) . . .	105	1.0	16.5	4.0	3	80	1.0 d
(Tastykake)	110	1.0	17.0	5.0	n.a.	75	m.q.
frozen, cinnamon:							
(Pepperidge Farm)	280	4.0	34.0	14.0	n.a.	190	m.q.
glazed (Weight Watchers)	180	4.0	31.0	5.0	5	170	m.q.
refrigerated:							
caramel, w/nuts (Pillsbury)	160	2.0	19.0	8.0	0	240	m.q.

Food and Measure	cal.	prot. (gms)	carbo. (gms)	fat (gms)	chol. (mgs)	sod. (mgs)	fiber (gms)
Roll, sweet, refrigerated *(cont.)*							
cinnamon, w/icing							
(Pillsbury)	110	1.0	17.0	5.0	0	260	m.q.
Roseapple, trimmed,							
1 oz.	7	.2	1.6	.1	0	tr.	.3 c
Roselle, 1 oz. or							
1/2 cup	14	.3	3.2	.2	0	2	.3 c
Rosemary, dried,							
1 tsp.	4	.1	.8	.2	0	1	.2 c
Rotini entree, frozen:							
cheddar *(Green Giant Garden Gourmet Right for Lunch),*							
9.5 oz.	230	9.0	32.0	10.0	20	570	4.5 d
cheese, three *(Weight Watchers),* 9 oz. . . .	270	14.0	34.0	8.0	5	500	m.q.
seafood *(Mrs. Paul's Light),* 8 oz.	240	12.0	34.0	6.0	25	570	m.q.
Roughy, orange, meat only:							
raw, 4 oz.	143	16.7	0	8.0	23	72	0
baked, broiled, or microwaved, 4 oz. . . .	101	21.4	0	1.0	29	92	0
Roy Rogers, 1 serving:							
breakfast items, see *"Hardee's"*							
burgers:							
cheeseburger . . .	563	29.5	27.4	37.3	95	1404	m.q.
cheeseburger, bacon	581	32.3	25.0	39.2	103	1536	m.q.
hamburger	456	23.8	26.6	28.3	73	495	m.q.
R Bar Burger . . .	611	36.1	28.0	39.4	115	1826	m.q.
Roy's Roasters:							
skin on, breast/wing	500	56.0	3.0	29.0	240	1450	0
skin on, thigh/leg quarter	490	43.0	2.0	34.0	225	1120	0
skin off, breast/wing	190	32.0	2.0	6.0	100	700	0

Food and Measure	cal.	prot. (gms)	carbo. (gms)	fat (gms)	chol. (mgs)	sod. (mgs)	fiber (gms)
skin off, thigh/leg quarter	190	24.0	1.0	10.0	110	400	0
roast beef sandwich:							
regular	317	27.2	29.1	10.2	55	785	m.q.
regular, w/cheese	424	32.9	29.9	19.2	77	1694	m.q.
large	360	33.9	29.6	11.9	73	1044	m.q.
large, w/cheese . .	467	39.6	30.3	20.9	95	1953	m.q.
french fries, regular	268	3.9	32.0	13.5	42	165	m.q.
baked/topped potato:							
plain	211	5.9	47.9	.2	0	65	m.q.
w/margarine	274	5.9	47.9	7.3	0	161	m.q.
broccoli & cheese	376	13.7	39.6	18.1	<19	523	m.q.
sour cream & chives	408	7.3	47.6	20.9	31	138	m.q.
Rum runner mixer*, w/rum *(Bacardi)*, 7 fl. oz.	210	0	33.0	0	0	15	n.a.
Rutabaga, 1/2 cup:							
fresh, cubed:							
raw	25	.8	5.7	.1	0	14	1.8 d
boiled, drained . .	33	1.1	7.4	.2	0	17	1.5 d
fresh, boiled, drained, mashed	47	1.6	10.5	.3	0	25	2.2 d
canned, diced *(Allens/ Sunshine)*, 1/2 cup	20	1.0	4.0	<1.0	0	260	m.q.
Rye, whole-grain:							
1 cup	567	25.0	117.9	4.2	0	10	24.7 d
(Arrowhead Mills), 2 oz.	190	7.0	42.0	1.0	0	tr.	7.6 d
Rye flakes *(Arrow- head Mills)*, 2 oz.	190	7.0	42.0	1.0	0	1	7.6 d
Rye flour, 1 cup:							
dark	415	18.0	88.0	3.4	0	2	m.q.
light	374	8.6	81.8	1.4	0	2	14.9 d
medium	361	9.9	79.0	1.8	0	3	14.9 d
medium *(Pillsbury's Best)*	400	12.0	83.0	2.0	0	0	9.0 d
and wheat *(Pillsbury's Best* Bohemian Style)*	400	11.0	86.0	1.0	0	0	m.q.

S

Food and Measure	cal.	prot. (gms)	carbo. (gms)	fat (gms)	chol. (mgs)	sod. (mgs)	fiber (gms)
Sablefish, meat only:							
raw, 4 oz.	222	15.2	0	17.4	56	64	0
baked, broiled, or microwaved, 4 oz. . .	284	19.5	0	22.2	71	82	0
smoked, 4 oz.	291	20.0	0	22.8	73	836	0
Safflower seed kernel, dried, 1 oz. . .	147	4.6	9.7	10.9	0	(0)	.7 c
Safflower seed meal, partially defatted, 1 oz.	97	10.1	13.8	.7	0	n.a.	2.2 c
Saffron, 1 tsp.	2	.1	.5	<.1	0	1	<.1 d
Sage, ground, 1 tsp.	2	.1	.4	.1	0	tr.	.1 d
Salad dip *(Nasoya Vegi-Dip),* 1 oz. . .	45	2.0	3.0	3.0	0	110	n.a.
Salad dressing, 1 tbsp., except as noted:							
bacon and tomato *(Kraft)*	70	0	1.0	7.0	0	130	n.a.
blue cheese:							
(Cains Country) . .	70	0	2.0	8.0	5	160	n.a.
(La Martinique), 2 tbsp.	160	2.0	0	17.0	5	450	0
(Marie's Lite & Luscious)	50	0	4.0	4.0	0	115	n.a.
(Roka Brand) . . .	60	1.0	1.0	6.0	10	170	n.a.
chunky *(Kraft)* . . .	60	1.0	2.0	6.0	<5	230	n.a.
chunky *(Marie's)* . .	100	1.0	2.0	10.0	10	85	n.a.
chunky *(Wish-Bone)*	70	0	<1.0	8.0	0	150	n.a.

Food and Measure	cal.	prot. (gms)	carbo. (gms)	fat (gms)	chol. (mgs)	sod. (mgs)	fiber (gms)
creamy *(Bernstein's Restaurant)* . . .	60	0	1.0	6.0	5	95	n.a.
buttermilk:							
(Hain Old Fashioned)	70	0	0	7.0	0	100	n.a.
(Seven Seas Buttermilk Recipe) . . .	80	0	1.0	8.0	5	130	n.a.
creamy *(Kraft)* . . .	80	0	1.0	8.0	<5	120	n.a.
Caesar:							
(Lawry's Classic), 1 oz.	130	.8	1.0	13.9	1	337	.1 c
creamy *(Hain)* . . .	60	0	1.0	6.0	<5	220	n.a.
creamy *(Lawry's Classic)*, 1 oz. . . .	142	.7	1.8	14.2	6	291	n.a.
creamy *(Marie's)* . .	100	0	2.0	10.0	10	85	n.a.
golden *(Kraft)* . . .	70	0	1.0	7.0	0	180	n.a.
w/olive oil *(Wish-Bone)*	45	0	5.0	<1.0	0	170	n.a.
Champagne *(Lawry's Classic)*, 1 oz. . . .	143	.2	2.3	14.7	0	511	n.a.
Chinese vinaigrette *(Lawry's* Classic), 1 oz.	145	.2	2.4	15.0	n.a.	325	0
citrus, tangy *(Hain Canola)*	50	0	1.0	5.0	0	75	n.a.
coleslaw:							
(Kraft)	70	0	4.0	6.0	10	200	n.a.
(Marie's), 1.05 oz.	140	0	6.0	13.0	n.a.	210	n.a.
(Miracle Whip) . . .	70	0	3.0	6.0	5	105	n.a.
cucumber:							
creamy *(Herb Magic)*, 2 tbsp.	15	0	4.0	0	0	270	n.a.
creamy *(Kraft)* . . .	70	0	1.0	8.0	0	190	n.a.
dill *(Hain)*	80	0	0	8.0	<5	210	n.a.
Dijon:							
creamy *(Light Fantastic)*	20	0	3.0	<1.0	0	135	n.a.

Food and Measure	cal.	prot. (gms)	carbo. (gms)	fat (gms)	chol. (mgs)	sod. (mgs)	fiber (gms)
Salad dressing, Dijon (cont.)							
golden (Lawry's							
Classic), 1 oz. . .	60	.1	4.0	4.0	0	400	0
vinaigrette (Hain)	50	0	0	5.0	0	180	n.a.
dill, creamy:							
(Light Fantastic) . .	16	0	3.0	1.0	0	150	n.a.
(Nasoya Vegi-Dress-							
ing)	40	0	1.0	4.0	0	95	n.a.
French:							
(Cains Country) . .	60	0	3.0	5.0	0	85	n.a.
(Catalina)	60	0	4.0	5.0	0	180	n.a.
(Kraft)	60	0	2.0	6.0	0	125	n.a.
(Kraft Miracle) . . .	70	0	3.0	6.0	0	240	n.a.
(Seven Seas French!							
Light)	35	0	2.0	3.0	0	210	n.a.
(Wish-Bone Deluxe)	60	0	2.0	6.0	0	85	n.a.
(Wish-Bone Sweet							
'N Spicy)	70	0	3.0	6.0	0	160	n.a.
creamy (Hain) . . .	60	0	0	6.0	0	80	n.a.
creamy (Marie's) . .	70	0	4.0	6.0	<2	125	n.a.
creamy (Seven							
Seas)	60	0	2.0	6.0	0	240	n.a.
vinaigrette, true (La							
Martinique),							
2 tbsp.	170	0	<1.0	19.0	<5	430	n.a.
fruit salad (Knott's)	50	0	3.0	5.0	n.a.	75	n.a.
garlic:							
creamy (Kraft) . . .	50	0	1.0	5.0	0	170	n.a.
and sour cream							
(Hain)	70	0	0	7.0	0	100	n.a.
herb:							
classic (Marie's							
Zesty Fat Free)	16	0	4.0	0	0	130	n.a.
garden (Nasoya							
Vegi-Dressing) . .	40	0	1.0	4.0	0	100	n.a.
Italian, and Romano							
(Marie's)	100	0	2.0	10.0	10	85	n.a.

Food and Measure	cal.	prot. (gms)	carbo. (gms)	fat (gms)	chol. (mgs)	sod. (mgs)	fiber (gms)
savory (Hain No Salt)	90	0	0	10.0	0	25	n.a.
herb and spice:							
(Seven Seas Viva)	60	0	1.0	6.0	0	170	n.a.
(Seven Seas Viva Herbs & Spices! Light)	30	0	1.0	3.0	0	200	n.a.
honey mustard:							
(Marie's)	80	0	4.0	7.0	m.q.	80	n.a.
(PeggyJane's) . . .	60	0	2.0	6.0	n.a.	40	n.a.
vinaigrette (Cain's Country)	45	0	3.0	4.0	5	110	n.a.
Italian:							
(Hain Canola) . . .	50	0	1.0	5.0	0	150	n.a.
(Hain Traditional) . .	80	0	0	8.0	0	330	n.a.
(Herb Magic)	5	0	2.0	0	0	400	n.a.
(Kraft House) . . .	60	0	1.0	6.0	0	115	n.a.
(Kraft Presto) . . .	70	0	1.0	7.0	0	150	n.a.
(Light Fantastic Classico)	18	0	3.0	<1.0	0	150	n.a.
(Marie's)	100	0	2.0	10.0	10	115	n.a.
(Marie's Zesty Fat Free)	16	0	4.0	0	0	150	n.a.
(Nasoya Vegi-Dressing)	40	0	1.0	4.0	0	95	n.a.
(Ott's), 1.1 oz. . . .	125	0	1.0	14.0	0	211	0
(Seven Seas Free Viva)	4	0	1.0	0	0	220	n.a.
(Seven Seas Viva)	50	0	1.0	5.0	0	240	n.a.
(Seven Seas Viva Italian! Light) . .	30	0	1.0	3.0	0	230	n.a.
(Wish-Bone)	45	0	2.0	5.0	0	290	n.a.
(Wish-Bone Robusto)	50	0	2.0	5.0	0	300	n.a.
blended (Wish-Bone)	35	0	1.0	4.0	0	210	n.a.
w/bleu cheese (Lawry's Classic), 1 oz.	186	.1	1.9	15.0	<1	385	.1 c

Food and Measure	cal.	prot. (gms)	carbo. (gms)	fat (gms)	chol. (mgs)	sod. (mgs)	fiber (gms)
Salad dressing, Italian *(cont.)*							
cheese and garlic *(Bernstein's)* . . .	50	0	1.0	5.0	0	170	n.a.
w/cheese *(Bernstein's* Reduced Calorie)	14	0	1.0	1.0	0	250	n.a.
w/cheese *(Bernstein's* Cheese Fantastico!)* . . .	60	0	1.0	6.0	0	170	n.a.
creamy *(Hain)* . . .	80	0	0	8.0	0	100	n.a.
creamy *(Seven Seas)*	70	0	1.0	7.0	0	240	n.a.
creamy *(Seven Seas Viva Creamy Italian Light)*	45	0	1.0	4.0	0	230	n.a.
creamy *(Weight Watchers)*	50	0	2.0	5.0	5	80	n.a.
creamy *(Wish-Bone)*	60	0	1.0	6.0	0	150	n.a.
creamy, w/basil *(Cains* Country)	80	0	1.0	8.0	5	105	n.a.
creamy, w/real sour cream *(Kraft)* . .	50	0	1.0	5.0	0	120	n.a.
garlic *(Marie's)* . . .	100	0	2.0	10.0	10	115	n.a.
garlic *(Marie's Lite & Luscious)*	40	0	3.0	3.0	0	120	n.a.
herb and Romano *(Marie's)*	100	0	2.0	10.0	10	85	n.a.
olive oil *(Wish-Bone* Classic)	35	0	2.0	3.0	0	200	n.a.
olive oil blend *(Cains* Country)	50	0	2.0	5.0	0	270	n.a.
w/Parmesan *(Lawry's* Classic), 1 oz.	156	.1	4.5	15.1	<1	178	.1 c
zesty *(Kraft)*	50	0	1.0	5.0	0	260	n.a.
lemon pepper *(Lawry's* Classic), 1 oz. . . .	123	.4	3.0	12.2	0	291	n.a.

Food and Measure	cal.	prot. (gms)	carbo. (gms)	fat (gms)	chol. (mgs)	sod. (mgs)	fiber (gms)
mayonnaise type (see also "Mayonnaise"):							
(Kraft Free)	12	0	3.0	0	0	190	0
(Miracle Whip) . . .	70	0	2.0	7.0	5	85	0
(Miracle Whip Free)	20	0	5.0	0	0	210	0
(Miracle Whip Light)	45	0	2.0	4.0	0	125	0
(Spin Blend)	60	0	3.0	5.0	10	110	0
(Spin Blend Cholesterol Free)	40	0	2.0	4.0	0	110	0
(Weight Watchers Fat Free)	12	0	4.0	0	0	125	0
(Weight Watchers Light)	50	0	1.0	5.0	5	100	0
(Weight Watchers Low Sodium) . .	50	0	1.0	5.0	5	45	0
whipped (Cains) . .	80	0	2.0	8.0	15	80	n.a.
whipped (Cains Fat Free)	14	0	3.0	0	0	120	n.a.
whipped (Weight Watchers Fat Free)	14	0	4.0	0	0	115	n.a.
mustard, spicy French (Hain Canola) . . .	50	1.0	1.0	5.0	5	190	n.a.
oil and vinegar (Kraft)	70	0	1.0	8.0	0	210	0
olive oil vinaigrette (Wish-Bone)	30	0	2.0	2.0	0	125	n.a.
Oriental (Light Fantastic)	25	0	5.0	1.0	0	150	n.a.
Oriental chicken salad (PeggyJane's) . . .	60	0	2.0	6.0	n.a.	105	n.a.
(Ott's Famous), 1.1 oz.	78	0	8.0	6.0	0	383	0
(Ott's Fat Free Famous), 1.1 oz. . . .	31	0	8.0	0	0	384	0
(Ott's Reduced Calorie Famous), 1.1 oz.	53	0	8.0	3.0	0	193	0
peppercorn, ground (PeggyJane's) . . .	80	0	1.0	8.0	n.a.	100	n.a.

Food and Measure	cal.	prot. (gms)	carbo. (gms)	fat (gms)	chol. (mgs)	sod. (mgs)	fiber (gms)
Salad dressing *(cont.)*							
peppercorn w/Parmesan *(Cains* Country)	80	0	1.0	8.0	5	150	n.a.
poppyseed:							
(Hain Rancher's) . .	60	0	0	7.0	<5	105	n.a.
(La Martinique Original), 2 tbsp.	170	0	8.0	15.0	5	330	0
(Marie's)	70	0	4.0	6.0	m.q.	100	n.a.
(Ott's Reduced Calorie)	85	0	8.0	6.0	0	197	0
(PeggyJane's) . . .	60	0	4.0	5.0	n.a.	90	n.a.
ranch:							
(Cains Country) . .	70	0	1.0	8.0	5	180	n.a.
(Herb Magic), 2 tbsp.	15	<1.0	4.0	0	n.a.	270	n.a.
(Kraft Free)	16	0	3.0	0	0	150	n.a.
(Light Fantastic) . .	25	0	3.0	2.0	0	140	n.a.
(Marie's)	100	0	1.0	10.0	10	95	n.a.
(Marie's Lite & Luscious)	45	0	4.0	3.0	0	110	n.a.
(Ott's), 1.1 oz. . . .	145	0	2.0	16.0	1	126	0
(Seven Seas Buttermilk Recipe Ranch! Light) . .	50	0	1.0	5.0	0	135	n.a.
(Seven Seas Free)	16	0	4.0	0	0	120	n.a.
(Seven Seas Viva)	80	0	1.0	8.0	5	135	n.a.
(Seven Seas Viva Ranch! Light) . .	50	0	2.0	5.0	5	125	n.a.
(Wish-Bone)	80	0	<1.0	8.0	5	105	n.a.
buttermilk spice *(Marie's)*	90	0	2.0	9.0	10	115	n.a.
creamy *(Marie's)* . .	100	0	1.0	10.0	10	95	n.a.
creamy *(Rancher's Choice)*	90	0	1.0	10.0	5	140	n.a.
Italian *(Bernstein's)*	70	0	2.0	7.0	0	120	n.a.
Parmesan garlic *(Light Fantastic)*	30	<1.0	2.0	2.0	<5	140	n.a.

Food and Measure	cal.	prot. (gms)	carbo. (gms)	fat (gms)	chol. (mgs)	sod. (mgs)	fiber (gms)
red wine vinaigrette:							
(Cains Country) . .	35	0	2.0	3.0	0	180	n.a.
(Lawry's Classic),							
1 oz.	138	.1	4.9	13.7	0	178	0
(Marie's Zesty Fat							
Free)	20	0	5.0	0	0	135	n.a.
red wine vinegar							
(Seven Seas Free)	6	0	1.0	0	0	190	n.a.
red wine vinegar and							
oil:							
(Kraft)	60	0	4.0	4.0	0	200	n.a.
(Seven Seas Viva)	70	0	1.0	7.0	0	290	n.a.
(Seven Seas Viva							
Red Wine! Vinegar							
& Oil Light) . . .	45	0	1.0	4.0	0	190	n.a.
olive oil (Wish-Bone)	35	0	2.0	3.0	0	190	n.a.
rice wine vinaigrette							
(Lawry's Classic),							
1 oz.	60	.1	6.0	4.0	0	480	0
Russian:							
(Kraft Reduced Cal-							
orie)	30	0	4.0	1.0	0	130	n.a.
(Weight Watchers)	50	0	2.0	5.0	5	80	n.a.
(Wish-Bone)	50	0	7.0	3.0	0	170	n.a.
creamy (Kraft) . . .	60	0	2.0	5.0	5	150	n.a.
w/honey (Kraft) . .	60	0	4.0	5.0	0	130	n.a.
San Francisco, w/Ro-							
mano (Lawry's Clas-							
sic), 1 oz.	136	.6	2.0	14.0	<1	547	.1 c
Santa Fe (Wish-Bone)	70	0	1.0	7.0	5	105	n.a.
sesame garlic (Nasoya							
Vegi-Dressing) . . .	40	0	1.0	4.0	0	90	m.q.
sesame seed	68	.5	1.3	6.9	0	153	.1 c
sour (Friendship Sour							
Treat), 1 oz.	36	1.0	2.0	3.0	0	15	n.a.
sour cream and dill:							
(Marie's)	100	1.0	10.0	6.0	10	90	n.a.

Food and Measure	cal.	prot. (gms)	carbo. (gms)	fat (gms)	chol. (mgs)	sod. (mgs)	fiber (gms)
Salad dressing, sour cream and dill *(cont.)*							
(Marie's Lite & Luscious)	50	0	4.0	4.0	0	120	n.a.
sun-dried tomato vinaigrette *(Peggy-Jane's)*	45	0	1.0	4.0	n.a.	100	n.a.
sweet/sour *(Old Dutch)*	25	0	6.5	0	n.a.	240	n.a.
Swiss cheese vinaigrette *(Hain)*	60	0	0	7.0	<5	160	n.a.
Thousand Island:							
(Hain)	50	0	0	5.0	<5	85	n.a.
(Herb Magic), 2 tbsp.	15	0	4.0	0	n.a.	170	n.a.
(Kraft)	60	0	2.0	5.0	5	150	n.a.
(Marie's)	80	0	3.0	8.0	10	115	n.a.
(Seven Seas Thousand Island! Light)	30	0	3.0	2.0	5	160	n.a.
(Weight Watchers)	50	0	2.0	5.0	5	80	n.a.
(Wish-Bone)	70	0	3.0	6.0	5	170	n.a.
and bacon *(Kraft)*	60	0	2.0	6.0	0	100	n.a.
creamy *(Seven Seas)*	50	0	2.0	5.0	5	150	n.a.
tomato, garden, vinaigrette *(Hain* Canola*)*	60	0	1.0	6.0	0	150	n.a.
vinaigrette *(Herb Magic)*	5	0	1.5	0	0	135	n.a.
vintage, w/sherry wine *(Lawry's* Classic*)*, 1 oz.	110	4.3	2.5	10.3	1	415	.1 c
white wine vinaigrette:							
(Lawry's Classic*)*, 1 oz.	153	.1	2.7	15.7	<1	178	.1 c
(Marie's Zesty Fat Free*)*	20	0	5.0	0	0	135	n.a.

Food and Measure	cal.	prot. (gms)	carbo. (gms)	fat (gms)	chol. (mgs)	sod. (mgs)	fiber (gms)
Salad dressing mix*							
(Good Seasons),							
1 tbsp.:							
bleu cheese and herbs							
or classic dill . . .	70	0	1.0	8.0	0	150	n.a.
buttermilk, farm style	60	1.0	1.0	6.0	5	135	n.a.
cheese:							
garlic	70	0	1.0	8.0	0	170	n.a.
Italian	70	0	1.0	8.0	0	125	n.a.
Italian, lite	25	0	1.0	3.0	0	130	n.a.
garlic and herbs . . .	70	0	1.0	8.0	0	190	n.a.
herb, zesty, fat free	6	0	1.0	0	0	150	n.a.
honey mustard	80	0	2.0	8.0	0	125	n.a.
honey mustard, fat							
free	10	0	2.0	0	0	130	n.a.
Italian:							
regular	70	0	1.0	8.0	0	170	n.a.
fat free	6	0	1.0	0	0	170	n.a.
lite	25	0	1.0	3.0	0	170	n.a.
creamy, fat free . .	8	0	2.0	0	0	140	n.a.
mild	70	0	1.0	8.0	0	190	n.a.
zesty	70	0	1.0	8.0	0	120	n.a.
zesty, lite	25	0	1.0	3.0	0	130	n.a.
lemon and herbs . .	70	0	1.0	8.0	0	140	n.a.
ranch	60	0	1.0	6.0	5	110	n.a.
ranch, lite	30	1.0	2.0	2.0	5	115	n.a.
Salad mix*, 1/2 cup:							
(Kraft Light Rancher's							
Choice)	170	5.0	23.0	7.0	0	350	m.q.
(Kraft Rancher's							
Choice)	250	5.0	21.0	16.0	10	350	m.q.
Caesar *(Suddenly*							
Salad)	170	4.0	22.0	7.0	n.a.	410	m.q.
pasta:							
(McCormick/Schill-							
ing Pasta Prima)	390	7.0	41.0	23.0	n.a.	822	m.q.
bacon vinaigrette							
(Country Recipe)	140	4.0	24.0	4.0	n.a.	210	m.q.

Food and Measure	cal.	prot. (gms)	carbo. (gms)	fat (gms)	chol. (mgs)	sod. (mgs)	fiber (gms)
Salad mix, pasta *(cont.)*							
broccoli, creamy *(Lipton)*	200	5.0	23.0	10.0	n.a.	190	m.q.
broccoli and vegetables *(Kraft)* . . .	210	4.0	15.0	16.0	10	290	m.q.
classic *(Suddenly Salad)*	150	4.0	23.0	5.0	n.a.	590	m.q.
Dijon, creamy *(Country Recipe)*	190	4.0	24.0	10.0	n.a.	310	m.q.
garden primavera *(Kraft)*	170	5.0	21.0	7.0	0	450	m.q.
homestyle *(Kraft)*	240	4.0	21.0	16.0	10	300	m.q.
Italian *(Kraft)*	130	5.0	20.0	3.0	0	420	m.q.
Italian *(Suddenly Salad)*	160	4.0	22.0	6.0	n.a.	480	m.q.
Italian, creamy *(Country Recipe)*	160	4.0	22.0	7.0	n.a.	340	m.q.
Italian, herb *(Fantastic)*	185	5.0	21.0	9.0	1	221	3.0 d
Italian, robust *(Lipton)*	190	5.0	25.0	8.0	n.a.	300	m.q.
Oriental, spicy *(Fantastic)*	190	4.0	20.0	10.0	0	213	3.0 d
ranch *(Country Recipe)*	140	4.0	19.0	5.0	n.a.	300	m.q.
primavera *(Suddenly Salad)*	180	4.0	20.0	9.0	n.a.	340	m.q.
ranch and bacon *(Suddenly Salad)*	200	5.0	24.0	9.0	n.a.	310	m.q.
Salad Savoy *(Frieda's)*, 1 cup . .	50	4.2	6.0	1.9	0	63	m.q.
Salad seasoning *(McCormick/Schilling Salad Supreme)*, 1 tsp.	11	.7	.5	.1	0	288	m.q.
Salami:							
(Oscar Mayer Salami for Beer), 2 slices	110	6.0	<1.0	9.0	30	580	0

Food and Measure	cal.	prot. (gms)	carbo. (gms)	fat (gms)	chol. (mgs)	sod. (mgs)	fiber (gms)
beef:							
(Hebrew National),							
1 oz.	80	7.0	<1.0	7.0	15	230	0
(Kahn's), 1 slice . .	70	3.0	1.0	6.0	m.q.	250	0
(Kahn's Family							
Pack), 1 slice . .	60	2.0	1.0	5.0	m.q.	190	0
(Oscar Mayer							
Machiaeh),							
2 slices	120	6.0	1.0	10.0	30	510	0
cooked *(Kahn's),*							
1 slice	60	4.0	1.0	4.0	m.q.	300	0
cotto:							
(Kahn's Family							
Pack), 1 slice . .	45	3.0	1.0	3.0	m.q.	230	0
(Oscar Mayer),							
2 slices	110	6.0	<1.0	9.0	35	570	0
beef *(Oscar Mayer),*							
2 slices	90	6.0	<1.0	7.0	35	590	0
dry or hard:							
(Hormel Homeland),							
1 oz.	117	6.0	<2.0	10.0	29	448	0
(Oscar Mayer),							
3 slices	100	6.0	0	9.0	25	510	0
Genoa:							
(Hormel DiLusso),							
1 oz.	88	6.0	1.0	7.0	26	512	0
(Hormel San Remo							
Brand), 1 oz. . .	104	6.0	<2.0	9.0	26	470	0
(Oscar Mayer),							
3 slices	100	5.0	0	9.0	25	490	0
"Salami," vegetarian,							
frozen *(Worthington),*							
2 slices	70	7.0	2.0	4.0	0	460	m.q.
Salisbury steak, see							
"Beef dinner" and							
"Beef entree"							

Food and Measure	cal.	prot. (gms)	carbo. (gms)	fat (gms)	chol. (mgs)	sod. (mgs)	fiber (gms)
Salmon, fresh, meat only:							
Atlantic, farmed:							
raw, 4 oz.	207	22.6	0	12.3	67	66	0
baked, broiled, or							
microwaved, 4 oz.	234	25.0	0	14.0	71	69	0
Atlantic, wild:							
raw, 4 oz.	161	22.5	0	7.2	62	50	0
baked, broiled, or							
microwaved, 4 oz.	206	28.8	0	9.2	81	64	0
Chinook:							
raw, 4 oz.	204	22.8	0	11.9	75	53	0
baked, broiled, or							
microwaved, 4 oz.	262	29.2	0	15.2	96	68	0
smoked, 4 oz.	133	20.7	0	4.9	26	889	0
lox, 4 oz.	133	20.7	0	4.9	26	2268	0
chum:							
raw, 4 oz.	136	22.8	0	4.3	84	112	0
baked, broiled, or							
microwaved, 4 oz.	175	29.3	0	5.5	108	73	0
coho, farmed:							
raw, 4 oz.	182	24.1	0	8.7	58	53	0
baked, broiled, or							
microwaved, 4 oz.	202	27.6	0	9.3	71	59	0
coho, wild:							
raw, 4 oz.	165	25.0	0	6.7	51	53	0
baked, broiled, or							
microwaved, 4 oz.	158	26.6	0	4.9	62	66	0
boiled, poached, or							
steamed, 4 oz.	209	31.0	0	8.5	65	60	0
pink:							
raw, 4 oz.	132	22.6	0	3.9	59	76	0
baked, broiled, or							
microwaved, 4 oz.	169	29.0	0	5.0	76	98	0
sockeye:							
raw, 4 oz.	191	24.2	0	9.7	70	53	0
baked, broiled, or							
microwaved, 4 oz.	245	31.0	0	12.4	99	75	0

Food and Measure	cal.	prot. (gms)	carbo. (gms)	fat (gms)	chol. (mgs)	sod. (mgs)	fiber (gms)
Salmon, canned:							
chum, drained, 4 oz.	160	24.3	0	6.2	44	552	0
keta:							
(Libby's), 3.7 oz. . . .	130	20.0	0	6.0	40	450	0
w/liquid (Bumble							
Bee), 3.5 oz. . .	160	20.0	0	8.0	60	490	0
pink:							
(Libby's), 3.7 oz. . . .	150	21.0	0	7.0	40	400	0
w/liquid (Bumble							
Bee), 3.5 oz. . .	160	20.0	0	8.0	50	490	0
skinless, boneless							
(Libby's), 3.25 oz.	110	16.0	1.0	4.0	50	420	0
skinless, boneless,							
w/liquid (Bumble							
Bee), 3.25 oz. . . .	120	17.0	0	5.0	25	420	0
red:							
w/liquid (Bumble							
Bee), 3.5 oz. . .	180	20.0	0	10.0	60	490	0
blueback (Rubin-							
stein's), 1/2 cup	170	20.0	0	9.0	m.q.	450	0
skinless, boneless,							
w/liquid (Bumble							
Bee), 3.25 oz. . . .	130	17.0	0	6.0	30	420	0
red, sockeye:							
(Icy Point), 1/2 cup	175	21.0	0	9.0	m.q.	480	0
(Libby's), 3.7 oz. . . .	150	21.0	0	7.0	40	380	0
Salmon seasoning **mix** (Old Bay Salmon Classic),							
1 pkg.	159	8.0	21.0	5.0	n.a.	415	m.q.
Salsa, 2 tbsp., except as noted:							
(La Victoria Suprema)	10	0	2.0	0	0	220	m.q.
all varieties (Tio Sancho), 1/4 cup . .	22	.9	4.0	.4	n.a.	549	m.q.
green chili:							
(La Victoria)	10	0	2.0	0	0	150	m.q.

Food and Measure	cal.	prot. (gms)	carbo. (gms)	fat (gms)	chol. (mgs)	sod. (mgs)	fiber (gms)
Salsa, green chili *(cont.)*							
(Old El Paso Thick 'n Chunky) . . .	3	0	1.0	0	0	270	0
hot:							
(Chi-Chi's), 1 oz.	8	<2.0	2.0	<2.0	<2	153	m.q.
(Frito-Lay's Chunky), 1 oz.	12	0	2.0	0	0	180	m.q.
(Hain), 1/4 cup . . .	20	1.0	4.0	0	0	480	m.q.
(Hain Thick & Chunky)	6	<1.0	1.0	0	0	110	m.q.
(Master Choice), 1 oz.	10	0	2.0	0	0	186	m.q.
(Rosarita), 3 tbsp.	25	1.0	6.0	<1.0	0	300	<1.0 d
hot, medium or mild							
(Old El Paso Thick 'n Chunky)	6	<1.0	1.0	<1.0	0	170	m.q.
medium:							
(Chi-Chi's), 1 oz.	7	<2.0	2.0	<2.0	<2	135	m.q.
(Frito-Lay's Chunky), 1 oz.	12	0	2.0	0	0	150	m.q.
(Hain Thick & Chunky)	6	<1.0	1.0	0	0	100	m.q.
(Master Choice Thick & Savory), 1 oz.	10	0	2.0	0	0	185	m.q.
(Rosarita), 3 tbsp.	25	1.0	6.0	<1.0	0	350	<1.0 d
mild:							
(Chi-Chi's), 1 oz.	7	<2.0	2.0	<2.0	<2	116	m.q.
(Frito-Lay's Chunky), 1 oz.	12	0	2.0	0	0	200	m.q.
(Hain), 1/4 cup . . .	20	1.0	4.0	0	0	410	m.q.
(Hain Thick & Chunky)	6	1.0	<1.0	0	0	90	m.q.
(Master Choice), 1 oz.	10	0	2.0	0	0	170	m.q.
(Rosarita), 3 tbsp.	25	1.0	6.0	<1.0	0	340	<1.0 d

Food and Measure	cal.	prot. (gms)	carbo. (gms)	fat (gms)	chol. (mgs)	sod. (mgs)	fiber (gms)
picante, (see also "Picante sauce"):							
all varieties (Old El Paso)	10	<1.0	2.0	<1.0	0	160	m.q.
medium (La Victoria)	5	0	1.0	0	0	180	m.q.
mild (La Victoria) . .	10	1.0	2.0	0	0	230	m.q.
ranchera (La Victoria)	10	0	1.0	0	0	140	m.q.
taco (see also "Taco sauce"), 3 tbsp.:							
medium (Rosarita)	25	1.0	6.0	<1.0	0	310	<1.0 d
mild (Rosarita) . . .	25	1.0	6.0	<1.0	0	300	<1.0 d
Texas (Hot Cha Cha), 1 oz.	6	.3	2.5	0	0	2	.4 d
verde (Old El Paso Thick 'n Chunky)	10	<1.0	2.0	<1.0	0	135	1.0 d
Victoria (La Victoria)	10	0	1.0	0	0	160	m.q.
Salsa seasoning mix (Lawry's Seasoning Blends), 1 pkg. . .	95	2.1	20.5	.5	0	2042	1.1 d
Salsify:							
raw, untrimmed, 1 lb.	325	13.0	73.4	.8	0	79	13.0 d
raw, sliced, 1/2 cup	55	2.2	12.5	.1	0	13	2.2 d
boiled, drained, sliced, 1/2 cup	46	1.9	10.5	.1	0	11	2.1 d
black, raw (Frieda's), 1 oz.	23	.9	5.3	tr.	0	6	m.q.
Salt, 1 tsp., except as noted:							
1 tbsp.	0	0	0	0	0	6589	0
(Morton Lite Salt) . .	<1	0	tr.	0	0	1110	0
kosher (Morton) . . .	0	0	0	0	0	1800	0
noniodized (Morton) .	0	0	.0	0	0	2300	0
sea (Hain)	0	0	0	0	0	2255	0
seasoned (see also specific listings):							
(Lawry's)	4	.1	.6	.1	0	1367	.1 c
(Lawry's Lite) . . .	8	.3	1.7	<.1	0	357	.1 c

Food and Measure	cal.	prot. (gms)	carbo. (gms)	fat (gms)	chol. (mgs)	sod. (mgs)	fiber (gms)
Salt, seasoned *(cont.)*							
(McCormick/Schilling)	4	.2	.6	n.a.	0	980	n.a.
(McCormick/Schilling Salt 'n Spice)	3	.2	.6	n.a.	0	939	n.a.
(Morton)	4	<1.0	<1.	<.1	0	1300	n.a.
(Morton Nature's Seasons)	3	<.1	<1.0	<.1	0	1400	n.a.
hot'n spicy *(Lawry's Spice Blends)*	3	.1	1.5	.1	0	864	.1 c
Salt substitute, 1 tsp.:							
(Lawry's Salt-Free 17)	10	.3	1.8	.2	0	2	.4 c
(Morton)	<1	0	.1	0	0	<1	n.a.
seasoned *(Lawry's Salt-Free)*	3	.1	.6	<.1	0	7	<.1 c
Salt pork, raw, 1 oz.	212	1.4	0	22.8	25	404	0
Sandwich, see specific listings							
Sandwich sauce (see also specific listings):							
(Hunt's Manwich Extra Thick & Chunky), 2.5 oz.	60	1.0	15.0	<1.0	0	640	2.0 d
(Hunt's Manwich Extra Thick & Chunky), 1 sandwich*	330	17.0	36.0	13.0	50	870	3.0 d
Mexican *(Hunt's Manwich)*, 2.5 oz.	35	1.0	9.0	1.0	0	460	1.0 d
Mexican *(Hunt's Manwich)*, 1 sandwich*	310	17.0	30.0	13.0	50	690	2.0 d
sloppy Joe:							
(Hormel Not-So-Sloppy Joe Sauce), 2.24 oz.	70	1.0	16.0	1.0	5	730	n.a.

Food and Measure	cal.	prot. (gms)	carbo. (gms)	fat (gms)	chol. (mgs)	sod. (mgs)	fiber (gms)
(Hunt's Manwich),							
2.5 oz.	40	1.0	10.0	<1.0	0	390	1.0 d
(Hunt's Manwich),							
1 sandwich* . . .	310	17.0	31.0	13.0	50	620	1.0 d
(Libby's), 2.5 oz. . .	45	1.0	10.0	<1.0	n.a.	440	m.q.
Sandwich seasoning mix:							
(Hunt's Manwich),							
.25 oz.	20	<1.0	5.0	<1.0	0	350	<1.0 d
(Hunt's Manwich),							
1 sandwich*	320	17.0	31.0	13.0	50	590	2.0 d
sloppy Joe:							
(Lawry's Seasoning							
Blends), 1 pkg.	126	2.8	27.7	.4	0	3442	.8 c
(Tone's), 1 tsp. . .	14	.3	3.1	.1	0	347	m.q.
(French's), 1/8 pkg.	14	0	3.0	0	0	420	m.q.
(McCormick/Schill-							
ing), 1/4 pkg. . .	26	.5	6.0	.1	0	750	m.q.
Sandwich spread:							
meatless:							
(Blue Plate), 1 tbsp.	75	0	3.0	7.0	5	105	0
(Hellman's/Best							
Foods), 1 tbsp.	50	0	2.0	5.0	5	170	m.q.
(Kraft), 1 tbsp. . . .	50	0	3.0	5.0	5	95	m.q.
(LaLoma), 3 tbsp.	70	4.0	4.0	4.0	0	300	m.q.
meat *(Oscar Mayer)*,							
2 oz.	140	4.0	9.0	10.0	20	530	0
Sapodilla:							
1 medium, 3" × 2½"	140	.7	33.9	1.9	0	20	9.0 d
½ cup	100	.5	24.1	1.3	0	15	6.4 d
Sapote:							
1 medium, 11.2 oz.	301	4.8	76.0	1.4	0	21	5.9 d
trimmed, 1 oz.	38	.6	9.6	.2	0	3	.7 d
white *(Frieda's)*, 1 oz.	35	.5	9.0	.2	0	m.q.	m.q.
Sardine, fresh, see "Herring"							

Food and Measure	cal.	prot. (gms)	carbo. (gms)	fat (gms)	chol. (mgs)	sod. (mgs)	fiber (gms)
Sardine, canned:							
Atlantic, in oil, drained:							
2 oz.	118	14.8	0	6.5	81	286	0
2 medium,							
3″ × 1″ × 1/2″ . . .	50	5.9	0	2.8	34	121	0
Norwegian, in oil,							
drained (Empress),							
3.75 oz.	260	19.0	1.0	20.0	m.q.	m.q.	0
Pacific, in tomato							
sauce, drained:							
2 oz.	101	9.3	n.a.	6.8	35	235	.1 c
1 medium,							
43/4″ × 11/8″ × 5/8″	68	6.2	n.a.	4.6	23	157	<.1 c
Portuguese, skinless							
and boneless, in oil							
(Empress), 4.375-oz.							
can	500	22.0	2.0	45.0	m.q.	630	0
kippered (Brunswick							
Kippered Snacks),							
3.53-oz. can	185	16.0	1.0	14.0	m.q.	610	0
in mustard sauce (Un-							
derwood), 3.75 oz.	220	16.0	2.0	16.0	m.q.	650	n.a.
in soya oil, drained							
(Underwood),							
3.75 oz.	230	16.0	1.0	18.0	m.q.	400	0
in tomato sauce (Un-							
derwood), 3.75 oz.	220	16.0	2.0	16.0	m.q.	500	n.a.
Sauce, see specific							
listings							
Sauerkraut, 1 oz., ex-							
cept as noted:							
w/liquid, 1/2 cup . . .	22	1.1	5.1	.2	0	780	3.0 d
(Claussen), 3 oz. . . .	20	<1.0	4.0	0	0	610	3.0 d
(New Morning Kozmic							
Kraut)	6	<1.0	1.0	0	0	200	m.q.
(New Morning Kozmic							
Kraut Low Sodium)	6	<1.0	1.0	0	0	125	m.q.
(Stokely), 1/2 cup . . .	20	1.0	4.0	0	0	810	m.q.

Food and Measure	cal.	prot. (gms)	carbo. (gms)	fat (gms)	chol. (mgs)	sod. (mgs)	fiber (gms)
(Vlasic Old Fashioned)	4	0	1.0	0	0	280	m.q.
Sausage (see also "Sausage stick" and specific listings), 1 link, except as noted:							
beef:							
(Jones Dairy Farm Golden Brown)	80	3.5	tr.	7.0	18	160	0
and cheddar *(Hillshire Farm* Flavorseal), 2 oz. . . .	190	8.0	1.0	15.0	m.q.	500	0
brown and serve:							
(Jones Dairy Farm)	100	2.5	tr.	10.0	19	160	0
(Jones Dairy Farm Light)	60	3.0	tr.	4.5	16	160	0
w/bacon *(Jones Dairy Farm)* . . .	90	3.0	tr.	8.0	19	140	0
beef *(Jones Dairy Farm)*	90	3.0	tr.	8.5	18	200	0
country recipe *(Hillshire Farm* Flavorseal), 2 oz.	180	7.0	2.0	16.0	m.q.	490	0
Italian:							
(Jones Dairy Farm), 2-oz. link	140	8.0	tr.	11.5	44	420	0
hot *(Hillshire Farm* Links), 2 oz. . . .	180	7.0	1.0	17.0	m.q.	m.q.	0
mild *(Hillshire Farm* Links), 2 oz. . . .	190	7.0	1.0	17.0	m.q.	m.q.	0
pork, cooked, 1 oz.	92	5.7	.4	7.3	22	261	0
pork:							
fresh, cooked, .5 oz. (1 oz. raw link)	48	2.6	.1	4.1	11	168	0
(Hormel Little Sizzlers), 1 oz. . . .	130	3.0	<2.0	13.0	19	192	0
(Jones Dairy Farm Dinner Link) . . .	280	5.5	tr.	28.0	48	310	0

Food and Measure	cal.	prot. (gms)	carbo. (gms)	fat (gms)	chol. (mgs)	sod. (mgs)	fiber (gms)
Sausage, pork *(cont.)*							
(Jones Dairy Farm Golden Brown Light)	60	3.0	1.0	4.5	16	130	0
(Jones Dairy Farm Light Little Link)	70	4.0	tr.	5.5	21	220	0
(Jones Dairy Farm Little Link)	140	2.5	tr.	14.0	24	170	0
(Oscar Mayer Little Friers), 2 links . .	170	9.0	1.0	14.0	40	420	0
mild *(Jones Dairy Farm Golden Brown)*	100	2.5	tr.	9.5	18	160	0
spicy *(Jones Dairy Farm Golden Brown)*	100	2.5	tr.	9.0	18	150	0
pork, patty, 1 patty:							
(Jones Dairy Farm)	180	4.5	tr.	18.0	36	280	0
plain or extra mild, cooked *(Jimmy Dean)*	120	4.0	<1.0	11.0	20	220	0
fresh, cooked, 1 oz. (2-oz. raw patty)	100	5.3	.3	8.4	22	349	0
mild *(Jones Dairy Farm Golden Brown)*	150	4.5	tr.	14.0	29	250	0
sage, cooked *(Jimmy Dean)* . .	140	5.0	<1.0	13.0	m.q.	300	0
pork roll, 1-oz. slice:							
(Jones Dairy Farm Cello Roll)	100	3.5	tr.	9.5	24	180	0
beef *(Jones Dairy Farm Cello Roll)*	130	3.0	tr.	12.5	25	160	0
hot *(Jones Dairy Farm Country Cello Roll)*	110	3.5	tr.	10.0	24	170	0

Food and Measure	cal.	prot. (gms)	carbo. (gms)	fat (gms)	chol. (mgs)	sod. (mgs)	fiber (gms)
smoked:							
(Hillshire Farm Bun Size), 2 oz. . . .	180	8.0	2.0	16.0	m.q.	570	0
(Hillshire Farm Flavorseal), 2 oz.	190	7.0	1.0	17.0	m.q.	500	0
(Hillshire Farm Links), 2 oz.	190	8.0	1.0	18.0	m.q.	520	0
(Hillshire Farm Flavorseal Lite), 2 oz.	130	8.0	1.0	11.0	m.q.	m.q.	0
(Oscar Mayer Little Smokies), 6 links	160	7.0	1.0	15.0	35	570	0
(Oscar Mayer Smokie Links) . .	130	5.0	<1.0	12.0	25	430	0
hot (Hillshire Farm Flavorseal), 2 oz.	180	7.0	2.0	16.0	m.q.	510	0
Italian seasoned (Hillshire Farm Flavorseal), 2 oz.	200	7.0	1.0	18.0	m.q.	500	0
smoked, beef:							
(Hillshire Farm Bun Size), 2 oz. . . .	180	8.0	2.0	16.0	m.q.	570	0
(Hillshire Farm Flavorseal), 2 oz.	180	7.0	2.0	16.0	m.q.	490	0
(Oscar Mayer Beef Smokies)	120	6.0	<1.0	11.0	25	430	0
smoked, cheese (Oscar Mayer Cheese Smokies)	130	6.0	<1.0	12.0	30	450	0
turkey, see "Turkey sausage							
Sausage, freeze-dried, patty (Mountain House), 1/2 pkg.	80	8.0	0	5.0	m.q.	250	0

Food and Measure	cal.	prot. (gms)	carbo. (gms)	fat (gms)	chol. (mgs)	sod. (mgs)	fiber (gms)
"Sausage," vegetarian, 2 links or patties, except as noted:							
.9-oz. link	64	4.6	2.5	4.5	0	222	.7 d
1.3-oz. patty	97	7.0	3.7	6.9	0	337	1.1 d
canned *(LaLoma Little Links)*	90	9.0	2.0	5.0	0	180	m.q.
canned *(Worthington Saucettes)*	150	10.0	3.0	11.0	0	430	m.q.
frozen:							
(Morningstar Farms Breakfast Links)	90	8.0	3.0	5.0	0	300	m.q.
(Morningstar Farms Breakfast Patties)	170	16.0	6.0	9.0	0	600	m.q.
(Worthington Prosage Links)	130	9.0	3.0	9.0	0	460	m.q.
(Worthington Prosage Patties)	210	18.0	4.0	14.0	0	780	m.q.
roll *(Worthington Prosage)*, 2.5 oz.	180	13.0	4.0	12.0	0	570	m.q.
Sausage breakfast biscuit, frozen:							
(Hormel Quick Meal), 3.7 oz.	350	10.0	29.0	22.0	40	870	m.q.
(Swanson), 3.2 oz. . .	300	11.0	23.0	19.0	m.q.	1170	m.q.
(Weight Watchers), 3 oz.	220	11.0	19.0	11.0	70	560	m.q.
and cheese *(Hormel Quick Meal)*, 4.3 oz.	420	13.0	31.0	27.0	60	1060	m.q.
"Sausage" breakfast biscuit, vegetarian, frozen *(Morningstar Farms)*, 3.5 oz. . .	280	13.0	31.0	11.0	0	570	m.q.
Sausage seasoning, pork *(Tone's)*, 1 tsp.	12	.4	2.7	.3	0	1	.7 d

Food and Measure	cal.	prot. (gms)	carbo. (gms)	fat (gms)	chol. (mgs)	sod. (mgs)	fiber (gms)
Sausage stick (see also "Beef jerky"), 1 piece, except as noted:							
beef, 1.64 oz.:							
pepperoni (Pemmican)	240	13.0	3.0	20.0	m.q.	740	0
Tabasco (Pemmican)	250	11.0	4.0	21.0	m.q.	880	0
teriyaki (Pemmican)	220	12.0	7.0	16.0	m.q.	610	0
pickled:							
(Penrose Firecracker), 1.2 oz.	100	5.0	1.0	8.0	m.q.	500	0
(Penrose Giant Firecracker), 1.7 oz.	130	7.0	1.0	11.0	m.q.	700	0
hot, red hot, Polish, beer or Firecracker (Penrose), .5 oz.	40	2.0	1.0	3.0	m.q.	220	0
smoked:							
(Slim Jim Big Slim)	70	3.0	1.0	6.0	15	190	0
(Slim Jim Giant Slim)	150	6.0	2.0	13.0	35	420	0
all varieties (Slim Jim Handi-Paks)	60	2.0	1.0	5.0	10	140	0
plain or Tabasco (Slim Jim Super Slim)	100	4.0	1.0	9.0	20	270	0
beef'n cheese (Slim Jim), 1 pkg. . . .	160	9.0	2.0	13.0	35	650	0
nacho (Slim Jim Super Slim) . . .	90	6.0	1.0	7.0	m.q.	320	0
summer sausage, plain or teriyaki (Slim Jim)	110	5.0	1.0	10.0	m.q.	410	0
Savory, ground:							
1 tsp.	4	.1	1.0	.1	0	tr.	.2 c
summer (Tone's), 1 tsp.	4	.1	1.0	.1	0	1	.2 c

Food and Measure	cal.	prot. (gms)	carbo. (gms)	fat (gms)	chol. (mgs)	sod. (mgs)	fiber (gms)
Scallion, see "Onion, green"							
Scallop, meat only:							
raw, 4 oz.	100	19.0	2.7	.9	38	183	0
raw, 2 large or 5 small, 1.1 oz. . . .	26	5.0	.7	.2	10	48	0
"Scallop," imitation:							
from surimi, 4 oz. . .	112	14.5	12.1	.5	25	902	0
"Scallop," vegetarian, canned, 1/2 cup:							
(Worthington Vegetable Skallops)	90	15.0	4.0	2.0	0	430	m.q.
(Worthington Vegetable Skallops No Salt)	80	13.0	4.0	1.0	0	80	m.q.
Scallop entree, fried, frozen *(Mrs. Paul's)*, 3.5 oz.	160	8.0	18.0	7.0	10	320	m.q.
Scallop squash:							
raw, sliced, 1/2 cup	12	.8	2.5	.1	0	1	1.2 d
boiled, drained:							
sliced, 1/2 cup . . .	14	.9	3.0	.2	0	1	1.1 d
mashed, 1/2 cup . .	19	1.2	4.0	.2	0	1	1.4 d
Scrapple *(Jones Dairy Farm)*, 1.5-oz. slice	90	4.0	5.0	6.0	24	230	n.a.
Scrod, fresh, see "Cod, Atlantic"							
Scup, meat only, raw:							
4 oz.	119	21.4	0	3.1	m.q.	48	0
baked, broiled, or microwaved, 4 oz. . . .	153	27.5	0	4.0	m.q.	61	0
Sea bass, meat only:							
raw, 4 oz.	110	20.9	0	2.3	47	77	0
baked, broiled, or microwaved, 4 oz. . .	141	26.8	0	2.9	60	99	0
Sea trout, meat only:							
raw, 4 oz.	118	19.0	0	4.1	94	66	0

Food and Measure	cal.	prot. (gms)	carbo. (gms)	fat (gms)	chol. (mgs)	sod. (mgs)	fiber (gms)
baked, broiled, or microwaved, 4 oz. . . .	151	24.3	0	5.3	120	84	0
Seafood, see specific listings							
Seafood entree, frozen:							
combination platter, breaded *(Mrs. Paul's)*, 9 oz.	600	19.0	55.0	33.0	85	408	m.q.
Creole, w/rice *(Swanson* Homestyle), 9 oz.	240	7.0	40.0	6.0	m.q.	810	m.q.
Newburg *(Healthy Choice)*, 8 oz. . . .	200	13.0	30.0	3.0	55	440	m.q.
Seafood sauce (see also "Cocktail sauce") *(Golden Dipt)*, 2 tbsp.:							
barbecue, Cajun style	90	0	5.0	8.0	0	360	n.a.
cooking sauce:							
Creole style	20	0	2.0	1.0	0	190	n.a.
Dijonnaise	52	0	2.0	4.0	0	130	n.a.
French white . . .	55	0	3.0	4.0	0	210	n.a.
lemon butter dill . .	100	0	4.0	9.0	0	190	n.a.
marinade:							
lemon herb	130	0	2.0	14.0	0	210	n.a.
teriyaki, ginger . . .	120	1.0	12.0	7.0	0	920	n.a.
Seafood seasoning, see "Fish seasoning and coating mix"							
Seasoning and coating mix (see also specific listings) *(Shake'n Bake):*							
country mild, 1/4 pkt.	80	1.0	10.0	4.0	0	500	m.q.
Italian herb, 1/4 pkt.	80	2.0	14.0	1.0	0	610	m.q.
Seaweed, 1 oz.:							
agar, raw	7	.2	1.9	tr.	0	3	.1 d

Food and Measure	cal.	prot. (gms)	carbo. (gms)	fat (gms)	chol. (mgs)	sod. (mgs)	fiber (gms)
Seaweed (cont.)							
agar, dried	87	1.8	22.9	.1	0	29	2.2 d
Irish moss, raw . . .	14	.4	3.5	<.1	0	19	.4 d
kelp, raw	12	.5	2.7	.2	0	66	.4 d
laver, raw	10	1.6	1.4	.1	0	14	.1 d
spirulina, raw	8	1.7	.7	.1	0	28	.1 c
spirulina, dried	82	16.3	6.8	2.2	0	297	1.0 d
wakame, raw	13	.9	2.6	.2	0	247	.1 d
Seitan mix (Arrowhead Mills), 2.5 oz.	160	22.0	14.0	1.0	n.a.	20	m.q.
Semolina, whole grain, 1 cup	602	21.2	121.6	1.8	0	2	6.5 d
Sesame butter (see also "Sesame paste"):							
(Roaster Fresh), 1 oz.	168	5.0	6.0	15.0	0	3	m.q.
(Erewhon), 2 tbsp. . . .	190	7.0	3.0	17.0	0	20	m.q.
Sesame flour, 1 oz.:							
high fat	149	8.7	7.6	10.5	0	12	1.8 c
partially defatted . . .	109	11.5	10.0	3.4	0	12	1.7 c
lowfat	95	14.2	10.1	.5	0	11	1.4 c
Sesame meal, partially defatted, 1 oz.	161	4.8	7.4	13.6	0	11	1.1 c
Sesame paste (see also "Tahini"), from whole sesame seeds, 1 tbsp.	95	2.9	4.1	8.1	0	2	.9 d
Sesame seasoning, all-purpose (McCormick/Schilling Parsley Patch), 1/2 tsp.	8	.3	.5	.5	0	1	n.a.
Sesame seeds:							
(Spice Islands), 1 tsp.	9	.5	.9	.4	0	1	.7 c
whole (Arrowhead Mills), 1 oz.	160	5.0	6.0	14.0	0	4	3.1 d
whole, roasted and toasted, 1 oz. . . .	161	4.8	7.3	13.6	0	3	4.0 d

Food and Measure	cal.	prot. (gms)	carbo. (gms)	fat (gms)	chol. (mgs)	sod. (mgs)	fiber (gms)
kernels, decorticated:							
(Arrowhead Mills),							
2 oz.	160	6.0	4.0	14.0	0	3	3.7 d
dried, 1 tsp.	16	.7	.3	1.5	0	0	.1 d
toasted, 1 oz. . . .	161	4.8	7.4	13.6	0	11	4.8 d
Sesbania flower:							
raw, 1 cup	5	.3	1.4	<.1	0	3	.3 c
steamed, 1/2 cup . .	11	.6	2.7	<.1	0	6	.8 c
Shad, American, meat only:							
raw, 4 oz.	223	19.2	0	15.6	m.q.	58	0
baked, broiled, or microwaved, 4 oz. . .	286	24.6	0	20.0	m.q.	74	0
Shallot:							
fresh or stored:							
peeled, 1 oz. . . .	20	.7	4.8	<.1	0	3	.2 c
chopped, 1 tbsp. .	7	.3	1.7	<.1	0	1	.1 c
freeze-dried, 1 tbsp.	3	.1	.7	tr.	0	1	<.1 c
Shark, meat only:							
raw, 4 oz.	148	23.8	0	5.1	58	90	0
batter-dipped, 4 oz.	259	21.1	7.2	15.7	67	138	.2 c
Sheepshead, meat only:							
raw, 4 oz.	123	22.9	0	2.7	m.q.	81	0
baked, broiled, or microwaved, 4 oz. . .	143	29.5	0	1.8	m.q.	83	0
Shellie bean, canned, w/liquid, 1/2 cup . .	37	2.1	7.6	.2	0	408	4.1 d
Shells, pasta, entree, frozen:							
stuffed:							
(Celentano), 6.25 oz.	330	17.0	32.0	15.0	70	500	7.0 d
(Celentano Great Choice), 10 oz.	250	16.0	41.0	2.5	15	650	5.0 d
broccoli *(Celentano* Great Choice),							
10 oz.	190	12.0	31.0	4.0	15	520	4.0 d

Food and Measure	cal.	prot. (gms)	carbo. (gms)	fat (gms)	chol. (mgs)	sod. (mgs)	fiber (gms)
Shells, pasta, entree, stuffed (cont.)							
cheese, w/tomato sauce (Stouffer's), 9.25 oz.	300	17.0	28.0	13.0	m.q.	820	m.q.
w/sauce (Celentano), 10 oz. . . .	400	23.0	34.0	20.0	90	840	m.q.
w/tomato sauce (Healthy Choice Extra Portion), 12 oz.	330	24.0	53.0	3.0	35	470	m.q.
Shells, pasta, mix*, and curry, w/tofu, 1/2 cup:							
(Tofu Classics)	119	7.0	16.0	3.0	0	235	3.0 d
w/butter (Tofu Classics)	155	7.0	16.0	7.0	m.q.	282	3.0 d
Sherbet (see also "Sorbet"):							
all flavors (Sealtest), 1/2 cup	130	1.0	28.0	1.0	5	30	n.a.
orange:							
1/2 cup	132	1.1	29.2	1.9	5	44	.3 c
(Blue Bell), 1/2 cup	130	1.0	29.0	1.0	4	30	n.a.
bar, orange, 2.75-fl.-oz. bar	91	.7	20.1	1.3	3	30	.2 c
Shoney's:							
breakfast, kitchen ordered:							
bacon, 3 strips . .	109	5.8	.1	9.4	16	303	0
biscuit, 1 piece . .	170	2.7	21.6	8.1	0	364	m.q.
blueberry muffin, 2 pieces	214	2.9	35.4	7.0	33	2	.9 d
country gravy, 3 oz.	114	1.2	5.7	9.8	2	358	0
croissant, 1 piece	260	5.0	22.0	16.0	2	260	m.q.
egg, fried, 1 egg	159	6.1	.6	14.7	274	69	0
grits, 3 oz.	57	.7	6.2	3.2	0	62	m.q.
ham, breakfast, 2 slices	59	7.2	.6	2.1	28	526	0
hash browns, 3 oz.	90	1.6	14.1	3.1	0	50	m.q.

Food and Measure	cal.	prot. (gms)	carbo. (gms)	fat (gms)	chol. (mgs)	sod. (mgs)	fiber (gms)
home fries, 3 oz.	115	2.0	18.7	3.7	0	53	m.q.
honey bun, 1 piece	265	4.0	32.0	14.0	3	33	m.q.
pancakes, 1 piece	91	1.8	19.9	.2	0	522	m.q.
sausage patty, 1 patty	103	3.7	.2	9.6	17	161	0
sirloin steak, char-broiled	357	31.9	0	24.5	99	160	0
syrup, low-cal, 2.2 oz.	98	0	24.4	0	0	0	0
toast, buttered, 2 slices	163	4.2	24.6	5.2	0	296	1.2 d
soups, 6 oz.:							
bean	63	3.8	9.8	1.1	4	479	1.4 d
beef cabbage . . .	86	6.1	9.4	3.0	13	503	2.3 d
broccoli, cream of	75	1.8	10.5	4.6	1	415	.4 d
broccoli/cauliflower	124	3.8	11.9	9.2	12	560	.5 d
cheddar chowder	91	3.0	14.4	2.3	n.a.	948	n.a.
cheese Florentine ham	110	3.7	11.8	7.8	11	890	.6 d
chicken, cream of	136	4.6	13.5	8.9	11	1164	.3 d
chicken gumbo . .	60	4.0	7.0	2.0	m.q.	1050	m.q.
chicken noodle . .	62	3.1	9.2	1.4	14	127	m.q.
chicken rice	72	3.0	13.3	.5	6	117	.5 d
chicken vegetable, cream of	79	3.5	13.4	1.3	m.q.	714	m.q.
clam chowder . . .	94	1.7	9.6	5.4	0	66	n.a.
corn chowder . . .	148	4.0	22.1	4.7	n.a.	510	m.q.
onion	29	1.1	1.5	2.0	1	88	.1 d
potato	102	1.4	16.8	3.4	0	335	1.6 d
tomato Florentine	63	2.3	11.0	1.1	0	683	0
tomato vegetable	46	1.9	9.8	.3	0	314	.4 d
vegetable beef . .	82	3.5	14.1	1.5	5	1254	.3 d
entrees, 1 serving[1]:							
beef patty, light . .	289	20.7	0	22.9	82	187	0
chicken tenders . .	388	34.9	16.6	20.4	64	239	0
fish, baked	170	34.6	2.4	1.4	83	1641	0

[1] Does not include potato, bread, or salad bar.

Food and Measure	cal.	prot. (gms)	carbo. (gms)	fat (gms)	chol. (mgs)	sod. (mgs)	fiber (gms)
Shoney's, entrees *(cont.)*							
fish, fried, light . .	297	19.8	21.5	14.4	65	536	.1 d
Fish N'Chips, w/fries	639	32.3	50.4	34.8	103	873	2.9 d
Fish N'Shrimp . . .	487	28.1	36.5	25.5	127	644	.3 d
Italian feast	500	37.5	43.8	19.6	74	369	1.1 d
lasagna	297	8.3	44.9	9.8	26	870	2.8 d
Liver n'Onions . . .	411	34.9	15.4	22.9	529	321	.8 d
seafood platter . .	566	32.8	45.7	28.0	127	893	.3 d
shrimp, bite size . .	387	16.4	24.7	24.7	140	1266	0
shrimp, boiled . . .	93	19.6	0	1.0	182	210	0
shrimp, charbroiled	138	24.7	3.0	3.0	162	170	0
shrimp sampler . .	412	25.5	26.1	22.7	217	783	.1 d
Shrimper's Feast	383	16.5	29.9	22.2	125	216	.3 d
Shrimper's Feast, large	575	24.8	44.9	33.3	188	324	.4 d
spaghetti	496	24.2	63.4	16.3	55	387	2.2 d
steak, country fried	449	19.4	33.9	27.2	27	1177	.9 d
steak, rib eye, 8 oz.	605	35.2	0	50.5	141	211	0
steak, sirloin, 6 oz.	357	31.9	0	24.5	99	160	0
Steak N'Shrimp (fried shrimp) . .	507	36.5	15.0	32.7	150	249	.1 d
Steak N'Shrimp (charbroiled shrimp)	361	36.5	1.0	22.6	141	198	0
burgers:							
All-American	501	25.0	26.8	32.6	86	597	.5 d
bacon	591	28.7	28.6	40.0	86	801	.5 d
mushroom/Swiss	616	31.6	28.8	41.7	106	1135	.7 d
Old Fashioned . . .	470	25.1	25.6	28.2	82	681	.6 d
Shoney	498	23.4	22.2	35.7	79	782	.2 d
sandwiches:							
bacon & cheese, grilled	440	18.2	27.9	28.2	36	1200	1.3 d
cheese, grilled . . .	302	12.4	25.1	16.9	36	880	1.4 d
chicken, charbroiled	451	43.2	28.1	17.0	90	1002	.5 d
chicken fillet	464	29.7	38.9	21.2	51	585	.5 d
country fried	588	24.5	67.0	25.8	29	1501	1.4 d
fish	323	12.2	41.0	12.7	21	740	.4 d

Food and Measure	cal.	prot. (gms)	carbo. (gms)	fat (gms)	chol. (mgs)	sod. (mgs)	fiber (gms)
ham, baked	290	19.2	28.2	10.3	42	1263	1.8 d
ham club, whole wheat	642	37.0	45.2	35.5	78	2105	10.2 d
Patty Melt	640	38.8	29.5	41.7	121	826	6.7 d
Philly steak	673	31.8	37.2	44.0	103	1242	.1 d
Reuben	596	32.7	31.5	34.7	138	3873	6.3 d
Slim Jim	484	27.4	40.4	23.9	57	1620	.5 d
turkey club, whole wheat	635	43.5	44.1	32.7	100	1289	10.2 d
side dishes, 1 serving:							
Grecian bread . . .	80	2.0	13.2	2.2	0	94	m.q.
mushrooms, sauteed	75	1.6	4.3	6.5	0	968	1.3 d
onion rings, 1 piece	52	.9	5.0	3.1	2	102	.4 d
onions, sauteed . .	37	.8	4.3	2.1	0	221	.5 d
potato, baked, 10 oz.	264	5.6	61.1	.3	0	16	6.8 d
french fries, 3 oz.	189	2.9	28.9	7.5	0	273	2.7 d
french fries, 4 oz.	252	3.9	38.6	9.9	0	364	3.6 d
rice	137	2.4	23.1	3.7	1	765	.1 d
salads, prepared, 1/4 cup:							
ambrosia	75	.8	11.5	3.3	0	167	.8 d
apple grape surprise	19	0	4.9	0	0	2	.1 d
beet onion	25	.6	3.0	1.3	0	167	.8 d
broccoli/cauliflower	98	2.3	4.0	8.5	0	478	.9 d
broccoli/cauliflower/ carrot	53	1.1	2.7	4.4	1	193	.9 d
broccoli/cauliflower/ ranch	65	.9	1.6	6.4	9	12	.9 d
carrot apple	99	.6	4.2	9.1	8	10	.9 d
coleslaw	69	1.1	5.1	5.1	7	106	.9 d
cucumber lite . . .	12	.2	2.7	.1	0	344	.2 d
fruit, glacé	51	.3	12.9	.1	0	5	.5 d
fruit, mixed	37	.4	9.3	.1	0	3	.2 d
fruit delight	54	.6	10.1	1.6	0	2	.7 d
kidney bean	55	2.6	6.8	2.1	2	154	1.9 d
macaroni	207	4.2	17.0	13.9	14	382	.2 d

Food and Measure	cal.	prot. (gms)	carbo. (gms)	fat (gms)	chol. (mgs)	sod. (mgs)	fiber (gms)
Shoney's, salads (cont.)							
Oriental . . . . ·	79	.7	13.3	2.7	1	32	.5 d
pea	73	2.5	3.5	5.5	42	89	2.4 d
pistachio pineapple	98	.7	19.6	2.5	0	39	m.q.
pasta, Don's	82	1.8	8.6	4.6	0	223	.2 d
pasta, rotelli	78	1.4	8.9	4.0	0	82	.2 d
Seigan	72	2.3	8.1	3.6	5	122	1.2 d
snow	72	.6	9.0	4.1	0	18	.1 d
spaghetti	81	1.6	8.7	4.6	0	20	.2 d
spring	38	.8	2.4	2.9	0	162	.7 d
squash, mixed . . .	49	1.1	2.3	4.1	0	230	.3 d
summer	114	1.1	2.2	11.6	0	233	.9 d
three bean	96	1.4	11.9	5.1	0	189	1.3 d
vegetable, Italian	11	.4	2.5	.1	0	110	.7 d
Waldorf	81	.9	8.5	5.2	2	68	.8 d
dressings, 2 tbsp.:							
Biscayne, lo-cal . .	62	6.0	1.0	1.0	0	334	0
blue cheese	113	0	0	13.0	15	109	0
French	124	2.0	2.0	12.0	12	204	0
French, Rue	122	5.0	2.0	10.0	0	364	0
honey mustard . .	165	2.4	2.4	17.0	18	5	0
Italian, creamy . . .	135	0	1.0	15.0	0	454	0
Italian, golden . . .	141	0	1.0	15.0	0	302	0
Italian, W.W.	10	0	2.4	0	0	615	0
ranch	95	0	0	10.0	15	10	0
Thousand Island . .	130	1.0	2.0	13.0	12	179	0
sauces, 1 soufflé cup:							
BBQ	41	.1	8.2	1.0	0	232	0
cocktail	36	.4	8.7	.1	0	260	0
Sweet N'Sour . . .	58	0	14.7	0	0	5	0
tartar	84	.2	3.6	7.7	11	177	0
desserts, 1 serving:							
apple pie à la mode	492	6.0	67.0	23.0	35	574	m.q.
carrot cake	500	9.0	56.0	26.0	37	476	m.q.
hot fudge cake . .	522	7.4	81.9	19.7	27	485	m.q.
hot fudge sundae	451	7.0	60.0	22.0	60	226	0
strawberry pie . . .	332	2.1	44.5	16.7	0	247	2.3 d
strawberry sundae	380	6.0	47.7	19.0	69	145	.3 d

Food and Measure	cal.	prot. (gms)	carbo. (gms)	fat (gms)	chol. (mgs)	sod. (mgs)	fiber (gms)
walnut brownie à la mode	576	9.6	60.6	33.7	35	435	m.q.
Shortening, 1 tbsp.:							
lard and vegetable oil	115	0	0	12.8	m.q.	(0)	0
hydrogenated soybean and cottonseed or palm	113	0	0	12.8	0	(0)	0
vegetable, regular or butter flavor (Crisco)	110	0	0	12.0	0	0	0
Shrimp, meat only:							
raw, 4 oz.	120	23.0	1.0	2.0	173	168	0
raw, 4 large, 1 oz. . . .	30	5.7	.3	.5	43	42	0
boiled or steamed:							
4 oz.	112	23.7	n.a.	1.2	221	254	0
4 large	22	4.6	n.a.	.2	43	49	0
Shrimp, canned, drained, 1 cup . . .	154	29.6	1.3	2.5	222	216	0
"Shrimp," imitation, from surimi, 4 oz.	115	14.1	10.4	1.7	41	800	0
Shrimp cocktail:							
(Sau-Sea), 4-oz. jar	100	8.0	17.0	0	85	1010	3.0 d
(Sau-Sea), 6-oz. jar	150	11.0	26.0	0	120	1510	4.0 d
Shrimp dinner, frozen:							
Creole (Armour Classics Lite), 11.25 oz.	260	6.0	53.0	2.0	45	900	m.q.
marinara (Healthy Choice), 10.5 oz.	260	10.0	51.0	1.0	60	320	m.q.
Shrimp dinner mix, Creole (Luzianne), 1/5 pkg.	150	3.0	34.0	.5	<5	810	<1.0 d
Shrimp entree, canned, chow mein:							
(La Choy), 3/4 cup . .	35	4.0	4.0	1.0	50	940	2.0 d
(La Choy Bi-Pack), 3/4 cup	70	7.0	6.0	1.0	19	860	1.0 d

Food and Measure	cal.	prot. (gms)	carbo. (gms)	fat (gms)	chol. (mgs)	sod. (mgs)	fiber (gms)
Shrimp entree, frozen:							
breaded:							
(Gorton's Original), 5 pieces	210	7.0	17.0	13.0	65	390	m.q.
(Gorton's Microwave), 2 oz.	150	5.0	14.0	8.0	25	350	m.q.
(Mrs. Paul's Special Recipe), 5.5 oz.	300	19.0	34.0	10.0	120	850	m.q.
butter flavor *(Mrs. Paul's),* 5.5 oz.	320	20.0	26.0	15.0	125	800	m.q.
garlic and herb *(Mrs. Paul's),* 5.5 oz.	250	19.0	11.0	14.0	130	960	m.q.
Oriental seasoned *(Gorton's),* 5 pieces	170	7.0	16.0	9.0	55	420	m.q.
popcorn style *(Gorton's),* 2.7 oz. . . .	220	7.0	18.0	13.0	60	580	m.q.
scampi seasoned *(Gorton's),* 5 pieces	240	8.0	17.0	15.0	65	410	m.q.
marinara, w/linguine *(Weight Watchers Smart Ones),* 8 oz.	150	8.0	26.0	<1.0	60	390	m.q.
and okra gumbo *(Bodin's),* 4 oz.	54	4.0	8.0	0	18	117	1.0 d
Shrimp spice *(Tone's* Craboil), 1 tsp. . .	10	.3	1.2	.6	1	1	.3 d
Skipper's:							
thick cut cod:							
3 piece, fries . . .	665	27.0	68.0	32.0	38	1054	m.q.
4 piece, fries . . .	759	34.0	74.0	36.0	50	1388	m.q.
5 piece, fries . . .	853	42.0	80.0	41.0	62	1723	m.q.
famous fish fillets:							
1 fish, fries	558	17.0	51.0	28.0	55	408	m.q.
2 fish, fries	733	28.0	71.0	38.0	108	765	m.q.
3 fish, fries	908	39.0	82.0	48.0	160	1122	m.q.

Food and Measure	cal.	prot. (gms)	carbo. (gms)	fat (gms)	chol. (mgs)	sod. (mgs)	fiber (gms)
seafood combo							
1 fish, w/fries:							
shrimp	728	24.0	77.0	37.0	105	943	m.q.
jumbo shrimp . . .	720	24.0	75.0	36.0	91	1268	m.q.
clam strips	868	25.0	81.0	54.0	61	667	m.q.
oysters	885	25.0	95.0	44.0	80	809	m.q.
seafood basket							
w/fries:							
shrimp	723	20.0	82.0	36.0	102	1121	m.q.
jumbo shrimp . . .	707	20.0	79.0	35.0	73	911	m.q.
clam strips	1003	22.0	90.0	70.0	14	569	m.q.
oysters	1038	28.0	118.0	51.0	52	853	m.q.
Skipper's Platter . .	1038	32.0	97.0	63.0	111	1202	m.q.
chicken tenderloin							
strips w/fries:							
5 piece	793	44.0	69.0	38.0	77	798	m.q.
3 piece, 1 fish . . .	805	80.0	72.0	40.0	100	858	m.q.
3 piece, shrimp . .	800	36.0	77.0	39.0	97	1036	m.q.
salads & lite catch:							
2 fish, small salad	409	25.0	27.0	23.0	119	937	m.q.
3 chicken, small							
salad	305	26.0	17.0	15.0	58	673	m.q.
1 fish, 2 chicken,							
small salad . . .	399	29.0	24.0	21.0	96	880	m.q.
small salad	59	3.0	6.0	3.0	13	223	m.q.
shrimp and seafood							
salad	167	23.0	15.0	3.0	80	657	m.q.
Create A Catch:							
chicken sandwich	606	31.0	44.0	32.0	82	976	m.q.
chicken strip	82	8.0	4.0	4.0	15	150	m.q.
fish sandwich . . .	524	19.0	43.0	33.0	86	1191	m.q.
fish sandwich,							
double	698	30.0	54.0	73.0	139	1548	m.q.
fish fillet	175	11.0	11.0	10.0	53	357	m.q.
fries	383	6.0	50.0	18.0	<2	51	m.q.
clam chowder cup	100	3.0	14.0	3.5	12	525	m.q.
clam chowder pint	200	5.0	19.0	7.0	24	1050	m.q.
coleslaw, 5 oz. . .	289	2.0	10.0	27.0	50	329	m.q.

Food and Measure	cal.	prot. (gms)	carbo. (gms)	fat (gms)	chol. (mgs)	sod. (mgs)	fiber (gms)
Skipper's (cont.)							
condiments, 1 tbsp.:							
barbecue sauce . .	25	0	5.0	1.0	0	226	n.a.
cocktail sauce . . .	20	0	5.0	0	0	216	n.a.
tartar sauce	65	0	0	7.0	4	102	n.a.
salad dressing, 1 pkt.:							
blue cheese, pre-							
mium	222	1.0	4.0	23.0	8	240	n.a.
Italian, gourmet . .	140	0	2.0	15.0	0	200	n.a.
Italian, lo-cal	17	0	2.0	1.0	0	680	n.a.
ranch house	188	1.0	2.0	20.0	0	302	n.a.
Thousand Island . .	160	0	8.0	14.0	6	415	n.a.
Sloppy Joe sauce, see "Sandwich sauce"							
Smelt, rainbow, meat only:							
raw, 4 oz.	110	20.0	0	2.8	80	68	0
baked, broiled, or mi- crowaved, 4 oz. . .	141	25.6	0	3.5	102	87	0
Snack bar (see also "Granola and cereal bar"), all varieties, 1 bar:							
(Health Valley Fat Free Bakes)	75	2.0	17.0	0	0	60	2.5 d
(Health Valley Fat Free Fruit Bars)	140	3.0	33.0	<1.0	0	10	3.7 d
Snack chips (see also specific listings), 1 oz., except as noted:							
(Sunchips Original) . .	150	2.0	18.0	8.0	0	100	m.q.
cheddar:							
(Pepperidge Farm Swirl), 1/2 oz. . .	70	2.0	7.0	4.0	20	125	m.q.
(Sunchips Harvest Cheddar)	140	2.0	18.0	7.0	0	125	m.q.

Food and Measure	cal.	prot. (gms)	carbo. (gms)	fat (gms)	chol. (mgs)	sod. (mgs)	fiber (gms)
and jack *(Supremos)*	140	4.0	17.0	6.0	0	180	m.q.
onion:							
(Supremos Cool Onion)	140	4.0	17.0	6.0	0	170	m.q.
French *(Sunchips)*	140	3.0	18.0	7.0	0	120	m.q.
Snack mix, 1 oz.:							
(Doo Dads Original)	130	3.0	17.0	6.0	0	360	m.q.
(Flavor House Party Mix)	150	5.0	11.0	10.0	0	220	2.0 d
(Pepperidge Farm Classic)	140	4.0	14.0	8.0	0	360	1.0 d
(Pepperidge Farm Goldfish Party Mix)	140	4.0	16.0	7.0	0	380	1.0 d
(Ritz Traditional)	130	2.0	18.0	6.0	0	300	m.q.
cheddar, super *(Pepperidge Farm* Goldfish Party Mix)	140	4.0	15.0	7.0	15	330	1.0 d
cheese *(Ritz)*	130	2.0	18.0	6.0	0	350	m.q.
herb, zesty *(Pepperidge Farm)*	150	3.0	14.0	9.0	0	250	1.0 d
nutty *(Pepperidge Farm)*	150	3.0	15.0	8.0	0	180	2.0 d
smoked, lightly *(Pepperidge Farm)*	150	4.0	13.0	9.0	0	350	1.0 d
spicy *(Pepperidge Farm)*	140	4.0	14.0	8.0	0	340	1.0 d
Snail, sea, see "Whelk"							
Snapper, meat only:							
raw, 4 oz.	113	23.3	0	1.5	42	73	0
baked, broiled, or microwaved, 4 oz.	145	3.0	0	2.0	53	65	0
Snow peas, see "Peas, edible-podded"							

Food and Measure	cal.	prot. (gms)	carbo. (gms)	fat (gms)	chol. (mgs)	sod. (mgs)	fiber (gms)
Soft drinks and mixers (see also specific listings), 12 fl. oz., except as noted:							
all varieties, except diet *(Crush)*	200	<1.0	52.0	<1.0	0	80	0
apple:							
(Slice)	173	0	46.3	0	0	1	0
(Welch's Sparkling)	200	0	56.0	0	0	26	0
cherry *(Sundrop)* . . .	200	<1.0	46.0	<1.0	0	70	0
cherry, black *(Shasta)*	160	0	40.0	0	0	52	0
cherry cola:							
(Coca-Cola)	152	0	40.0	0	0	8	0
(Shasta)	148	0	37.0	0	0	47	0
cherry-lime *(Spree)*	176	0	44.0	0	0	24	0
citrus mist *(Shasta)*	192	0	48.0	0	0	48	0
club soda:							
(Schweppes)	0	0	0	0	0	100	0
(Shasta)	0	0	0	0	0	68	0
cola:							
(Coca-Cola Classic)	144	0	38.0	0	0	14	0
(Coke II)	154	0	40.0	0	0	8	0
(R.W. Knudsen) . .	140	<1.0	33.0	<1.0	0	m.q.	0
(Pepsi Regular/Free)	157	0	40.8	0	0	0	0
(Shasta/Shasta Caffeine Free)	160	0	40.0	0	0	24	0
(Shasta Low Sodium)	108	0	26.0	0	0	16	0
(Spree)	176	0	44.0	0	0	24	0
collins mixer *(Schweppes)*	140	<1.0	36.0	<1.0	0	80	0
cream:							
(A&W), 1 fl. oz. . .	15	<.1	3.8	<.1	0	2	0
(Hires)	180	<1.0	48.0	<1.0	0	80	0
(I.B.C.)	180	0	42.0	0	0	30	0
(Mug)	184	0	47.3	0	0	31	0
(Shasta Creme) . .	164	0	41.0	0	0	47	0

Food and Measure	cal.	prot. (gms)	carbo. (gms)	fat (gms)	chol. (mgs)	sod. (mgs)	fiber (gms)
vanilla (Crush) . . .	180	<1.0	44.0	<1.0	0	80	0
(Dr. Diablo)	156	0	39.0	0	0	38	0
(Dr Pepper Regular/ Free)	156	0	39.6	0	0	18	0
fruit punch:							
(Minute Maid) . . .	172	0	44.0	0	0	28	0
(Welch's Sparkling)	210	0	53.0	0	0	28	0
ginger ale:							
(Fanta)	126	0	32.0	0	0	28	0
(R.W. Knudsen) . .	155	<1.0	37.0	<1.0	0	m.q.	0
(R.W. Knudsen Organic)	155	1.0	36.0	<1.0	0	m.q.	0
(Schweppes)	140	<1.0	34.0	<1.0	0	70	0
(Shasta)	132	0	33.0	0	0	47	0
(Shasta Low Sodium)	89	0	22.0	0	0	28	0
(Spree)	132	0	33.0	0	0	24	0
raspberry (R.W. Knudsen)	140	1.0	32.0	<1.0	0	m.q.	0
raspberry (Schweppes)	160	<1.0	38.0	<1.0	0	70	0
ginger beer (Schweppes)	140	<1.0	36.0	<1.0	0	110	0
grape:							
(Fanta)	172	0	44.0	0	0	14	0
(Minute Maid) . . .	178	0	46.0	0	0	12	0
(Schweppes)	200	<1.0	48.0	<1.0	0	80	0
(Shasta)	176	0	44.0	0	0	58	0
(Welch's Sparkling)	200	0	51.0	0	0	38	0
grapefruit:							
(Schweppes)	160	<1.0	40.0	<1.0	0	110	0
(Spree)	176	0	44.0	0	0	24	0
(Wink), 8 fl. oz. . . .	120	0	30.0	0	0	19	0
kiwi-strawberry (Shasta)	176	0	44.0	0	0	44	0
lemon, bitter (Schweppes)	160	<1.0	42.0	<1.0	0	69	0

Food and Measure	cal.	prot. (gms)	carbo. (gms)	fat (gms)	chol. (mgs)	sod. (mgs)	fiber (gms)
Soft drinks and mixers *(cont.)*							
lemon sour *(Schweppes)*	160	<1.0	38.0	<1.0	0	80	0
lemon-lime:							
(Schweppes)	140	<1.0	38.0	<1.0	0	110	0
(Shasta)	148	0	37.0	0	0	78	0
(Shasta Low Sodium)	100	0	24.0	0	0	16	0
(Slice)	150	0	38.6	0	0	16	0
(Spree)	172	0	43.0	0	0	24	0
lemon tangerine *(Spree)*	188	0	47.0	0	0	24	0
lime:							
Mandarin *(Spree)*	176	0	44.0	0	0	24	0
tropical *(R.W. Knudsen)*	120	1.0	40.0	1.0	0	m.q.	0
(Mello Yello)	174	0	44.0	0	0	28	0
mineral water, sparkling, all flavors *(A Santé)*, 10 fl. oz. . . .	0	0	0	0	0	48	0
(Mountain Dew) . . .	178	0	44.4	0	0	31	0
(Mr. Pibb)	142	0	38.0	0	0	20	0
orange:							
(Fanta)	176	0	46.0	0	0	14	0
(Minute Maid) . . .	174	0	44.0	0	0	<1	0
(Shasta)	184	0	46.0	0	0	52	0
(Welch's Sparkling)	200	0	51.0	0	0	25	0
mandarin *(Slice)* . .	192	0	50.0	0	0	16	0
peach:							
(Shasta)	176	0	44.0	0	0	52	0
(Welch's Sparkling)	220	0	52.0	0	0	10	0
pineapple:							
(Shasta)	212	0	53.0	0	0	42	0
(Welch's Sparkling)	210	0	53.0	0	0	52	0
pineapple-orange *(Shasta)*	188	0	47.0	0	0	44	0
pop, red *(Shasta)* . .	176	0	44.0	0	0	44	0

Food and Measure	cal.	prot. (gms)	carbo. (gms)	fat (gms)	chol. (mgs)	sod. (mgs)	fiber (gms)
raspberry creme							
(Shasta)	180	0	45.0	0	0	44	0
root beer:							
(A&W), 1 fl. oz. . .	15	<.1	3.8	<.1	0	3	0
(Fanta)	156	0	40.0	0	0	20	0
(Hires)	180	<1.0	46.0	<1.0	0	110	0
(I.B.C.)	168	0	42.0	0	0	16	0
(Mug)	211	0	42.8	0	0	38	0
(Ramblin')	176	0	46.0	0	0	34	0
(Shasta)	160	0	40.0	0	0	52	0
(Spree)	172	0	43.0	0	0	24	0
seltzer, all flavors							
(Schweppes)	0	0	0	0	0	0	0
(7Up)	156	0	36.3	0	0	32	0
(7Up Cherry)	148	0	38.7	0	0	32	0
(Slice Red)	192	0	49.8	0	0	16	0
(Sprite)	142	0	36.0	0	0	46	0
spritzer:							
apple (R.W. Knud-sen)	165	<1.0	42.0	<1.0	0	m.q.	0
boysenberry (R.W. Knudsen)	160	<1.0	41.0	<1.0	0	m.q.	0
cherry, black (R.W. Knudsen)	120	<1.0	31.0	<1.0	0	15	0
cranberry (R.W. Knudsen)	120	<1.0	25.0	<1.0	0	15	0
grape (R.W. Knud-sen)	120	<1.0	28.0	<1.0	0	22	0
grape, Concord (R.W. Knudsen)	135	<1.0	35.0	<1.0	0	m.q.	0
lemon-lime (R.W. Knudsen)	120	<1.0	30.0	<1.0	0	30	0
lemonade, Jamaican (R.W. Knudsen)	150	<1.0	36.0	<1.0	0	m.q.	0
lime, mandarin (R.W. Knudsen)	120	<1.0	31.0	<1.0	0	m.q.	0
orange (R.W. Knud-sen)	150	1.0	37.0	1.0	0	m.q.	0

Food and Measure	cal.	prot. (gms)	carbo. (gms)	fat (gms)	chol. (mgs)	sod. (mgs)	fiber (gms)
Soft drinks and mixers, spritzer *(cont.)*							
orange–passion-fruit *(R.W. Knudsen)*	140	<1.0	36.0	<1.0	0	m.q.	0
peach *(R.W. Knudsen)*	150	<1.0	38.0	<1.0	0	m.q.	0
raspberry, red *(R.W. Knudsen)*	145	<1.0	37.0	<1.0	0	m.q.	0
strawberry *(R.W. Knudsen)*	120	<1.0	30.0	<1.0	0	26	0
tangerine *(R.W. Knudsen)*	130	<1.0	34.0	<1.0	0	30	0
tangerine-orange *(R.W. Knudsen)*	150	<1.0	39.0	<1.0	0	m.q.	0
tango mango *(R.W. Knudsen)*	90	<1.0	24.0	<1.0	0	m.q.	0
(Squirt), 1 fl. oz. . . .	13	<.1	3.2	<.1	0	2	0
strawberry:							
(Minute Maid) . . .	180	0	46.0	0	0	12	0
(Shasta)	152	0	38.0	0	0	77	0
(Welch's Sparkling)	200	0	51.0	0	0	26	0
strawberry-peach *(Shasta)*	172	0	43.0	0	0	44	0
(Sundrop)	200	<1.0	46.0	<1.0	0	70	0
tonic:							
(Schweppes)	140	<1.0	34.0	<1.0	0	60	0
(Shasta)	128	0	32.0	0	0	41	0
tropical blend *(Spree)*	160	0	40.0	0	0	24	0
(Vernors), 1 fl. oz. . .	12	<.1	2.8	<.1	0	1	0
Sole:							
fresh, see "Flatfish"							
frozen *(Van de Kamp's Natural),* 4 oz. . . .	100	22.0	0	2.0	35	105	0
Sole dinner, frozen:							
au gratin *(Healthy Choice),* 11 oz. . .	270	16.0	40.0	5.0	55	470	m.q.

Food and Measure	cal.	prot. (gms)	carbo. (gms)	fat (gms)	chol. (mgs)	sod. (mgs)	fiber (gms)
Sole entree, frozen:							
breaded:							
(Mrs. Paul's Light), 4.25 oz.	240	16.0	20.0	10.0	50	450	m.q.
(Van de Kamp's Light), 1 piece . .	250	17.0	18.0	12.0	45	480	m.q.
country herb *(Gorton's)*, 2 pieces . .	110	20.0	<1.0	3.0	75	340	0
w/lemon butter sauce *(Healthy Choice)*, 8.25 oz.	230	16.0	33.0	4.0	45	430	m.q.
seafood stuffed *(Gorton's)*, 1 piece . . .	170	18.0	17.0	3.0	55	730	m.q.
Sorbet (see also "Sherbet" and "Ice"):							
orange, mandarin *(Dole)*, 4 oz.	110	.5	28.0	.1	0	9	n.a.
orange, and vanilla ice cream *(Häagen-Dazs)*, 1/2 cup . . .	200	3.0	30.0	8.0	60	30	n.a.
peach *(Dole)*, 4 oz.	120	.6	28.0	.6	0	11	n.a.
pineapple *(Dole)*, 4 oz.	120	.5	28.0	.1	0	11	n.a.
raspberry:							
(Dole), 4 oz.	110	.4	28.0	<.1	0	12	n.a.
(Frusen Glädjé), 1/2 cup	140	0	36.0	0	0	10	n.a.
and vanilla ice cream *(Häagen-Dazs)*, 1/2 cup . .	180	3.0	26.0	7.0	60	30	n.a.
strawberry *(Dole)*, 4 oz.	110	.5	28.0	.1	0	11	n.a.
bar, orange, and cream *(Häagen-Dazs)*, 1 bar	130	2.0	18.0	6.0	40	25	m.q.
Sorghum, whole-grain, 1 cup	650	21.7	143.3	6.3	0	n.a.	4.6 c

Food and Measure	cal.	prot. (gms)	carbo. (gms)	fat (gms)	chol. (mgs)	sod. (mgs)	fiber (gms)
Sorghum syrup:							
¹/₂ cup	479	0	123.7	0	0	13	0
1 tbsp.	61	0	15.7	0	0	2	0
Sorrel, see "Dock"							
Soufflé see specific listings							
Soup, canned, ready-to-serve, 9.5 oz., except as noted:							
bean:							
(Grandma Brown's), 1 cup	190	9.0	30.9	3.4	<1	700	9.8 d
w/bacon'n ham *(Campbell's* Microwave), 8 oz.	200	9.0	31.0	5.0	m.q.	790	m.q.
w/ham *(Campbell's* Chunky Old Fashioned), 9.65 oz.	260	13.0	33.0	8.0	m.q.	970	m.q.
and ham *(Campbell's* Home Cookin')	180	12.0	26.0	3.0	m.q.	850	m.q.
and ham *(Healthy Choice),* 7.5 oz.	220	12.0	35.0	4.0	5	480	m.q.
and ham *(Hormel Hearty),* 7.5 oz.	190	9.0	29.0	4.0	23	640	m.q.
bean, black:							
(Hain 99% Fat Free)	120	10.0	29.0	1.0	0	620	10.5 d
(Progresso Hearty)	140	9.0	33.0	2.0	<5	820	11.0 d
and carrots *(Health Valley* Fat Free), 7.5 oz.	70	9.0	9.0	<1.0	0	290	17.0 d
beef:							
(Campbell's Chunky)	180	13.0	21.0	5.0	m.q.	1000	m.q.
(Progresso)	160	13.0	15.0	5.0	30	760	m.q.
hearty *(Healthy Choice),* 7.5 oz.	120	9.0	17.0	1.0	20	580	m.q.
beef barley *(Progresso)*	130	12.0	15.0	4.0	30	870	4.0 d

Food and Measure	cal.	prot. (gms)	carbo. (gms)	fat (gms)	chol. (mgs)	sod. (mgs)	fiber (gms)
beef broth:							
(Health Valley Natural Fat Free),							
6.9 oz.	10	1.0	2.0	<1.0	0	290	0
(Swanson), 7.25 oz.	18	2.0	1.0	1.0	m.q.	750	0
beef minestrone (Progresso)	160	13.0	16.0	5.0	30	910	m.q.
beef noodle:							
(Campbell's Chunky)	180	24.0	8.0	6.0	m.q.	900	m.q.
(Progresso)	160	15.0	17.0	4.0	35	1020	m.q.
beef Stroganoff style (Campbell's Chunky), 10.75-oz. can	320	16.0	28.0	16.0	m.q.	1200	m.q.
beef vegetable:							
(Hormel Hearty), 7.5 oz.	90	6.0	15.0	1.0	5	730	m.q.
(Progresso)	140	14.0	14.0	3.0	30	820	m.q.
chunky (Healthy Choice), 7.5 oz.	110	10.0	14.0	1.0	20	490	m.q.
and pasta (Campbell's Home Cookin')	120	11.0	15.0	2.0	m.q.	920	m.q.
borscht, 1 cup:							
(Gold's)	100	4.0	21.0	0	0	1280	m.q.
w/beets (Manischewitz)	80	1.0	20.0	0	0	660	m.q.
low calorie (Gold's)	20	1.0	5.0	<1.0	0	1160	m.q.
low calorie (Manischewitz)	20	1.0	4.0	0	0	725	m.q.
chickarina (Progresso)	130	8.0	13.0	5.0	20	820	m.q.
chicken:							
(Campbell's Chunky Old Fashioned)	150	11.0	18.0	4.0	m.q.	1040	m.q.
(Progresso Homestyle)	110	10.0	11.0	3.0	20	790	m.q.
hearty (Healthy Choice), 7.5 oz.	150	9.0	17.0	5.0	35	530	m.q.

Food and Measure	cal.	prot. (gms)	carbo. (gms)	fat (gms)	chol. (mgs)	sod. (mgs)	fiber (gms)
Soup, canned, ready-to-serve, chicken *(cont.)*							
hearty *(Progresso)*	130	12.0	11.0	4.0	25	1000	m.q.
chicken barley							
(Progresso), 9.25 oz.	110	10.0	14.0	3.0	20	790	4.0 d
chicken broth:							
(Campbell's Low							
Sodium), 10.5 oz.	30	3.0	2.0	1.0	m.q.	85	n.a.
(Hain), 9 oz.	30	2.0	0	3.0	5	950	0
(Hain No Salt), 9 oz.	45	3.0	2.0	3.0	<5	105	n.a.
(Health Valley Fat							
Free), 7.5 oz. . .	20	4.0	1.0	<1.0	0	290	n.a.
(Swanson), 7.25 oz.	30	2.0	2.0	2.0	m.q.	900	n.a.
clear *(Swanson* Nat-							
ural Goodness),							
7.25 oz.	20	2.0	1.0	1.0	m.q.	580	n.a.
chicken corn chowder							
(Campbell's Chunky)	270	11.0	19.0	17.0	m.q.	1020	m.q.
chicken gumbo,							
w/sausage *(Camp-*							
bell's Home Cookin')*	110	9.0	13.0	3.0	m.q.	950	m.q.
chicken minestrone:							
(Campbell's Home							
Cookin')	150	12.0	14.0	5.0	m.q.	790	m.q.
(Progresso)	130	11.0	13.0	4.0	20	860	m.q.
chicken mushroom,							
creamy *(Campbell's*							
Chunky), 9.4 oz. . .	250	10.0	12.0	18.0	m.q.	1130	m.q.
chicken noodle:							
(Campbell's Chunky)	170	12.0	16.0	6.0	m.q.	940	m.q.
(Campbell's Chunky							
Classic)	140	10.0	17.0	4.0	m.q.	960	m.q.
(Campbell's Home							
Cookin')	110	11.0	10.0	3.0	m.q.	1010	m.q.
(Campbell's Low							
Sodium),							
10.75 oz.	170	13.0	17.0	5.0	m.q.	90	m.q.
(Campbell's Micro-							
wave), 7.75 oz.	90	5.0	10.0	3.0	m.q.	1090	m.q.

Food and Measure	cal.	prot. (gms)	carbo. (gms)	fat (gms)	chol. (mgs)	sod. (mgs)	fiber (gms)
(Hain), 8 oz.	110	8.0	11.0	4.0	20	800	m.q.
(Hain No Salt), 8 oz.	100	7.0	9.0	4.0	20	75	m.q.
(Healthy Choice Old Fashioned), 7.5 oz.	90	5.0	9.0	3.0	20	520	m.q.
(Hormel Hearty), 7.5 oz.	110	7.0	14.0	3.0	18	690	m.q.
(Progresso)	90	11.0	9.0	2.0	25	870	m.q.
(Progresso Healthy Classics), 8 oz.	80	7.0	10.0	2.0	15	460	m.q.
hearty (Campbell's Healthy Request), 8 oz.	80	9.0	7.0	2.0	25	470	m.q.
and vegetable (Healthy Choice), 7.5 oz.	160	12.0	18.0	4.0	45	500	m.q.
chicken nuggets w/vegetables and noodles (Campbell's Chunky)	180	9.0	22.0	6.0	m.q.	920	m.q.
chicken w/rice: (Campbell's Chunky)	140	10.0	16.0	4.0	m.q.	1040	m.q.
(Campbell's Home Cookin')	150	8.0	21.0	4.0	m.q.	890	m.q.
(Campbell's Microwave), 7.75 oz.	110	3.0	15.0	4.0	m.q.	1030	m.q.
(Healthy Choice), 7.5 oz.	140	5.0	18.0	4.0	15	510	m.q.
(Hormel Hearty), 7.5 oz.	110	5.0	17.0	2.0	6	890	m.q.
(Progresso)	120	8.0	14.0	3.0	20	800	m.q.
hearty (Campbell's Healthy Request), 8 oz.	110	7.0	15.0	3.0	10	480	m.q.
w/vegetables (Progresso Healthy Classics), 8 oz.	80	7.0	11.0	2.0	10	440	m.q.

Food and Measure	cal.	prot. (gms)	carbo. (gms)	fat (gms)	chol. (mgs)	sod. (mgs)	fiber (gms)
Soup, canned, ready-to-serve, chicken w/rice *(cont.)*							
wild rice *(Progresso)*	120	6.0	17.0	3.0	20	850	m.q.
chicken vegetable:							
(Campbell's Chunky)	170	10.0	20.0	6.0	m.q.	1040	m.q.
(Campbell's Home Cookin')	160	9.0	22.0	4.0	m.q.	850	m.q.
(Hain), 8 oz.	110	7.0	13.0	3.0	10	790	m.q.
(Hain No Salt), 8 oz.	100	7.0	12.0	3.0	10	85	m.q.
(Progresso)	130	9.0	16.0	3.0	20	820	m.q.
hearty *(Campbell's* Healthy Request), 8 oz.	120	7.0	16.0	3.0	10	420	m.q.
chili beef:							
(Campbell's Chunky), 9.75 oz.	260	18.0	33.0	6.0	m.q.	960	m.q.
(Campbell's Microwave), 8 oz. . . .	190	7.0	32.0	4.0	m.q.	870	m.q.
clam chowder, Manhattan:							
(Campbell's Chunky)	150	7.0	22.0	4.0	m.q.	990	m.q.
(Progresso)	120	13.0	13.0	2.0	10	800	m.q.
clam chowder, New England:							
(Campbell's Chunky)	260	8.0	23.0	15.0	m.q.	1070	m.q.
(Campbell's Home Cookin')	230	7.0	13.0	16.0	m.q.	1090	m.q.
(Campbell's Microwave), 7.75 oz.	200	5.0	15.0	13.0	m.q.	890	m.q.
(Hormel Hearty), 7.5 oz.	130	5.0	16.0	5.0	30	790	m.q.
(Progresso), 9.25 oz.	190	6.0	18.0	11.0	15	930	m.q.
hearty *(Campbell's* Healthy Request), 8 oz.	100	4.0	14.0	3.0	10	490	m.q.
corn chowder *(Progresso)*, 9.25 oz.	200	5.0	22.0	10.0	10	840	m.q.

Food and Measure	cal.	prot. (gms)	carbo. (gms)	fat (gms)	chol. (mgs)	sod. (mgs)	fiber (gms)
corn and vegetable, country (Health Valley Fat Free), 7.5 oz.	70	4.0	13.0	<1.0	0	290	3.0 d
Creole style (Campbell's Chunky) . . .	230	11.0	29.0	8.0	n.a.	780	m.q.
escarole in chicken broth (Progresso), 9.25 oz.	30	2.0	2.0	1.0	<5	1100	m.q.
gazpacho, 1 cup . . .	57	8.7	.8	2.2	0	1183	3.7 d
ham and bean (Progresso)	130	11.0	26.0	3.0	15	990	10.0 d
ham and butter bean (Campbell's Chunky), 10.75-oz. can	280	13.0	34.0	10.0	m.q.	1170	m.q.
lentil:							
(Progresso)	130	10.0	24.0	2.0	0	840	7.0 d
(Progresso Healthy Classics), 8 oz.	120	7.0	19.0	1.0	0	420	m.q.
and carrots (Health Valley Fat Free), 7.5 oz.	70	8.0	10.0	<1.0	0	290	15.0 d
hearty (Campbell's Home Cookin')	140	9.0	25.0	1.0	n.a.	840	m.q.
w/sausage (Progresso) . . .	170	8.0	21.0	8.0	20	840	5.0 d
vegetarian (Hain 99% Fat Free) . .	150	9.0	25.0	1.0	0	740	5.5 d
vegetarian (Hain 99% Fat Free No Salt)	140	11.0	22.0	1.0	0	60	5.5 d
macaroni and bean (Progresso)	140	8.0	25.0	5.0	0	1070	6.5 d
minestrone:							
(Campbell's Chunky)	160	6.0	24.0	4.0	n.a.	860	m.q.
(Campbell's Home Cookin')	120	4.0	21.0	3.0	n.a.	1080	m.q.
(Hain)	160	7.0	26.0	3.0	0	930	m.q.

Food and Measure	cal.	prot. (gms)	carbo. (gms)	fat (gms)	chol. (mgs)	sod. (mgs)	fiber (gms)
Soup, canned, ready-to-serve, minestrone *(cont.)*							
(Hain No Salt) . . .	160	7.0	26.0	4.0	0	75	m.q.
(Health Valley),							
7.5 oz.	120	4.0	18.0	3.0	0	80	5.8 d
(Healthy Choice),							
7.5 oz.	160	6.0	30.0	2.0	0	520	m.q.
(Hormel Hearty),							
7.5 oz.	100	5.0	17.0	1.0	5	460	m.q.
(Progresso)	120	7.0	21.0	3.0	0	910	7.0 d
(Progresso Healthy							
Classics), 8 oz.	120	4.0	19.0	2.0	0	490	m.q.
hearty *(Campbell's*							
Healthy Request),							
8 oz.	90	4.0	13.0	2.0	2	420	m.q.
hearty *(Progresso),*							
9.25 oz.	90	7.0	16.0	2.0	<5	760	4.0 d
real Italian *(Health*							
Valley Fat Free),							
7.5 oz.	80	6.0	12.0	<1.0	0	230	4.0 d
zesty *(Progresso)*	150	7.0	19.0	8.0	10	1130	4.0 d
mushroom, cream of:							
(Campbell's Low							
Sodium), 10.5 oz.	210	3.0	18.0	14.0	n.a.	55	m.q.
(Progresso), 9.25 oz.	160	4.0	14.0	10.0	15	1120	m.q.
mushroom barley							
(Hain 99% Fat Free)	90	4.0	14.0	2.0	5	640	m.q.
pea, split:							
(Campbell's Low							
Sodium),							
10.75 oz.	230	12.0	37.0	4.0	n.a.	30	m.q.
(Grandma Brown's),							
1 cup	208	11.7	31.0	4.1	<1	522	5.8 d
and carrots *(Health*							
Valley Fat Free),							
7.5 oz.	80	9.0	17.0	<1.0	0	290	12.5 d
green *(Progresso)*	160	11.0	27.0	3.0	<5	1050	5.0 d
w/ham *(Campbell's*							
Chunky)	210	11.0	29.0	5.0	m.q.	950	m.q.

Food and Measure	cal.	prot. (gms)	carbo. (gms)	fat (gms)	chol. (mgs)	sod. (mgs)	fiber (gms)
w/ham (Campbell's Home Cookin')	190	13.0	29.0	2.0	m.q.	1040	m.q.
and ham (Healthy Choice), 7.5 oz.	170	10.0	25.0	3.0	10	460	m.q.
w/ham (Progresso)	140	10.0	22.0	5.0	15	930	6.0 d
vegetarian (Hain 99% Fat Free) . .	160	12.0	30.0	1.0	0	820	4.0 d
vegetarian (Hain 99% Fat Free No Salt)	150	13.0	27.0	1.0	0	70	4.0 d
pepper steak (Campbell's Chunky) . . .	160	13.0	21.0	3.0	m.q.	930	m.q.
schav (Gold's), 8 oz.	25	2.0	4.0	0	15	1380	n.a.
sirloin burger (Campbell's Chunky) . . .	210	11.0	21.0	9.0	m.q.	1050	m.q.
steak and potato (Campbell's Chunky)	180	13.0	21.0	5.0	m.q.	990	m.q.
tomato: (Progresso)	90	4.0	18.0	2.0	0	1120	4.0 d
garden (Campbell's Home Cookin')	140	3.0	24.0	3.0	n.a.	800	m.q.
garden (Healthy Choice), 7.5 oz.	130	4.0	22.0	3.0	5	510	m.q.
w/tomato pieces (Campbell's Low Sodium), 10.5 oz.	190	4.0	30.0	6.0	n.a.	45	m.q.
tomato beef, w/rotini (Progresso)	160	12.0	17.0	5.0	25	910	m.q.
tomato tortellini (Progresso), 9.25 oz.	130	5.0	16.0	5.0	10	1040	m.q.
tomato vegetable (Health Valley Fat Free), 7.5 oz. . . .	50	5.0	8.0	<1.0	0	290	3.0 d
tortellini: (Progresso)	80	5.0	12.0	2.0	5	870	2.0 d
creamy (Progresso), 9.25 oz.	240	5.0	17.0	16.0	35	910	m.q.

Food and Measure	cal.	prot. (gms)	carbo. (gms)	fat (gms)	chol. (mgs)	sod. (mgs)	fiber (gms)
Soup, canned, ready-to-serve (cont.)							
turkey rice, 8 oz.:							
(Hain)	80	7.0	8.0	3.0	15	820	m.q.
(Hain No Salt) . . .	100	6.0	11.0	3.0	10	65	m.q.
turkey vegetable (Campbell's Chunky), 9.4 oz. . . .	160	10.0	16.0	6.0	m.q.	1050	m.q.
vegetable:							
(Campbell's Chunky)	150	4.0	25.0	4.0	n.a.	960	m.q.
(Campbell's Microwave), 7.75 oz.	100	3.0	17.0	2.0	n.a.	910	m.q.
(Progresso)	90	3.0	19.0	1.0	<5	810	3.0 d
(Progresso Healthy Classics), 8 oz.	80	4.0	13.0	1.0	5	450	m.q.
country (Campbell's Home Cookin')	130	4.0	25.0	2.0	n.a.	760	m.q.
country (Healthy Choice), 7.5 oz.	120	3.0	23.0	1.0	0	540	m.q.
country (Hormel Hearty), 7.5 oz.	90	4.0	14.0	2.0	2	730	m.q.
14 garden (Health Valley Fat Free), 7.5 oz.	50	4.0	9.0	<1.0	0	260	3.0 d
5 bean (Health Valley Fat Free), 7.5 oz.	100	8.0	14.0	<1.0	0	260	3.0 d
hearty (Campbell's Healthy Request), 8 oz.	90	3.0	17.0	3.0	0	480	m.q.
Mediterranean (Campbell's Chunky)	170	5.0	24.0	6.0	n.a.	940	m.q.
vegetarian (Hain)	150	4.0	22.0	4.0	0	790	m.q.
vegetarian (Hain No Salt)	150	5.0	23.0	5.0	0	80	m.q.
vegetable barley (Health Valley Fat Free), 7.5 oz. . . .	60	4.0	11.0	<1.0	0	270	4.0 d

Food and Measure	cal.	prot. (gms)	carbo. (gms)	fat (gms)	chol. (mgs)	sod. (mgs)	fiber (gms)
vegetable beef:							
(Campbell's Chunky Old Fashioned)	170	11.0	18.0	6.0	m.q.	970	m.q.
(Campbell's Home Cookin')	120	11.0	15.0	2.0	m.q.	1020	m.q.
(Campbell's Micro-wave), 7.75 oz.	100	7.0	14.0	2.0	m.q.	930	m.q.
(Healthy Choice), 7.5 oz.	130	8.0	21.0	1.0	15	530	m.q.
chunky (Campbell's Low Sodium), 10.75 oz.	180	14.0	19.0	5.0	m.q.	90	m.q.
hearty (Campbell's Healthy Request), 8 oz.	120	8.0	17.0	2.0	15	460	m.q.
vegetable broth, vege-tarian, 9.25 oz.:							
(Hain 99% Fat Free)	40	1.0	8.0	0	0	690	n.a.
(Hain 99% Fat Free No Salt)	40	1.0	9.0	0	0	95	n.a.
vegetable w/pasta (Progresso Hearty)	100	5.0	22.0	1.0	0	830	4.0 d
wild rice (Hain 99% Fat Free)	80	3.0	16.0	2.0	0	770	3.0 d
Soup, canned, con-densed*[1], 8 oz., ex-cept as noted:							
asparagus, cream of:							
(Campbell's)	120	2.0	10.0	8.0	5	820	m.q.
(Campbell's)[2] . . .	170	5.0	15.0	10.0	10	870	m.q.
barley and bean (Rokeach), 1 cup	90	5.0	15.0	1.5	0	740	5.0 d
bean (Campbell's Home-style)	130	5.0	25.0	1.0	5	700	6.0 d

[1] Prepared with water, except as noted.

[2] Prepared with 2% lowfat milk.

Food and Measure	cal.	prot. (gms)	carbo. (gms)	fat (gms)	chol. (mgs)	sod. (mgs)	fiber (gms)
Soup, canned, condensed, bean (cont.)							
w/bacon (Campbell's)	130	7.0	22.0	4.0	5	780	6.0 d
w/bacon (Campbell's Healthy Request)	150	6.0	22.0	4.0	5	470	6.0 d
beef:							
(Campbell's)	80	5.0	10.0	2.0	10	830	m.q.
broth or bouillon (Campbell's) . . .	14	2.0	1.0	0	5	820	n.a.
consommé (Campbell's)	25	4.0	2.0	0	5	750	n.a.
beef noodle:							
(Campbell's)	60	4.0	7.0	2.0	15	840	m.q.
(Campbell's Homestyle)	90	6.0	8.0	4.0	20	810	m.q.
broccoli, cream of:							
(Campbell's)	80	1.0	8.0	5.0	5	680	m.q.
(Campbell's)[1] . . .	140	5.0	14.0	7.0	10	740	m.q.
broccoli cheese (Campbell's)	110	2.0	9.0	7.0	n.a.	800	m.q.
celery, cream of (Campbell's)	100	2.0	8.0	7.0	5	820	m.q.
cheese:							
cheddar (Campbell's)	130	3.0	10.0	8.0	15	750	n.a.
nacho (Campbell's)	110	4.0	8.0	8.0	15	740	n.a.
nacho (Campbell's)[2]	160	7.0	11.0	10.0	20	800	n.a.
chicken, cream of:							
(Campbell's)	110	2.0	9.0	7.0	15	820	n.a.
(Campbell's Healthy Request)	70	2.0	11.0	2.0	10	490	n.a.
chicken alphabet (Campbell's)	70	3.0	10.0	2.0	10	800	m.q.

[1] Prepared with 2% lowfat milk.

[2] Prepared with whole milk.

Food and Measure	cal.	prot. (gms)	carbo. (gms)	fat (gms)	chol. (mgs)	sod. (mgs)	fiber (gms)
chicken barley *(Campbell's)*	70	3.0	10.0	2.0	5	850	m.q.
chicken broth:							
(Campbell's)	30	1.0	2.0	2.0	5	710	n.a.
and noodles *(Campbell's)*	60	2.0	8.0	2.0	10	870	m.q.
chicken 'n dumplings *(Campbell's)*	80	4.0	9.0	3.0	25	950	m.q.
chicken gumbo *(Campbell's)*	50	2.0	8.0	1.0	5	890	m.q.
chicken mushroom, creamy *(Campbell's)*	120	3.0	10.0	8.0	15	920	m.q.
chicken noodle:							
(Campbell's)	60	2.0	8.0	2.0	10	870	m.q.
(Campbell's Healthy Request)	60	2.0	8.0	2.0	10	460	m.q.
(Campbell's Homestyle)	60	3.0	8.0	2.0	10	880	m.q.
(Campbell's Noodle-O's)	70	3.0	9.0	2.0	10	860	m.q.
double noodle *(Campbell's)*	90	4.0	13.0	2.0	m.q.	700	m.q.
chicken w/pasta *(Campbell's* Souperstars)	70	2.0	11.0	2.0	5	850	m.q.
chicken w/rice:							
(Campbell's)	60	2.0	8.0	2.0	5	770	m.q.
(Campbell's Healthy Request)	60	2.0	7.0	3.0	10	480	m.q.
chicken and stars *(Campbell's)*	60	3.0	9.0	2.0	5	830	m.q.
chicken vegetable *(Campbell's)*	70	3.0	11.0	2.0	10	820	m.q.
chili beef *(Campbell's)*	150	6.0	21.0	5.0	10	820	m.q.
clam chowder, Manhattan:							
(Campbell's)	70	2.0	11.0	2.0	0	820	m.q.

Food and Measure	cal.	prot. (gms)	carbo. (gms)	fat (gms)	chol. (mgs)	sod. (mgs)	fiber (gms)
Soup, canned, condensed, clam chowder, Manhattan *(cont.)*							
(Doxsee/Snow's), 7.5 oz.	70	3.0	11.0	2.0	<5	780	m.q.
clam chowder, New England:							
(Campbell's)	80	4.0	11.0	2.0	5	880	m.q.
(Campbell's)[1] . . .	130	7.0	17.0	3.0	10	940	m.q.
(Gorton's), 1/4 can[2]	140	7.0	17.0	5.0	20	740	m.q.
(Doxsee/Snow's), 7.5 oz.	70	5.0	8.0	2.0	10	620	m.q.
corn, golden:							
(Campbell's)	110	2.0	18.0	3.0	5	700	m.q.
(Campbell's)[1] . . .	160	6.0	23.0	5.0	10	760	m.q.
minestrone *(Campbell's)*	80	3.0	13.0	2.0	5	890	m.q.
mushroom:							
beefy *(Campbell's)*	60	4.0	5.0	3.0	5	930	m.q.
golden *(Campbell's)*	70	2.0	9.0	3.0	5	850	m.q.
mushroom, cream of:							
(Campbell's)	100	2.0	9.0	7.0	5	800	m.q.
(Campbell's Healthy Request)	60	1.0	9.0	2.0	5	480	m.q.
noodles:							
and ground beef *(Campbell's)* . . .	90	4.0	10.0	4.0	20	820	m.q.
curly, w/chicken *(Campbell's)* . . .	70	2.0	11.0	2.0	15	800	m.q.
onion, French *(Campbell's)*	60	2.0	9.0	2.0	5	890	m.q.
onion, cream of:							
(Campbell's)	100	2.0	12.0	5.0	15	830	m.q.
(Campbell's)[3] . . .	140	4.0	15.0	7.0	25	860	m.q.
oyster stew:							
(Campbell's)	80	2.0	6.0	5.0	15	840	m.q.

[1] *Prepared with 2% lowfat milk.*
[2] *Prepared with whole milk.*
[3] *Prepared with equal parts 2% lowfat milk and water.*

Food and Measure	cal.	prot. (gms)	carbo. (gms)	fat (gms)	chol. (mgs)	sod. (mgs)	fiber (gms)
(Campbell's)[1] . . .	130	6.0	10.0	7.0	20	900	m.q.
pea:							
green (Campbell's)	150	8.0	25.0	3.0	5	800	4.0 d
split (Rokeach),							
1 cup	80	6.0	13.0	.5	0	820	4.0 d
split, w/ham and ba-							
con (Campbell's)	160	9.0	24.0	3.0	5	760	4.0 d
pepper pot (Camp-							
bell's)	90	5.0	9.0	4.0	25	970	m.q.
potato, cream of:							
(Campbell's)	80	1.0	12.0	3.0	10	840	m.q.
(Campbell's)[2] . . .	120	3.0	15.0	4.0	20	900	m.q.
Scotch broth (Camp-							
bell's)	80	4.0	9.0	3.0	10	870	m.q.
shrimp, cream of:							
(Campbell's)	90	2.0	8.0	6.0	20	810	m.q.
(Campbell's)[3] . . .	140	5.0	13.0	10.0	20	870	m.q.
tomato:							
(Campbell's)	90	1.0	17.0	2.0	0	670	m.q.
(Campbell's)[3] . . .	140	5.0	22.0	4.0	10	730	m.q.
(Campbell's Healthy							
Request)	90	1.0	17.0	2.0	0	410	m.q.
(Campbell's Healthy							
Request)[3]	140	5.0	22.0	3.0	5	490	m.q.
(Rokeach), 1 cup	50	2.0	9.0	1.0	0	680	2.0 d
bisque (Campbell's)	120	1.0	22.0	3.0	0	820	m.q.
Italian (Campbell's)	90	1.0	21.0	2.0	n.a.	740	m.q.
zesty (Campbell's)	90	1.0	21.0	2.0	n.a.	760	m.q.
tomato, cream of:							
(Campbell's Home-							
style)	110	1.0	19.0	2.0	5	730	m.q.
(Campbell's Home-							
style[1]	180	5.0	25.0	7.0	15	860	m.q.

[1] Prepared with whole milk.
[2] Prepared with equal parts 2% lowfat milk and water.
[3] Prepared with 2% lowfat milk.

Food and Measure	cal.	prot. (gms)	carbo. (gms)	fat (gms)	chol. (mgs)	sod. (mgs)	fiber (gms)
Soup, canned, condensed *(cont.)*							
tomato rice:							
(Campbell's Old							
Fashioned) . . .	110	1.0	22.0	2.0	0	720	m.q.
(Rokeach), 1 cup	90	2.0	21.0	0	0	582	2.0 d
turkey noodle *(Campbell's)*	70	3.0	9.0	2.0	15	880	m.q.
turkey vegetable							
(Campbell's)	70	3.0	9.0	2.0	10	770	m.q.
vegetable:							
(Campbell's)	90	3.0	14.0	2.0	5	830	m.q.
(Campbell's Dinosaur)	100	4.0	18.0	2.0	5	670	m.q.
(Campbell's Healthy							
Request)	90	3.0	14.0	2.0	5	500	m.q.
(Campbell's Homestyle)	60	2.0	9.0	2.0	0	880	m.q.
(Campbell's Old							
Fashioned) . . .	60	2.0	9.0	2.0	5	870	m.q.
(Rokeach), 1 cup	60	2.0	13.0	0	0	542	3.0 d
vegetable beef:							
(Campbell's)	70	5.0	9.0	2.0	5	740	m.q.
(Campbell's Healthy							
Request)	70	5.0	9.0	2.0	5	490	m.q.
vegetable, vegetarian							
(Campbell's)	80	2.0	13.0	2.0	0	790	m.q.
wonton *(Campbell's)*	40	3.0	5.0	1.0	15	850	m.q.
Soup, frozen							
(Tabatchnick),							
7.5 oz., except as							
noted:							
barley and bean . . .	130	6.0	22.0	2.0	0	760	m.q.
bean, northern	164	8.0	29.0	2.0	0	510	m.q.
broccoli, cream of . .	90	4.0	10.0	4.0	5	600	m.q.
cabbage	110	2.0	21.0	2.0	0	390	m.q.
chicken	65	2.0	10.0	2.0	0	540	n.a.
lentil	170	11.0	27.0	2.0	0	670	m.q.
minestrone	145	8.0	24.0	2.0	0	600	m.q.

Food and Measure	cal.	prot. (gms)	carbo. (gms)	fat (gms)	chol. (mgs)	sod. (mgs)	fiber (gms)
mushroom, cream of, 6 oz.	75	3.0	11.0	2.0	3	1000	m.q.
mushroom barley . .	100	2.0	16.0	2.0	0	690	m.q.
mushroom barley, no salt	97	4.0	18.0	1.0	0	165	m.q.
New England chowder	98	6.0	14.0	2.0	4	540	m.q.
pea	175	10.0	31.0	1.0	0	615	m.q.
pea, no salt	175	10.0	31.0	1.0	0	170	m.q.
potato	95	2.0	19.0	1.0	0	690	m.q.
spinach, cream of . .	85	5.0	12.0	2.0	4	425	m.q.
tomato rice, 6 oz. . . .	73	2.0	14.0	1.0	0	950	m.q.
vegetable	97	4.0	18.0	1.0	0	400	m.q.
vegetable, no salt . .	92	2.0	16.0	2.0	0	165	m.q.
zucchini, cream of 6 oz.	80	3.0	12.0	2.0	3	640	m.q.
Soup base *(Soup Starter),* 1/8 mix:							
beef barley	80	3.0	17.0	<1.0	0	800	m.q.
beef vegetable	90	3.0	18.0	<1.0	0	790	m.q.
chicken noodle . . .	70	3.0	14.0	<1.0	0	720	m.q.
chicken and rice . . .	70	2.0	14.0	<1.0	0	730	m.q.
Soup mix*:							
barley:							
better *(Aunt Patsy's Pantry),* 8 oz. . .	208	14.0	46.0	6.0	29	377	5.0 d
vegetable *(Fantastic Bouncin'),* 10 oz.	180	7.0	38.0	1.0	0	480	8.0 d
bean:							
black *(Fantastic Jumpin' Black Beans),* 10 oz. . . .	170	12.0	40.0	1.0	0	490	13.0 d
black *(Knorr Cup-a-Soup),* 1 serving	200	11.3	37.8	.8	0	680	m.q.
many *(Aunt Patsy's Pantry),* 8 oz.	125	7.0	24.0	1.0	n.a.	157	4.0 d

Food and Measure	cal.	prot. (gms)	carbo. (gms)	fat (gms)	chol. (mgs)	sod. (mgs)	fiber (gms)
Soup mix, bean *(cont.)*							
navy *(Aunt Patsy's Pantry)*, 8 oz. . .	224	20.0	24.0	5.0	30	942	3.0 d
navy *(Knorr* Cup-a-Soup), 1 serving	140	7.3	26.9	.5	0	870	m.q.
7, and barley *(Arrowhead Mills)*, 1 oz. dry	90	6.0	19.0	<1.0	0	0	12.5 d
broccoli:							
in cheddar *(Fantastic Dancin' Broccoli)*, 10 oz.	120	7.0	18.0	2.0	6	480	2.0 d
and cheese *(Lipton Cup-a-Soup)*, 6 fl. oz.	70	2.0	10.0	3.0	5	550	1.0 d
cheddar, creamy, w/noodles *(Fantastic Noodles)*, 7 oz. . .	178	7.0	21.0	8.0	n.a.	578	m.q.
chicken flavor:							
creamy *(Lipton Cup-a-Soup)*, 6 fl. oz.	80	<1.0	12.0	3.0	0	700	m.q.
supreme *(Lipton Cup-a-Soup Hearty)*, 6 fl. oz.	80	<1.0	12.0	3.0	0	700	m.q.
thyme *(Aunt Patsy's Pantry)*, 8 oz. . .	122	12.0	17.0	1.0	22	266	2.0 d
chicken noodle:							
(Campbell's Quality Soup & Recipe), 1 cup	100	5.0	16.0	2.0	n.a.	700	m.q.
(Lipton Hearty), 1 cup	80	5.0	14.0	1.0	n.a.	790	m.q.
(Lipton Cup-a-Soup Hearty), 6 fl. oz.	70	3.0	12.0	1.0	15	630	m.q.
(Mrs. Grass Homestyle), 1 cup . . .	70	3.0	11.0	1.0	n.a.	760	m.q.

Food and Measure	cal.	prot. (gms)	carbo. (gms)	fat (gms)	chol. (mgs)	sod. (mgs)	fiber (gms)
w/white meat (Campbell's Cup 2 Minute Soup), .7 oz. dry	80	4.0	11.0	2.0	m.q.	890	n.a.
chicken rice:							
(Lipton Cup-a-Soup), 6 fl. oz.	45	2.0	8.0	<1.0	5	620	m.q.
(Mrs. Grass), 1 cup	60	1.0	12.0	1.0	0	780	m.q.
chicken vegetable:							
(Lipton Cup-a-Soup), 6 fl. oz.	60	2.0	10.0	<1.0	10	560	m.q.
creamy (Lipton Cup-a-Soup), 1 pouch	100	2.0	12.0	5.0	0	690	1.0 d
clam chowder, Manhattan (Golden Dipt), 1/4 pkg. dry	80	2.0	13.0	2.0	3	700	n.a.
clam chowder, New England (Golden Dipt), 1/4 pkg. dry	24	2.0	12.0	2.0	2	680	n.a.
corn and potato chowder (Fantastic Jammin'), 10 oz. . .	180	8.0	34.0	2.0	4	490	2.0 d
herb, savory, w/garlic (Lipton Recipe Secrets), 1 cup . .	35	<1.0	7.0	<1.0	0	490	m.q.
lentil:							
(Fantastic Laughin' Lentils), 10 oz.	230	15.0	42.0	2.0	0	480	12.0 d
(Knorr Cup-a-Soup), 1 serving	220	13.1	40.4	.5	0	900	m.q.
red (Aunt Patsy's Pantry), 8 oz.	99	6.0	19.0	1.0	n.a.	254	3.0 d
lobster bisque (Golden Dipt), 1/4 pkg. dry	30	1.0	5.0	1.0	2	560	n.a.

Food and Measure	cal.	prot. (gms)	carbo. (gms)	fat (gms)	chol. (mgs)	sod. (mgs)	fiber (gms)
Soup mix *(cont.)*							
minestrone:							
(Manischewitz),							
6 fl. oz.	50	3.0	9.0	<1.0	n.a.	160	m.q.
w/pasta *(Fantastic*							
Seradin'), 10 oz.	190	9.0	38.0	2.0	2	480	5.0 d
mushroom:							
beef *(Lipton Recipe*							
Secrets), 1 cup	35	1.0	7.0	n.a.	n.a.	810	m.q.
cream of *(Fantastic*							
Marchin' Cream of							
Mushroom),							
10 oz.	90	4.0	14.0	2.0	2	480	2.0 d
creamy *(Lipton*							
Cup-a-Soup),							
6 fl. oz.	70	<1.0	10.0	3.0	0	670	<1.0 d
noodle:							
(Campbell's Quality							
Soup & Recipe),							
1 cup	110	4.0	20.0	2.0	n.a.	740	m.q.
(Lipton), 1 cup . . .	80	4.0	12.0	2.0	n.a.	810	m.q.
(Lipton Cup-a-Soup							
Ring Noodle),							
6 fl. oz.	60	2.0	10.0	<1.0	5	620	m.q.
beef *(Campbell's*							
Cup Microwave),							
1.35 oz. dry . . .	140	6.0	25.0	2.0	n.a.	1330	m.q.
beef *(Campbell's*							
Ramen), 1.25 oz.							
dry	140	4.0	27.0	2.0	2	430	m.q.
beef *(Campbell's*							
Ramen Block),							
1.5 oz. dry . . .	160	5.0	32.0	1.0	n.a.	890	m.q.
beef *(La Choy),*							
1 cup	225	6.0	33.0	8.0	0	865	4.0 d
beef *(Maruchan* In-							
stant Lunch),							
2.25 oz. dry . . .	290	7.0	37.0	14.5	0	1030	m.q.

Food and Measure	cal.	prot. (gms)	carbo. (gms)	fat (gms)	chol. (mgs)	sod. (mgs)	fiber (gms)
beef (Maruchan Instant Picante), 2.25 oz. dry . . .	290	7.0	37.0	14.5	0	950	3.0 d
beef (Maruchan Ramen Supreme), 1.5 oz. dry . . .	190	4.0	26.0	8.5	<1	770	m.q.
beef, w/vegetables (Campbell's Cup-A-Ramen), 1 cup	270	6.0	38.0	10.0	n.a.	1530	m.q.
cheddar, creamy (Fantastic Noodles), 7 oz. . . .	186	6.0	18.0	10.0	8	495	2.5 d
chicken (Campbell's Cup Microwave), 1.35 oz. dry . . .	140	7.0	24.0	2.0	n.a.	1370	m.q.
chicken (Campbell's Ramen), 1.25 oz. dry	140	4.0	27.0	2.0	2	420	m.q.
chicken (Campbell's Ramen Block), 1.5 oz. dry . . .	160	5.0	32.0	1.0	n.a.	940	m.q.
chicken (La Choy), 1 cup	200	6.0	29.0	7.0	0	740	4.0 d
chicken (Maruchan Instant Lunch), 2.25 oz. dry . . .	290	7.0	35.0	15.5	<5	1050	m.q.
chicken (Maruchan Instant Picante), 2.25 oz. dry . . .	290	7.0	38.0	14.0	5	920	3.0 d
chicken (Maruchan Ramen Supreme), 1.5 oz. dry . . .	190	4.0	25.0	8.5	<1	780	m.q.
w/chicken broth (Campbell's Cup Microwave), 1.35 oz. dry . . .	140	6.0	25.0	2.0	n.a.	1400	m.q.

Food and Measure	cal.	prot. (gms)	carbo. (gms)	fat (gms)	chol. (mgs)	sod. (mgs)	fiber (gms)
Soup mix, noodle (cont.)							
w/chicken broth (Campbell's Cup 2 Minute Soup), 1.35 oz. dry . . .	90	4.0	15.0	2.0	n.a.	950	m.q.
w/real chicken broth (Lipton), 1 cup	60	2.0	10.0	1.0	m.q.	710	m.q.
w/real chicken broth (Lipton Ring-O-Noodle), 1 cup	70	2.0	11.0	2.0	m.q.	710	m.q.
w/chicken broth (Mrs. Grass), 1 cup	70	2.0	10.0	2.0	n.a.	900	m.q.
chicken, w/vegetables (Campbell's Cup-A-Ramen), 2.2 oz. dry . . .	270	6.0	38.0	10.0	n.a.	1470	m.q.
chili (Maruchan Ramen Supreme), 1.5 oz. dry . . .	190	4.0	26.0	8.5	n.a.	710	m.q.
curry vegetable (Fantastic Noodles), 7 oz. . . .	180	5.0	22.0	8.0	0	435	3.2 d
double (Campbell's Quality Soup & Recipe), 1 cup	200	8.0	36.0	2.0	n.a.	770	m.q.
hearty (Campbell's Quality Soup & Recipe), 1 cup	90	4.0	15.0	1.0	n.a.	980	m.q.
hearty, w/vegetables (Campbell's Cup Microwave), 1.7 oz. dry . . .	180	7.0	32.0	2.0	n.a.	1310	m.q.
hearty, w/vegetables (Lipton), 1 cup	80	3.0	12.0	2.0	n.a.	690	m.q.
miso vegetable (Fantastic Noodles), 7 oz. . . .	172	5.0	20.0	8.0	0	495	3.0 d

Food and Measure	cal.	prot. (gms)	carbo. (gms)	fat (gms)	chol. (mgs)	sod. (mgs)	fiber (gms)
mushroom *(Maruchan* Instant Lunch), 2.25 oz. dry	290	6.0	37.0	14.0	0	1170	m.q.
mushroom *(Maruchan* Ramen Supreme), 1.5 oz. dry	190	4.0	25.0	8.5	0	910	m.q.
Oriental *(Campbell's* Ramen), 1.25 oz. dry	140	4.0	27.0	2.0	2	440	m.q.
Oriental *(Campbell's* Ramen Block), 1.5 oz. dry . . .	150	5.0	31.0	1.0	n.a.	940	m.q.
Oriental *(Maruchan* Ramen Supreme), 1.5 oz. dry . . .	190	4.0	26.0	8.5	0	860	m.q.
Oriental, w/vegetables *(Campbell's* Cup-A-Ramen), 2.2 oz. dry . . .	270	6.0	38.0	10.0	n.a.	1210	m.q.
pork *(Campbell's* Ramen), 1.25 oz. dry	140	4.0	27.0	2.0	2	450	m.q.
pork *(Campbell's* Ramen Block), 1.5 oz. dry . . .	140	4.0	27.0	2.0	n.a.	450	m.q.
pork *(Maruchan* Instant Lunch), 2.25 oz. dry . . .	290	7.0	37.0	14.5	0	1240	m.q.
pork *(Maruchan* Ramen Supreme), 1.5 oz. dry . . .	190	4.0	25.0	9.0	<1	980	m.q.
shrimp *(Maruchan* Instant Lunch), 2.25 oz. dry . . .	290	7.0	36.0	15.0	5	940	m.q.

Food and Measure	cal.	prot. (gms)	carbo. (gms)	fat (gms)	chol. (mgs)	sod. (mgs)	fiber (gms)
Soup mix, noodle *(cont.)*							
shrimp *(Maruchan Instant Picante)*, 2.25 oz. dry . . .	300	7.0	36.0	15.5	5	1120	4.0 d.
shrimp *(Maruchan Ramen Supreme)*, 1.5 oz. dry . . .	190	4.0	26.0	8.5	<1	820	m.q.
shrimp, w/vegetables *(Campbell's Cup-A-Ramen)*, 2.2 oz. dry . . .	280	6.0	40.0	10.0	n.a.	1190	m.q.
tomato vegetable *(Fantastic Noodles)*, 7 oz. . . .	188	5.0	24.0	8.0	0	434	3.2 d
vegetable, California *(Maruchan Instant Picante)*, 2.25 oz. dry	280	7.0	37.0	14.0	0	1220	4.0 d
vegetable beef *(Maruchan Instant Lunch)*, 2.25 oz. dry	290	7.0	37.0	14.0	0	1250	m.q.
vegetable curry *(Fantastic Noodles)*, 7 oz. . . .	150	5.0	18.0	7.0	n.a.	472	m.q.
whole wheat *(Fantastic Rockin' ABC's)*, 10 oz.	130	6.0	24.0	1.0	0	460	4.0 d
onion:							
(Campbell's Quality Soup & Recipe), 1 cup	30	1.0	7.0	1.0	n.a.	650	m.q.
(Lipton Recipe Secrets), 1 cup	20	<1.0	4.0	0	0	630	m.q.
(Mrs. Grass Soup & Dip Mix), .4 oz. dry	35	1.0	6.0	<1.0	0	1070	m.q.

Food and Measure	cal.	prot. (gms)	carbo. (gms)	fat (gms)	chol. (mgs)	sod. (mgs)	fiber (gms)
beefy (Lipton Recipe Secrets), 1 cup	30	<1.0	5.0	<1.0	0	640	m.q.
golden (Lipton Recipe Secrets), 1 cup	60	1.0	11.0	1.0	n.a.	730	m.q.
mushroom (Lipton Recipe Secrets), 1 cup	60	1.0	11.0	1.0	n.a.	730	m.q.
mushroom (Mrs. Grass Soup & Dip Mix), .6 oz. dry	60	2.0	10.0	1.0	0	1120	m.q.
pea:							
green (Lipton Cup-a-Soup), 6 fl. oz.	110	3.0	17.0	4.0	0	660	2.0 d
plentiful (Aunt Patsy's Pantry), 8 oz.	135	10.0	24.0	1.0	n.a.	363	6.0 d
split (Fantastic Splittin' Peas), 10 oz.	145	13.0	31.0	1.0	0	490	3.0 d
split (Manischewitz), 6 fl. oz.	45	3.0	9.0	<1.0	0	320	m.q.
Virginia (Lipton Cup-a-Soup), 6 fl. oz.	150	4.0	21.0	5.0	0	700	3.0 d
potato leek (Knorr Cup-a-Soup), 1 serving	120	4.1	24.2	.4	0	970	m.q.
seafood chowder (Golden Dipt),1/4 pkg. dry	70	2.0	12.0	2.0	2	730	m.q.
shrimp bisque (Golden Dipt), 1/4 pkg. dry	30	1.0	5.0	1.0	2	570	m.q.
tomato:							
(Lipton Cup-a-Soup), 6 fl. oz.	110	2.0	21.0	3.0	0	520	1.0 d
basil (Knorr), 1 serving	80	2.0	14.1	2.2	0	840	m.q.

Food and Measure	cal.	prot. (gms)	carbo. (gms)	fat (gms)	chol. (mgs)	sod. (mgs)	fiber (gms)
Soup mix, tomato *(cont.)*							
herb *(Lipton Recipe Secrets)*, 1 cup	50	<1.0	12.0	<1.0	0	490	m.q.
vegetable:							
(Campbell's Quality Soup & Recipe), 1 cup	40	1.0	8.0	0	n.a.	710	m.q.
(Lipton Recipe Secrets), 1 cup	35	1.0	7.0	n.a.	0	680	m.q.
(Manischewitz), 6 fl. oz.	50	3.0	9.0	<1.0	0	65	m.q.
(Mrs. Grass Soup & Dip Mix), .4 oz. dry	35	1.0	7.0	<1.0	0	930	m.q.
country *(Lipton Cook Up)*, 1 cup	70	2.0	13.0	1.0	0	790	2.0 d
harvest *(Lipton Cup-a-Soup Hearty)*, 6 fl. oz.	100	2.0	19.0	2.0	0	510	2.0 d
miso, w/noodles *(Fantastic Noodles)*, 7 oz. . . .	152	5.0	19.0	7.0	n.a.	434	m.q.
spring *(Lipton Cup-a-Soup)*, 6 fl. oz.	50	2.0	9.0	<1.0	5	520	<1.0 d
tomato, w/noodles *(Fantastic Noodles)*, 7 oz. . . .	158	5.0	20.0	7.0	n.a.	434	m.q.
vegetable beef *(Mrs. Grass)*, 1 cup . . .	60	3.0	10.0	1.0	0	930	m.q.
wonton, 1.49 oz. dry, except as noted:							
beef *(Maruchan)*, .68 oz. dry . . .	90	2.0	8.0	5.0	n.a.	890	m.q.
chicken *(Maruchan)*, .67 oz. dry . . .	90	2.0	8.0	5.0	n.a.	810	m.q.
chicken *(Maruchan* Instant)	200	5.0	19.0	12.0	n.a.	1440	m.q.

Food and Measure	cal.	prot. (gms)	carbo. (gms)	fat (gms)	chol. (mgs)	sod. (mgs)	fiber (gms)
Oriental (Maruchan Instant)	190	5.0	19.0	11.5	n.a.	1340	m.q.
pork (Maruchan), .68 oz. dry . . .	90	2.0	9.0	5.0	n.a.	930	m.q.
pork (Maruchan Instant)	200	5.0	19.0	12.0	n.a.	1450	m.q.
shrimp (Maruchan Instant)	200	6.0	19.0	12.0	n.a.	1120	m.q.
vegetable (Maruchan), .7 oz. dry	90	2.0	9.0	5.5	n.a.	980	m.q.
Sour cream, see "Cream, sour"							
Sour cream sauce mix (McCormick/ Schilling), 1/4 pkg.	44	1.3	4.0	2.8	n.a.	272	n.a.
Soursop, 1/2 cup . .	75	1.1	18.9	.3	0	16	3.7 d
Souse loaf:							
(Jesse Jones), 2 oz.	150	6.0	2.0	13.0	m.q.	790	0
(Kahn's), 1 slice . . .	90	4.0	1.0	7.0	m.q.	190	0
Soy beverage:							
(EdenSoy Original), 8.45 fl. oz.	140	10.0	14.0	4.0	0	120	n.a.
(Soy Moo Fat Free), 8 fl. oz.	110	7.0	19.0	0	0	25	0
carob (EdenSoy), 8.45 fl. oz.	160	6.0	30.0	5.0	0	125	n.a.
vanilla (EdenSoy), 8.45 fl. oz.	150	6.0	25.0	2.0	0	120	n.a.
mix* (Soyagen), 1/4 cup:							
all purpose	130	6.0	14.0	6.0	0	150	m.q.
carob	140	6.0	16.0	6.0	0	160	m.q.
no sucrose	130	6.0	14.0	6.0	0	210	m.q.
Soy flour:							
(Arrowhead Mills), 2 oz.	250	20.0	18.0	11.0	0	1	8.1 d
stirred, 1 cup:							
full fat, raw	371	29.4	29.9	17.6	0	11	8.2 d

Food and Measure	cal.	prot. (gms)	carbo. (gms)	fat (gms)	chol. (mgs)	sod. (mgs)	fiber (gms)
Soy flour, stirred, 1 cup *(cont.)*							
full fat, roasted . .	375	29.6	28.6	18.6	0	11	1.9 c
defatted	329	47.0	38.4	1.2	0	20	17.5 d
lowfat	287	40.9	33.4	2.4	0	16	9.0 d
Soy meal, defatted,							
raw, 1 cup	414	54.8	49.0	2.9	0	3	14.0 d
Soy milk:							
fluid, 8 fl. oz.	79	6.6	4.3	4.6	0	30	3.1 d
powder *(Soyamel)*,							
1 oz.	130	6.0	11.0	7.0	0	150	m.q.
Soy nuggets *(Love*							
Natural Foods),							
2 oz.	220	28.0	20.0	3.0	0	9	m.q.
Soy protein, concen-							
trate, 1 oz.:							
w/alcohol	94	16.5	8.8	.1	0	1	1.1 c
acid/water wash . . .	94	16.5	8.8	.1	0	255	1.1 c
Soy sauce, 1/2 tsp.,							
except as noted:							
(La Choy)	2	<1.0	<1.0	<1.0	0	230	<1.0 d
(La Choy Lite)	1	<1.0	<1.0	<1.0	0	110	<1.0 d
tamari, 1 tbsp.	11	1.9	1.0	<.1	0	1005	.1 d
tamari *(Eden)*	2	0	0	0	0	160	0
shoyu, 1 tbsp.	9	.9	1.5	tr.	0	1029	.1 d
shoyu *(Eden/Eden*							
Naturally Brewed)	2	0	0	0	0	140	0
shoyu *(Eden* Reduced							
Sodium)	2	0	0	0	0	80	0
Soybean, 1/2 cup:							
green:							
raw, shelled	188	16.6	14.1	8.7	0	n.a.	5.4 d
boiled, drained . .	127	11.1	10.0	5.8	0	n.a.	3.8 d
dry:							
raw	387	33.9	28.1	18.5	0	2	8.6 d
raw *(Arrowhead*							
Mills), 2 oz. . . .	230	19.0	19.0	10.0	0	2	13.2 d
boiled	149	14.3	8.5	7.7	0	1	5.2 d
dry-roasted	387	34.0	28.1	18.6	0	2	7.0 d

Food and Measure	cal.	prot. (gms)	carbo. (gms)	fat (gms)	chol. (mgs)	sod. (mgs)	fiber (gms)
roasted	405	30.3	28.9	21.8	0	140	4.0 c
Soybean, fermented, see "Miso" and "Natto"							
Soybeam, sprouted:							
raw, 1/2 cup	45	4.6	3.9	2.3	0	5	.8 c
steamed, 1/2 cup . .	38	4.0	3.1	2.1	0	5	.4 d
Soybean cake or curd, see "Tofu"							
Soybean flakes *(Arrowhead Mills)*, 2 oz.	250	20.0	18.0	11.0	0	2	8.1 d
Soybean kernels, roasted, toasted:							
1 oz. or 95 kernels	129	10.5	8.7	6.8	0	1	1.0 d
whole, 1 cup	490	40.0	33.0	25.9	0	4	3.9 d
salted, whole, 1 cup	490	40.0	33.0	25.9	0	176	3.9 d
Spaghetti, see "Pasta"							
Spaghetti dinner, and meatballs, frozen *(Swanson)*, 12.5 oz.	280	10.0	35.0	11.0	m.q.	1090	m.q.
Spaghetti dishes, mix*, 1 cup, except as noted:							
(Kraft American Dinner)	300	10.0	50.0	7.0	0	630	m.q.
w/meat sauce *(Kraft* Dinner)	360	12.0	47.0	14.0	15	880	m.q.
tangy *(Kraft* Italian Style Dinner)	310	11.0	49.0	8.0	5	670	m.q.
whole wheat *(Fantastic All-O-Round Spaghetti)*, 10 oz. . . .	200	8.0	40.0	1.0	2	490	5.0 d

Food and Measure	cal.	prot. (gms)	carbo. (gms)	fat (gms)	chol. (mgs)	sod. (mgs)	fiber (gms)
Spaghetti entree, canned or packaged, 7.5 oz., except as noted:							
in tomato sauce:							
w/cheese (Franco-American), 7.35 oz.	180	5.0	35.0	2.0	n.a.	840	m.q.
and cheese sauce (Franco-American SpaghettiO's) . .	160	4.0	31.0	2.0	n.a.	880	m.q.
w/franks (Franco-American SpaghettiO's), 7.35 oz.	210	8.0	26.0	8.0	m.q.	1000	m.q.
w/meat sauce:							
(Healthy Choice) . .	150	10.0	21.0	3.0	20	390	m.q.
(Hormel Top Shelf), 10 oz.	260	14.0	37.0	6.0	20	980	m.q.
w/meatballs:							
(Franco-American), 7.35 oz.	220	9.0	28.0	8.0	m.q.	870	m.q.
(Franco-American SpaghettiO's), 7.35 oz.	210	9.0	25.0	8.0	m.q.	940	m.q.
(Hormel Micro Cup)	210	10.0	27.0	7.0	20	930	m.q.
(Libby's Diner), 7.75 oz.	190	10.0	31.0	3.0	15	870	m.q.
rings (Healthy Choice)	140	5.0	30.0	0	0	460	m.q.
Spaghetti entree, freeze-dried,							
w/meat and sauce (Mountain House), 1 cup*	220	10.0	27.0	8.0	m.q.	940	m.q.

Food and Measure	cal.	prot. (gms)	carbo. (gms)	fat (gms)	chol. (mgs)	sod. (mgs)	fiber (gms)
Spaghetti entree, frozen:							
(Dining Lite), 9 oz. . .	220	12.0	25.0	8.0	20	440	m.q.
w/meat sauce:							
(Banquet Entree Express), 8.5 oz. . . .	220	11.0	35.0	4.0	m.q.	1180	m.q.
(Healthy Choice Quick Meal), 10 oz.	280	14.0	42.0	6.0	20	480	m.q.
(Lean Cuisine), 11.5 oz.	290	15.0	45.0	6.0	20	500	m.q.
(Stouffer's), 12⁷/8 oz.	320	16.0	38.0	12.0	m.q.	560	m.q.
(Weight Watchers), 10 oz.	240	16.0	28.0	7.0	5	490	m.q.
w/meatballs:							
(Stouffer's), 12⁵/8 oz.	440	22.0	53.0	16.0	m.q.	960	m.q.
and sauce *(Lean Cuisine)*, 9.5 oz. .	290	20.0	36.0	7.0	30	550	m.q.
w/tomato and meat sauce *(The Budget Gourmet* Light and Healthy), 10 oz. . .	300	18.0	44.0	8.0	35	470	m.q.
Spaghetti sauce, see "Pasta sauce"							
Spaghetti sauce seasoning mix *(French's):*							
Italian, 1/5 pkg.	20	0	5.0	0	0	360	n.a.
mushroom, 1/5 pkg.	20	0	4.0	0	0	810	n.a.
thick, 1/6 pkg.	18	0	4.0	0	0	640	n.a.
Spaghetti squash:							
raw, strands *(Frieda's)*, 1 oz.	6	.3	2.8	m.q.	0	<1	m.q.
baked or boiled, drained, 1/2 cup . .	23	.5	5.0	.2	0	14	1.1 d
Spareribs, see "Pork"							

Food and Measure	cal.	prot. (gms)	carbo. (gms)	fat (gms)	chol. (mgs)	sod. (mgs)	fiber (gms)
Spelt:							
flakes *(Arrowhead Mills)*, 1 oz.	100	4.0	21.0	1.0	0	60	3.0 d
flour *(Arrowhead Mills)*, 2 oz.	170	7.0	40.0	1.0	0	0	8.0 d
Spice loaf, 1 slice:							
(Kahn's Family Pack)	70	3.0	1.0	6.0	m.q.	180	0
beef *(Kahn's* Family Pack)	60	2.0	1.0	5.0	m.q.	200	0
Spinach:							
fresh, 1/2 cup:							
raw, chopped . . .	6	.8	1.0	.1	0	22	.8 d
boiled, drained . .	21	2.7	3.4	.2	0	63	2.2 d
canned, 1/2 cup:							
w/liquid	22	2.5	3.4	.4	0	373	2.6 d
(Allens/Popeye) . .	30	2.0	3.0	<1.0	0	330	m.q.
(Allens Low Sodium)	30	2.0	3.0	<1.0	0	50	m.q.
(Stokely)	30	2.0	3.0	0	0	420	m.q.
chopped *(Allens/ Popeye)*	30	3.0	2.0	<1.0	0	250	m.q.
frozen, 1/2 cup, except as noted:							
(Green Giant) . . .	25	3.0	6.0	0	0	100	5.0 d
(Green Giant Harvest Fresh) . . .	25	4.0	5.0	0	0	170	3.0 d
whole *(Frosty Acres)*, 3.3 oz.	20	3.0	4.0	0	0	75	1.0 c
au gratin *(The Budget Gourmet* Side Dish), 5.5 oz. . .	160	5.0	9.0	11.0	25	600	m.q.
creamed *(Birds Eye)*, 3 oz.	60	2.0	5.0	4.0	0	310	1.0 d
creamed *(Green Giant)*	70	3.0	10.0	3.0	2	480	2.0 d
creamed *(Stouffer's)*, 4.5 oz.	190	4.0	8.0	16.0	n.a.	400	m.q.
in butter sauce, cut *(Green Giant)* . .	40	3.0	6.0	2.0	5	380	3.5 d

Food and Measure	cal.	prot. (gms)	carbo. (gms)	fat (gms)	chol. (mgs)	sod. (mgs)	fiber (gms)
Spinach, New Zealand, see "New Zealand spinach"							
Spinach soufflé, frozen *(Stouffer's),* 6 oz.	220	9.0	11.0	15.0	n.a.	820	m.q.
Spiny lobster, meat only:							
raw, 4 oz.	127	23.4	2.8	1.7	80	201	0
boiled or steamed, 2-lb. lobster	233	43.1	5.1	3.2	146	370	0
boiled or steamed, 4 oz.	138	29.9	3.5	2.2	102	257	0
Split peas:							
boiled, 1/2 cup	116	8.2	20.7	.4	0	2	8.1 d
green, dry *(Arrowhead Mills),* 2 oz.	200	14.0	35.0	1.0	0	7	7.5 d
Spot, meat only:							
raw, 4 oz.	140	21.0	0	5.6	m.q.	33	0
baked, broiled, or microwaved, 4 oz. . .	179	26.9	0	7.1	m.q.	42	0
Spring onion, see "Onion, green"							
Sprouts, see also specific listings):							
bean:							
(Frieda's), 1 oz. . .	10	1.1	1.9	.1	0	1	m.q.
stir-fry *(Frieda's Sprout Munchies),* 1 oz.	10	1.1	1.9	.1	0	m.q.	m.q.
canned *(La Choy),* 2/3 cup	8	1.0	1.0	<1.0	0	20	<1.0 d
mixed *(Shaw's Premium),* 2 oz.	9	2.0	0	<1.0	0	40	2.0 d
Squab, fresh, raw:							
meat w/skin, 4 oz. . .	333	20.9	0	27.0	m.q.	m.q.	0
breast meat only, 4 oz.	161	19.8	0	8.5	m.q.	m.q.	0

Food and Measure	cal.	prot. (gms)	carbo. (gms)	fat (gms)	chol. (mgs)	sod. (mgs)	fiber (gms)
Squash, fresh, see specific listings							
Squash, frozen (see also specific listings) *(Frosty Acres),*							
3.3 oz.	18	1.0	4.0	0	0	1	1.0 c
Squid, meat only, raw,							
4 oz.	104	17.7	3.5	1.6	265	50	0
Star fruit, see "Carambola"							
Steak, see "Beef"							
Steak biscuit sandwich, frozen *(Hormel Quick Meal),*							
4.2 oz.	330	13.0	36.0	15.0	55	830	m.q.
Steak sauce, 1 tbsp.:							
(A.1.)	12	0	3.0	0	0	280	n.a.
(French's)	25	0	6.0	0	0	150	n.a.
(Heinz 57)	16	0	4.0	0	0	190	0
(Heinz Traditional) . .	12	0	3.0	0	0	190	n.a.
(Lea & Perrins)	25	0	6.0	0	0	135	0
(Maull's)	20	0	5.0	0	0	250	0
hickory smoke *(Heinz 57)*	16	0	4.0	0	0	180	0
sweet & mild *(Maull's)*	20	0	4.0	0	0	190	0
Steak seasoning:							
(McCormick/Schilling Grillmates), 1 tsp.	7	0	1.0	0	n.a.	420	n.a.
blackened *(Tone's),* 1 tsp.	9	.4	1.6	.3	0	486	n.a.
broiled *(McCormick/ Schilling Spice Blends),* 1/4 tsp. . .	1	.1	.1	n.a.	0	273	n.a.
Stir-fry entree mix:							
(Tyson Stir-Fry Kit): meat/vegetable mix,							
9 oz.	230	22.0	15.0	9.0	80	480	m.q.

Food and Measure	cal.	prot. (gms)	carbo. (gms)	fat (gms)	chol. (mgs)	sod. (mgs)	fiber (gms)
Yoshida sauce, 1.6 oz.	100	2.0	22.0	1.0	0	1260	n.a.
Stir-fry seasoning *(Gilroy)*, 1 tsp. . . .	6	.2	1.0	0	0	5	n.a.
Stomach, pork, raw, 1 oz.	44	4.7	0	2.7	55	15	0
Strawberry:							
fresh:							
1 pint	97	2.0	22.5	1.2	0	4	7.4 d
1/2 cup	23	.5	5.2	.3	0	1	1.7 d
canned in heavy syrup, 1/2 cup . . .	117	.7	29.9	.3	0	5	2.2 d
freeze-dried *(Mountain House Fruit Crisps),* 1/4 cup	60	1.0	13.0	1.0	0	0	m.q.
frozen:							
unsweetened, 1/2 cup	26	.3	6.8	.1	0	1	1.6 d
in syrup *(Birds Eye Lite),* 5 oz.	100	1.0	25.0	0	0	0	2.0 d
Strawberry colada mixer, frozen*, w/rum *(Bacardi),* 7 fl. oz.	230	0	34.0	1.0	0	15	n.a.
Strawberry drink mix*, 8 fl. oz.:							
(Kool-Aid)	100	0	25.0	0	0	25	0
(Kool-Aid Presweet- ened)	70	0	18.0	0	0	0	0
(Wylers)	80	(0)	21.0	(0)	0	35	(0)
split *(Wylers)*	80	(0)	20.0	(0)	0	15	(0)
Strawberry milk drink:							
chilled, 1 cup:							
(Nestlé Quik)	230	8.0	32.0	8.0	m.q.	140	(0)
lowfat *(Nestlé Quik)*	200	8.0	33.0	4.0	m.q.	120	(0)
mix, powder:							
1 oz.	110	<.1	28.1	.1	0	11	<.1 c

Food and Measure	cal.	prot. (gms)	carbo. (gms)	fat (gms)	chol. (mgs)	sod. (mgs)	fiber (gms)
Strawberry milk drink, mix, powder *(cont.)*							
(Carnation Instant Breakfast), 1 pkt.	130	4.0	29.0	0	3	160	m.q.
(Nestlé Quik), 3/4 oz. or 12/3 heaping tsp. . . .	100	0	24.0	0	0	0	m.q.
(Pillsbury Instant Breakfast), 1 pkt.	130	6.0	27.0	0	0	100	m.q.
Strawberry float							
(R.W. Knudsen), 8 fl. oz.	130	2.0	32.0.	<1.0	0	(0)	n.a.
Strawberry fruit roll, see "Fruit snack"							
Strawberry nectar:							
(Kern's), 6 fl. oz. . . .	110	0	28.0	0	0	0	m.q.
(R.W. Knudsen), 8 fl. oz.	105	<1.0	29.0	<1.0	0	(0)	m.q.
(Libby's), 6 fl. oz. . .	110	0	27.0	0	0	0	m.q.
(Libby's Ripe), 8 fl. oz.	150	0	36.0	0	0	5	m.q.
Strawberry topping:							
(Kraft), 1 tbsp.	50	0	14.0	0	0	5	n.a.
(Smucker's), 2 tbsp.	120	0	30.0	0	0	0	n.a.
Strawberry-banana nectar:							
(Kern's), 6 fl. oz. . . .	110	0	28.0	0	0	0	m.q.
(Libby's Ripe), 8 fl. oz.	150	0	37.0	0	0	5	m.q.
Strawberry-guava juice *(R.W. Knudsen),* 8 fl. oz. . . .	105	<1.0	26.0	<1.0	0	(0)	m.q.
Strawberry-guava nectar *(Santa Cruz Natural),* 8 fl. oz. . .	90	<1.0	24.0	<1.0	0	(0)	m.q.
String bean, see "Green bean"							

Food and Measure	cal.	prot. (gms)	carbo. (gms)	fat (gms)	chol. (mgs)	sod. (mgs)	fiber (gms)
Stroganoff entree, vegetarian, mix*:							
(Natural Touch), 4 oz.	90	4.0	10.0	3.0	0	700	m.q.
creamy, 1/2 cup:							
w/tofu (Tofu Classics)	103	6.0	13.0	3.0	2	206	1.9 d
w/tofu and butter (Tofu Classics) . .	139	6.0	13.0	7.0	m.q.	245	1.9 d
Stroganoff sauce mix:							
(Lawry's), 1 pkg. . . .	123	4.5	25.5	.3	0	2814	.8 c
(Natural Touch), 4 oz.*	90	4.0	10.0	3.0	n.a.	n.a.	n.a.
Stroganoff seasoning (French's), 1/4 pkg.	50	2.0	6.0	2.0	10	230	n.a.
Stuffing, 1 oz., except as noted:							
apple and raisin (Pepperidge Farm Distinctive)	110	3.0	21.0	1.0	n.a.	410	m.q.
chicken, classic (Pepperidge Farm Distinctive)	110	4.0	20.0	1.0	n.a.	410	m.q.
corn (Arnold)	100	4.0	18.0	2.0	0	280	2.0 d
cornbread:							
(Brownberry)	100	4.0	18.0	2.0	0	280	2.0 d
(Pepperidge Farm)	110	3.0	22.0	1.0	n.a.	320	m.q.
honey pecan (Pepperidge Farm Distinctive)	120	2.0	19.0	4.0	0	330	m.q.
country style (Pepperidge Farm)	100	4.0	21.0	1.0	n.a.	400	m.q.
cube:							
(Pepperidge Farm)	110	3.0	22.0	1.0	n.a.	400	m.q.
unspiced (Arnold), .5 oz.	50	2.0	9.0	<1.0	0	110	1.0 d
herb, country garden (Pepperidge Farm Distinctive)	120	4.0	18.0	4.0	n.a.	300	m.q.

Food and Measure	cal.	prot. (gms)	carbo. (gms)	fat (gms)	chol. (mgs)	sod. (mgs)	fiber (gms)
Stuffing *(cont.)*							
herb seasoned:							
(Arnold/Brownberry),							
.5 oz.	50	2.0	10.0	<1.0	0	150	1.0 d
(Pepperidge Farm)	110	3.0	22.0	1.0	n.a.	380	m.q.
sage and onion							
(Arnold/Brownberry),							
.5 oz.	50	2.0	9.0	<1.0	0	230	1.0 d
(Pepperidge Farm							
Distinctive) . . .	100	4.0	21.0	1.0	0	520	2.0 d
seasoned *(Arnold),*							
.5 oz.	50	2.0	9.0	<1.0	0	200	1.0 d
vegetable, harvest,							
and almond *(Pep-*							
peridge Farm Dis-							
tinctive)	110	4.0	19.0	3.0	n.a.	250	m.q.
wild rice and mush-							
room *(Pepperidge*							
Farm Distinctive)	130	4.0	17.0	5.0	n.a.	310	m.q.
Stuffing mix, 1/2 cup*:							
(Stove Top Americana							
San Francisco) . .	170	4.0	20.0	9.0	0	640	m.q.
beef *(Stove Top)* . . .	180	4.0	21.0	9.0	0	590	m.q.
broccoli and cheese							
(Stove Top Micro-							
wave)	170	4.0	20.0	8.0	5	570	m.q.
chicken:							
(Betty Crocker) . .	180	4.0	21.0	9.0	n.a.	620	m.q.
(Stove Top)	180	4.0	20.0	9.0	0	500	m.q.
(Stove Top Flexible							
Serving)	170	4.0	20.0	9.0	0	580	m.q.
(Stove Top Micro-							
wave)	160	4.0	20.0	8.0	0	480	m.q.
w/rice *(Stove Top)*	180	4.0	22.0	9.0	0	580	m.q.
cornbread:							
(Stove Top)	180	3.0	21.0	9.0	0	560	m.q.
(Stove Top Flexible							
Serving)	180	4.0	22.0	9.0	0	590	m.q.

Food and Measure	cal.	prot. (gms)	carbo. (gms)	fat (gms)	chol. (mgs)	sod. (mgs)	fiber (gms)
homestyle (Stove Top Microwave)	160	3.0	20.0	7.0	0	450	m.q.
herb:							
homestyle (Stove Top Flexible Serving)	170	4.0	20.0	9.0	0	510	m.q.
savory (Stove Top)	180	4.0	20.0	9.0	0	580	m.q.
traditional (Betty Crocker)	180	4.0	22.0	8.0	n.a.	640	m.q.
long grain and wild rice (Stove Top) . .	180	4.0	22.0	9.0	0	550	m.q.
mushroom and onion:							
(Stove Top)	180	4.0	20.0	9.0	0	480	m.q.
(Stove Top Microwave)	170	4.0	21.0	7.0	0	500	m.q.
pork:							
(Stove Top)	180	4.0	20.0	9.0	0	560	m.q.
(Stove Top Flexible Serving)	170	3.0	20.0	9.0	0	630	m.q.
turkey (Stove Top) . .	180	4.0	20.0	9.0	0	630	m.q.
Sturgeon, meat only:							
raw, 4 oz.	120	18.3	0	4.6	m.q.	m.q.	0
baked, broiled, or microwaved, 4 oz. . .	153	23.5	0	5.9	m.q.	m.q.	0
smoked, 4 oz.	196	35.4	0	5.0	m.q.	m.q.	0
Succotash: fresh, boiled, drained, ½ cup	111	4.9	23.4	.8	0	16	1.3 c
canned, ½ cup:							
w/cream-style corn	102	3.5	23.4	.7	0	325	1.7 c
w/whole kernel . .	81	3.3	17.9	.6	0	283	6.9 d
frozen, boiled, drained, ½ cup	79	3.7	17.0	.8	0	38	4.6 d
frozen (Frosty Acres), 3.3 oz.	100	4.0	19.0	0	0	47	1.0 c
Sucker, white, meat only:							
raw, 4 oz.	105	19.0	0	2.6	47	45	0

Food and Measure	cal.	prot. (gms)	carbo. (gms)	fat (gms)	chol. (mgs)	sod. (mgs)	fiber (gms)
Sucker *(cont.)*							
baked, broiled, or microwaved, 4 oz. . . .	135	24.4	0	3.4	60	58	0
Sugar, beet or cane:							
brown:							
1 oz.	107	0	27.6	0	0	11	0
1 cup, not packed	546	0	141.0	0	0	57	0
1 cup, packed . . .	828	0	214.0	0	0	86	0
cane baton *(Frieda's)*, 1 oz.	21	<.1	49.9	.1	0	n.a.	(0)
granulated:							
1 oz.	110	0	28.3	0	0	<1	0
1 cup	773	0	199.8	0	0	<1	0
1 tbsp.	46	0	12.0	0	0	tr.	0
1 tsp.	15	0	4.0	0	0	tr.	0
powdered or confectioner's:							
1 oz.	110	0	28.2	0	0	<1	0
1 cup, sifted	389	0	99.5	0	0	1	0
1 tbsp., unsifted . .	31	0	8.0	0	0	tr.	0
Sugar, maple, 1 oz.	99	0	25.5	0	0	4	0
"Sugar" substitute:							
(Equal), 1 pkt.	4	0	<1.0	0	0	0	0
(NutraSweet), 1 tsp.	2	0	<1.0	0	0	0	0
(Sweet'N Low), 1 pkt.	4	0	1.0	0	0	0	0
Sugar apple:							
1 medium, 9.9 oz. . .	146	3.2	36.6	.5	0	15	6.8 d
1/2 cup	118	2.6	29.6	.4	0	12	5.5 d
Sugar snap peas, see "Peas, ediblepodded"							
Summer sausage (see also "Thuringer cervelat"):							
(Hillshire Farm), 2 oz.	180	9.0	1.0	16.0	m.q.	670	0
beef *(Oscar Mayer)*, 2 slices	140	7.0	<1.0	12.0	35	640	0

Food and Measure	cal.	prot. (gms)	carbo. (gms)	fat (gms)	chol. (mgs)	sod. (mgs)	fiber (gms)
beef *(Hillshire Farm),* 2 oz.	190	9.0	1.0	17.0	m.q.	m.q.	0
(Oscar Mayer), 2 slices	140	7.0	0	13.0	40	650	0
w/cheese *(Hillshire Farm),* 2 oz.	200	9.0	1.0	18.0	m.q.	m.q.	0
Sunburst squash, raw *(Frieda's),* 1 oz. . .	4	.3	.9	<.1	0	<1	m.q.
Sunfish, pumpkin-seed, meat only:							
raw, 4 oz.	101	22.0	0	.8	76	91	0
baked, broiled, or microwaved, 4 oz. . . .	129	28.2	0	1.0	98	117	0
Sunflower seed, 1 oz.:							
(Arrowhead Mills) . .	160	7.0	6.0	13.0	0	3	4.4 d
(Frito-Lay's)	160	7.0	6.0	14.0	0	265	m.q.
dried, kernels	162	6.5	5.3	14.1	0	1	3.0 d
dry-roasted, in shell *(Fisher)*	170	6.0	6.0	15.0	0	110	m.q.
dry-roasted, kernels:							
unsalted	165	5.5	6.8	14.1	0	1	2.6 d
salted	165	5.5	6.8	14.1	0	221	2.6 d
(Fisher)	170	6.0	6.0	15.0	0	200	5.0 d
(Flavor House) . . .	150	8.0	8.0	11.0	0	200	3.0 d
oil-roasted, kernels:							
unsalted	175	6.1	4.2	16.3	0	1	1.9 d
salted	175	6.1	4.2	16.3	0	171	1.9 d
(Fisher)	170	6.0	4.0	16.0	0	170	m.q.
salted, in shell *(Fisher)*	170	6.0	6.0	14.0	0	110	m.q.
toasted, kernels:							
unsalted	176	4.9	5.9	16.1	0	1	.5 c
salted	176	4.9	5.9	16.1	0	174	.5 c
unsalted *(Fisher)* . . .	170	6.0	6.0	14.0	0	0	m.q.
Sunflower seed butter:							
1 oz.	165	5.6	7.8	13.6	0	1	1.4 d
1 tbsp.	93	3.2	4.4	7.6	0	1	.8 d
salted, 1 oz.	165	5.6	7.8	13.6	0	147	1.4 d

Food and Measure	cal.	prot. (gms)	carbo. (gms)	fat (gms)	chol. (mgs)	sod. (mgs)	fiber (gms)
Sunflower seed butter *(cont.)*							
(Erewhon), 2 tbsp. . .	200	7.0	3.0	18.0	0	20	m.q.
(Roaster Fresh), 1 oz.	160	6.0	5.0	13.6	0	1	m.q.
Sunflower seed flour, partially defatted,							
1 cup	261	38.5	28.7	1.3	0	2	4.2 d
Surimi[1], 4 oz.	112	17.2	7.8	1.0	34	162	0
Swamp cabbage:							
raw, .6-oz. shoot . .	2	.3	.4	<.1	0	15	.3 d
boiled, drained,							
chopped, 1/2 cup	10	1.0	1.8	.1	0	60	.9 d
Sweet potato:							
raw, 1 medium, 5″×2″							
diam.	136	2.1	31.6	.4	0	17	3.9 d
baked in skin:							
1 medium	118	2.0	27.7	.1	0	12	3.4 d
mashed, 1/2 cup . .	103	1.7	24.3	.1	0	10	3.0 d
boiled w/out skin:							
4 oz.	119	1.9	27.5	.3	0	15	2.8 d
mashed, 1/2 cup . .	172	2.7	39.8	.5	0	21	4.1 d
Sweet potato, canned, 1/2 cup:							
whole *(Pride of Louisiana* Yams)	90	2.0	20.0	<1.0	0	40	m.q.
cut *(Allens* Yams) . .	90	2.0	20.0	<1.0	0	20	m.q.
in syrup, w/liquid . .	101	1.1	23.9	.2	0	50	2.1 d
in syrup, drained . . .	106	1.3	24.9	.3	0	38	1.8 d
vacuum pack, pieces	92	1.7	21.1	.2	0	54	3.0 d
vacuum pack, mashed	117	2.1	26.9	.3	0	68	3.8 d
Sweet potato, frozen:							
baked, cubed, 1/2 cup	88	1.5	20.6	.1	0	7	2.6 d
candied:							
(Mrs. Paul's), 4 oz.	190	1.0	46.0	1.0	n.a.	140	m.q.
w/apples *(Mrs. Paul's* Sweets 'N Apples), 4 oz. . .	160	1.0	38.0	0	0	55	m.q.

[1] *Processed from walleye (Alaska) pollock.*

Food and Measure	cal.	prot. (gms)	carbo. (gms)	fat (gms)	chol. (mgs)	sod. (mgs)	fiber (gms)
patty *(Stilwell* Yam Patties), 2 pieces	150	1.0	33.0	1.0	0	200	3.0 d
Sweet potato leaf:							
raw, chopped, 1/2 cup	6	.7	1.1	.1	0	2	.2 c
steamed, 1/2 cup . .	11	.7	2.3	.1	0	4	.6 d
Sweet and sour drink mixer, bottled *(Holland House),* 3 fl. oz.	96	<1.0	24.0	<1.0	0	321	(0)
Sweet and sour sauce, 1 tbsp., except as noted:							
(Bennett's)	30	0	7.0	0	0	70	n.a.
(Contadina), 1/2 cup	150	<1.0	32.0	3.0	0	430	n.a.
(La Choy)	25	<1.0	7.0	<1.0	0	40	<1.0 d
(Sauceworks)	25	0	5.0	0	0	50	n.a.
(Woody's), 2 tbsp. . . .	70	0	17.0	0	0	610	<1.0 d
duck sauce *(La Choy)*	25	<1.0	7.0	<1.0	0	40	<1.0 d
Sweetbreads, see "Pancreas" and "Thymus"							
Swiss chard:							
raw, chopped, 1/2 cup	3	.3	.7	<.1	0	38	.3 d
boiled, drained, chopped, 1/2 cup	18	1.7	3.6	.1	0	158	1.8 d
Swiss steak, see "Beef dinner"							
Swiss steak seasoning mix:							
(French's Roasting Bag), 1/5 pkg. . . .	20	0	5.0	0	0	580	n.a.
(McCormick/Schilling Bag'n Season), 1 pkg.	81	1.9	17.0	.4	n.a.	2651	m.q.
Swordfish, fresh, meat only:							
raw, 4 oz.	137	22.5	0	4.6	45	102	0

Food and Measure	cal.	prot. (gms)	carbo. (gms)	fat (gms)	chol. (mgs)	sod. (mgs)	fiber (gms)
Swordfish *(cont.)*							
baked, broiled, or microwaved, 4 oz. . .	176	28.8	0	5.8	57	130	0
Syrup, see specific listings							
Szechwan sauce *(La Choy),* 1 oz.	48	.1	12.0	.2	0	141	0

T

Food and Measure	cal.	prot. (gms)	carbo. (gms)	fat (gms)	chol. (mgs)	sod. (mgs)	fiber (gms)
Tabbouleh mix*:							
(Casbah Tabouli), 1 oz.							
dry	90	3.0	19.0	m.q.	0	340	m.q.
w/oil *(Fantastic*							
Tabouli), 1/2 cup . .	152	3.0	17.0	9.0	0	265	5.0 d
w/out oil *(Fantastic*							
Tabouli), 1/2 cup . .	85	3.0	17.0	.5	0	265	5.0 d
Taco dip:							
(Wise), 2 tbsp.	12	0	3.0	0	0	115	n.a.
and sauce *(Hain),*							
4 tbsp.	25	1.0	5.0	1.0	5	350	n.a.
Taco John's, 1 serving:							
apple grande	257	5.0	44.0	8.0	n.a.	231	m.q.
beans, refried	331	19.0	79.0	6.0	n.a.	1195	m.q.
burrito:							
bean	249	10.0	36.0	6.0	n.a.	636	m.q.
beef	355	16.0	25.0	18.0	m.q.	666	m.q.
combo	302	11.0	30.0	12.0	m.q.	651	m.q.
super	434	17.0	66.0	11.0	m.q.	1022	m.q.
w/green chili	405	18.0	38.0	24.0	n.a.	995	m.q.
w/Texas chili	518	23.0	48.0	24.0	n.a.	746	m.q.
chili, Texas	430	23.0	35.0	22.0	m.q.	1580	m.q.
chimi	487	16.0	54.0	19.0	m.q.	1226	m.q.
churro	122	1.7	12.0	7.0	n.a.	153	m.q.
enchilada	379	19.0	33.0	18.0	m.q.	431	m.q.
nachos	407	11.0	42.0	19.0	m.q.	307	m.q.
nachos, super	657	23.0	57.0	34.0	m.q.	857	m.q.

Food and Measure	cal.	prot. (gms)	carbo. (gms)	fat (gms)	chol. (mgs)	sod. (mgs)	fiber (gms)
Taco John's *(cont.)*							
Potato Olé Large . .	414	6.0	96.0	6.0	n.a.	1595	m.q.
taco:							
burger	332	14.0	31.0	14.0	m.q.	660	m.q.
Bravo, super	485	18.0	51.0	20.0	m.q.	1006	m.q.
regular	228	11.0	15.0	13.0	m.q.	347	m.q.
soft shell	276	13.0	23.0	13.0	m.q.	505	m.q.
taco salad, super . .	450	16.0	48.0	18.0	n.a.	880	m.q.
tostada	228	11.0	15.0	13.0	n.a.	347	m.q.
Taco mix:							
(Old El Paso), 1 taco*	67	2.0	8.0	3.0	n.a.	423	n.a.
(Tio Sancho Dinner Kit):							
sauce, 2 oz.	62	1.6	13.4	.2	n.a.	750	.5 c
seasoning, 1.25 oz.	104	2.1	20.9	1.4	n.a.	2500	1.7 c
shell	64	1.1	8.1	3.1	n.a.	1	.5 c
vegetarian *(Natural Touch),* 2 tbsp. . .	90	10.0	6.0	2.0	0	210	m.q.
Taco sauce:							
(Chi-Chi's Thick & Chunky), 1 oz. . . .	12	<2.0	3.0	<2.0	<2	140	m.q.
(Lawry's Sauce'n Seasoner), 1/4 cup . . .	40	.7	7.6	.6	0	636	0
(Old El Paso), 2 tbsp.	15	1.0	3.0	0	0	130	1.0 d
chunky *(Lawry's),* 1/4 cup	22	.9	4.0	.4	0	549	.4 c
hot:							
(Chi-Chi's), 1 oz.	18	<2.0	4.0	<2.0	1	254	m.q.
(Ortega), 1 oz. . . .	12	0	3.0	0	0	210	m.q.
mild *(Ortega),* 1 oz.	12	0	3.0	0	0	220	m.q.
red *(La Victoria),* 1 tbsp.	5	0	1.0	0	0	80	m.q.
red, mild *(El Molino),* 2 tbsp.	10	0	2.0	0	0	170	m.q.
western style *(Ortega),* 1 oz. . .	8	0	2.0	0	0	180	m.q.
Taco seasoning mix:							
(French's), 1/12 pkg.	8	0	2.0	0	0	180	m.q.

Food and Measure	cal.	prot. (gms)	carbo. (gms)	fat (gms)	chol. (mgs)	sod. (mgs)	fiber (gms)
(Hain), 1/10 pkg. . . .	10	1.0	2.0	0	0	200	m.q.
(Lawry's Seasoning Blends), 1.25 oz.	118	3.4	23.6	1.1	0	1441	1.0 c
(McCormick/Schilling), 1/4 pkg.	31	1.0	6.0	.5	0	675	m.q.
(Old El Paso), 1/12 pkg.	8	<1.0	2.0	<1.0	0	240	m.q.
(Tio Sancho), 1.51 oz.	132	2.9	26.0	1.7	0	2623	2.0 c
onion, real *(French's)*, 1/12 pkg.	12	0	3.0	0	0	130	m.q.
salad *(Lawry's* Seasoning Blends), 1 pkg.	124	4.0	24.7	.9	0	1451	1.6 c
Taco shell, 1 piece, except as noted:							
(Chi-Chi's)	140	2.0	17.0	7.0	0	5	m.q.
(Gebhardt)	50	1.0	7.0	2.0	0	<1	<1.0 d
(Lawry's)	50	.8	8.0	3.0	0	123	.2 c
(Lawry's Super) . . .	86	1.4	13.0	4.1	0	210	.4 c
(Old El Paso)	50	0	6.0	3.0	0	50	.5 d
(Old El Paso Super)	100	1.0	11.0	6.0	0	95	1.5 d
(Ortega)	50	0	8.0	2.0	0	5	m.q.
(Rosarita)	50	1.0	7.0	2.0	0	<1	<1.0 d
(Tio Sancho)	64	1.1	8.1	3.1	0	1	.5 c
(Tio Sancho Super)	94	1.6	11.3	4.7	0	2	.7 c
corn *(Azteca)*	60	1.0	7.0	3.0	0	65	m.q.
mini *(Old El Paso)*, 3 pieces	70	1.0	7.0	4.0	0	60	.5 d
salad, flour *(Azteca)*	200	3.0	18.0	12.0	n.a.	130	m.q.
Tahini, 1 oz., except as noted:							
from unroasted kernels, 1 tbsp.	85	2.5	2.5	7.9	0	tr.	1.3 d
from roasted, toasted kernels, 1 tbsp. . . .	89	2.6	3.2	8.1	0	17	1.4 d
(Arrowhead Mills) . .	170	6.0	4.0	17.0	0	<1	2.6 d
(Erewhon), 2 tbsp. . . .	200	6.0	3.0	18.0	0	65	m.q.
(Joyva)	200	6.0	3.0	18.0	0	65	m.q.
imported *(Krinos)* . .	200	7.0	2.0	18.0	0	0	2.0 d

Food and Measure	cal.	prot. (gms)	carbo. (gms)	fat (gms)	chol. (mgs)	sod. (mgs)	fiber (gms)
Tahini sauce mix*							
(Casbah), 1/4 cup	150	5.0	10.0	11.0	0	160	0
Tamale, canned:							
(Derby), 2 pieces . . .	160	8.0	15.0	7.0	24	570	1.0 d
(Gebhardt), 2 pieces	290	5.0	19.0	22.0	54	730	2.0 d
(Gebhardt Jumbo),							
2 pieces	400	7.0	26.0	30.0	75	1025	3.0 d
(Old El Paso), 2 pieces	190	5.0	16.0	12.0	20	380	m.q.
beef, regular or hot							
(Hormel), 7.5 oz. . . .	280	6.0	19.0	20.0	35	990	m.q.
Tamalito, in chili							
gravy, canned (Den-							
nison's), 7.5 oz. . . .	310	6.0	37.0	16.0	m.q.	1395	m.q.
Tamari, see "Soy							
sauce"							
Tamarind:							
1 fruit, 3" × 1"	5	.1	1.3	<.1	0	1	.1 d
pulp, 1/2 cup	144	1.7	37.5	.4	0	17	3.1 d
pulp (Frieda's							
Tamarindo), 1 oz.	68	.8	17.7	.2	0	14	m.q.
Tangerine:							
fresh:							
1 medium, 23/8"							
diam.	37	.5	9.4	.2	0	1	1.9 d
sections w/out							
membrane,							
1/2 cup	43	.6	10.9	.2	0	2	2.2 d
canned, 1/2 cup:							
(Dole Mandarin) . .	70	0	19.0	<1.0	0	10	m.q.
in juice	46	.8	11.9	<.1	0	7	.9 d
in light syrup . . .	76	.6	20.4	.1	0	8	.9 d
Tangerine juice,							
6 fl. oz.:							
fresh	80	.9	18.7	.4	0	2	.4 d
chilled or frozen* (Min-							
ute Maid)	90	1.0	22.0	0	0	0	m.q.
Tapioca, pearl, dry,							
1 oz.	97	<.1	25.1	tr.	0	tr.	.3 d

Food and Measure	cal.	prot. (gms)	carbo. (gms)	fat (gms)	chol. (mgs)	sod. (mgs)	fiber (gms)
Taramosalata (Krinos),							
1 tbsp.	90	1.0	0	10.0	15	115	0
Taro:							
raw, sliced, 1/2 cup	56	.8	13.8	.1	0	6	2.1 d
cooked, sliced, 1/2 cup	94	.3	22.8	.1	0	10	3.4 d
cooked (Frieda's),							
5 oz.	150	1.0	36.0	m.q.	0	10	4.0 d
Taro chips:							
1 oz.	141	.7	19.3	7.1	0	97	.3 c
1/2 cup	57	.3	8.1	3.1	0	44	.1 c
Taro leaf:							
raw, 1/2 cup	6	.7	.9	.1	0	1	.5 d
steamed, 1/2 cup . .	18	2.0	3.0	.3	0	2	.4 c
Taro shoots:							
raw, sliced, 1/2 cup	5	.4	1.0	<.1	0	<1	.3 c
cooked, sliced, 1/2 cup	10	.5	2.2	.1	0	1	.4 c
Taro, Tahitian:							
raw, sliced, 1/2 cup	25	1.7	4.3	.6	0	31	1.1 c
cooked, sliced, 1/2 cup	30	2.8	4.7	.5	0	37	1.6 c
Tarragon, ground,							
1 tsp.	5	.4	.8	.1	0	1	.1 d
Tart shell, see "Pastry dough"							
Tartar sauce, 1 tbsp.:							
(Bennett's)	70	0	<1.0	7.0	5	100	n.a.
(Golden Dipt)	70	0	2.0	7.0	10	100	n.a.
(Golden Dipt Lite) . .	50	0	4.0	4.0	5	40	n.a.
(Heinz)	70	0	2.0	7.0	3	240	n.a.
(Hellmann's/Best Foods)	70	0	0	8.0	5	220	n.a.
(Lyon)	40	0	3.0	3.0	5	86	0
(Lyon Lite)	21	0	2.0	1.0	4	92	0
(Sauceworks)	50	0	2.0	5.0	5	85	n.a.
natural lemon and herb flavor							
(Sauceworks) . . .	70	0	0	8.0	5	85	n.a.

Food and Measure	cal.	prot. (gms)	carbo. (gms)	fat (gms)	chol. (mgs)	sod. (mgs)	fiber (gms)
Tea*, 8 fl. oz.:							
caffeine-free *(Celestial Seasonings)*	8	0	.1	0	0	1	0
instant:							
(Nestea 100%) . .	2	0	0	0	0	0	0
lemon flavor *(Nestea)*	4	0	1.0	0	0	0	0
w/sugar and lemon *(Tetley)*	90	0	21.0	0	0	10	0
Tea,* flavored, 8 fl. oz.:							
all flavors *(Celestial Seasonings Distinctive)*	<5	0	<.2	0	0	<2	0
blackberry, peach, or raspberry *(Lipton)*	2	0	0	0	0	0	0
lemon, orange, or cinnamon, with honey *(Lipton)*	4	0	<1.0	0	0	0	0
Tea,* herbal, 8 fl. oz.:							
all flavors *(Lipton)* . .	2	0	0	0	0	0	0
all flavors, except lemon and mint *(Celestial Seasonings)*	<5	0	<2.0	0	0	<7	0
(Celestial Seasonings Lemon Zinger) . . .	<7	0	<1.0	0	0	2	0
(Celestial Seasonings Mint Magic)	2	0	.4	0	0	13	0
Tea, iced:							
brewed, herbal *(Celestial Seasonings Iced Delight)*, 8 fl. oz. . . .	<4	0	<.7	0	0	14	0
boxed, lemon or orange *(Boku)*, 12 fl. oz.	180	0	44.0	0	0	35	0
canned, 12 fl. oz.:							
(Lipton Brisk) . . .	160	0	39.0	0	0	10	0
(Shasta)	136	0	34.0	0	0	58	0

Food and Measure	cal.	prot. (gms)	carbo. (gms)	fat (gms)	chol. (mgs)	sod. (mgs)	fiber (gms)
canned w/fruit juice, 12 fl. oz.: *(Fruit Teazers)*:							
cherry spice	110	1.0	25.0	<1.0	0	n.a.	0
ginger peach . . .	120	1.0	27.0	<1.0	0	n.a.	0
hibiscus blossom or raspberry rose	115	1.0	26.0	<1.0	0	n.a.	0
chilled, 8 fl. oz.:							
no lemon *(Lipton)*	80	0	20.0	0	0	15	0
w/lemon *(Lipton)*	80	0	20.0	0	0	10	0
mix*, 8 fl. oz., except as noted:							
all flavors *(Nestea Ice Teasers)* . . .	6	0	1.0	0	0	0	0
citrus or lemon-lime, w/sugar *(Lipton)*	60	0	14.0	0	0	0	0
lemon flavor *(Lipton Multi Pack)*, 6 fl. oz.	60	0	14.0	0	0	0	0
w/lemon *(Nestea Presweetened)*	70	0	19.0	0	0	0	0
Teff seed or flour *(Arrowhead Mills)*, 2 oz.	200	7.0	41.0	1.0	0	6	7.7 d
Tempeh:							
1 oz.	56	5.4	4.8	2.2	0	2	.8 c
1/2 cup	165	15.7	14.1	6.4	0	5	2.5 c
quinoa-sesame *(Lightlife)*, 4 oz.	198	19.0	14.0	8.0	0	2	m.q.
Tempura batter mix *(Golden Dipt)*, 1 oz.	100	3.0	22.0	0	0	130	m.q.
Teriyaki marinade:							
(Lawry's), 2 tbsp. . .	72	6.4	11.0	.4	0	7100	.2 c
barbecue *(Lawry's)*, 1/4 cup	164	8.2	27.4	2.3	n.a.	12330	.2 c
seafood, see "Seafood sauce"							

Food and Measure	cal.	prot. (gms)	carbo. (gms)	fat (gms)	chol. (mgs)	sod. (mgs)	fiber (gms)
Teriyaki sauce, 1/2 tsp.:							
(La Choy)	5	<1.0	1.0	<1.0	0	290	<1.0 d
(La Choy Lite)	5	<1.0	1.0	<1.0	0	85	<1.0 d
basting (La Choy) . .	2	<1.0	<1.0	<1.0	0	110	<1.0 d
Thirst quencher drink, 8 fl. oz., except as noted:							
all flavors (PowerAde), 6 fl. oz.	54	0	14.0	0	0	21	(0)
all flavors (10-K) . . .	60	0	15.0	0	0	55	(0)
lemon (Recharge) . .	60	<1.0	14.0	<1.0	0	n.a.	(0)
lemon (Recharge Organic)	45	<1.0	11.0	<1.0	0	n.a.	(0)
orange (Recharge) . .	50	<1.0	13.0	<1.0	0	n.a.	(0)
tropical (Recharge) . .	60	<1.0	13.0	<1.0	0	n.a.	(0)
Thuringer cervelat (see also "Summer sausage") (Hillshire Farm), 2 oz.	180	9.0	1.0	15.0	m.q.	650	0
Thyme, ground, 1 tsp.	4	.1	.9	.1	0	1	.3 d
Thymus, 4 oz.:							
beef, braised	362	24.8	0	28.3	333	132	0
veal, braised	197	35.8	0	4.9	532	75	0
Tilefish, meat only:							
raw, 4 oz.	108	19.9	0	2.6	m.q.	60	0
baked, broiled, or microwaved, 4 oz. . .	167	27.8	0	5.3	m.q.	67	0
Toaster muffins and pastries, 1 piece:							
apple:							
(Pillsbury Toaster Strudel)	200	3.0	26.0	9.0	5	190	m.q.
cinnamon (Kellogg's Pop-Tarts)	210	2.0	37.0	6.0	0	170	1.0 d
cinnamon (Pepperidge Farm Croissant Toaster Tarts)	170	3.0	25.0	7.0	0	120	m.q.

Food and Measure	cal.	prot. (gms)	carbo. (gms)	fat (gms)	chol. (mgs)	sod. (mgs)	fiber (gms)
spice (Toaster Muffins)	130	2.0	21.0	5.0	n.a.	100	m.q.
banana nut:							
(Thomas' Toast-r-Cakes)	110	2.0	17.0	4.0	10	200	1.0 d
(Toaster Muffins) . .	130	2.0	19.0	6.0	n.a.	85	m.q.
blueberry:							
(Kellogg's Pop-Tarts)	210	2.0	37.0	6.0	0	210	0
(Pillsbury Toaster Strudel)	190	3.0	26.0	9.0	5	210	m.q.
(Thomas' Toast-r-Cakes)	100	2.0	17.0	3.0	10	170	<1.0 d
frosted (Kellogg's Pop-Tarts)	200	2.0	37.0	5.0	0	210	0
wild Maine (Toaster Muffins)	120	2.0	23.0	3.0	n.a.	135	m.q.
brown sugar-cinnamon:							
(Kellogg's Pop-Tarts)	210	3.0	33.0	8.0	0	200	0
frosted (Kellogg's Pop-Tarts)	210	3.0	34.0	7.0	0	190	0
cheese (Pepperidge Farm Croissant Toaster Tarts) . . .	190	5.0	22.0	10.0	10	180	m.q.
cherry:							
(Kellogg's Pop-Tarts)	210	2.0	37.0	6.0	0	220	0
frosted (Kellogg's Pop-Tarts)	200	2.0	37.0	5.0	0	220	0
chocolate chip (Thomas' Toast-r-Cakes)	100	2.0	15.0	4.0	n.a.	150	2.0 d
chocolate fudge, frosted (Kellogg's Pop-Tarts)	200	3.0	37.0	5.0	0	220	0
chocolate graham (Kellogg's Pop-Tarts)	210	3.0	37.0	6.0	0	220	0

Food and Measure	cal.	prot. (gms)	carbo. (gms)	fat (gms)	chol. (mgs)	sod. (mgs)	fiber (gms)
Toaster muffins and pastries (cont.)							
chocolate-vanilla creme, frosted (Kellogg's Pop-Tarts)	200	3.0	37.0	5.0	0	230	0
cinnamon (Pillsbury Toaster Strudel) . .	200	5.0	23.0	10.0	5	200	m.q.
corn:							
(Thomas' Toast-r-Cakes)	120	2.0	20.0	4.0	10	190	<1.0 d
old fashioned (Toaster Muffins)	120	2.0	17.0	5.0	n.a.	200	m.q.
grape, frosted (Kellogg's Pop-Tarts)	200	2.0	37.0	5.0	0	200	0
oat bran w/raisins (Awrey's Toastums)	130	3.0	17.0	5.0	0	310	1.0 d
raisin bran:							
(Toaster Muffins) . .	120	3.0	16.0	5.0	n.a.	220	m.q.
(Thomas' Toast-r-Cakes)	100	2.0	18.0	3.0	10	180	1.0 d
raspberry, frosted (Kellogg's Pop-Tarts)	200	2.0	37.0	5.0	0	210	0
strawberry:							
(Kellogg's Pop-Tarts)	210	2.0	37.0	6.0	0	200	0
(Pepperidge Farm Croissant Toaster Tarts)	190	3.0	28.0	7.0	0	120	m.q.
(Pillsbury Toaster Strudel)	190	3.0	26.0	9.0	5	200	m.q.
frosted (Kellogg's Pop-Tarts)	200	2.0	37.0	5.0	0	190	1.0 d
Tofu:							
raw:							
1 oz.	22	2.3	.5	1.4	0	2	.3 d
1/2 cup	94	10.0	2.3	5.9	0	9	1.5 d
extra firm (Nasoya), 4 oz.	110	12.1	1.1	6.7	0	19	m.q.
firm, 1 oz.	41	4.5	1.2	2.5	0	4	.7 d
firm, 1/2 cup	183	19.9	5.4	11.0	0	17	2.9 d

Food and Measure	cal.	prot. (gms)	carbo. (gms)	fat (gms)	chol. (mgs)	sod. (mgs)	fiber (gms)
pasteurized							
(Frieda's), 4.2 oz.	86	9.6	2.9	m.q.	0	8	m.q.
silken (Nasoya),							
4 oz.	59	6.0	2.3	2.9	0	20	m.q.
soft (Nasoya), 4 oz.	90	8.8	1.7	5.1	0	20	m.q.
dried-frozen (koya-dofu), 1 oz.	136	13.6	4.1	8.6	0	2	<.1 c
flavored:							
Chinese 5-spice							
(Nasoya), 4 oz.	110	12.0	2.0	6.0	0	90	m.q.
French country herb							
(Nasoya), 4 oz.	110	12.0	1.0	7.0	0	280	m.q.
fried, 1 oz.	77	4.9	3.0	5.7	0	5	1.1 d
okara, 1 oz.	22	.9	3.6	.5	0	3	1.2 c
okara, 1/2 cup	47	2.0	7.7	1.1	0	6	2.5 c
salted and fermented							
(fuyu), 1 oz.	33	2.3	1.5	2.3	0	814	.1 c
Tofu dishes, see specific listings							
Tofu patty, frozen, 1 patty:							
(Natural Touch Okara)	160	11.0	7.0	10.0	0	420	m.q.
garden (Natural Touch)	120	11.0	8.0	4.0	0	300	m.q.
Tofu "yogurt," see " 'Yogurt,' tofu"							
Tom collins mixer (Holland House):							
bottled, 3 fl. oz. . . .	132	<1.0	33.0	<1.0	0	288	n.a.
instant, .56 oz. dry . .	64	<1.0	16.0	<1.0	0	14	n.a.
Tomatillo:							
1 medium, 15/8" diam.	11	.3	2.0	.4	0	tr.	.6 d
chopped, 1/2 cup . .	21	.6	3.8	.7	0	1	1.3 d
Tomato:							
raw:							
2³/5"-diam. tomato	26	1.0	5.7	.4	0	11	1.4 d
chopped, 1/2 cup	19	.8	4.2	.3	0	8	1.0 d

Food and Measure	cal.	prot. (gms)	carbo. (gms)	fat (gms)	chol. (mgs)	sod. (mgs)	fiber (gms)
Tomato *(cont.)*							
boiled, 1/2 cup	32	1.3	7.0	.5	0	13	1.2 d
sun-dried:							
1 oz.	73	4.0	15.8	.8	0	594	3.5 d
1 piece (32 per cup)	5	.3	1.1	.1	0	42	.3 d
1/2 cup	70	3.8	15.1	.8	0	566	3.3 d
no salt added							
(Frieda's), 1 oz.	86	3.7	21.2	.1	0	38	m.q.
Tomato, canned (see also "Tomato sauce"), 1/2 cup, except as noted:							
whole:							
(Contadina)	25	1.0	5.0	<1.0	0	260	m.q.
(Contadina Pasta Ready)*	50	1.0	8.0	2.0	0	560	m.q.
(Contadina Recipe Ready)*	25	1.0	5.0	.2	0	570	m.q.
(Del Monte)	25	1.0	6.0	0	0	160	2.0 d
(Hunt's), 4 oz. . . .	20	1.0	5.0	<1.0	0	330	<1.0 d
(Hunt's No Salt)*, 4 oz.	20	1.0	5.0	<1.0	0	15	<1.0 d
Italian, pear *(Contadina)*	25	1.0	5.0	<1.0	0	220	m.q.
Italian flavored *(Hunt's)*, 4 oz. . .	25	1.0	6.0	<1.0	0	420	<1.0 d
chunky *(Del Monte)*:							
chili style	30	1.0	6.0	0	0	580	m.q.
pasta style	40	1.0	9.0	0	0	500	m.q.
pizza style	40	1.0	8.0	0	0	560	m.q.
cut, peeled *(Hunt's* Choice-Cut)*, 4 oz.	20	1.0	5.0	<1.0	0	460	1.0 d
diced:							
in tomato juice *(Del Monte)*	25	1.0	6.0	0	0	160	2.0 d
w/olive oil, herbs *(Master Choice)*	110	1.0	20.0	3.0	0	240	m.q.

Food and Measure	cal.	prot. (gms)	carbo. (gms)	fat (gms)	chol. (mgs)	sod. (mgs)	fiber (gms)
crushed:							
(Contadina)	30	1.0	6.0	<1.0	0	350	m.q.
(Eden No Salt Added)	35	2.0	6.0	0	0	0	m.q.
(Hunt's Angela Mia), 4 oz.	35	1.0	7.0	<1.0	0	260	<1.0 d
w/basil (Master Choice)	40	1.0	9.0	0	0	330	m.q.
Italian flavored (Hunt's), 4 oz. . . .	40	2.0	9.0	<1.0	0	460	<1.0 d
w/green chilies (Old El Paso), 1/4 cup . . .	14	<1.0	3.0	<1.0	0	480	m.q.
w/jalapeños:							
(Old El Paso), 1/4 cup	11	1.0	2.0	<1.0	0	150	0
(Ortega), 1 oz. . . .	8	0	1.0	0	0	120	m.q.
paste, see "Tomato paste"							
puree:							
1/2 cup	51	2.1	12.5	.1	0	499	2.9 d
(Contadina)	40	2.0	8.0	<1.0	0	35	m.q.
(Del Monte), 1/4 cup	30	1.0	7.0	0	0	25	1.0 d
(Hunt's), 4 oz. . . .	45	2.0	10.0	<1.0	0	150	2.0 d
(Progresso)	45	2.0	10.0	0	0	35	m.q.
heavy concentrate (Progresso) . . .	50	2.0	11.0	0	0	35	m.q.
stewed:							
1/2 cup	34	1.2	8.3	.2	0	325	.9 d
(Contadina)	35	1.0	8.0	<1.0	0	330	m.q.
(Del Monte)	35	1.0	9.0	0	0	360	2.0 d
(Del Monte No Salt)	35	1.0	9.0	0	0	50	2.0 d
(Hunt's), 4 oz. . . .	35	1.0	8.0	<1.0	0	400	<1.0 d
(Hunt's No Salt), 4 oz.	35	1.0	8.0	<1.0	0	20	<1.0 d
Italian flavored (Hunt's), 4 oz. . . .	40	2.0	9.0	<1.0	0	370	<1.0 d
Italian recipe (Del Monte)	30	1.0	7.0	0	0	360	m.q.

Food and Measure	cal.	prot. (gms)	carbo. (gms)	fat (gms)	chol. (mgs)	sod. (mgs)	fiber (gms)
Tomato, canned, stewed *(cont.)*							
Italian style *(Contadina)*	35	1.0	8.0	<1.0	0	250	m.q.
Italian style *(Del Monte)*	30	1.0	8.0	0	0	420	2.0 d
Mexican style *(Contadina)*	35	1.0	8.0	.3	0	230	m.q.
Mexican style *(Del Monte)*	35	1.0	9.0	0	0	400	2.0 d
pizza style *(Del Monte)*	35	1.0	9.0	0	0	670	2.0 d
sliced *(Libby's)* . .	35	1.0	9.0	0	0	355	m.q.
sliced *(Master Choice)*	35	1.0	9.0	0	0	300	m.q.
wedges:							
in tomato juice . .	34	1.0	8.3	.2	0	285	.6 c
(Del Monte)	35	1.0	9.0	0	0	380	2.0 d
Tomato, green, 2³/₅″-diam.	30	1.5	6.3	.3	0	16	1.8 d
Tomato, pickled *(Claussen)*, 3 oz. . .	15	<1.0	3.0	0	0	960	2.0 d
Tomato, sun-dried, see "Tomato"							
Tomato juice, 6 fl. oz., except as noted:							
regular	32	1.4	7.7	.1	0	658	.7 d
low-sodium	32	1.4	7.7	.1	0	18	1.5 d
(Campbell's)	40	1.0	8.0	0	0	490	1.0 d
(Hunt's)	30	1.0	7.0	<1.0	0	520	2.0 d
(Hunt's No Salt Added)	35	1.0	8.0	<1.0	0	25	2.0 d
(R.W. Knudsen Organic)	50	<1.0	10.0	<1.0	0	412	m.q.
(Libby's)	35	1.0	8.0	0	0	450	m.q.
(Welch's)	35	1.0	7.0	0	0	550	0

Food and Measure	cal.	prot. (gms)	carbo. (gms)	fat (gms)	chol. (mgs)	sod. (mgs)	fiber (gms)
Tomato paste, canned, 2 oz., except as noted:							
1 oz.	24	1.1	5.3	.3	0	224	1.2 d
(Contadina)	50	2.0	11.0	<1.0	0	40	m.q.
(Del Monte), 2 tbsp.	30	1.0	7.0	0	0	23	2.0 d
(Hunt's)	45	2.0	11.0	<1.0	0	135	2.0 d
(Hunt's No Salt) . . .	45	2.0	11.0	<1.0	0	25	2.0 d
w/garlic *(Hunt's)* . . .	50	2.0	11.0	<1.0	0	440	2.0 d
Italian *(Contadina)* . .	65	2.0	12.0	1.0	0	520	m.q.
Italian *(Hunt's)*	50	2.0	11.0	<1.0	0	430	2.0 d
Tomato sauce, canned (see also "Tomato, canned" and "Pasta sauce"):							
1/2 cup	37	1.6	8.8	.2	0	738	1.7 d
(Contadina), 1/2 cup	30	1.0	7.0	<1.0	0	580	m.q.
(Contadina Thick & Zesty)*, 1/2 cup . . .	40	2.0	8.0	<1.0	0	650	m.q.
(Del Monte), 1/4 cup	20	0	4.0	0	0	320	0
(Del Monte No Salt)*, 1/4 cup	20	0	4.0	0	0	20	0
(Hunt's), 4 oz.	30	1.0	7.0	<1.0	0	650	2.0 d
(Hunt's No Salt)*, 4 oz.	35	1.0	8.0	<1.0	0	20	2.0 d
(Hunt's Special)*, 4 oz.	35	1.0	8.0	<1.0	0	280	2.0 d
(Progresso), 1/2 cup	40	2.0	9.0	0	0	620	m.q.
w/garlic *(Hunt's)*, 4 oz.	70	2.0	10.0	2.0	0	480	2.0 d
herb flavored *(Hunt's)*, 4 oz.	70	2.0	12.0	2.0	<1	470	2.0 d
Italian style:							
(Contadina), 1/2 cup	30	1.0	7.0	<1.0	0	670	m.q.
(Hunt's), 4 oz. . . .	60	2.0	10.0	2.0	<1	460	2.0 d
(Rokeach), 3 oz. . . .	60	1.0	8.0	2.0	0	243	m.q.
marinara:							
1/2 cup	86	2.0	12.7	4:2	0	786	.8 c
(Rokeach), 3 oz. . . .	60	1.0	9.0	2.0	0	257	m.q.

Food and Measure	cal.	prot. (gms)	carbo. (gms)	fat (gms)	chol. (mgs)	sod. (mgs)	fiber (gms)
Tomato sauce *(cont.)*							
for meat loaf *(Hunt's Meatloaf Fixin's)*,							
2 oz.	20	<1.0	5.0	<1.0	0	580	<1.0 d
w/mushrooms:							
1/2 cup	42	1.8	10.3	.2	0	552	1.0 c
(Hunt's), 4 oz. . . .	25	1.0	6.0	<1.0	0	710	2.0 d
(Rokeach), 1 cup	110	4.0	16.0	3.0	0	846	6.0 d
w/onions:							
1/2 cup	52	1.9	12.1	.2	0	672	1.0 c
(Hunt's), 4 oz. . . .	40	1.0	9.0	<1.0	0	650	2.0 d
w/tomato bits:							
(Hunt's), 4 oz. . . .	30	1.0	7.0	<1.0	0	620	2.0 d
low-sodium, 1/2 cup	39	1.6	8.7	.5	0	18	1.3 c
Tomato-beef cocktail							
(Beefamato), 6 fl. oz.	80	1.0	19.0	<1.0	<1	240	m.q.
Tomato-chile cocktail							
(Snap-E-Tom),							
6 fl. oz.	40	2.0	7.0	0	0	980	m.q.
Tomato-clam juice							
cocktail *(Clamato)*,							
6 fl. oz.	77	1.6	17.9	.2	m.q.	701	m.q.
Tongue, braised:							
beef, 4 oz.	321	25.1	.4	23.5	121	68	0
lamb, 4 oz.	312	24.5	0	23.0	214	76	0
pork, 4 oz.	307	27.3	0	21.1	166	124	0
veal (calf), 4 oz. . . .	229	29.3	0	11.5	m.q.	73	0
Tortellini *(Contadina)*							
refrigerated, 3 oz.:							
cheese and herb . . .	270	13.0	37.0	8.0	40	230	m.q.
chicken	270	12.0	39.0	7.0	60	240	m.q.
chicken and proscuitto	290	13.0	36.0	10.0	65	390	m.q.
Tortellini dishes,							
cheese, frozen *(The Budget Gourmet Side Dish)*, 5.5 oz.	200	8.0	25.0	8.0	20	530	m.q.

Food and Measure	cal.	prot. (gms)	carbo. (gms)	fat (gms)	chol. (mgs)	sod. (mgs)	fiber (gms)
Tortellini entree, frozen:							
(Weight Watchers),							
9 oz.	310	14.0	50.0	6.0	15	570	m.q.
in Alfredo sauce							
(Stouffer's), 8⅞ oz.	580	26.0	35.0	37.0	m.q.	830	m.q.
w/tomato sauce							
(Stouffer's), 9¼ oz.	360	18.0	39.0	15.0	m.q.	720	m.q.
Provençale *(Green Giant Garden Gourmet Right for Lunch),*							
9.5 oz.	260	10.0	44.0	6.0	15	840	3.0 d
Tortilla, 1 piece:							
corn, enchilada style							
(Tyson)	54	1.0	11.0	.4	0	4	m.q.
flour:							
(Old El Paso) . . .	150	4.0	27.0	3.0	0	360	m.q.
burrito style *(Tyson)*	173	5.0	29.0	4.0	0	40	m.q.
burrito style, hand stretched *(Tyson)*	106	3.0	19.0	2.0	0	50	m.q.
burrito style, heat pressed *(Tyson)*	182	5.0	33.0	4.0	0	90	m.q.
fajita style *(Tyson)*	84	3.0	18.0	2.0	0	20	m.q.
soft taco *(Tyson)* . .	121	4.0	20.0	3.0	0	30	m.q.
whole wheat *(Tyson)*	120	4.0	20.0	3.0	0	32	m.q.
Tortilla chips, 1 oz.:							
corn:							
(Doritos)	140	2.0	19.0	7.0	0	80	1.5 d
(Doritos Jumpin' Jack)	140	2.0	18.0	7.0	0	220	1.5 d
(Hain Taco Style)	160	2.0	15.0	11.0	<5	320	m.q.
(Lafamous)	140	2.0	18.0	7.0	0	200	m.q.
(NaChips)	150	2.0	18.0	7.0	0	80	1.5 d
(Tostitos)	140	2.0	18.0	8.0	0	160	1.5 d
(Tostitos Bite Size)	150	2.0	18.0	8.0	0	110	1.5 d
(Tyson Mexican Original Traditional)	140	2.0	17.0	7.0	0	95	m.q.

Food and Measure	cal.	prot. (gms)	carbo. (gms)	fat (gms)	chol. (mgs)	sod. (mgs)	fiber (gms)
Tortilla chips, corn *(cont.)*							
(Tyson Mexican Original Unsalted)	140	2.0	17.0	7.0	0	7	m.q.
blue *(Kettle Tias Lightly Salted)* . .	140	3.0	18.0	6.0	0	80	2.0 d
blue *(Kettle Tias No Salt)*	140	3.0	18.0	6.0	0	2	2.0 d
lime'n chile, restaurant style *(Tostitos)*	150	2.0	18.0	7.0	0	190	1.5 d
nacho *(Doritos)* . .	140	1.0	18.0	7.0	0	160	1.5 d
nacho *(Eagle* Thins)	150	2.0	17.0	8.0	0	200	m.q.
nacho *(Tom's)*, 1¼-oz. pkg. . .	180	3.0	22.0	9.0	0	250	m.q.
nacho *(Tyson* Mexican Original) . .	140	2.0	17.0	7.0	0	145	m.q.
ranch *(Doritos Cool Ranch)*	140	2.0	18.0	7.0	0	170	1.5 d
ranch *(Eagle* Thins)	150	2.0	17.0	8.0	0	150	m.q.
ranch *(Tyson* Mexican Original) . .	140	2.0	17.0	2.0	0	m.q.	m.q.
salsa flavor *(Doritos Salsa Rio)*	140	2.0	18.0	7.0	0	190	1.5 d
sesame *(Hain)* . . .	140	2.0	19.0	7.0	0	190	m.q.
sesame *(Hain* No Salt)*	140	2.0	19.0	7.0	0	<5	m.q.
sesame cheese *(Hain)*	160	2.0	20.0	8.0	<5	270	m.q.
taco flavor *(Doritos)*	140	2.0	18.0	7.0	0	250	1.5 d
white, restaurant style *(Tostitos)* . .	130	2.0	20.0	6.0	0	75	1.5 d
white, round *(NaChips* Low Sodium)*	160	2.0	17.0	9.0	0	5	m.q.
flour *(Chacho's)*:							
original	140	3.0	18.0	7.0	<5	180	m.q.
cheesy quesadilla	140	3.0	17.0	7.0	0	230	m.q.
cinnamon crispana	140	2.0	19.0	7.0	0	70	m.q.

Food and Measure	cal.	prot. (gms)	carbo. (gms)	fat (gms)	chol. (mgs)	sod. (mgs)	fiber (gms)
Tortilla mix, corn *(Albers Ricamasa),* 1/3 cup dry	140	3.0	28.0	1.0	0	5	5.0 d
Tostaco shell *(Old El Paso),* 1 piece . . .	100	1.0	11.0	5.0	0	10	1.0 d
Tostada shell, 1 piece:							
(Lawry's)	73	1.2	9.5	3.0	0	147	.4 d
(Old El Paso)	55	<1.0	6.0	3.0	0	65	.5 d
(Ortega)	50	0	8.0	2.0	0	5	m.q.
(Pancho Villa)	55	<1.0	6.0	3.0	0	65	m.q.
(Rosarita)	60	1.0	8.0	3.0	0	<1	<1.0 d
(Tio Sancho)	67	1.2	8.4	3.2	0	1	.5 c
Tree fern, cooked, chopped, 1/2 cup	28	.2	7.8	.1	0	3	2.6 d
Triticale, whole grain, 1 cup	646	25.1	138.5	4.0	0	10	34.8 d
Triticale flour, whole grain, 1 cup	440	17.1	95.1	2.4	0	3	19.0 d
Tropical nectar *(Kern's),* 6 fl. oz. . . .	110	0	27.0	0	0	5	m.q.
Tropical punch, see "Fruit punch"							
Trout, meat only:							
mixed species:							
raw, 4 oz.	168	23.6	0	7.5	66	59	0
baked, broiled, or microwaved, 4 oz.	215	30.2	0	9.6	84	76	0
rainbow, farmed:							
raw, 4 oz.	156	23.7	0	6.1	67	40	0
baked, broiled, or microwaved, 4 oz.	192	27.5	0	8.2	77	48	0
rainbow, wild:							
raw, 4 oz.	135	23.2	0	3.9	67	35	0
baked, broiled, or microwaved, 4 oz.	170	26.0	0	6.6	78	64	0
sea, see "Sea trout"							

Food and Measure	cal.	prot. (gms)	carbo. (gms)	fat (gms)	chol. (mgs)	sod. (mgs)	fiber (gms)
Tuna, meat only:							
bluefin:							
raw, 4 oz.	163	26.5	0	5.6	43	44	0
baked, broiled, or							
microwaved, 4 oz.	209	33.9	0	7.1	56	57	0
skipjack:							
raw, 4 oz.	117	25.0	0	1.2	53	42	0
baked, broiled, or							
microwaved, 4 oz.	150	32.0	0	1.5	68	53	0
yellowfin:							
raw, 4 oz.	123	26.5	0	1.1	51	42	0
baked, broiled, or							
microwaved, 4 oz.	158	34.0	0	1.4	66	53	0
Tuna, canned,							
drained, 2 oz., ex-							
cept as noted:							
solid light, in oil:							
(Progresso), 1/3 cup	150	13.0	<1.0	13.0	m.q.	400	0
(Star-Kist Prime							
Catch)	150	13.0	<1.0	13.0	25	250	0
solid light, in water:							
(Empress)	60	12.0	0	1.0	m.q.	310	0
(Star-Kist/Star-Kist							
Prime Catch) . .	60	14.0	<1.0	<1.0	25	250	0
chunk light, in oil:							
(Bumble Bee) . . .	160	12.0	0	12.0	30	310	0
(Star-Kist)	150	12.0	<1.0	13.0	25	250	0
chunk light, in water:							
(Star-Kist)	60	12.0	<1.0	<1.0	25	250	0
(Star-Kist Diet) . . .	65	14.0	<1.0	<1.0	25	35	0
(Star-Kist Select—							
60% Less Salt)	65	14.0	<1.0	1.0	25	120	0
(Weight Watchers)	60	13.0	<1.0	<1.0	25	210	0
hickory smoke flavor							
(Star-Kist)	50	12.0	<1.0	<1.0	25	250	0
(Bumble Bee) . .	60	12.0	0	1.0	30	310	0

Food and Measure	cal.	prot. (gms)	carbo. (gms)	fat (gms)	chol. (mgs)	sod. (mgs)	fiber (gms)
solid white, albacore, in oil:							
(Bumble Bee) . . .	130	14.0	0	8.0	30	310	0
(Star-Kist)	140	14.0	<1.0	10.0	25	250	0
solid white, albacore, in water:							
(Bumble Bee) . . .	70	14.0	0	2.0	30	310	0
(Master Choice Line Caught)	70	14.0	<1.0	1.0	25	250	0
(Star-Kist)	70	14.0	<1.0	1.0	25	250	0
(Weight Watchers)	70	15.0	<1.0	1.0	25	210	0
hickory smoke flavor (Star-Kist)	60	13.0	<1.0	<1.0	25	250	0
chunk white, in oil:							
(Bumble Bee) . . .	160	12.0	0	12.0	30	310	0
(Star-Kist)	140	14.0	<1.0	10.0	25	250	0
chunk white, in water:							
(Bumble Bee) . . .	70	12.0	0	2.0	30	310	0
(Star-Kist)	70	14.0	<1.0	1.0	25	250	0
(Star-Kist Diet) . . .	70	15.0	<1.0	1.0	25	35	0
(Star-Kist Select— 60% Less Salt)	70	15.0	<1.0	<1.0	25	120	0
"Tuna," vegetarian, frozen (Worthington Tuno), 2 oz.	100	5.0	3.0	7.0	0	310	m.q.
Tuna entree, frozen, noodle casserole:							
(Stouffer's), 10 oz. . .	340	17.0	33.0	15.0	m.q.	1090	m.q.
(Weight Watchers), 9 oz.	230	15.0	27.0	7.0	20	550	m.q.
Tuna entree, packaged, noodle casserole (Dinty Moore American Classics), 10 oz.	240	16.0	28.0	7.0	65	1280	m.q.

Food and Measure	cal.	prot. (gms)	carbo. (gms)	fat (gms)	chol. (mgs)	sod. (mgs)	fiber (gms)
Tuna entree mix*[1]:							
au gratin (Tuna Helper), 6 oz. . . .	280	14.0	30.0	11.0	m.q.	960	m.q.
fettucine Alfredo (Tuna Helper), 7 oz. . . .	300	15.0	28.0	14.0	m.q.	930	m.q.
garden & herb, zesty tomato or classic Italian (Bumble Bee Tuna Mix-Ins), 1 oz. dry	25	0	5.0	0	0	5	m.q.
lemon herb (Bumble Bee Tuna Mix-Ins), 1 oz. dry	25	0	6.0	0	0	5	m.q.
mushroom, creamy (Tuna Helper), 7 oz.	210	12.0	28.0	6.0	m.q.	720	m.q.
noodles:							
cheesy (Tuna Helper), 7.75 oz.	240	14.0	27.0	8.0	m.q.	960	m.q.
creamy (Tuna Helper), 8 oz. . .	300	14.0	29.0	14.0	m.q.	940	m.q.
pot pie (Tuna Helper), 5.1 oz.	420	12.0	31.0	27.0	m.q.	870	m.q.
rice, buttery (Tuna Helper), 6 oz. . . .	270	11.0	32.0	11.0	m.q.	1020	m.q.
Romanoff (Tuna Helper), 8 oz. . . .	280	14.0	38.0	8.0	m.q.	800	m.q.
salad (Tuna Helper), 5.5 oz.	410	12.0	29.0	27.0	m.q.	850	m.q.
tetrazzini (Tuna Helper), 6 oz. . . .	230	14.0	26.0	8.0	m.q.	780	m.q.
Tuna salad:							
(Longacre), 1 oz. . . .	64	2.7	4.1	4.1	7	158	m.q.
spread (Libby's Spreadables), 1.9 oz.	80	5.0	5.0	5.0	m.q.	220	1.0 d

[1] Prepared with water-packed tuna.

Food and Measure	cal.	prot. (gms)	carbo. (gms)	fat (gms)	chol. (mgs)	sod. (mgs)	fiber (gms)
Tuna seasoning mix							
(Old Bay Tuna Classic), 1 pkg.	117	7.0	15.0	3.0	n.a.	349	m.q.
Turbot, European, meat only:							
raw, 4 oz.	108	18.2	0	3.4	m.q.	170	0
baked, broiled, or microwaved, 4 oz. . .	138	23.3	0	4.3	m.q.	218	0
Turkey, fresh, all classes, roasted:							
meat w/skin, 4 oz. . .	236	31.9	0	11.0	93	77	0
meat only:							
4 oz.	193	33.2	0	5.6	86	79	0
diced, 1 cup	238	41.0	0	7.0	107	99	0
skin only, 1 oz. . . .	125	5.6	0	11.2	32	15	0
dark meat:							
w/skin, 4 oz.	251	31.2	0	13.1	101	86	0
meat only, 4 oz. . .	212	32.4	0	8.2	96	90	0
meat only, diced, 1 cup	262	40.0	0	10.1	119	110	0
light meat:							
w/skin, 4 oz.	223	32.4	0	9.4	86	71	0
meat only, 4 oz. . .	178	33.9	0	3.7	78	73	0
meat only, diced, 1 cup	219	41.9	0	4.5	97	89	0
back, meat w/skin, 4 oz.	276	30.2	0	16.3	103	83	0
breast, meat w/skin:							
1/2 breast, 1.9 lb., (4.2 lbs. raw w/bone)	1637	248.1	0	64.1	643	541	0
4 oz.	214	32.6	0	8.4	84	71	0
leg, meat w/skin:							
1 leg, 1.2 lb. (1.5 lbs. raw w/bone)	1133	152.2	0	53.6	466	420	0
4 oz.	236	31.6	0	11.1	96	87	0

Food and Measure	cal.	prot. (gms)	carbo. (gms)	fat (gms)	chol. (mgs)	sod. (mgs)	fiber (gms)
Turkey *(cont.)*							
wing, meat w/skin:							
1 wing, 6.6 oz.							
(9.9 oz. raw w/							
bone)	426	50.9	0	23.1	150	114	0
4 oz.	260	31.0	0	14.1	92	69	0
Turkey, boneless and luncheon meat (see also "Turkey ham," etc.), 1 oz., except as noted:							
breast:							
(Healthy Deli Gourmet)	26	4.5	.6	.5	9	240	0
(Hormel Bread Ready)	29	6.0	1.0	<2.0	11	410	0
(Hormel Deli No Salt)	33	8.0	<2.0	<2.0	13	18	0
(Hormel Deli Petite)	25	6.0	<2.0	<2.0	11	243	0
(Norbest Blue Label)	23	5.1	<1.0	.5	10	201	0
(Norbest Orange Label)	26	5.5	<1.0	.4	10	230	0
(Norbest Sliced) . .	43	6.8	<1.0	1.7	13	252	0
(Norbest Yellow Label)	28	4.8	<1.0	.8	11	230	0
(Tyson), 1 slice . .	20	4.0	.3	.4	m.q.	136	0
Black Forest *(Healthy Deli)* . .	31	6.0	.5	.5	12	220	0
browned, glazed *(Longacre* Gourmet)	31	5.3	.5	.7	12	227	0
browned, roasted *(Longacre* Gourmet)	35	5.8	.7	.7	12	232	0
cooked *(Healthy Deli* Lessalt)	25	4.5	.7	.5	10	150	0

Food and Measure	cal.	prot. (gms)	carbo. (gms)	fat (gms)	chol. (mgs)	sod. (mgs)	fiber (gms)
honey (Healthy Deli)	35	5.5	2.0	.5	9	280	0
honey roasted (Louis Rich) . . .	32	4.9	1.2	.8	12	319	0
mini (Longacre Gourmet)	34	5.8	.6	.8	11	241	0
oven cooked (Healthy Deli) . .	25	3.7	1.2	.3	8	290	0
oven roasted (Hillshire Farm Deli Select)	31	6.0	<1.0	.2	m.q.	340	0
oven roasted (Longacre Lean-Lite)	34	6.5	0	.7	14	155	0
oven roasted (Louis Rich), .4-oz. slice	12	1.9	.4	.3	4	123	0
oven roasted (Louis Rich)	30	4.9	1.0	.7	11	312	0
oven roasted (Weight Watchers)	30	5.0	<1.0	<1.0	10	240	0
prebrowned (Norbest Orange Label)	28	6.2	<1.0	.5	12	187	0
roast (Oscar Mayer Deli-Thin), 5 slices	60	11.0	2.0	1.5	25	500	0
roll (Longacre Sliced)	37	5.2	.6	1.4	11	215	0
breast, skinless: (Hormel Deli Premium)	25	6.0	<2.0	<2.0	10	240	0
(Longacre Gourmet)	28	5.5	.7	.2	13	254	0
(Longacre Lean-Lite)	31	6.7	0	.3	15	161	0
(Longacre No Salt)	31	6.6	0	.3	12	12	0
(Longacre Premium)	25	4.6	.7	.2	10	260	0
(Longacre Salt Watchers)	33	6.7	0	.5	13	18	0
(Norbest Blue Label)	27	5.4	<1.0	.6	10	190	0
(Norbest Blue Label Salt Free)	34	8.5	<1.0	.2	10	15	0

Food and Measure	cal.	prot. (gms)	carbo. (gms)	fat (gms)	chol. (mgs)	sod. (mgs)	fiber (gms)
Turkey, boneless and luncheon meat, breast, skinless *(cont.)*							
(Norbest Extra Tan Label)	31	5.0	1.1	.7	9	258	0
(Norbest Orange Label)	26	5.6	<1.0	.2	9	207	0
(Norbest Tan Label)	26	4.5	.7	.6	7	244	0
(Norbest Yellow Label)	26	5.4	<1.0	.5	11	227	0
caramel *(Norbest* Yellow Label) . .	30	5.4	<1.0	.9	10	198	0
breast, smoked:							
(Healthy Deli Gourmet)	28	5.0	.6	.5	9	240	0
(Hillshire Farm Deli Select)	31	6.0	<1.0	.2	m.q.	290	0
(Longacre Gourmet)	30	5.7	.6	.5	13	244	0
(Longacre Lean-Lite)	34	6.6	0	.7	16	168	0
(Longacre Sliced)	28	5.3	.9	.2	10	352	0
(Louis Rich), .4-oz. slice	11	2.3	.1	.1	5	111	0
(Louis Rich), .7-oz. slice	21	4.4	.1	.3	9	212	0
(Louis Rich)	33	5.7	.2	1.0	11	263	0
(Norbest Orange Label)	30	5.9	<1.0	.7	13	232	0
(Oscar Mayer) . . .	25	6.0	0	0	10	280	0
(Oscar Mayer Deli-Thin), 5 slices . .	60	12.0	0	.5	25	590	0
(Oscar Mayer Healthy Favorites), 5 slices	60	12.0	<1.0	0	25	400	0
(Weight Watchers)	30	5.0	<1.0	1.0	10	260	0
breast and white, skinless *(Longacre* Deli Chef)	38	4.9	.8	1.5	12	195	0
dark, smoked, cured *(Longacre/Longacre* Chunk)	45	4.4	.4	2.7	21	312	0

Food and Measure	cal.	prot. (gms)	carbo. (gms)	fat (gms)	chol. (mgs)	sod. (mgs)	fiber (gms)
luncheon loaf *(Louis Rich)*	45	4.6	.4	2.8	16	271	0
roll:							
combination *(Long-acre)*	44	3.9	.5	2.9	17	187	0
white *(Longacre)* . .	44	3.8	.7	2.7	13	196	0
smoked *(Louis Rich)*	31	5.4	.3	1.0	15	291	0
Turkey, canned, chunk, 2.5 oz.:							
(Hormel)	80	13.0	1.0	3.0	45	420	0
(Swanson Premium)	90	15.0	2.0	3.0	m.q.	270	0
white *(Swanson Pre-mium)*	80	17.0	1.0	1.0	m.q.	260	0
Turkey, frozen or re-frigerated, 1 oz.:							
breast, raw:							
(Longacre Cook-In-The-Bag)	27	5.9	.4	.2	13	124	0
cutlets *(Norbest Tasti-Lean)* . . .	28	6.4	<1.0	.3	14	20	0
cutlets or tenders *(Norbest Saddle Pack)*	28	6.5	<1.0	.4	15	20	0
roast *(Norbest)* . .	26	4.9	<1.0	.6	11	122	0
roast *(Norbest Sweetheart)* . . .	27	5.5	<1.0	.5	12	88	0
steaks *(Norbest Saddle Pack)* . .	27	7.0	<1.0	.2	14	10	0
steaks, cubed *(Norbest/Norbest Tasti-Lean)* . . .	27	7.0	<1.0	.2	14	10	0
strips or tips *(Norbest Tasti-Lean)*	28	6.4	<1.0	.3	14	20	0
tenders *(Norbest Tasti-Lean)* . . .	31	6.5	<1.0	.4	15	20	0

Food and Measure	cal.	prot. (gms)	carbo. (gms)	fat (gms)	chol. (mgs)	sod. (mgs)	fiber (gms)
Turkey, frozen or refrigerated (cont.)							
breast, cooked:							
(Louis Rich)	45	8.3	0	1.3	21	22	0
barbecued (Louis Rich)	30	5.7	.7	.5	12	336	0
hen, w/out wing (Louis Rich) . . .	51	7.9	0	2.1	21	19	0
hickory smoked (Louis Rich) . . .	28	5.7	.6	.3	13	372	0
honey roasted (Louis Rich) . . .	29	5.4	1.2	.3	12	340	0
oven roasted (Louis Rich)	26	5.5	.3	.3	12	319	0
roast (Louis Rich)	42	8.3	.2	.8	19	20	0
slices (Louis Rich)	39	8.5	0	.5	18	24	0
steaks (Louis Rich)	38	8.5	0	.5	18	24	0
tenderloins (Louis Rich)	38	8.5	0	.4	19	23	0
dark meat, roast, raw (Longacre)	39	5.1	0	2.1	17	122	0
drumstick, cooked (Louis Rich)	56	8.0	0	2.6	37	27	0
ground, see "Turkey, ground"							
roast, w/out gravy (Norbest)	38	4.9	<1.0	2.0	14	108	0
thigh, cooked (Louis Rich)	63	7.5	0	3.6	34	22	0
whole, cooked:							
browned and roasted (Long- acre)	55	6.7	0	2.7	20	100	0
w/out giblets (Louis Rich)	52	7.7	0	2.3	24	24	0
smoked (Longacre)	50	6.5	0	2.5	24	228	0
wing, cooked:							
(Louis Rich)	53	7.3	0	2.6	32	23	0

Food and Measure	cal.	prot. (gms)	carbo. (gms)	fat (gms)	chol. (mgs)	sod. (mgs)	fiber (gms)
(Louis Rich Drumettes)	51	7.8	0	2.2	32	22	0
portion *(Louis Rich)*	54	7.0	0	2.9	31	19	0
Turkey, ground (see also "Turkey patties"), 1 oz.:							
1 oz.	42	4.9	0	2.3	22	27	0
(Longacre)	60	4.0	0	4.3	30	25	0
(Norbest), 1 oz. . . .	51	5.5	<1.0	3.1	19	21	0
cooked:							
1 oz.	67	7.8	0	3.7	29	30	0
(Louis Rich)	59	6.8	0	3.5	28	30	0
(Louis Rich 90% Fat Free)	52	6.7	0	2.7	27	32	0
(Perdue)	38	6.0	0	2.0	25	15	0
breast meat *(Perdue)*	32	7.0	0	<1.0	14	13	0
w/natural flavoring *(Louis Rich* 90% Fat Free)	49	7.3	0	2.2	25	33	0
"Turkey," vegetarian:							
canned *(Worthington* Turkee), 2 slices . .	130	9.0	3.0	9.0	0	430	m.q.
frozen, smoked *(Worthington),* 4 slices	180	13.0	5.0	12.0	0	820	m.q.
Turkey bacon, 1 slice:							
(Louis Rich)	35	2.0	0	2.5	15	210	0
(Oscar Mayer)	20	2.0	0	1.0	10	140	0
Turkey bologna, 1 oz., except as noted:							
(Longacre)	62	3.6	0	5.2	21	294	0
(Longacre Sliced) . .	62	3.6	0	5.1	21	294	0
(Louis Rich)	60	3.5	.6	4.9	23	244	0
mild *(Louis Rich)* . . .	60	3.7	.7	4.7	17	301	0
Turkey burger, see "Turkey patty"							

Food and Measure	cal.	prot. (gms)	carbo. (gms)	fat (gms)	chol. (mgs)	sod. (mgs)	fiber (gms)
Turkey and corned beef *(Healthy Deli Doubledecker),* 1 oz.	30	5.1	.6	.7	12	195	0
Turkey dinner, frozen:							
(Banquet Extra Helping), 17 oz.	460	23.0	64.0	12.0	70	2030	m.q.
(Swanson), 11.5 oz.	340	20.0	43.0	11.0	m.q.	980	m.q.
(Swanson Hungry Man), 16.5 oz. . . .	510	33.0	59.0	16.0	m.q.	1220	m.q.
breast of *(Healthy Choice),* 10.5 oz.	260	21.0	41.0	3.0	40	560	m.q.
breast, stuffed:							
(The Budget Gourmet Light and Healthy),* 11 oz.	250	21.0	31.0	6.0	35	570	m.q.
(Weight Watchers), 8.5 oz.	270	18.0	31.0	8.0	60	520	m.q.
w/dressing and gravy *(Armour Classics),* 11.5 oz.	320	19.0	34.0	12.0	50	1280	m.q.
w/gravy *(Tyson Premium),* 9.5 oz. . . .	320	19.0	34.0	12.0	35	900	m.q.
sliced *(Freezer Queen),* 9.25 oz.	190	13.0	24.0	4.0	20	970	m.q.
tetrazzini *(Healthy Choice),* 12.6 oz.	340	23.0	49.0	6.0	40	490	m.q.
Turkey entree, canned, and dressing, w/gravy *(Libby's Diner),* 7 oz.	170	11.0	15.0	7.0	35	830	m.q.
Turkey entree, freeze-dried*, tetrazzini *(Mountain House),* 1 cup . . .	210	13.0	21.0	8.0	m.q.	1150	m.q.

Food and Measure	cal.	prot. (gms)	carbo. (gms)	fat (gms)	chol. (mgs)	sod. (mgs)	fiber (gms)
Turkey entree, frozen:							
breast:							
nuggets *(Perdue Done It!)*, 1 piece	54	3.0	3.0	3.0	7	112	n.a.
roast, w/mushrooms, in gravy *(Healthy Choice)*, 8.5 oz.	200	18.0	26.0	3.0	40	380	m.q.
roast, w/stuffing *(Stouffer's Homestyle)*, 7⅞ oz.	270	19.0	27.0	9.0	m.q.	920	m.q.
sliced, w/dressing *(Lean Cuisine)*, 7⅞ oz.	200	15.0	22.0	6.0	30	540	m.q.
sliced, in mushroom sauce w/rice pilaf *(Lean Cuisine)*, 8 oz.	230	17.0	24.0	7.0	35	540	m.q.
croquettes:							
(On-Cor), 8 oz. . .	237	12.0	23.0	10.0	m.q.	1339	m.q.
gravy and *(Freezer Queen* Family), 7 oz.	250	13.0	19.0	13.0	m.q.	940	m.q.
Dijon *(Lean Cuisine)*, 9.5 oz.	210	20.0	20.0	6.0	45	590	m.q.
w/dressing:							
(Freezer Queen), 9 oz.	210	15.0	27.0	5.0	20	950	m.q.
(On-Cor), 8 oz. . .	238	14.0	24.0	10.0	m.q.	1225	m.q.
glazed *(The Budget Gourmet* Light and Healthy), 9 oz. . . .	260	16.0	38.0	5.0	30	710	m.q.
and gravy:							
(Banquet Meals), 9.25 oz.	260	15.0	31.0	10.0	45	1110	m.q.
(On-Cor), 8 oz. . .	129	9.0	10.0	6.0	m.q.	1385	n.a.

Food and Measure	cal.	prot. (gms)	carbo. (gms)	fat (gms)	chol. (mgs)	sod. (mgs)	fiber (gms)
Turkey entree *(cont.)*							
and gravy, w/dressing:							
(Banquet Healthy Balance),							
11.25 oz.	270	17.0	40.0	5.0	35	760	m.q.
(Freezer Queen Family), 7 oz. . .	150	12.0	14.0	5.0	m.q.	1190	m.q.
(Swanson), 9 oz. . .	290	18.0	29.0	10.0	m.q.	940	m.q.
sliced *(Healthy Choice Homestyle Classic),* 10 oz.	270	27.0	30.0	4.0	50	530	m.q.
gravy and:							
(Banquet Cookin' Bag), 5 oz. . . .	100	7.0	5.0	6.0	m.q.	m.q.	n.a.
(Banquet Family), 6 oz.	120	9.0	6.0	6.0	m.q.	m.q.	n.a.
(Freezer Queen Family), 7 oz. . .	110	9.0	8.0	5.0	m.q.	1160	n.a.
w/dressing *(Banquet Entree Express),* 7 oz.	220	12.0	26.0	8.0	m.q.	1410	m.q.
medallions, roast *(Weight Watchers Smart Ones),* 8.5 oz.	200	13.0	35.0	1.0	25	440	m.q.
pie:							
(Stouffer's), 10 oz.	410	16.0	33.0	24.0	m.q.	750	m.q.
(Swanson), 7 oz. . . .	390	11.0	38.0	21.0	m.q.	720	m.q.
(Swanson Hungry Man), 14 oz. . . .	660	24.0	58.0	37.0	m.q.	1570	m.q.
tetrazzini *(Stouffer's),* 10 oz.	400	22.0	26.0	23.0	m.q.	960	m.q.
w/vegetables, home-style *(Healthy Choice),* 9.5 oz. . .	230	24.0	28.0	3.0	35	470	m.q.
w/vegetables and pasta, homestyle *(Lean Cuisine),* 9³/8 oz.	230	21.0	25.0	5.0	50	550	m.q.

Food and Measure	cal.	prot. (gms)	carbo. (gms)	fat (gms)	chol. (mgs)	sod. (mgs)	fiber (gms)
Turkey entree, packaged, w/dressing and gravy *(Dinty Moore American Classics)*, 10 oz. . . .	290	28.0	33.0	5.0	40	910	m.q.
Turkey entree, refrigerated *(Turkey By George)*, 5 oz.:							
hickory barbecue . .	190	28.0	8.0	5.0	65	840	n.a.
lemon pepper	160	28.0	4.0	4.0	60	830	n.a.
mustard tarragon . .	180	29.0	3.0	6.0	80	830	n.a.
Parmesan, Italian . .	170	28.0	3.0	5.0	70	860	n.a.
Turkey fat, 1 tbsp.	115	0	0	12.8	13	0	0
Turkey frankfurter:							
(Longacre), 1 oz. . . .	67	3.7	0	5.7	25	290	0
(Louis Rich), 1 link . .	98	5.7	1.3	7.8	41	512	0
(Louis Rich Bun Length)*, 1 link . . .	125	7.2	1.7	9.9	52	648	0
(Perdue), 1.6-oz. link	106	6.0	2.0	8.0	107	519	0
cheese *(Louis Rich)*, 1 link	108	6.1	1.3	8.8	44	526	0
Turkey giblets:							
simmered, 4 oz. . . .	189	30.1	2.4	5.8	474	67	0
simmered, chopped or diced, 1 cup	243	38.5	3.0	7.4	606	85	0
Turkey gravy:							
canned, 2 oz., 1/4 cup:							
(Franco-American)	30	(0)	3.0	2.0	m.q.	290	n.a.
(Heinz HomeStyle)	25	1.0	3.0	1.0	<1	370	0
seasoned *(Pepperidge Farm)* . . .	30	1.0	4.0	1.0	m.q.	320	n.a.
mix:							
(French's), 1/4 pkg.	25	0	5.0	0	0	190	n.a.
(Lawry's), 1 cup*	98	3.2	14.9	2.9	2	1380	.2 c
(McCormick/Schilling), 1/4 cup* . .	22	.5	4.0	.5	n.a.	353	n.a.

Food and Measure	cal.	prot. (gms)	carbo. (gms)	fat (gms)	chol. (mgs)	sod. (mgs)	fiber (gms)
Turkey ham, 1 oz., except as noted:							
(Healthy Deli)	35	4.4	.7	1.6	14	200	0
(Longacre Sliced) . .	35	5.6	0	1.3	22	319	0
(Louis Rich)	35	4.9	.3	1.6	20	317	0
(Louis Rich Round) . .	34	5.3	.4	1.2	20	303	0
(Louis Rich Square), .7-oz. slice	22	3.9	.2	.5	15	233	0
(Louis Rich Thin Sliced), 1 slice . . .	11	2.1	.1	.3	8	122	0
(Norbest/Norbest Sliced)	33	5.0	<1.0	1.4	17	275	0
(Norbest Canadian Style)	35	5.5	<1.0	1.4	17	318	0
(Norbest Tavern Ham)	34	5.3	<1.0	1.5	22	292	0
(Tyson), 1 slice	23	3.1	1.0	.2	m.q.	182	0
baked (Longacre, 12% Water Added) . . .	26	4.7	0	1.4	20	320	0
baked (Longacre, 20% Water Added) . . .	42	4.3	1.5	2.0	18	389	0
chopped (Louis Rich)	42	4.9	.3	2.3	22	291	0
cured (Norbest Gourmet)	40	5.0	<1.0	2.2	20	281	0
honey cured (Louis Rich), .7-oz. slice	22	3.8	.5	.6	15	222	0
roll (Norbest)	31	4.6	.5	1.1	m.q.	346	0
Turkey ham salad (Longacre), 1 oz.	53	2.1	2.9	3.7	12	186	m.q.
Turkey luncheon meat, see "Turkey, boneless and luncheon meat"							
Turkey nuggets, breaded, heated* (Louis Rich), 1 piece	63	3.2	4.0	3.6	9	151	m.q.

Food and Measure	cal.	prot. (gms)	carbo. (gms)	fat (gms)	chol. (mgs)	sod. (mgs)	fiber (gms)
Turkey pastrami, 1 oz.:							
(Healthy Deli)	35	4.1	1.4	1.4	14	280	0
(Longacre Sliced) . .	36	5.5	0	1.4	22	276	0
(Norbest Sliced) . . .	31	4.8	<1.0	1.2	17	286	0
Turkey patty:							
breaded, heated* (Louis Rich), 1 patty	217	11.5	13.3	13.0	35	564	m.q.
frozen, 1 oz.:							
(Longacre)	60	4.0	0	4.3	30	25	0
barbecued (Longacre)	59	4.5	1.0	4.0	30	70	0
Turkey pie, see "Turkey entree"							
Turkey salad:							
(Longacre), 1 oz. . . .	59	2.5	3.0	4.1	73	142	m.q.
spread (Libby's Spreadables), 1.9 oz.	100	5.0	6.0	6.0	15	260	1.0 d
Turkey salami, 1 oz.:							
(Longacre)	46	4.8	.6	2.6	25	340	0
(Louis Rich)	43	4.5	0	2.7	21	285	0
cooked	56	4.6	.2	3.9	23	285	0
cotto (Louis Rich) . .	42	4.3	.1	2.7	22	289	0
Turkey sandwich, pocket, frozen:							
w/broccoli 'n cheese (Lean Pockets), 4.5 oz.	260	12.0	31.0	9.0	35	750	m.q.
w/ham 'n cheese (Hot Pockets), 4.5 oz.	300	14.0	40.0	9.0	40	800	m.q.
Turkey sausage, 1 oz., except as noted:							
(Longacre Chub or Patties)	60	4.3	0	4.5	20	75	0
(Norbest Chub) . . .	42	4.6	<1.0	2.3	22	159	0

Food and Measure	cal.	prot. (gms)	carbo. (gms)	fat (gms)	chol. (mgs)	sod. (mgs)	fiber (gms)
Turkey sausage *(cont.)*							
(Norbest Links)	44	4.8	<1.0	2.6	23	162	0
breakfast, cooked:							
(Louis Rich)	51	5.4	0	3.2	25	262	0
(Louis Rich), 1 link	46	5.5	.3	2.5	18	234	0
(Perdue), 1 link . .	40	4.0	<1.0	4.0	19	106	0
(Perdue), 1 patty	61	6.0	<1.0	3.0	27	175	0
Italian, hot or sweet, cooked *(Perdue)*, 2-oz. link	94	10.0	0	6.0	43	348	0
Polish *(Louis Rich Polska)*	40	4.5	.5	2.2	19	250	0
smoked:							
(Louis Rich)	42	4.4	.8	2.3	18	252	0
w/cheese *(Louis Rich)*	46	4.7	.7	2.7	18	270	0
Turkey and pork sausage, cooked *(Jimmy Dean Light)*:							
1 oz.	80	6.0	<1.0	7.0	25	230	0
hot, 1 oz.	80	6.0	<1.0	6.0	25	220	0
sage, 1 oz.	80	6.0	<1.0	6.0	25	210	0
Turkey seasoning and coating mix, roast *(McCormick/ Schilling Bag'n Season)*, 1 pkg.	146	6.0	20.0	5.0	n.a.	1935	m.q.
Turkey spread, canned, chunky *(Underwood Light)*, 2 1/8 oz.	75	11.0	2.0	2.0	25	330	n.a.
Turkey sticks, breaded, heated* *(Louis Rich)*, 1 piece	80	4.2	4.5	5.0	12	204	m.q.
Turkey summer sausage *(Louis Rich)*, 1 oz.	44	5.1	.4	2.4	28	340	0

Food and Measure	cal.	prot. (gms)	carbo. (gms)	fat (gms)	chol. (mgs)	sod. (mgs)	fiber (gms)
Turmeric, ground,							
1 tsp.	8	.2	1.4	.2	0	1	.5 d
Turnip:							
fresh or stored:							
raw, cubed, 1/2 cup	18	.6	4.1	.1	0	44	1.2 d
boiled, drained,							
cubed, 1/2 cup	14	.6	3.8	.1	0	39	1.6 d
boiled, drained,							
mashed, 1/2 cup	21	.8	5.6	.1	0	58	2.3 d
frozen, boiled, drained,							
4 oz.	26	1.7	4.9	.3	0	41	.8 c
Turnip greens:							
fresh:							
raw, untrimmed,							
1 lb.	85	4.8	18.2	1.0	0	126	7.6 d
raw, chopped,							
1/2 cup	7	.4	1.6	.1	0	11	.7 d
boiled, drained,							
chopped, 1/2 cup	15	.8	3.1	.2	0	21	2.2 d
canned, 1/2 cup:							
w/liquid	17	1.6	2.8	.4	0	325	1.5 d
(Allens/Sunshine)	20	2.0	3.0	<1.0	0	15	1.0 d
chopped, w/diced							
turnips (Allens/							
Sunshine)	20	2.0	1.0	<1.0	0	20	1.0 d
frozen:							
boiled, drained,							
w/turnips, 4 oz.	19	2.4	3.3	.2	0	17	3.5 d
chopped (Frosty							
Acres), 3.3 oz.	20	2.0	4.0	0	0	10	1.0 c
chopped, w/diced							
turnips (Sea-							
brook), 3.3 oz.	20	3.0	3.0	0	0	n.a.	m.q.
Turnover, frozen or							
refrigerated, 1 piece:							
apple:							
(Pepperidge Farm)	280	3.0	33.0	15.0	0	210	m.q.
flaky (Pillsbury) . .	170	2.0	23.0	8.0	0	330	m.q.

Food and Measure	cal.	prot. (gms)	carbo. (gms)	fat (gms)	chol. (mgs)	sod. (mgs)	fiber (gms)
Turnover (cont.)							
blueberry (Pepperidge Farm)	280	4.0	32.0	15.0	0	210	m.q.
cherry:							
(Pepperidge Farm)	290	3.0	33.0	17.0	0	210	m.q.
flaky (Pillsbury) . .	170	2.0	24.0	8.0	0	330	m.q.
peach (Pepperidge Farm)	310	3.0	34.0	18.0	n.a.	260	m.q.
raspberry (Pepperidge Farm)	310	4.0	36.0	17.0	n.a.	260	m.q.

V

Food and Measure	cal.	prot. (gms)	carbo. (gms)	fat (gms)	chol. (mgs)	sod. (mgs)	fiber (gms)
Vanilla extract *(Virginia Dare)*, 1 tsp.	10	0	.3	0	0	0	0
Vanilla flavor drink:							
canned *(Sego* Very Vanilla), 10 fl. oz.	225	11.0	34.0	5.0	n.a.	360	n.a.
mix *(Carnation* Instant Breakfast), 1 pkt.	130	4.0	28.0	0	3	100	m.q.
mix *(Pillsbury* Instant Breakfast), 1 pkt.	130	6.0	28.0	0	0	100	n.a.
Veal, meat only, 4 oz.:							
cubed, lean only, braised or stewed	213	39.6	0	4.9	164	105	0
ground, broiled . . .	195	27.6	0	8.6	117	94	0
leg:							
braised, lean w/fat	239	41.0	0	7.2	152	76	0
braised, lean only	230	41.6	0	5.8	159	76	0
roasted, lean w/fat	181	31.4	0	5.3	117	77	0
roasted, lean only	170	31.8	0	3.8	117	77	0
loin:							
braised, lean w/fat	322	34.2	0	19.5	134	91	0
braised, lean only	256	38.1	0	10.4	142	95	0
roasted, lean w/fat	246	28.1	0	14.0	117	105	0
roasted, lean only	198	29.8	0	7.9	120	109	0
rib:							
braised, lean w/fat	285	36.8	0	14.2	158	108	0
braised, lean only	247	39.1	0	8.9	163	112	0
roasted, lean w/fat	259	27.2	0	15.8	125	104	0
roasted, lean only	201	29.2	0	8.4	130	110	0
shoulder, whole:							
braised, lean w/fat	259	36.4	0	11.5	143	108	0

Food and Measure	cal.	prot. (gms)	carbo. (gms)	fat (gms)	chol. (mgs)	sod. (mgs)	fiber (gms)
Veal, shoulder, whole (cont.)							
braised, lean only	226	38.2	0	6.9	147	110	0
roasted, lean w/fat	209	28.7	0	9.5	128	109	0
roasted, lean only	193	29.3	0	7.5	129	110	0
shoulder, arm:							
braised, lean w/fat	268	38.1	0	11.6	168	99	0
braised, lean only	228	40.5	0	6.0	176	102	0
roasted, lean w/fat	208	28.9	0	9.4	122	102	0
roasted, lean only	186	29.6	0	6.6	124	103	0
shoulder, blade:							
braised, lean w/fat	255	35.4	0	11.4	174	111	0
braised, lean only	224	37.0	0	7.3	179	115	0
roasted, lean w/fat	211	28.5	0	9.8	133	113	0
roasted, lean only	194	29.1	0	7.8	135	116	0
sirloin:							
braised, lean w/fat	286	35.4	0	14.9	122	90	0
braised, lean only	231	38.5	0	7.4	128	92	0
roasted, lean w/fat	229	28.5	0	11.9	116	94	0
roasted, lean only	191	29.8	0	7.1	118	96	0
"Veal," vegetarian, frozen (Worthington Veelets), 1 patty . .	230	14.0	12.0	14.0	0	390	m.q.
Veal dinner, parmigiana, frozen:							
(Armour Classics), 11.25 oz.	400	18.0	34.0	22.0	55	1320	m.q.
(Freezer Queen), 9 oz.	290	21.0	44.0	4.0	20	700	m.q.
(Swanson), 11.5 oz.	400	21.0	40.0	18.0	m.q.	1070	m.q.
(Swanson Hungry Man), 18.25 oz. . .	590	32.0	57.0	26.0	m.q.	1840	m.q.
Veal entree, parmigiana, frozen:							
(Banquet Meals), 9 oz.	300	12.0	35.0	15.0	30	970	m.q.
(On-Cor), 8 oz.	350	16.0	29.0	19.0	m.q.	1373	m.q.
(Swanson), 10 oz. . . .	320	19.0	33.0	12.0	m.q.	980	m.q.
w/pasta Alfredo (Stouffer's Homestyle), 9.25 oz.	350	28.0	26.0	15.0	m.q.	1060	m.q.

Food and Measure	cal.	prot. (gms)	carbo. (gms)	fat (gms)	chol. (mgs)	sod. (mgs)	fiber (gms)
patty (Banquet Family), 7 oz.	320	16.0	29.0	16.0	m.q.	m.q.	m.q.
patty (Weight Watchers Ultimate 200), 8.2 oz.	150	22.0	5.0	4.0	50	550	m.q.
Vegetable chips:							
exotic (Terra), 1 oz.	150	1.0	18.0	8.0	0	70	m.q.
sea (Eden), 1 oz. . . .	130	1.0	22.0	5.0	0	200	m.q.
Vegetable entree, canned:							
chow mein, meatless (La Choy), 3/4 cup	25	1.0	5.0	<1.0	0	860	2.0 d
stew (Dinty Moore), 8 oz.	155	5.0	20.0	6.0	14	850	m.q.
Vegetable entree, freeze-dried, stew, w/beef (Mountain House), 1 cup* . .	230	11.0	27.0	7.0	m.q.	580	m.q.
Vegetable entree, frozen:							
Chinese, and chicken (The Budget Gourmet Light and Healthy), 10 oz. . .	280	11.0	47.0	7.0	10	590	m.q.
Italian, and chicken (The Budget Gourmet Light and Healthy), 10.25 oz.	310	14.0	50.0	8.0	30	690	m.q.
and pasta mornay, w/ham (Lean Cuisine), 93/8 oz. . . .	280	15.0	29.0	11.0	35	970	m.q.
pot pie, 7 oz:							
w/beef (Banquet)	510	12.0	39.0	33.0	25	870	m.q.
w/beef (Morton) . .	430	11.0	27.0	31.0	30	740	m.q.
w/chicken (Banquet)	550	15.0	39.0	36.0	35	860	m.q.
w/chicken (Morton)	420	14.0	27.0	28.0	35	740	m.q.
w/turkey (Banquet)	510	16.0	39.0	31.0	40	860	m.q.
w/turkey (Morton)	420	14.0	27.0	28.0	40	740	m.q.

Food and Measure	cal.	prot. (gms)	carbo. (gms)	fat (gms)	chol. (mgs)	sod. (mgs)	fiber (gms)
Vegetable juice cocktail, 8 fl. oz., except as noted:							
(R.W. Knudsen Very Veggie Low Sodium)	40	2.0	8.0	<1.0	0	32	2.0 d
("V-8"), 6 fl. oz.	35	1.0	8.0	0	0	490	1.0 d
("V-8" Light 'N Tangy), 6 fl. oz.	40	1.0	8.0	0	0	240	1.0 d
("V-8" Low Sodium), 6 fl. oz.	40	1.0	8.0	0	0	70	1.0 d
hearty *(Smucker's)* . .	58	.6	13.0	<.1	0	714	m.q.
hot & spicy *(Smucker's)*	58	.6	13.0	<.1	0	650	m.q.
original or spicy *(R.W. Knudsen Very Veggie)*	40	2.0	8.0	<1.0	0	560	2.0 d
spicy hot *("V-8"),* 6 fl. oz.	35	1.0	8.0	0	0	590	1.0 d
Vegetable oyster, see "Salsify"							
Vegetable pie, see "Vegetable entree"							
Vegetable sandwich, pocket, frozen *(Veggie Pockets),* 5 oz.:							
Bar-B-Q	320	11.0	50.0	10.0	0	560	1.5 d
broccoli cheddar . . .	275	11.0	37.0	9.0	0	540	.2 d
Greek	270	11.0	35.0	10.0	0	500	<.1 d
Indian	300	9.6	41.0	12.0	0	500	.9 d
Oriental	295	9.6	40.8	12.0	0	572	.9 d
pizza	315	12.0	42.0	12.0	0	620	1.2 d
Tex-Mex	310	11.0	43.0	11.0	0	595	.3 d
Vegetable protein, 1 oz.:							
(Naturade Original) . .	105	25.0	1.0	0	0	290	m.q.
chocolate *(Naturade)*	105	24.0	1.0	0	0	290	m.q.
soy free *(Naturade)*	105	23.0	3.0	0	0	290	m.q.

Food and Measure	cal.	prot. (gms)	carbo. (gms)	fat (gms)	chol. (mgs)	sod. (mgs)	fiber (gms)
Vegetable sticks, frozen *(Stilwell)*, 5 pieces	180	3.0	24.0	9.0	0	480	2.0 d
Vegetables, see specific listings							
Vegetables, mixed, canned or packaged, 1/2 cup:							
(Green Giant Garden Medley)	35	1.0	9.0	0	0	350	1.0 d
(Green Giant Pantry Express)	35	1.0	8.0	<1.0	0	300	1.0 d
(La Choy Fancy Mix)	12	1.0	2.0	<1.0	0	30	1.0 d
(Stokely)	40	2.0	8.0	0	0	300	m.q.
chop suey *(La Choy)*	10	1.0	2.0	<1.0	0	320	<1.0 d
Dijon *(Del Monte Vegetable Classics)* . .	70	1.0	8.0	4.0	n.a.	420	m.q.
Vegetables, mixed, frozen, 1/2 cup, except as noted:							
(Frosty Acres), 3.3 oz.	65	3.0	13.0	0	0	50	1.0 c
(Green Giant)	40	2.0	9.0	0	0	40	2.0 d
(Green Giant Harvest Fresh)	40	2.0	9.0	0	0	125	2.0 d
(Seabrook), 3.3 oz. . .	65	3.0	13.0	0	0	50	1.0 c
(Southern), 3.5 oz. . .	69	3.2	13.9	0	0	60	m.q.
Austrian style *(Birds Eye International)*	70	4.0	6.0	3.0	10	390	m.q.
Bavarian style *(Birds Eye International)*	90	3.0	10.0	5.0	25	280	m.q.
for beef, 7 oz.[1]:							
Burgundy *(Birds Eye Easy Recipe)* . .	120	4.0	17.0	5.0	0	670	4.0 d
Italiano *(Birds Eye Easy Recipe)* . .	150	5.0	28.0	2.0	0	580	3.0 d

[1] *Without added ingredients.*

Food and Measure	cal.	prot. (gms)	carbo. (gms)	fat (gms)	chol. (mgs)	sod. (mgs)	fiber (gms)
in butter sauce *(Green Giant)*	60	2.0	11.0	2.0	5	300	2.0 d
California style *(Green Giant)*	25	2.0	6.0	0	0	40	2.0 d
for chicken, 7 oz.[1]:							
Alfredo *(Birds Eye Easy Recipe)* . .	160	6.0	22.0	7.0	0	430	3.0 d
glazed *(Birds Eye Easy Recipe)* . .	150	4.0	30.0	2.0	0	440	4.0 d
primavera *(Birds Eye Easy Recipe)* . .	80	4.0	14.0	3.0	0	540	7.0 d
teriyaki *(Birds Eye Easy Recipe)* . .	160	7.0	28.0	4.0	0	600	4.0 d
Dutch style *(Frosty Acres)*, 3.2 oz. . . .	30	2.0	5.0	0	0	30	m.q.
heartland style *(Green Giant)*	25	1.0	6.0	0	0	35	2.5 d
Japanese style *(Birds Eye Stir-Fry)*	30	2.0	6.0	0	0	360	m.q.
mandarin *(The Budget Gourmet* Side Dish), 5.25 oz.	160	3.0	13.0	11.0	10	440	m.q.
Manhattan style *(Green Giant)* . . .	25	2.0	5.0	0	0	15	2.0 d
medley, breaded *(Ore-Ida)*, 3 oz.	160	3.0	16.0	9.0	<5	490	m.q.
New England recipe *(The Budget Gourmet* Side Dish), 5.5 oz.	230	5.0	21.0	13.0	25	380	m.q.
New England style:							
(Birds Eye International)	130	3.0	12.0	5.0	10	280	m.q.
(Green Giant) . . .	70	3.0	14.0	1.0	0	75	4.0 d

[1] *Without added ingredients.*

Food and Measure	cal.	prot. (gms)	carbo. (gms)	fat (gms)	chol. (mgs)	sod. (mgs)	fiber (gms)
San Francisco style (Green Giant) . . .	25	1.0	7.0	0	0	35	2.5 d
Santa Fe style (Green Giant)	70	2.0	16.0	1.0	0	0	2.0 d
Seattle style (Green Giant)	25	2.0	7.0	0	0	35	2.0 d
soup mix (Frosty Acres), 3 oz.	45	4.0	11.0	0	0	35	m.q.
spring, cheese sauce (The Budget Gourmet Side Dish), 5 oz.	130	5.0	9.0	8.0	20	370	m.q.
stew:							
(Frosty Acres), 3 oz.	42	3.0	10.0	0	0	21	m.q.
(Kohl's), 3.3 oz. . .	50	1.0	10.0	<1.0	0	30	m.q.
(Ore-Ida), 3 oz. . .	50	1.0	11.0	<1.0	0	35	m.q.
Western style (Green Giant)	60	2.0	12.0	2.0	0	25	2.0 d
Vegetables, mixed, pickled, hot and spicy (Vlasic Garden Mix), 1 oz.	4	0	1.0	0	0	480	m.q.
Vegetarian burger, see " 'Hamburger,' vegetarian"							
Vegetarian entree, (see also specific listings):							
frozen (Natural Touch Dinner Entree), 3-oz. patty	230	20.0	6.0	14.0	0	300	m.q.
mix*, 1/2 cup, except as noted:							
chow mein, mandarin, w/tofu:							
(Tofu Classics) . .	123	7.0	17.0	3.0	0	192	2.7 d
w/butter (Tofu Classics)	150	7.0	17.0	6.0	0	192	2.7 d

Food and Measure	cal.	prot. (gms)	carbo. (gms)	fat (gms)	chol. (mgs)	sod. (mgs)	fiber (gms)
Vegetarian entree, mix, 1/2 cup *(cont.)*							
loaf *(Natural Touch)*, 4 oz.	180	18.0	12.0	7.0	0	670	m.q.
Vegetarian foods, see specific listings							
Venison, meat only, roasted, 4 oz. . . .	179	34.3	0	3.6	127	61	0
Vienna sausage, canned:							
(Hormel), 1 oz.	69	3.0	<2.0	7.0	15	225	0
in barbecue sauce *(Libby's)*, 2.5 oz. . . .	180	8.0	2.0	15.0	m.q.	420	n.a.
in beef broth *(Libby's, 5 oz.)*, 2 oz.	160	6.0	1.0	15.0	m.q.	390	0
beef and pork, 2" link, .6-oz.	45	1.7	.3	4.0	8	152	0
chicken:							
(Hormel), 1 oz.	56	3.0	1.0	5.0	27	220	0
in beef broth *(Libby's)*, 2 oz.	130	7.0	3.0	10.0	m.q.	560	0
Vine spinach, raw, untrimmed, 1 lb. . .	86	8.2	15.4	1.4	0	m.q.	3.2 c
Vinegar, 1 tbsp., except as noted:							
apple cider:							
(Heinz)	2	0	0	0	0	1	0
(White House), 1 fl. oz.	4	0	2.0	0	0	5	0
raw unpasteurized *(Hain)*	2	0	<1.0	0	0	0	0
malt *(Heinz Gourmet)*	4	0	0	0	0	5	0
salad or tarragon *(Heinz Gourmet)* . .	2	0	0	0	0	0	0
white, distilled *(Heinz)*	2	0	0	0	0	0	0
wine:							
all varieties *(Regina)*, 1 fl. oz.	4	0	0	0	0	0	0
plain or garlic *(Heinz Gourmet)*	4	0	0	0	0	0	0

W

Food and Measure	cal.	prot. (gms)	carbo. (gms)	fat (gms)	chol. (mgs)	sod. (mgs)	fiber (gms)
Waffle, frozen,							
1 piece, except as noted:							
(Aunt Jemima Low Fat)	80	3.0	16.0	<1.0	0	280	4.7 d
(Downyflake)	60	1.5	10.0	1.5	0	210	m.q.
(Downyflake Hot-N-Buttery) . . .	90	2.0	13.5	3.0	n.a.	310	m.q.
(Downyflake Jumbo)	85	2.0	15.0	2.0	0	285	m.q.
(Eggo Homestyle) . .	120	3.0	16.0	5.0	15	250	0
(Eggo Minis), 4 pieces	90	2.0	14.0	3.0	10	190	0
(Eggo Nutri-Grain), 2 pieces	180	6.0	28.0	6.0	0	430	3.0 d
(Kellogg's Special K)	80	3.0	16.0	0	0	120	0
plain or apple cinnamon (Downyflake Crisp & Healthy) . .	80	2.0	16.0	1.0	0	180	1.0 d
apple (Eggo Fruit Top), 3.1 oz.	190	3.0	32.0	6.0	0	250	m.q.
apple cinnamon (Eggo)	130	3.0	18.0	5.0	15	250	0
Belgian (Belgian Chef)	70	2.0	11.0	1.0	0	230	6.0 d
blueberry:							
(Downyflake)	90	2.0	16.0	2.0	0	285	m.q.
(Eggo)	130	3.0	18.0	5.0	15	250	0
(Eggo Fruit Top), 3.1 oz.	190	3.0	32.0	6.0	0	250	m.q.
(Eggo Minis), 4 pieces	90	2.0	13.0	3.0	10	170	n.a.
buttermilk:							
(Downyflake Jumbo)	85	2.0	15.0	2.0	n.a.	315	m.q.

Food and Measure	cal.	prot. (gms)	carbo. (gms)	fat (gms)	chol. (mgs)	sod. (mgs)	fiber (gms)
Waffle, frozen, buttermilk *(cont.)*							
(Eggo)	120	3.0	16.0	5.0	15	220	0
or cinnamon (Aunt Jemima)	110	3.0	16.0	4.0	n.a.	330	m.q.
multibran (Eggo Nutri-Grain), 2 pieces . .	180	5.0	30.0	6.0	0	380	5.0 d
nut and honey (Eggo)	130	3.0	17.0	6.0	15	250	0
oat bran, 2 pieces:							
(Eggo Common Sense)	190	6.0	27.0	7.0	0	350	3.0 d
w/fruit and nut (Eggo Common Sense)	220	6.0	32.0	8.0	0	340	4.0 d
peach (Eggo Fruit Top), 3.1 oz.	190	3.0	30.0	6.0	0	240	m.q.
raisin and bran (Eggo Nutri-Grain), 2 pieces	200	5.0	33.0	6.0	0	400	4.0 d
sticks (Swanson Breakfast Blast), 2.75 oz.	280	4.0	34.0	14.0	n.a.	220	m.q.
strawberry (Eggo) . .	130	3.0	18.0	5.0	15	250	0
strawberry (Eggo Fruit Top), 3.1 oz.	190	3.0	31.0	6.0	0	230	m.q.
whole grain (Roman Meal)	140	2.5	16.5	7.0	10	340	1.5 d
Waffle breakfast, frozen, w/sausage (Swanson Budget), 2.25 oz.	230	5.0	21.0	14.0	m.q.	310	m.q.
Waffle mix, see "Pancake and waffle mix"							
Walnut, dried:							
black:							
shelled, 1 oz. . . .	172	6.9	3.4	16.1	0	tr.	1.4 d
chopped, 1 cup . .	759	30.4	15.1	70.7	0	2	6.3 d
(Fisher), 1 oz. . . .	170	7.0	3.0	16.0	0	0	m.q.

Food and Measure	cal.	prot. (gms)	carbo. (gms)	fat (gms)	chol. (mgs)	sod. (mgs)	fiber (gms)
English or Persian, dried:							
shelled, 1 oz. . . .	182	4.1	5.2	17.6	0	3	1.4 d
pieces, 1 cup . . .	770	17.2	22.0	74.2	0	12	5.8 d
halves, 1 cup . . .	642	14.3	18.3	61.9	0	10	4.8 d
raw, chopped or ground (Fisher), 1 oz.	180	4.0	5.0	18.0	0	0	m.q.
Walnut topping, in syrup (Smucker's), 2 tbsp.	130	2.0	27.0	1.0	0	0	m.q.
Waterchestnut, Chinese:							
fresh:							
4 medium, 2″ diam.	38	.5	8.6	<.1	0	5	1.1 d
sliced, 1/2 cup . . .	66	.9	14.8	.1	0	9	1.9 d
(Frieda's), 1 oz. . .	22	.4	5.4	.1	0	6	m.q.
canned:							
4 medium or 1 oz.	14	.3	3.5	<.1	0	2	.7 d
w/liquid, sliced, 1/2 cup	35	.6	8.7	<.1	0	6	1.8 d
whole (La Choy), 4 medium	14	<1.0	4.0	<1.0	0	2	<1.0 d
sliced (La Choy), 1/4 cup	18	<1.0	4.0	<1.0	0	3	<1.0 d
Watercress:							
10 sprigs, 111/4″ . . .	3	.6	.3	<.1	0	10	.6 d
chopped, 1/2 cup . .	2	.4	.2	<.1	0	7	.4 d
Watermelon:							
1 slice, 10″ diam. × 1″ thick	152	3.0	34.6	2.0	0	10	2.4 d
diced, 1/2 cup	25	.5	5.7	.3	0	2	.4 d
seedless (Frieda's), 1 oz.	7	.1	1.8	.1	0	<1	m.q.
Watermelon seed, dried, 1 oz.	158	8.1	4.4	13.5	0	28	.9 c

Food and Measure	cal.	prot. (gms)	carbo. (gms)	fat (gms)	chol. (mgs)	sod. (mgs)	fiber (gms)
Wax beans:							
fresh, see "Green bean"							
canned, 1/2 cup:							
golden, all cuts *(Del Monte)*	20	0	4.0	0	0	360	m.q.
frozen, 3 oz.:							
(Frosty Acres) . . .	25	2.0	5.0	0	0	1	1.0 c
cut *(Seabrook)* . . .	25	2.0	5.0	0	0	1	1.0 c
Wax gourd, boiled, drained, cubed, 1/2 cup	11	.4	2.6	.2	0	93	.9 d
Welsh rarebit:							
canned *(Snow's),* 1/2 cup	170	9.0	10.0	11.0	n.a.	460	n.a.
frozen *(Stouffer's),* 5 oz.	270	13.0	9.0	20.0	n.a.	460	n.a.
Wendy's, 1 serving:							
sandwiches:							
bacon cheeseburger, Jr.	440	22.0	33.0	25.0	65	870	m.q.
Big Classic	480	27.0	44.0	23.0	75	850	m.q.
cheeseburger, Jr. .	320	18.0	34.0	13.0	45	760	m.q.
cheeseburger, Kid's Meal	310	18.0	33.0	13.0	45	760	m.q.
cheeseburger deluxe, Jr.	390	18.0	36.0	20.0	50	800	m.q.
chicken, grilled . .	290	24.0	35.0	7.0	60	670	m.q.
chicken, breaded	450	26.0	44.0	20.0	60	740	m.q.
chicken club	520	30.0	44.0	25.0	75	980	m.q.
fish	460	18.0	42.0	25.0	55	780	m.q.
hamburger, single, plain	350	25.0	31.0	15.0	70	510	m.q.
hamburger, single, w/everything . .	440	26.0	36.0	23.0	75	850	m.q.
hamburger, Jr. . . .	270	15.0	34.0	9.0	35	590	m.q.
hamburger, Kid's Meal	270	15.0	33.0	9.0	35	590	m.q.

Food and Measure	cal.	prot. (gms)	carbo. (gms)	fat (gms)	chol. (mgs)	sod. (mgs)	fiber (gms)
steak, country fried	460	15.0	45.0	26.0	35	880	m.q.
chicken nuggets, 6 pieces	280	14.0	12.0	20.0	50	600	n.a.
nuggets sauces, 1 pkt.:							
barbecue	50	1.0	11.0	0	0	100	n.a.
honey	45	0	12.0	0	0	tr.	0
sweet mustard . .	50	1.0	9.0	1.0	0	140	n.a.
sweet and sour . .	45	<1.0	11.0	0	0	55	n.a.
chili, small, 8 oz. . . .	190	19.0	21.0	6.0	40	670	m.q.
chili, large, 12 oz. . . .	290	28.0	31.0	9.0	60	1000	m.q.
baked potato:							
plain	300	6.0	69.0	<1.0	0	20	m.q.
bacon and cheese	510	17.0	75.0	17.0	15	1170	m.q.
broccoli and cheese	450	9.0	77.0	14.0	0	450	m.q.
cheese	550	14.0	74.0	24.0	30	640	m.q.
chili and cheese . .	600	21.0	80.0	25.0	45	740	m.q.
sour cream w/chives	370	8.0	71.0	6.0	15	35	m.q.
salads/side dishes:							
breadstick	130	4.0	24.0	3.0	5	250	m.q.
Caesar salad, side	160	10.0	18.0	6.0	10	700	m.q.
chicken salad, grilled, to go . .	200	25.0	9.0	8.0	55	690	m.q.
fries, Biggie	450	6.0	62.0	22.0	0	280	m.q.
fries, medium . . .	360	5.0	50.0	17.0	0	220	m.q.
fries, small	240	3.0	33.0	12.0	0	150	m.q.
garden salad, deluxe, to go . .	110	7.0	9.0	5.0	0	380	m.q.
side salad, to go	60	4.0	6.0	3.0	0	200	m.q.
taco salad, to go	640	34.0	70.0	30.0	80	960	m.q.
dressing, 2 tbsp.:							
bacon and tomato, reduced calorie	90	<1.0	5.0	7.0	0	350	n.a.
blue cheese	180	1.0	<1.0	19.0	20	200	n.a.
blue cheese, re- duced fat/calorie	65	1.0	1.0	7.0	13	260	n.a.
celery seed	130	<1.0	6.0	11.0	5	120	n.a.
French	120	<1.0	6.0	10.0	0	330	n.a.

Food and Measure	cal.	prot. (gms)	carbo. (gms)	fat (gms)	chol. (mgs)	sod. (mgs)	fiber (gms)
Wendy's, dressing, 2 tbsp. *(cont.)*							
French, sweet red	130	<1.0	9.0	10.0	0	230	n.a.
Hidden Valley Ranch	100	1.0	1.0	10.0	10	220	n.a.
Italian, golden . . .	90	<1.0	6.0	7.0	0	460	n.a.
Italian, reduced fat/							
calorie	40	0	2.5	3.5	0	340	n.a.
Italian Caesar . . .	150	1.0	1.0	16.0	10	260	n.a.
ranch, fat free . . .	35	0	8.0	0	0	180	n.a.
Thousand Island . .	130	<1.0	3.0	13.0	15	200	n.a.
desserts:							
chocolate chip							
cookie	280	3.0	39.0	13.0	15	260	m.q.
frosty, dairy:							
small	340	9.0	57.0	10.0	40	200	n.a.
medium	460	12.0	76.0	13.0	55	260	n.a.
large	570	15.0	95.0	17.0	70	330	n.a.
pudding, 1/4 cup:							
chocolate, ...	90	n.a.	12.0	4.0	tr.	70	n.a.
butterscotch . .	90	1.0	11.0	4.0	tr.	85	n.a.
Western dinner, frozen *(Swanson),*							
11.5 oz.	430	22.0	43.0	19.0	m.q.	1060	m.q.
Western entree, frozen *(Banquet Meals),* 9.5 oz. . . .	320	12.0	30.0	17.0	35	1360	m.q.
Wheat, whole-grain:							
durum, 1 cup	650	26.3	136.6	4.7	0	3	m.q.
hard red:							
spring, 1 cup . . .	631	29.6	130.6	3.7	0	4	24.2 d
spring or winter *(Arrowhead Mills),*							
2 oz.	190	8.0	41.0	1.0	0	1	8.3 d
winter, 1 cup . . .	628	24.2	136.7	3.0	0	4	24.2 d
soft red:							
for pastry *(Arrowhead Mills),* 2 oz.	190	8.0	41.0	1.0	0	1	8.3 d
hard white, 1 cup . .	656	21.7	145.7	3.3	0	n.a.	m.q.
soft white, 1 cup . . .	571	18.0	126.6	3.3	0	n.a.	m.q.

Food and Measure	cal.	prot. (gms)	carbo. (gms)	fat (gms)	chol. (mgs)	sod. (mgs)	fiber (gms)
winter, 1 cup	556	17.4	124.7	2.6	0	4	2.9 c
Wheat, parboiled, see "Bulgur"							
Wheat, sprouted, 1 cup	214	8.1	45.9	1.4	0	18	1.1 d
Wheat bran (see also "Cereal"):							
crude, 1 oz.	61	4.4	18.3	1.2	0	<1	12.1 d
crude, 2 tbsp.	15	1.1	4.5	.3	0	tr.	3.0 d
toasted (Kretschmer), 1 oz. or 1/3 cup . .	57	5.7	14.8	2.3	0	2	11.4 d
Wheat flakes (Arrowhead Mills), 2 oz.	210	8.0	42.0	1.0	0	1	6.7 d
Wheat flour, 1 cup, except as noted:							
pastry (Arrowhead Mills), 2 oz.	180	6.0	41.0	1.0	0	1	6.8 d
whole-grain:							
1 cup	407	16.4	87.1	2.2	0	1	15.1 d
(Gold Medal)	350	16.0	78.0	2.0	0	0	m.q.
(Pillsbury's Best) . .	400	15.0	80.0	2.0	0	10	12.0 d
blend (Gold Medal)	380	14.0	84.0	2.0	0	0	m.q.
stone ground (Arrowhead Mills), 2 oz.	200	8.0	40.0	1.0	0	1	6.7 d
white, all-purpose:							
1 cup	455	12.9	95.4	1.2	0	2	4.1 d
(Ballard/Pillsbury's Best)	400	11.0	87.0	1.0	0	0	2.0 d
regular or unbleached (Gold Medal)	400	11.0	87.0	1.0	0	0	m.q.
unbleached (Pillsbury's Best) . . .	400	12.0	86.0	1.0	0	0	3.0 d
white, bread (Gold Medal Better for Bread)	400	14.0	83.0	1.0	0	0	m.q.
(Pillsbury's Best) . .	400	14.0	83.0	2.0	0	0	2.0 d

Food and Measure	cal.	prot. (gms)	carbo. (gms)	fat (gms)	chol. (mgs)	sod. (mgs)	fiber (gms)
Wheat flour *(cont.)*							
white, cake	395	8.9	85.1	.9	0	2	1.8 d
white, presifted:							
(Pillsbury Shake &							
Blend), 2 tbsp.	50	1.0	11.0	0	0	0	m.q.
(Wondra)	400	11.0	87.0	1.0	0	0	m.q.
white, self-rising:							
1 cup	442	12.4	92.8	1.2	0	1587	4.0 d
(Pillsbury's Best) . .	380	9.0	84.0	1.0	0	1290	2.0 d
(Gold Medal)	380	10.0	83.0	1.0	0	1520	m.q.
tortilla mix	449	10.7	74.5	11.8	0	751	m.q.
Wheat germ:							
(Kretschmer), 1 oz.	103	9.3	12.3	3.4	0	2	3.3 d
crude	102	6.6	14.7	2.8	0	3	3.7 d
honey crunch							
(Kretschmer), 1 oz.	105	7.6	15.2	2.8	0	2	3.0 d
raw *(Arrowhead Mills),*							
2 oz.	210	15.0	26.0	6.0	0	1	6.5 d
toasted, 1 oz.	108	8.3	14.1	3.0	0	1	3.7 d
Wheat gluten, vital							
(Arrowhead Mills),							
1 oz.	100	15.0	9.0	1.0	0	1	.9 d
Whelk, meat only,							
raw, 4 oz.	156	27.0	8.8	.5	74	234	0
Whey:							
acid, dry, 1 oz. . . .	96	3.3	20.8	.2	(0)	274	0
acid, fluid, 1 cup . . .	59	1.9	12.6	.2	(0)	118	0
sweet, dry, 1 oz. . . .	100	3.7	21.1	.3	2	306	0
sweet, fluid, 1 cup . .	66	2.1	12.6	.9	5	132	0
Whipped topping, see							
"Cream" and							
"Cream topping,							
nondairy"							
Whiskey, see "Li-							
quor"							
Whiskey sour mixer							
(Holland House):							
bottled, 3 fl. oz. . . .	108	<1.0	27.0	<1.0	0	315	n.a.

Food and Measure	cal.	prot. (gms)	carbo. (gms)	fat (gms)	chol. (mgs)	sod. (mgs)	fiber (gms)
instant, .56 oz. dry . .	64	<1.0	16.0	<1.0	0	4	n.a.
White beans, 1/2 cup:							
dried, boiled	125	8.6	22.6	.3	0	6	5.7 d
dried, small, boiled	127	8.1	23.2	.6	0	2	3.7 d
canned, w/liquid . . .	153	9.5	28.7	.4	0	595	6.3 d
White beans, mix*, and rice *(Fantastic Italiano),* 10 oz. . .	190	10.0	40.0	2.0	1	490	8.0 d
White Castle, 1 serving:							
cheeseburger	200	7.8	15.5	11.2	m.q.	361	2.7 d
chicken sandwich . .	186	8.0	20.5	7.5	m.q.	497	1.7 d
fish sandwich, w/out tartar sauce	155	5.8	20.9	5.0	m.q.	201	1.4 d
hamburger	161	5.9	15.4	7.9	m.q.	266	2.1 d
sausage sandwich . .	196	6.7	13.3	12.3	m.q.	488	2.0 d
sausage w/egg sandwich	322	12.6	16.1	22.0	m.q.	698	3.0 d
side dishes:							
french fries	301	2.5	37.7	14.7	n.a.	193	4.6 d
onion chips	329	3.7	38.8	16.6	n.a.	823	3.5 d
onion rings	245	2.9	26.6	13.4	n.a.	566	2.6 d
White sauce mix:							
1 3/4-oz. pkt.	230	5.4	25.1	13.2	tr.	1691	.1 c
(McCormick/Schilling McCormick Collection), 1/4 cup* . . .	59	3.0	3.0	3.0	n.a.	296	n.a.
Whitefish, meat only:							
raw, 4 oz.	153	21.7	0	6.7	68	58	0
baked, broiled, or microwaved, 4 oz. . .	195	27.7	0	8.5	87	74	0
smoked, 4 oz.	122	26.5	0	1.1	37	1156	0
Whiting, meat only:							
raw, 4 oz.	102	20.8	0	1.5	76	82	0
baked, broiled, or microwaved, 4 oz. . .	130	26.6	0	1.9	95	150	0
Wiener, see "Frankfurters"							

Food and Measure	cal.	prot. (gms)	carbo. (gms)	fat (gms)	chol. (mgs)	sod. (mgs)	fiber (gms)
Wild rice (see also "Rice dishes"):							
raw, 1 oz.	101	4.2	21.2	.3	0	2	1.7 d
cooked, 1 cup	166	6.5	35.0	.6	0	6	1.5 d
(Fantastic Foods),							
1/2 cup	84	3.0	18.0	.3	0	3	2.0 d
precooked, cooked							
(Master Choice							
Texmati), 1/2 cup . .	76	3.0	16.0	0	0	0	.3 d
Wine, 1 fl. oz.:							
dessert or apertif[1] . .	41	tr.	2.3	0	0	1	0
dry or table[2]	25	tr.	1.2	0	0	1	0
Wine, cooking *(Holland House),* 1 fl. oz., except as noted:							
Marsala	9	0	2.3	0	0	186	0
red	6	0	1.5	0	0	186	0
sherry	5	0	1.2	0	0	186	0
vermouth or white . .	2	0	<1.0	0	0	186	0
Wine cooler, *(Bartles & Jaymes),* 6 fl. oz.:							
premium	99	.1	14.0	.1	0	2	0
premium light	67	.1	12.0	.1	0	0	0
berry	107	.1	16.8	.1	0	2	0
berry, light	75	.1	16.0	.1	0	0	0
cherry, black	104	.1	16.1	.1	0	2	0
peach	107	.1	16.8	.1	0	3	0
sangria, red	107	.1	14.9	.1	0	2	0
strawberry	107	<.1	16.2	.1	0	2	0
tropical	115	.1	18.6	.1	0	2	0
tropical, light	76	.1	16.8	.1	0	0	0

[1] *Includes wines containing more than 15% alcohol (sherry, port, vermouth, etc.).*
[2] *Includes wines containing less than 15% alcohol (Burgundy, Chablis, Champagne, rosé, etc.).*

Food and Measure	cal.	prot. (gms)	carbo. (gms)	fat (gms)	chol. (mgs)	sod. (mgs)	fiber (gms)
Wine marinade (Holland House), 1 fl. oz.:							
herb, garden	27	<1.0	5.0	<1.0	<1	352	n.a.
hot & spicy	29	<1.0	5.0	<1.0	<.1	397	n.a.
lemon & herb	16	<1.0	2.0	<1.0	<1	382	n.a.
red wine & herb . . .	19	<1.0	3.0	<1.0	<1	384	n.a.
teriyaki	36	1.0	6.0	<1.0	<1	536	n.a.
Winged bean, 1/2 cup:							
fresh, raw, sliced . .	11	1.5	1.0	.2	0	1	.6 c
fresh, boiled, drained	12	1.6	1.0	.2	0	1	.4 c
dry, raw	372	27.0	38.0	14.9	0	35	14.1 d
dry, boiled	126	9.1	12.8	5.0	0	11	2.1 c
Winged bean leaves, trimmed, 1 oz. . . .	21	1.7	4.0	.3	0	n.a.	.7 c
Winged bean tuber, trimmed, 1 oz. . . .	45	3.3	8.0	.3	0	n.a.	2.1 c
Wolf fish, Atlantic, meat only:							
raw, 4 oz.	109	19.9	0	2.7	52	97	0
baked, broiled, or microwaved, 4 oz. . . .	139	25.4	0	3.5	67	124	0
Wonton wrapper:							
(Azumaya), 1 oz. . . .	78	2.8	15.9	.3	0	126	m.q.
(Frieda's), 1 piece . .	31	1.0	7.0	.1	0	68	m.q.
(Nasoya), 1 piece . .	90	3.0	20.0	0	0	35	m.q.
Worcestershire sauce:							
(Heinz), 1 tbsp. . . .	6	0	1.0	0	0	170	0
(Lea & Perrins), 1 tsp.	4	0	1.0	0	0	50	0
regular or hickory (French's), 1 tbsp.	8	<1.0	2.0	<1.0	0	180	(0)
white wine (Lea & Perrins), 1 tsp.	4	0	1.0	0	0	25	0

Y

Food and Measure	cal.	prot. (gms)	carbo. (gms)	fat (gms)	chol. (mgs)	sod. (mgs)	fiber (gms)
Yam, 1/2 cup:							
baked or boiled . .	79	1.0	18.8	.1	0	6	2.7 d
canned or frozen, see "Sweet potato"							
Yam, mountain, Hawaiian, 1/2 cup:							
raw, cubed	46	.9	11.1	.1	0	9	.3 c
steamed, cubed . . .	59	1.2	14.4	.1	0	9	.4 c
Yam bean tuber:							
raw, sliced, 1/2 cup	23	.4	5.3	.1	0	3	m.q.
boiled, drained, 4 oz.	43	.8	10.0	.1	0	5	m.q.
Yard-long bean, 1/2 cup:							
fresh, raw, sliced . .	22	1.3	3.8	.2	0	2	m.q.
fresh, boiled, drained, sliced	25	1.3	4.8	.1	0	2	.8 c
dried, raw	292	20.4	52.0	1.1	0	14	4.0 c
dried, boiled	102	7.1	18.1	.4	0	4	1.4 c
Yeast, baker's:							
(Fleischmann's Active Dry/RapidRise), 1/4 oz.	20	3.0	3.0	0	0	10	m.q.
(Red Star Active Dry), 1/4 oz.	20	3.0	2.7	.3	0	4	1.2 c
fresh (Fleischmann's), .6 oz.	15	2.0	2.0	0	0	5	m.q.
household (Fleischmann's), .5 oz. . . .	15	2.0	2.0	0	0	5	m.q.
Yellow beans, dry, boiled, 1/2 cup . . .	126	8.1	22.2	1.0	0	4	1.0 c

Food and Measure	cal.	prot. (gms)	carbo. (gms)	fat (gms)	chol. (mgs)	sod. (mgs)	fiber (gms)
Yellow squash, see "Crookneck squash"							
Yellow squash, breaded, frozen (*Stilwell*), 6 pieces	80	2.0	17.0	0	0	470	1.0 d
Yellowtail, meat only:							
raw, 4 oz.	166	26.3	0	6.0	m.q.	44	0
baked, broiled, or microwaved, 4 oz. . .	212	33.6	0	7.6	m.q.	57	0
Yogurt, 8 oz. or 1 cup, except as noted:							
plain:							
(*Bison* Lowfat) . . .	150	12.0	17.0	4.0	20	180	0
(*Bison* Nonfat) . . .	120	12.0	16.0	0	n.a.	170	0
(*Breyers* Lowfat) . .	140	12.0	16.0	3.0	20	170	0
(*Colombo*)	160	9.0	13.0	8.0	m.q.	160	0
(*Colombo* Nonfat Lite)	110	11.0	17.0	<1.0	5	160	0
(*Friendship* Lowfat)	150	12.0	17.0	3.0	14	190	0
(*Knudsen*)	200	12.0	16.0	9.0	35	170	0
(*Knudsen* Lowfat)	160	12.0	17.0	5.0	25	180	0
(*Yoplait* Fat Free)	120	13.0	17.0	0	10	170	0
(*Yoplait* Original 98% Fat Free), 6 oz.	120	10.0	15.0	2.0	15	150	0
all fruit flavors:							
(*Bison* Nonfat), 6 oz.	80	7.0	13.0	0	<5	100	m.q.
(*Colombo* Fruit on the Bottom) . . .	230	7.0	36.0	6.0	m.q.	140	m.q.
(*Colombo* Fruit on the Bottom Nonfat)	190	8.0	33.0	<1.0	5	140	m.q.
(*Yoplait* Custard Style), 6 oz. . . .	180	7.0	30.0	3.0	15	110	m.q.
(*Yoplait* Fat Free), 6 oz.	160	8.0	32.0	0	5	110	m.q.

Food and Measure	cal.	prot. (gms)	carbo. (gms)	fat (gms)	chol. (mgs)	sod. (mgs)	fiber (gms)
Yogurt, all fruit flavors *(cont.)*							
(Yoplait Light), 6 oz.	80	6.0	13.0	0	<5	85	m.q.
(Yoplait Original 99% Fat Free), 6 oz.	180	8.0	33.0	2.0	10	120	m.q.
(Yoplait Parfait Style), 6 oz. . . .	200	8.0	34.0	3.0	m.q.	120	m.q.
except lemon *(Bison Lowfat)*	240	10.0	44.0	3.0	15	150	m.q.
except strawberry *(Knudsen Lowfat)*	240	11.0	43.0	4.0	15	135	m.q.
except strawberry fruit cup *(Light n' Lively Free)*, 4.4 oz.	50	4.0	8.0	0	0	60	m.q.
apple crisp granola *(Bison Astro)*, 4.4 oz.	160	7.0	24.0	4.0	10	100	m.q.
berry, mixed:							
(Yoplait Breakfast Yogurt), 6 oz. . . .	200	8.0	39.0	2.0	m.q.	125	m.q.
crunch *(Bison Astro)*, 4.4 oz.	170	6.0	28.0	4.0	m.q.	115	m.q.
or blueberry *(Breyers Lowfat)*	250	9.0	48.0	2.0	10	120	m.q.
blueberry:							
(Knudsen Cal 70), 6 oz.	70	6.0	11.0	0	5	80	m.q.
(Light n' Lively) . .	240	8.0	46.0	2.0	10	130	m.q.
(Light n' Lively 100 Calorie)	90	8.0	15.0	0	0	110	m.q.
cherry, black:							
(Breyers Lowfat) . .	260	9.0	49.0	3.0	10	120	m.q.
(Knudsen Cal 70), 6 oz.	70	5.0	12.0	0	5	75	m.q.
(Light n' Lively) . .	230	9.0	44.0	2.0	10	125	m.q.
(Light n' Lively 100 Calorie)	100	8.0	17.0	0	0	100	m.q.

Food and Measure	cal.	prot. (gms)	carbo. (gms)	fat (gms)	chol. (mgs)	sod. (mgs)	fiber (gms)
cherry almond (Yoplait Breakfast Yogurt), 6 oz.	210	9.0	41.0	2.0	m.q.	100	m.q.
chocolate fudge crunch (Bison Astro), 4.4 oz.	180	7.0	27.0	5.0	10	130	m.q.
coffee:							
(Bison Lowfat) . . .	210	11.0	33.0	4.0	20	160	0
(Friendship Lowfat)	210	11.0	35.0	3.0	14	125	0
date-walnut-raisin (Bison Lowfat)	240	10.0	44.0	3.0	15	150	m.q.
fruit, tropical (Yoplait Breakfast Yogurt), 6 oz.	220	8.0	41.0	3.0	m.q.	110	m.q.
grape (Light n' Lively), 4.4 oz.	130	6.0	24.0	1.0	10	70	n.a.
lemon:							
(Bison Lowfat) . . .	210	11.0	33.0	4.0	20	160	n.a.
(Knudsen Cal 70), 6 oz.	70	6.0	12.0	0	0	125	n.a.
(Light n' Lively 100 Calorie)	100	9.0	16.0	0	5	150	n.a.
oat bran raisin (Bison Astro), 4.4 oz. . . .	160	7.0	27.0	4.0	10	110	m.q.
peach:							
(Breyers)	250	9.0	48.0	2.0	10	120	m.q.
(Knudsen Cal 70), 6 oz.	70	6.0	11.0	0	0	95	m.q.
(Light n' Lively) . .	240	9.0	46.0	2.0	15	120	m.q.
(Light n' Lively 100 Calorie)	100	9.0	16.0	0	5	115	m.q.
peanut butter crunch (Bison Astro), 4.4 oz.	200	9.0	29.0	7.0	10	80	m.q.
pecan toffee crunch (Bison Astro), 4.4 oz.	190	6.0	29.0	6.0	m.q.	80	m.q.

Food and Measure	cal.	prot. (gms)	carbo. (gms)	fat (gms)	chol. (mgs)	sod. (mgs)	fiber (gms)
Yogurt *(cont.)*							
pineapple:							
(Breyers Lowfat) . .	250	9.0	50.0	2.0	10	120	m.q.
(Knudsen Cal 70),							
6 oz.	70	6.0	12.0	0	0	125	m.q.
(Light n' Lively) . .	230	9.0	47.0	2.0	10	120	m.q.
raspberry, red:							
(Knudsen Cal 70),							
6 oz.	70	6.0	11.0	0	5	80	m.q.
(Light n' Lively) . .	230	9.0	43.0	2.0	10	130	m.q.
or strawberry							
(Breyers Lowfat)	250	9.0	48.0	2.0	10	120	m.q.
or strawberry (Light							
n' Lively 100 Cal-							
orie)	90	8.0	15.0	0	0	105	m.q.
strawberry:							
(Colombo)	210	8.0	29.0	7.0	m.q.	140	m.q.
(Knudsen Cal 70),							
6 oz.	70	6.0	11.0	0	0	85	m.q.
(Knudsen Lowfat)	250	10.0	45.0	4.0	15	135	m.q.
(Light n' Lively) . .	240	9.0	45.0	2.0	15	130	m.q.
fruit basket (Knud-							
sen Cal 70), 6 oz.	70	6.0	11.0	0	5	75	m.q.
fruit cup (Light n'							
Lively)	240	9.0	47.0	2.0	15	120	m.q.
fruit cup (Light n'							
Lively Free),							
4.4 oz.	50	4.0	8.0	0	0	55	m.q.
fruit cup (Light n'							
Lively 100 Calorie)	90	8.0	15.0	0	0	100	m.q.
strawberry-almond							
(Yoplait Breakfast							
Yogurt), 6 oz. . . .	200	9.0	38.0	2.0	m.q.	105	m.q.
strawberry-banana:							
(Breyers Lowfat) . .	250	9.0	50.0	2.0	10	120	m.q.
(Knudsen Cal 70),							
6 oz.	70	6.0	12.0	0	0	80	m.q.
(Light n' Lively) . .	260	9.0	52.0	2.0	10	120	m.q.

Food and Measure	cal.	prot. (gms)	carbo. (gms)	fat (gms)	chol. (mgs)	sod. (mgs)	fiber (gms)
(Light n' Lively 100 Calorie)	100	8.0	15.0	0	0	105	m.q.
(Yoplait Breakfast Yogurt), 6 oz. . . .	200	8.0	40.0	2.0	m.q.	110	m.q.
vanilla:							
(Bison Lowfat) . . .	210	11.0	33.0	4.0	20	160	0
(Colombo Nonfat Lite)	160	10.0	30.0	<1.0	5	140	0
(Friendship Lowfat)	210	11.0	35.0	3.0	14	125	0
(Knudsen Cal 70), 6 oz.	70	6.0	11.0	0	0	90	0
(Knudsen Lowfat)	240	11.0	43.0	4.0	15	135	0
(Yoplait Fat Free)	180	11.0	34.0	0	10	160	0
(Yoplait Original 99% Fat Free), 6 oz.	170	9.0	30.0	2.0	10	130	0
(Yoplait Custard Style), 6 oz. . . .	180	7.0	30.0	3.0	15	110	0
bean *(Breyers* Lowfat)	230	11.0	41.0	3.0	20	150	0
French *(Colombo)*	215	8.0	30.0	7.0	m.q.	140	0
Yogurt, frozen, 1/2 cup, except as noted:							
all flavors *(Borden/ Meadow Gold)* . . .	100	2.0	19.0	2.0	10	50	n.a.
almond praline *(Edy's Inspirations)*	130	3.0	22.0	4.0	10	100	m.q.
banana nut chocolate chunk *(Colombo Gourmet),* 3 fl. oz.	130	3.0	17.0	4.0	10	45	m.q.
banana split *(Colombo Gourmet),* 3 fl. oz.	100	2.0	20.0	1.0	<5	50	(0)
banana-strawberry *(Häagen-Dazs)* . . .	170	6.0	27.0	4.0	60	50	(0)
Black Forest cake *(Swensen's)*	95	3.0	21.0	<1.0	5	130	n.a.

Food and Measure	cal.	prot. (gms)	carbo. (gms)	fat (gms)	chol. (mgs)	sod. (mgs)	fiber (gms)
Yogurt, frozen *(cont.)*							
boysenberry-vanilla swirl *(Edy's Inspirations)*	110	3.0	19.0	3.0	10	45	(0)
Brownie Nut Blast (Häagen-Dazs Exträas)	220	8.0	29.0	9.0	55	60	m.q.
cappuccino coffee bean *(Colombo Gourmet)*, 3 fl. oz.	120	2.0	19.0	4.0	10	45	n.a.
caramel fudge sundae *(Colombo* Gourmet), 3 fl. oz.	100	3.0	21.0	1.0	5	60	(0)
caramel pecan chunk *(Colombo* Gourmet), 3 fl. oz.	120	2.0	19.0	4.0	10	110	m.q.
cheesecake, wild raspberry *(Colombo* Gourmet), 3 fl. oz.	100	2.0	18.0	2.0	10	40	(0)
cherry:							
black *(Sealtest Free)*	110	2.0	24.0	0	0	50	(0)
black-vanilla swirl *(Edy's Inspirations Nonfat)*	90	4.0	19.0	<1.0	0	80	n.a.
Bordeaux *(Swensen's)*	105	5.0	21.0	0	0	65	n.a.
cherry-almond chunk *(Colombo* Gourmet), 3 fl. oz.	110	3.0	17.0	4.0	5	65	m.q.
chocolate:							
(Edy's Inspirations)	110	3.0	18.0	3.0	10	45	(0)
(Edy's Inspirations Nonfat)	90	4.0	18.0	<1.0	0	80	(0)
(Häagen-Dazs)	170	8.0	26.0	4.0	40	45	(0)
(Sealtest Free)	110	3.0	24.0	0	0	55	(0)
brownie chunk *(Edy's Inspirations)*	130	3.0	20.0	4.0	10	70	n.a.

Food and Measure	cal.	prot. (gms)	carbo. (gms)	fat (gms)	chol. (mgs)	sod. (mgs)	fiber (gms)
chunk, Bavarian *(Colombo Gourmet)*, 3 fl. oz. . .	120	3.0	18.0	4.0	10	50	(0)
sundae *(Edy's Inspirations)*	120	3.0	21.0	3.0	10	50	(0)
white, almond *(Colombo Gourmet)*, 3 fl. oz.	140	3.0	19.0	6.0	10	55	m.q.
chocolate chip, strawberry *(Edy's Inspirations)*	130	3.0	21.0	5.0	10	40	n.a.
citrus heights *(Edy's Inspirations)*	120	2.0	20.0	3.0	10	40	n.a.
coffee *(Häagen-Dazs)*	180	8.0	28.0	4.0	40	60	n.a.
cookies n' cream *(Edy's Inspirations)*	130	3.0	22.0	4.0	10	55	n.a.
Heath bar crunch: *(Colombo Gourmet)*, 3 fl. oz.	130	2.0	19.0	5.0	10	75	n.a.
(Edy's Inspirations) . .	130	3.0	20.0	4.0	15	75	n.a.
marble fudge *(Edy's Inspirations)*	120	3.0	20.0	3.0	10	55	(0)
mocha chip *(Swensen's)*	100	5.0	20.0	0	0	120	n.a.
mocha Swiss almond *(Colombo Gourmet)*, 3 fl. oz.	120	5.0	17.0	5.0	10	45	m.q.
Orange Tango *(Häagen-Dazs Exträas)*	130	4.0	26.0	2.0	20	30	(0)
orange-vanilla swirl *(Edy's Inspirations)*	110	3.0	19.0	3.0	10	50	n.a.
peach: *(Blue Bell Lowfat)*	120	3.0	22.0	2.0	9	70	(0)
(Edy's Inspirations)	110	3.0	19.0	3.0	10	40	(0)
(Häagen-Dazs) . . .	170	6.0	26.0	4.0	40	45	(0)
(Sealtest Free) . . .	100	2.0	23.0	0	0	35	(0)

Food and Measure	cal.	prot. (gms)	carbo. (gms)	fat (gms)	chol. (mgs)	sod. (mgs)	fiber (gms)
Yogurt, frozen *(cont.)*							
peanut butter cup *(Colombo* Gourmet),							
3 fl. oz.	150	4.0	16.0	8.0	5	95	(0)
Praline Pandemonium (Häagen-Dazs Exträas)	240	7.0	33.0	9.0	45	115	n.a.
raspberry:							
(Edy's Inspirations)	110	3.0	19.0	3.0	10	40	(0)
(Edy's Inspirations Nonfat)	90	3.0	20.0	<1.0	0	70	(0)
red *(Sealtest Free)*	100	2.0	23.0	0	0	40	(0)
Raspberry Rendezvous (Häagen-Dazs Exträas)	130	4.0	26.0	2.0	20	25	(0)
rasberry-vanilla swirl							
(Edy's Inspirations)	110	3.0	19.0	3.0	10	45	(0)
strawberry:							
(Blue Bell Nonfat)	100	3.0	20.0	0	0	45	(0)
(Edy's Inspirations)	110	2.0	18.0	3.0	10	40	(0)
(Edy's Inspirations Nonfat)	90	3.0	20.0	<1.0	0	70	(0)
(Häagen-Dazs) . . .	170	6.0	27.0	4.0	50	45	(0)
(Sealtest Free) . . .	100	2.0	22.0	0	0	35	(0)
passion *(Colombo* Gourmet), 3 fl. oz.	100	2.0	18.0	2.0	10	40	(0)
Strawberry Cheesecake Craze, (Häagen-Dazs Exträas)	210	7.0	31.0	7.0	50	100	n.a.
vanilla:							
(Edy's Inspirations)	110	3.0	19.0	3.0	10	50	0
(Edy's Inspirations Nonfat)	90	4.0	18.0	<1.0	0	80	0
(Häagen-Dazs) . . .	170	8.0	26.0	4.0	50	50	0
(Sealtest Free) . . .	100	2.0	23.0	0	0	45	0
dream *(Colombo* Gourmet), 3 fl. oz.	100	3.0	16.0	3.0	10	45	0

Food and Measure	cal.	prot. (gms)	carbo. (gms)	fat (gms)	chol. (mgs)	sod. (mgs)	fiber (gms)
vanilla almond crunch (Häagen-Dazs) . . .	200	8.0	29.0	6.0	50	65	m.q.
vanilla-chocolate swirl (Edy's Inspirations Nonfat)	90	4.0	19.0	<1.0	0	85	(0)
Yogurt, frozen, soft-serve, all flavors: (Bresler's Gourmet), 1 oz.	29	.9	5.5	.5	2	15	(0)
(Bresler's Lite), 1 oz.	27	1.1	6.0	0	0	11	(0)
"Yogurt," tofu, (Stir Fruity), 6 oz.:							
apple, spiced	161	5.6	29.5	2.2	0	43	m.q.
berry, mixed	149	5.9	26.0	2.5	0	34	m.q.
blueberry	140	6.0	25.7	1.5	0	43	m.q.
cherry, black	141	5.7	25.1	2.0	0	51	m.q.
lemon chiffon	149	5.3	25.9	2.7	0	43	m.q.
orange, mandarin . .	143	6.4	25.7	1.6	0	51	m.q.
peach	153	6.1	25.8	2.9	0	34	m.q.
piña colada	154	5.9	27.6	2.2	0	43	m.q.
raspberry	151	5.6	27.5	2.1	0	34	m.q.
strawberry	140	6.2	24.8	1.8	0	51	m.q.
vanilla	143	6.5	22.8	2.8	0	51	m.q.
Yogurt bar, frozen, 1 bar:							
all flavors (Frozfruit Nonfat)	90	3.0	20.0	0	0	55	n.a.
cherry chocolate fudge (Häagen-Dazs)	230	5.0	28.0	12.0	35	50	n.a.
crunch, vanilla/chocolate (Häagen-Dazs)	210	5.0	23.0	11.0	25	45	n.a.
crunch, chocolate/coffee (Häagen-Dazs)	210	5.0	24.0	11.0	20	50	n.a.
orange passion, tropical (Häagen-Dazs)	100	2.0	21.0	1.0	20	30	n.a.
peach (Häagen-Dazs)	100	2.0	19.0	1.0	15	20	n.a.
piña colada (Häagen-Dazs)	100	2.0	21.0	1.0	15	25	n.a.

Food and Measure	cal.	prot. (gms)	carbo. (gms)	fat (gms)	chol. (mgs)	sod. (mgs)	fiber (gms)
Yogurt bar *(cont.)*							
raspberry *(Häagen-Dazs)*	100	3.0	19.0	1.0	15	20	n.a.
strawberry daiquiri *(Häagen-Dazs)*	100	2.0	20.0	1.0	20	20	n.a.
Yogurt shake, frozen: chocolate *(Weight Watchers Sweet Celebrations),* 7.5 fl. oz.	220	8.0	44.0	1.0	5	140	n.a.
Yuca, boiled, drained *(Frieda's),* 4 oz.	77	1.2	38.6	.2	0	2	m.q.

Z

Food and Measure	cal.	prot. (gms)	carbo. (gms)	fat (gms)	chol. (mgs)	sod. (mgs)	fiber (gms)
Ziti dinner, frozen:							
ribbed *(Swanson Hungry Man),* 17.25 oz.	550	31.0	51.0	25.0	n.a.	1580	m.q.
ribbed, in meat sauce *(Swanson),* 11 oz.	340	17.0	45.0	11.0	m.q.	1060	m.q.
Ziti dishes, frozen, in marinara sauce *(The Budget Gourmet Side Dish),* 6.25 oz.	200	7.0	23.0	9.0	10	600	m.q.
Ziti entree, frozen, w/zesty tomato sauce *(Healthy Choice Pasta Classics),* 12 oz.	350	16.0	59.0	5.0	30	530	m.q.
Zucchini:							
fresh, raw:							
sliced, 1/2 cup . . .	9	.8	1.9	.1	0	2	.8 d
baby, 1 large, 31/8" long, 5/8" diam.	3	.4	.5	.1	0	tr.	m.q.
fresh, boiled, drained:							
sliced, 1/2 cup . . .	14	.6	3.5	.1	0	2	1.3 d
mashed, 1/2 cup . .	19	.8	4.7	.1	0	3	1.7 d
canned, 1/2 cup:							
Italian style *(Progresso)* . . .	50	1.0	8.0	2.0	<1	540	2.0 d
w/tomato juice . .	33	1.2	7.8	.1	0	424	.6 c
frozen:							
(Seabrook), 3.3 oz. .	16	1.0	3.0	0	0	2	1.0 c
battered *(Stilwell),* 8 sticks	150	3.0	17.0	8.0	0	180	2.0 d

Food and Measure	cal.	prot. (gms)	carbo. (gms)	fat (gms)	chol. (mgs)	sod. (mgs)	fiber (gms)
Zucchini, frozen *(cont.)*							
breaded:							
(Ore-Ida), 3 oz.	150	3.0	17.0	8.0	<5	340	m.q.
(Qwik Krisp),							
6 pieces . . .	190	3.0	20.0	11.0	25	840	4.0 d
(Stilwell), 8 sticks	110	3.0	18.0	2.5	5	450	2.0 d

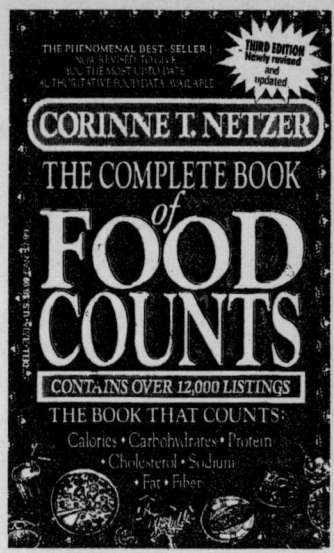
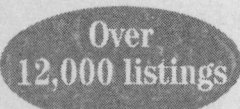
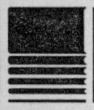